P9-BZB-907

PSYCHIATRY

1982 The American Psychiatric Association
Annual Review

Edited by Lester Grinspoon, M.D.

American
Psychiatric
Press, Inc.

Washington, D.C. 1982

American
Psychiatric
Press, Inc.

1700 18TH STREET, N.W.
WASHINGTON, D.C. 20009

Copyright 1982 © American Psychiatric Association
ALL RIGHTS RESERVED.
Printed and bound in the United States of America.

ISBN 0-88048-000-9

CONTENTS

Part

V

**Borderline and Narcissistic
Personality Disorders**

Introduction
Psychiatry
1982

Psychiatry
1982

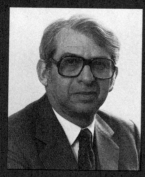

Lester Grinspoon, M.D.,
Editor

Associate Professor of Psychiatry
Harvard Medical School
Massachusetts Mental Health Center

Introduction

by Lester Grinspoon, M.D., Editor

As the boundaries of psychiatry expand and its knowledge base grows, the mental health professional is increasingly challenged to keep abreast of developments in the many facets of his or her specialty. Mindful of this, shortly after I accepted the Chair of the Scientific Program Committee, I wrote to almost 400 members of the American Psychiatric Association to ask them to share their thoughts about what should be included in the program and how. The sample of psychiatrists covered the full range of professional roles, from academic to general practice. The thoughts, feelings, and ideas reaped from this effort were carefully compiled and studied.

One theme which emerged was that while the scientific program of the Annual Meeting presented a diversity of fine trees, it was difficult for a participant to get a sense of the forest. The annual review program was thus designed to provide a fresh panorama of the forest, a view of one large area at a time.

The areas chosen for the first year were those that constitute the Parts of this volume. For each of the areas, a well-recognized authority was invited to act as the Preceptor. He or she would have the responsibility for selecting the faculty for that Part and for organizing non-overlapping presentations which together would provide the comprehensive review of that area.

Only after several of the Preceptors were selected did it occur to me that it might be a useful extension of this idea to provide an even more comprehensive articulation of the annual reviews in the form of a book. This *Annual Review* would both mirror and magnify the reviews presented at the Annual Meeting. With the acceptance of this idea, the Preceptors then became *de facto* associate editors, a responsibility which all accepted graciously and which several assumed enthusiastically.

The Preceptors and Parts for this year's *Annual Review* are Virginia A. Sadock, "Psychiatric Aspects of Sexuality;" Robert Cancro, "The Schizophrenic Disorders;" Henry H. Work, "Depression in Childhood and Adolescence;" Alan A. Stone, "Law and Psychiatry;" and Otto F. Kernberg, "Borderline and Narcissistic Personality Disorders." Our good fortune is not simply that these preeminent authorities agreed to be Preceptors, but also that they were so successful in assembling such impressive faculties. This volume is the fruition of much work on the part of the Preceptors and their faculties. Their only reward is the pleasure they take in sharing knowledge with their colleagues. All of us who profit from what they have written are indebted to them.

Planning for next year's *Annual Review* is already underway. Again, there will be five Parts, and the titles and Preceptors will be as follows: "New Issues in Psychoanalysis," with Arnold M. Cooper as Preceptor; "Family Psychiatry," with Henry U. Grunebaum as Preceptor; "Bipolar Disorders," with Paula J. Clayton as Preceptor; "Major Depression," with Gerald L. Klerman as Preceptor; and "Geriatric Psychiatry," with Ewald W. Busse as Preceptor.

Finally, I should like to express gratitude to those who helped make it possible to launch this idea and to produce the first volume. Melvin Sabshin was most supportive of the idea and contributed to the solution of some of the various problems that any new project of this magnitude is bound to encounter. Ron McMillen, Hermine Dlesk, and the staff of the newly created American Psychiatric Press had to hit the ground running with such a large and complicated book as their first product. They did so with great skill and spirit. The members of the Scientific Program Committee as a whole, and particularly those of the Long-Range Planning Subcommittee, were most generous in sharing their thoughts and suggestions with me. I am most indebted to Nancy Palmer for the creative energy and effectiveness which she brought to the myriad administrative details connected with introducing a new format into the scientific program of the Annual Meeting and producing this book on such a tight schedule. And finally, it must be said, if this book enjoys the success that I hope it will, much of the credit belongs to Carolyn Mercer-McFadden, whose exceptional intelligence and caring attention to detail were focused on every sentence of the manuscript.

It is my pleasure to introduce *Psychiatry 1982,* the first of the *Annual Review* series from the American Psychiatric Association.

Part I

The Psychiatric Aspects of Sexuality

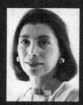

Avodah K. Offit, M.D.
Clinical Assistant Professor of
  Psychiatry
Cornell University Medical College
  at the New York Hospital-Cornell
  University Medical Center

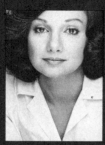

***Virginia A. Sadock, M.D.,
Preceptor***

Clinical Associate Professor of
  Psychiatry and Director,
  Graduate Education in
  Human Sexuality
New York University School of
  Medicine

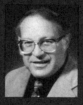

Ira B. Pauly, M.D.
Professor and Chairman
Department of Psychiatry and
  Behavioral Sciences
University of Nevada
  School of Medicine

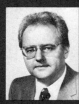

Alexander N. Levay, M.D.
Associate Clinical Professor
of Psychiatry
Columbia University
College of Physicians and Surgeons

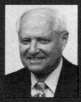

Robert Dickes, M.D.
Professor of Psychiatry, Director
Center for Human Sexuality
State University of New York
Downstate Medical Center

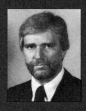

Jon K. Meyer, M.D.
Associate Professor of Psychiatry
Department of Psychiatry and
Behavioral Science
The Johns Hopkins University
School of Medicine and
Director, Consultation Unit
The Johns Hopkins Medical
Institutions

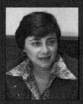

Carol C. Nadelson, M.D.
Professor and Vice-chairman
Department of Psychiatry
Tufts University School of Medicine
and Director of Training and
Education
Department of Psychiatry
Tufts-New England Medical Center
Hospital

I

The Psychiatric Aspects of Sexuality

Introduction
by Virginia A. Sadock, M.D.

The history of Western civilization reveals that social attitudes toward expressions of human sexuality vary greatly across time and cultures. In the sphere of religion, for instance, some cultures have positively associated sex with the ritual activity, while others have idealized asceticism and celibacy. There have been periods of liberality and periods of puritanism, and there have been periods when both flourished in apparent contradiction to one another. In the Victorian era, for example, sex was socially taboo, while prostitution and pornography were rife.

During the past several decades American society has radically changed so many of its prevalent sexual attitudes that the period has been called an era of sexual revolution. The Kinsey reports of 1948 and 1953 made public the degree, type, and frequency of sexual activity occurring in this country, bringing sexual practices from the realm of inference and secrecy into accepted, if still private, reality. In the early 1970's the Presidential Commission on Pornography advised against sexual repression, encouraging the candid discussion of sexuality in society and the acceptance of frank and sexually stimulating material. The advent of effective birth control methods and legalized abortion clearly differentiated the pleasure of sexual activity from its procreative function. The feminist movement attacked the double standard in what was considered acceptable sexual behavior for men and women, encouraged women to accept sexual responsibility for the gratification of their needs, and challenged society to reevaluate stereotyped male and female roles. The women's movement also focused attention on rape and incest. Gerontologists and elderly people alike have drawn attention to the sexual needs of the aged. Few of these issues have been fully resolved in the form of new social mores, however, and it may be that sexual attitudes will swing back to the puritanical and prohibitive.

Concurrent with the cultural changes of the sexual revolution has been a growth in scientific research into sexual practices and sexual dysfunctions. Masters and Johnson published their pioneering work on the physiology of sexual response in 1966 and reported on their program to treat sexual complaints in 1970. Most medical centers now have programs specifically geared to the treatment of sexual dysfunctions. The significant new studies of gender development are becoming even more important as people are more frequently requesting gender-altering surgery.

With the advent of sex therapy programs and the flourishing of sex therapists, organizations have evolved to disseminate information to professionals, to establish criteria for adequate training, and to maintain ethics and standards. These organizations include the Sex Information and Education Council of the United States (SIECUS), the Society for Sex Therapy and Research (SSTAR), and the American Association of Sex Educators, Counselors and Therapists (AASECT).

In addition, most medical schools now include lectures on sexuality in their curricula. The American Medical Association has published the volume *Human Sexuality*, and several medical textbooks include sections on the medical aspects of sexuality. Physicians are becoming more alert to the side effects of medication which alter sexual responses.

Historically, psychiatry has always treated problems arising from sexual conflict or presenting as sexual dysfunctions. Pioneers like Havelock Ellis, Krafft-Ebing, and Freud focused broadly on human sexuality. More recent workers have focused more intensively on sexual physiology and dysfunctions. Recent studies suggest that psychosexual dysfunctions may occur as the only disorder (Maurice and Guze, 1970), or in conjunction with other psychopathology (Derogatis et al., 1981).

In the current *Diagnostic and Statistical Manual,* Third Edition, (DSM-III) psychosexual dysfunctions are recognized as distinct syndromes and impairments. They may, where relevant, be diagnosed in conjunction with personality disorders and physical conditions (American Psychiatric Association, 1980).

Various corrective therapies are now used or combined to treat psychosexual dysfunctions. Some significant new techniques are available, and psychiatrists are eminently well qualified to incorporate the recently developed techniques of sex therapy into their practices. This simply follows the general history of psychiatry, which has modified and absorbed any number of specialized techniques into its treatment repertoire. Where the dysfunction occurs alone, an unmodified sex therapy approach seems to be the treatment of choice. For patients with accompanying personality disorders or physical conditions, it is but one of many techniques to be considered. Whatever the technique, it is important to remember that all of the treatment options are forms of psychotherapy.

The results of these developments in the area of human sexuality and in the treatment of psychosexual dysfunctions are dealt with in the chapters which follow. The first chapter, by the Preceptor, reviews sexual physiology and anatomy, as a knowledge of these subjects is a necessary prerequisite to the appropriate treatment of psychosexual dysfunctions. Dr. Avodah Offit illustrates the uses of DSM-III in diagnosing these dysfunctions, and the Preceptor discusses the major treatment approaches. Dr. Alexander Levay places in excellent perspective the problems presented by and the methods most effective in treating difficult cases.

Dr. Robert Dickes discusses the psychosexual outcomes of medical conditions and surgical procedures, focusing on the interplay between organic and functional problems. Dr. Ira Pauly, on the other hand, deals with the effect of cultural factors on sexuality in his thoughtful chapter on the sexual behavior and adaptation of people who are separated, divorced, or widowed and the special issues associated with aging and sexuality. These populations make up a significant portion of the general population in this country, as well as of the psychiatrist's patient population, but they have often been neglected in previous discussions of sexual mores and practices.

Dr. Jon Meyer discusses gender disturbances, dealing incisively with the manifestation of dysphoria in childhood, adolescence, and adulthood and with treatment approaches. Although Gender Identity Disorders are considered psychosexual disorders rather than psychosexual dysfunctions in DSM-III, they are too important to omit from this work. The degree of disturbance coincident with problems in this area and the drastic treatment requested by patients with these problems warrant the discussion of the disorders in this Part. Similarly, Dr. Carol Nadelson's chapter on the repercussions of rape and incest provides a timely review of problems not strictly considered psychosexual dysfunctions. These, too, have only recently begun to receive attention and are of great importance to the practicing psychiatrist.

The topic of psychosexual dysfunctions has particular importance for contemporary psychiatry. Problems of dysfunction are particularly distressing to patients and have often been resistant to treatment. The current emphasis on human sexuality reflects the cultural and scientific developments of recent years, new hope for the treatment of these problems, the historical interest of psychiatry in this area, and the recognition of its importance in psychiatric practice.

Chapter 1

Sexual Anatomy and Physiology
by Virginia A. Sadock, M.D.

INTRODUCTION

The diagnosis and treatment of psychosexual dysfunctions require a working knowledge of anatomy and physiology as well as of psychology. To the psychiatrist who is evaluating a person's psychosexual development and dysfunction, anatomical, neurological, or endocrinological factors may be as crucial for understanding the problem as the individual's personality and social environment. A discussion of the organs of sexuality and the physiological sequence of male and female responses forms the basis for reviewing endocrinology and considering the physiological basis for the DSM-III typology of psychosexual dysfunctions.

ANATOMY OF THE MALE

The external genitalia of the normal adult male include the penis, scrotum, testes, epididymis, and parts of the vas deferens. Internal components include the vas deferens, seminal vesicles, ejaculatory ducts, and the prostate gland.

Freud referred to the penis as the executive organ of sexuality. Since antiquity culture after culture has represented the penis in a variety of art forms. In ancient Greece, the cults of Dionysus, Priapus, and the Satyrs used the phallus as a recurrent symbol of fertility and rejuvenation. The word *penis* has been traced from the Latin, meaning variously "tail" or "to hang" and referring to the pendant position of the organ in its resting or flaccid state. The size of the penis varies within a fairly constant range, but sex researchers over the years have disagreed on the dimensions of the range. All agree, however, that concern over the size of the penis is practically universal among men. Masters and Johnson (1966) report a range of seven to 11 cm in the flaccid state and 14 to 18 cm in the erect state. Of particular interest was their observation that the flaccid dimension bears little relation to the erect dimension; the smaller penis erects to a proportionally greater size than does the larger penis.

Circumcision, in which the prepuce is surgically removed, has been practiced for centuries as a religious rite by Jews and Moslems and is a common medical procedure in the United States today. It was once believed that the circumcised penis, with its exposed glans, was less sensitive due to cornification of the epithelium. In laboratory studies, however, researchers have found no difference in tactile threshold between the circumcised penis and the uncircumcised penis. Intravaginally, they have found, the prepuce of the uncircumcised penis remains retracted behind the glans during penile thrusting, dispelling the myth that premature ejaculation may be more common in uncircumcised men because of increased stimulation caused by preputial movements (Masters and Johnson, 1966).

The parasympathetic nervous system activates the process of erection. The pelvic splanchnic nerves (S2, S3, and S4) stimulate the blood vessels of the area to dilate, causing the penis to become erect. In ejaculation, the sympathetic nervous system is involved. Through its hypogastric plexus, the sympathetic nervous system innervates the urethral crest and the muscles of the epididymis, vas deferens, seminal vesicles, and prostate. Stimulation of the plexus causes ejaculation of seminal fluid from those glands and ducts into the urethra. That passage of fluid into the urethra provides the man with a sensation of impending climax. Indeed, once the prostate contracts, ejaculation is inevitable. The ejaculate is propelled through the penis by urethral contractions. It consists of about one teaspoon of fluid (2.5 ml) and contains about 120 million sperm cells.

ANATOMY OF THE FEMALE

The external genitalia of the normal female are also called the vulva and include the mons pubis, major and minor lips, clitoris, glans, vestibule of the vagina, and the vaginal orifice. The internal system includes the ovaries, fallopian tubes, uterus, and vagina.

The word *vagina* comes from the Latin word meaning "sheath." It is usually in a collapsed state, a potential rather than an actual space. About eight cm long, it extends from the cervix of the uterus above to the vestibule of the vagina or the vaginal opening below. In most virgins a membranous fold, the hymen, separates the vestibule and opening from the rest of the vaginal canal. The mucous membrane lining the vaginal walls rests in numerous transverse folds. To accommodate the penis during sexual intercourse, the vagina expands in both length and width. After menopause, due to decreased circulating estrogen levels, the vagina loses much of its elasticity.

Hippocrates first described the clitoris in the medical literature, referring to it as the site of sexual excitation. More recently, Masters and Johnson (1966) described the clitoris as the primary female sexual organ, because orgasm depends physiologically on adequate clitoral stimulation. Anatomically the clitoris has a nerve net that is proportionally three times as large as that of the penis.

Kinsey found that when women masturbate most prefer clitoral stimulation to any other (1953). This finding was refined further by Masters and Johnson, who reported that women prefer the shaft of the clitoris to the glans, since the glans is hypersensitive if stimulated excessively (1966).

An important anatomical finding is that the clitoral prepuce is contiguous with the labia minora and that during coitus the penis does not stimulate the clitoris directly. Rather, the penile thrusting exerts traction on the minor lips which in turn stimulate the clitoris sufficiently for orgasm to occur. Masters and Johnson (1966) also note that during the plateau phase (before orgasm) the clitoris retracts under the clitoral hood as a result of the ischiocavernosi muscles contracting. Retracting thus, the clitoris moves away from the vaginal barrel, which makes clitoral-penile contact impossible. The size of the clitoris varies considerably and is unrelated to the degree of sexual responsiveness of a particular female.

Many of Masters and Johnson's findings regarding female sexuality were revolutionary. That all orgasms, whether precipitated by masturbation or intercourse, involve stimulation (direct or indirect) of the clitoris, that there is no physiological difference between a clitoral or vaginal orgasm, and that the penis does not directly stimulate the clitoris are especially germane. Based on their work, we ought to reconsider Freud's postulation that women must give up clitoral sensitivity in favor of vaginal sensitivity in order to be considered sexually mature. However, some women state they feel a special sense of satisfaction with an orgasm precipitated by coitus. Some workers attribute this to the psychological feeling of closeness engendered by the act of coitus, but others maintain that a coital orgasm is a physiologically different experience (Sadock, 1980; Perry and Whipple, 1978).

ENDOCRINOLOGY

From the time of conception, hormones play a major role in human sexual development. Unlike the fetal gonads, which are under chromosomal influence, the fetal external genitalia are very susceptible to hormones. Exogenous hormonal administration can cause external genital development inconsistent with the fetal sex gland development. For instance, if the pregnant mother receives sufficient exogenous androgen, a female fetus, possessing an ovary, can develop external genitalia resembling those of a male. Fetal, maternal, or exogenous hormones administered to a pregnant woman may all affect the development of the external genitalia of the fetus. Deprived of male and female gonads and the respective hormones, testosterone and estrogen, the human adult does not develop normal secondary sexual characteristics, is incapable of reproduction, and, in the case of the female, does not develop a menstrual cycle.

Testosterone is the hormone believed to be connected with libido in both men and women. In men there is an inverse correlation between stress and the testosterone blood level. Other factors, such as sleep, mood, and lifestyle, are being studied to evaluate their relationship to circulating levels of this hormone.

The administration of androgens to patients complaining of sexual dysfunctions is usually futile if normal hormonal function is present. Androgen administered to men complaining of loss of potency and loss of libido has usually been unsuccessful, and administration to women results in disturbing virilizing side effects. Many clinicians correct the hormone deficiency of the postmenopausal period with estrogen replacement therapy. Although this therapy is effective in relieving much of the physiological stress of the period, prolonged administration of estrogens increases risk of endometrial cancer.

PHYSIOLOGICAL RESPONSES

Normal men and women experience a sequence of physiological responses to sexual stimulation. In the first detailed description of these responses, Masters and Johnson (1966) observed that the physiological process involves increasing levels of vasocongestion and myotonia (tumescence) and the subsequent rapid release of the vascular activity and muscle tone as a result of orgasm (detumescence). The process occurs in the four phases of excitement, plateau, orgasm, and resolution. DSM-III makes some variations in the definition of these phases, and these are discussed following the physiological discussion.

Phase I: Excitement

This phase is brought on by psychological stimulation (fantasy, the presence of a love object), or physiological stimulation (stroking, kissing), or by a combination of the two. Occurring within ten to thirty seconds after effective stimulation, it is characterized by penile erection in the man and vaginal lubrication in the woman. The nipples of both sexes become erect, although nipple erection is more common in the woman than in the man. The woman's clitoris becomes hard and turgid, and her labia minora become thicker as a result of venous engorgement. The excitement phase may last several minutes to several hours.

Phase II: Plateau

With continued stimulation the man's testes increase in size fifty percent and elevate. The woman's vaginal barrel shows a characteristic constriction along the outer third known as the orgasmic platform. The clitoris elevates and retracts behind the symphysis pubis. As a result, the clitoris is not easily accessible. As the area is stimulated, though, traction on the labia minora and the prepuce occur, and there is intrapreputial movement of the clitoral shaft. Breast size in the woman increases 25 percent. Continued engorgement of the penis and vagina produces specific color changes, most marked in the labia minora, which become bright or deep red. Voluntary contractions of large muscle groups occur, rate of heartbeat and respiration increase, and blood pressure rises. The plateau stage lasts thirty seconds to several minutes.

Phase III: Orgasm

A subjective sense of ejaculatory inevitability triggers the man's orgasm. The forceful emission of semen follows. The male orgasm is also associated with four to five rhythmic spasms of the prostate, seminal vesicles, vas, and urethra. In the woman, orgasm is characterized by three to 15 involuntary contractions of the lower third of the vagina and by strong, sustained contractions of the uterus, flowing from the fundus downward to the cervix. Both men and women have involuntary contractions of the internal and external anal sphincter. These and the other contractions during orgasm occur at intervals of 0.8 second. Other manifestations include voluntary and involuntary movements of the large muscle groups, including facial grimacing and carpopedal spasm. Blood pressure rises 20 to 40 mm (systolic and diastolic, respectively), and the heart rate increases up to 160 beats a minute. Orgasm lasts from three to 15 seconds and is associated with a slight clouding of consciousness.

Phase IV: Resolution

Resolution consists of the disgorgement of blood from the genitalia (detumescence), and this brings the body back to its resting state. If orgasm occurs, resolution is rapid; if it does not occur, resolution may take two to six hours and be associated with irritability and discomfort. Resolution, through orgasm, is characterized by a subjective sense of well-being.

Refractory Period

After orgasm, men have a refractory period that may last from several minutes to many hours; in that period they cannot be stimulated to further orgasm. The refractory period does not exist in women, who are capable of multiple and successive orgasms.

THE DSM-III PHASES OF THE SEXUAL RESPONSE CYCLE

Sexual response is a true psychophysiological experience. Arousal is triggered by both psychological and physical stimuli, levels of tension are experienced both physiologically and emotionally, and, with orgasm, there is normally a subjective perception of a peak of physical reaction and release. Psychosexual development, psychological attitude toward sexuality, and attitudes toward one's sexual partner are directly involved with and affect the physiology of human sexual response.

Because the process is truly psychophysiological, DSM-III incorporates the four physiological phases as the basis for its classification of psychosexual dysfunctions. DSM-III, however, consolidates the excitement and plateau phases into a single excitement phase and precedes it with its unique *appetitive* phase.

DSM-III Phase 1. Appetitive

This phase is distinct from any identified solely through physiology and reflects the psychiatrist's fundamental concern with motivations, drives, and personality. The phase is characterized by sexual fantasies and the desire to have sexual activity.

DSM-III Phase 2. Excitement

This phase consists of a subjective sense of sexual pleasure and accompanying physiological changes. All the physiologic responses noted in Masters and Johnson's excitement and plateau phases are combined under this phase.

DSM-III Phase 3. Orgasm

This phase consists of a peaking of sexual pleasure, with release of sexual tension and rhythmic contraction of the perineal muscles and pelvic reproductive organs. The phase is identical to Masters and Johnson's Phase III.

DSM-III Phase 4. Resolution

This phase entails a sense of general relaxation, well-being, and muscular relaxation. This phase, as defined, does not differ from the Masters and Johnson resolution phase.

CONCLUSION

Building on the concept of phases in the process of physiological sexual activity, DSM-III newly categorizes some familiar psychosexual dysfunctions to parallel the appetitive, excitement, and orgasm phases. Inhibitions in these areas are now first-order concerns. With the multiaxial framework of DSM-III, the practicing psychiatrist can more readily diagnose and treat sexual problems in the psychophysiological context which is their true domain.

Chapter 2 # The Psychosexual Dysfunctions: Diagnostic Complexities
by Avodah K. Offit, M.D.

REVIEW AND HISTORICAL NOTES

Psychosexual Dysfunctions as Clinical Syndromes

Psychiatrists have opened their minds to the pains and pleasures of sexuality as important psychotherapeutic issues. Under the scheme of DSM-III, sexual dysfunctions rank on the first line of diagnosis (American Psychiatric Association, 1980). They may now be designated on Axis I as clinical syndromes. No previous psychiatric classification scheme had considered sexual disturbances to be primary contributors to mental distress or results of it.

In the second *Diagnostic and Statistical Manual of Mental Disorders* (DSM-II), American classifiers gave sex but brief mention (American Psychiatric Association, 1968). The joys and sorrows of the reproductive system did not warrant a category of their own but were combined with the problems of the excretory system.

ICD-9 advanced considerably over DSM-II (World Health Organization, 1978). Sexual disorders achieved a status and a number of their own (302.7). However, frigidity, impotence, and dyspareunia were the only difficulties listed. Problems related to orgasm in both men and women were not then recognized as important or as separate dysfunctions.

At last, with DSM-III, sex has begun to emerge as the significant informer of human happiness that early practitioners of psychoanalysis believed it to be. Sexual dysfunction is becoming an increasingly important symptom and diagnostic tool in all clinical medicine, as researchers discover how the biochemical paths of sex, depression, and disease intersect one another.

Personality Disorders

Experienced clinicians are grateful to the creators of DSM-III for making it possible to include both personality disorders and personality traits in a multiaxial diagnosis. Although sexual dysfunctions and particular personality disorders do not appear correlated on the basis of the frequency with which they appear together, the psychological paths that individual personality types will take to the differing dysfunctions are noteworthy for their similarity. For example, a man of the avoidant personality type may become impotent or premature under threat of intimacy. He will not risk closeness. A man or a woman of the passive-aggressive type often becomes sexually dysfunctional when performance is demanded. He or she will passively resist fulfilling sexual expectations. Identifying the personality trait or disorder is frequently the most crucial key to treatment.

Physical Disorders and Conditions

The enumeration of possible physical etiologies for sexual dysfunction is a significant responsibility of the psychiatrist who deals in sexual dilemmas, and DSM-III allows for this in Axis III. (It is critical to note that diseases not considered relevant to the Axis I problem are not listed in the diagnosis.) The roster of ailments that may initiate a sexual dysfunction increases daily. Also, the anxiety engendered by disease may create greater havoc in a person's sexual abilities than the organic disease itself.

Psychosocial Stressors and Adaptive Functioning

The importance of precipitating stressors and a person's general level of functioning are well known to the clinician. Variations in sexual patterns in response to emotional trauma, and in light of a person's overall effectiveness, have been well documented. DSM-III enables the consideration of such factors in Axis IV and Axis V.

Some Comments on DSM-III

DSM-III conceives of psychosexual dysfunctions as "inhibitions" of sexuality. This word is used in its broadest sense to include those impediments to sexual happiness that have always been present in a person's constellation of traits, as well as those that arise in the course of life. Some "sexual problems," however, are not included. Hypersexuality, for instance, is not listed as a dysfunction. In clinical practice we find that conditions where sexual hyperactivity occurs are usually tied to another clinical syndrome, such as a Manic Episode.

DSM-III does require some sophistication of its users. The line between a practical nomenclature and scientific classification is often difficult to draw. For example, what aspect of sexuality is being inhibited in premature ejaculation and vaginismus? To what broad category do they belong? The answer is that both dysfunctions are related to an inhibited excitement phase. In prematurity, the excitement phase is inhibited from developing to its full potential. (In some who are premature, the orgasm phase is diminished or abbreviated as well.) In vaginismus, there is an inhibition of vaginal relaxation and accommodation, anatomical changes that are manifestations of a normal female excitement phase. It takes considerable sophistication to see these disorders as related to an inhibition of excitement.

As helpful and progressive as DSM-III seems, many of us regret some omissions. The manual divides the "sexual response cycle" into four phases: appetitive, excitement, orgasm, and resolution. Many clinicians feel that since male orgasm and male ejaculation may occur separately, men have five phases, rather than four. (And some linguists wonder why the first phase is an adjective while the other three are nouns.)

DSM-III also states that the resolution phase is rarely of clinical significance. Since many women want to go on to multiorgasmic experience, this period has become or should become increasingly important to the clinician. Postejaculation and postorgasmic difficulties in handling conflicting physical, emotional, and affectional states occupy more and more psychiatric time. As inhibition of the resolution phase becomes a significant area for presenting complaints, it should achieve prominence in our diagnostic manual.

THE PSYCHOSEXUAL DYSFUNCTIONS

The psychosexual dysfunctions themselves now possess their own individual numbers and decimal points. They are:

302.71	Inhibited sexual desire
302.72	Inhibited sexual excitement
302.73	Inhibited female orgasm
302.74	Inhibited male orgasm
302.75	Premature ejaculation
302.76	Functional dyspareunia
306.51	Functional vaginismus
302.70	Atypical psychosexual dysfunction

The following discussion covers each of these disorders, by referring especially to the diagnostic dilemmas they present. In considering cases where the diagnosis is complex or difficult, the beauty of the multiaxial system emerges. The clinician can consider and readily convey the entire spectrum of contributing factors, revealing not only the diagnosis but also his or her feelings about the case.

Inhibited Sexual Desire

Difficulties in the diagnosis of psychosexual dysfunction often involve whether to place the psychosexual syndrome along Axis I. In the case of Major Depression, for example, the answer depends on which came first, the sexual problem or the depression.

CASE HISTORY Emily G., a 42-year-old housewife and graphic designer, began to experience a lack of sexual desire for her husband approximately three years prior to seeking psychiatric help. Ms. G. rarely became excited and had ceased to have orgasms. She and her husband had intercourse less and less frequently and finally not at all. She sought help from a local "sex therapist," a woman who gave classes in having orgasms with vibrators, but Ms. G. gained no relief. She then sought psychiatric help for the relief of depressive symptoms which had begun a few weeks prior to her first visit: sleeplessness with early morning awakening; loss of appetite; agitation and crying jags; lack of motivation; and aversion to her husband's sexual advances.

Two years before consultation, after the lack of desire had first begun, Ms. G., a quiet, timid artist, had decided to leave the safe routine of her home life at the urging of a feminist neighbor. She went back to the work which she had left ten years previously. At that time she had wanted to devote herself entirely to her husband's comfort. They had had no children. Her talent was so obvious that, on seeking work again, she was immediately employed by a large advertising agency. While the work absorbed and excited her, her husband's attitude became increasingly critical and derogatory. He missed her company in the evenings, as well as the home services she had ungrudgingly provided. He told her so. Soon thereafter, a competitive worker at the office initiated a campaign to damage Ms. G.'s reputation and self-esteem. Unable to cope with negative relationships both at home and at work, she rapidly entered a depressive decline.

In this case, Ms. G.'s sexual dysfunction began three years before she experienced depression. Her sexual dysfunction was related to the personality problems activated by considering separating from home and returning to work. At the time her dependency dilemma had caused a minor depression, of which the only symptom was inhibited sexual desire. Later, her inability to use her anger constructively precipitated a major depression.

DSM-III guidelines state that if another Axis I mental disorder, for example Major Depression, is the primary cause of a disturbance in sexual functioning, such as loss of sexual desire, a Psychosexual Dysfunction should not be diagnosed. As the manual further states, in some instances it will not be clear whether the disturbance in sexual functioning antedates the other mental disorder (in which case both the sexual dysfunction and the other disorder should be diagnosed), or whether the sexual dysfunction is secondary to the other disorder (in which case it should not be diagnosed).

Since the sexual dysfunction in the case described above antedated the Major Depression as a characterological problem, the case could be diagnosed as follows:

Axis I: 296.23 Major Depression, with Melancholia
          302.71 Inhibited Sexual Desire
Axis II: 301.60 Dependent Personality Disorder
Axis III: No diagnosis on Axis III.
Axis IV: Psychosocial stressors: occupational, returning
          to work, marital discord
          Severity: 4—Moderate
Avis V: Highest level of adaptive functioning past year:
          3—Good.

Another diagnostic difficulty with inhibitions of desire can arise from situational factors. For example, a woman may want to have sexual relations with a lover but not with her husband. In that instance, one would make an Axis I diagnosis of Inhibited Sexual Desire, Situational.

Inhibited Sexual Excitement

CASE STUDY   John D. is a 44-year-old male executive who has noted gradual diminution in erectile ability for the past three years, subsequent to a diagnosis of diabetes mellitus, maturity onset. Within the past year, he has entirely lost the ability to have intercourse, his erections failing at entry.

Married for seven years, John D. and his wife had their first child two years ago. They have since been in regular conflict over the care of the child, as previously they had clashed on almost every other issue. Mr. D. is meticulous in all his endeavors, running both business and household with orderly, dictatorial, and irrational passion. His wife considers his extreme control and regularity to be signs of illness. She has not enjoyed sex with him for many years, not only because of the decreasing erections, but also because of the monotonous ritual of the act.

The diagnostic question is whether Mr. D.'s sexual dysfunction is due to the diabetes or to mental factors. Should the sexual diagnosis be made along Axis I when a physical condition is so strongly implicated? In this case, the sexual dysfunction is both psychological and physical in origin. While the gradual loss of erectile ability is probably organic in origin, the sudden loss of erection prior to entry is probably psychological. Therefore, since a major cause of the particular dysfunction is very likely emotional, the physical dysfunction is noted on Axis III, as follows:

Axis I: 302.72 Inhibited Sexual Excitement
Axis II: 301.40 Compulsive Personality Disorder
Axis III: Diabetes Mellitus, Maturity Onset
Axis IV: Psychological stressors: becoming a parent,
           marital discord
           Severity: 4—Moderate
Axis V: Highest level of adaptive functioning past year:
           3—Good.

Inhibited Female Orgasm

Is it a normal variant or a pathological condition when a woman can reach orgasms with masturbation but not through intercourse? An assessment of personality traits can sometimes assist the clinician in making a difficult diagnosis.

CASE STUDY   Erica S. is a 46-year-old computer programmer. Her work is solitary. She does not enjoy the stress of human contact. Alone, she has always been able to masturbate to climax and does so frequently. She has had a lover for twenty years and sees him once a week. But she has never been able to climax with intercourse, even though his stimulation is apparently adequate. She fears that if she is orgasmic with intercourse, she will be required to marry, even though her lover has assured her that he has no wish to become legally bound to anyone. Ms. S. says that she "never feels free when someone else is around," no matter what the relationship. Although she is able to socialize through her company's sports and recreation program, she does little to seek spontaneous friendship on her own for fear or rejection.

The first three axes of the diagnosis for Ms. S. would read:

Axis I: 302.73 Inhibited Female Orgasm
Axis II: 301.82 Avoidant Personality Disorder
Axis III: No diagnosis on Axis III.

Some cases are extremely challenging. Reaching a diagnosis can be difficult, given today's limited physical diagnostic tools. For example, although we do know that certain diseases impair the ability to appreciate touch, we do not yet have a widely accepted test for tactile sensitivity in either a man's penis or a female's clitoris. Therefore, when a woman with a histrionic personality disorder and diabetes mellitus presents a recent onset of inhibited orgasm, we have no way of knowing precisely whether the disorder is physical or psychological in its origin. If her personality disorder is sufficiently marked, however, we assume it has an effect on sexual function. In this case, the first three axes would become:

Axis I: 302.73 Inhibited Female Orgasm
Axis II: 301.50 Histrionic Personality Disorder
Axis III: Diabetes Mellitus, Maturity Onset

Inhibited Male Orgasm

In cases where male orgasm is slow to result from either manual stimulation or intercourse, the diagnosis is often difficult to make. Is the problem physical or psychological? Will therapy merely teach the person to bypass a lack of physical or tactile sensitivity, or will it truly help to resolve a personality problem? Will the patient be at all amenable to therapy?

CASE HISTORY   Roger F. was a 52-year-old male advertising executive who had suffered inhibited orgasms since the age of twenty. Until that time, he had no difficulty. After a severe back strain, which received no treatment, he noted that he was unable to have orgasm as easily on masturbation as previously. When he first had intercourse at 22, he was unable to have an orgasm or to ejaculate. Thereafter, only during self-stimulation and by focusing intently on fantasy was Mr. F. able to experience climax. The climaxes he did achieve were brief and not particularly gratifying.

After examining all the vascular, nerve conduction, and muscle parameters, a urologist deemed them normal. Because of a possible deficit of tactile sensation at the glans and a questionable loss of sensation along the lateral aspect of the left foot, some physical cause of impairment was strongly suspected, and further neurological testing was advised.

Mr. F. refused the testing summarily, stating that he had no time. He became distant, uncommunicative, and even rude to the psychiatrist in whom he had previously expressed belief and confidence. In a reaction similar to his reported pattern of rejecting women after three to five sexual encounters, he abruptly discontinued the treatment he had so eagerly sought.

Mr. F.'s wife described him as intense, unstable, and prone to impulsive sexual affairs that frequently embarrassed her. He suffered severe mood swings, was unable to tolerate isolation, and was confused about his long-term goals. In spite of all this, Mr. F. maintained a high level of functioning in the advertising business, an occupation that was suited to his "inspired" approach.

Mr. F.'s physical problem may have contributed to his numerous abnormal personality responses. Conversely, his personality problem may have caused Mr. F. to withhold his orgasm and fail to enjoy it. Because there is such a pronounced personality disturbance in this case, the diagnoses on the first three axes could appropriately read:

Axis I: 302.74 Inhibited Male Orgasm
Axis II: 301.83 Borderline Personality Disorder
Axis III: Rule out Neurological Impairment

Premature Ejaculation

Whether rapid and uncontrolled ejaculation is an abnormal psychological state or a normal physical condition that simply needs control, the diagnosis is usually made after one or both parties to the sexual act have a complaint. A complaint is unlikely when a young woman, slow to reach orgasm herself, is pleased by the lubrication and excitement of her young lover's first quick release. She may later be able to have her orgasm along with his second climax, which is usually slower to evolve. Only when a man is older and unable to sustain a second erection is the prematurity likely to lead to his or his partner's seeking help.

Lifelong premature ejaculation is one condition often unaccompanied by an Axis II diagnosis. The personality constellation is frequently quite normal. Such early onset cases are, perhaps, sustained by some as yet undiscovered neurological facilitator.

Functional Dyspareunia, Functional Vaginismus, and Atypical Psychosexual Dysfunctions

In addition to functional dyspareunia, there exists a common syndrome involving the fear of vaginal pain when pain has been experienced in the past but the physical cause for such pain is no longer present. This is particularly true in patients after childbirth. In males, a similar phenomenon stems from the fear of pain they experience when recovering from prostatitis. The pain, no longer there, causes such fear that pleasure is inhibited. In such cases it is, of course, still essential to rule out any other physical reason for inhibition.

Miscellaneous cases include the rapidly orgasmic female, whose climaxes would be stronger if she could tell her partner to slow his stimulation, or would be more frequent if she could tell him to continue after she has had her first orgasm. In both of these instances, a failure of sexual assertiveness, supported by the woman's cultural conditioning to accept a single orgasm as the measure, may be the problem.

CONCLUSION

Using DSM-III in the diagnosis of sexual dysfunctions does require us to work through some difficult puzzles, but the effort is worthwhile. In the area of sexual dysfunction, the multiaxial diagnosis is most effective; it provides a perspective on the patient's accompanying psychiatric, social, and adaptive functioning and a format for expressing thoughts about a patient, even when the psychiatrist must operate on inference and clinical judgment.

By attending to proper diagnosis in this way, the clinician approaches a treatment outline easily and comprehensively. Does the woman with inhibited orgasm have a dependency disorder? Then we may help her to become more independent in both her life style and sexual style. Does the man with inhibited excitement have compulsive traits? Then we may help him to lessen his controls and, perhaps, to give up trying to be so perfectly pleasing. By conscientiously composing a DSM-III diagnosis, a physician can learn much about a patient. The discerning therapist may even infer with reasonable clarity which treatment or mediation offers the best possibility for relieving pain or enhancing joy in a range of life spheres.

Chapter *3*

The Treatment of Psychosexual Dysfunctions: An Overview
by Virginia A. Sadock, M.D.

INTRODUCTION

Patient complaints of sexual dysfunction and dissatisfaction are not new to the psychiatrist. Recently, our changing cultural mores, Kinsey's sociological study of sexual behavior, and Masters and Johnson's pioneering investigations into the anatomy and physiology of human sexual response have led to the development of new techniques specifically labeled sex therapy. A variety of approaches are now available for treating the complaints which DSM-III calls psychosexual dysfunctions. Therapies include dual-sex therapy (Masters and Johnson's technique), analytically oriented sex therapy, hypnotherapy, behavior therapy, individual psychotherapy, and group therapy. In all cases of sexual dysfunction, the diagnostic workup should include a thorough medical history, a physical examination, and appropriate laboratory studies to determine if an organic cause is implicated in the dysfunction. If that is the case, treatment should include measures directed toward the underlying physiological condition. In the majority of instances, however, sexual dysfunction has a predominantly psychological basis.

DUAL-SEX THERAPY

The new techniques, those specifically labeled sex therapy, began with Masters and Johnson's essentially behavioral approach. The theoretical basis of this treatment, also called dual-sex therapy, is that the couple, rather than the dysfunctional individual, is the focus of therapy. Rather than viewing the couple as having one sick half, the therapist sees both as being involved in a relationship in which there is sexual distress. Both people, therefore, participate in the therapy program. Often the couple's major problems are misinformation or lack of information and fear of performance.

Dual-sex therapy is intensive and short-term, occurring as often as daily and lasting for as short a time as two weeks. Basic to treatment, a dual-sex therapy team consists of male and female co-therapists. They act as educators and role models for the patients. They prescribe exercises which patients practice in private to relieve their guilt and anxiety and to allow them to confront a previously threatening situation in a new, more confident way. Intercourse is forbidden in the early part of therapy to relieve the patients of performance anxiety and to allow patients to benefit fully from the initial exercises. Beginning exercises have a sensate focus: they heighten the sensory awareness of touch, sight, sound, and smell. Genital stimulation is eventually included as part of exercises which entail general body stimulation.

Discussion periods with the co-therapy team follow each new exercise period, and problems and satisfactions in sexual and in other life areas are discussed. The aim of the therapy is to establish or reestablish communication within the couple. In this context, sex is treated as a natural function that flourishes in the appropriate domestic climate, where communication is open. As the couple progresses, the co-therapy team introduces new exercises. Gradually the couple gains confidence and learns to communicate both verbally and sexually.

Before they may proceed with intercourse, couples learn and practice a variety of stimulating techniques. Exercises vary according to presenting complaints, and special techniques are used to treat the various dysfunctions.

In cases of vaginismus, for instance, part of the woman's therapy is to dilate her vaginal opening with her fingers or with size-graduated dilators. In cases of primary anorgasmia the woman is directed to masturbate, sometimes using a vibrator. When a man is impotent, the woman may be instructed to stimulate or tease his penis. This same technique is used with men who suffer from retarded ejaculation, and, in this case, stimulation sometimes involves a vibrator.

Dual-sex therapy has been most successful in the treatment of premature ejaculation. Therapy often includes an exercise known as the squeeze technique which raises and prolongs the threshold of penile excitability. In this exercise the man or the woman stimulates the erect penis until the man feels the earliest sensations of impending orgasm and ejaculation. Penile stimulation is then abruptly stopped, and the coronal ridge of the penis is forcibly squeezed by the woman for several seconds. Repeated several times, this technique raises the threshold of excitability to a more tolerant stimulation level. Communication between the partners improves, since the man must let his partner know the degree of his sexual excitement so that she can squeeze the penis before the ejaculatory process begins.

ANALYTICALLY ORIENTED SEX THERAPY

Integrating sex therapy and psychodynamic, psychoanalytically oriented psychotherapy enables us to treat patients whose sexual disorders are associated with other psychopathology. Analytically oriented sex therapy lasts over a longer time period than dual-sex therapy. The total number of sessions may exceed the number of sessions usual in dual-sex therapy (around 15 sessions), and patients are seen once or twice a week instead of daily. Another modification is to use one therapist or collaborative therapists rather than a sex-therapy team.

Although patients do not get the same impetus of concentrated treatment and the relief from daily pressures obtained by staying away from home, they benefit from the extended therapy schedule. Over the longer time period they can learn or relearn sexual satisfaction within the realistic conditions of their day-to-day lives. Couples who are prone to use family and work pressures in the service of avoiding sexual contact must confront resistance directly. The pressure and momentum which inevitably build up in the last few days of a strictly time-limited program are not present in the extended schedule, so the couple can learn to deal with occasional regression while still in treatment.

The themes and dynamics that emerge in a couple seen in sex therapy are often the same as those which arise in psychoanalytic therapy: relevant dreams, fear of punishment, difficulty trusting the partner, aggressive feelings, fear of intimacy, oedipal feelings, fear of genital mutilation, and so on. The meshing of the couple's unconscious fantasies and dynamics is often strikingly apparent.

From the original Masters and Johnson protocol, this form of therapy usually adopts two important parameters of treatment. The couple is the patient unit, and the treatment incorporates a series of exercises which gradually but directly enable the couple to work out the sexual problems. The general psychiatrist who uses the combined approach of analytically oriented sex therapy must choose the best time to introduce the sex therapy and carefully appraise the couple's joint and individual ability to tolerate the directive approach and to focus on sexual difficulties.

HYPNOTHERAPY

Hypnosis is a useful addition to basic individual psychotherapy programs, including programs focusing on sexual dysfunctions. It can accelerate the impact of psychotherapeutic intervention. Before beginning hypnotherapy the therapist must encourage the patient's co-operation during a series of nonhypnotic sessions. The aims of these sessions are to develop a secure doctor-patient relationship, to achieve a sense of physical and psychological comfort on the part of the patient, and to establish mutual goals for the treatment. During these initial meetings, the therapist also assesses the patient's capacity for the trance experience. Before any of the sessions involve hypnosis, the clinician takes a careful psychiatric history and performs a mental status examination.

Hypnotherapy generally focuses on symptom removal and attitude alteration. Used successfully, hypnosis enables the patient to gain control over the symptom that has been lowering self-esteem and disrupting psychological equilibrium. Focusing specifically on the symptom, the sexual dysfunction, the hypnotherapist instructs the patient on alternative means of dealing with the sexual encounter which provokes anxiety.

For example, a woman suffering from vaginismus receives the post-hypnotic suggestions that she will not feel pain during intercourse and that she will be able to relax her vagina and accept her partner's penis. She is also taught new attitudes, such as being entitled to sexual pleasure. Under hypnosis she can examine her fear or anger at sexual contact, and she learns how she expresses her emotions through her involuntary and symbolic bodily responses.

Patients are also taught techniques for relaxing before having sexual relations. Relaxed and relieved of anxiety, the patient's physiological responses to sexual stimulation can more readily result in pleasurable excitation and discharge. Psychological impediments to vaginal lubrication, erection, or orgasm are removed, and normal sexual functioning ensues.

BEHAVIOR THERAPY

Behavioral approaches were initially designed for the treatment of phobias. When the case involves sexual dysfunction, the behavioral therapist sees the patient as phobic of sexual interaction. Under a traditional behavioral model, a therapist sets up a hierarchy of anxiety-provoking situations for the patient, ranging from the least threatening to the most threatening. For example, a patient might experience minimal anxiety at the thought of caressing and overwhelming anxiety when imagining penile penetration. The behavior therapist then enables the patient to master the anxiety through a program of systematic desensitization. The program is designed to inhibit the patient's learned, maladaptive response by encouraging behaviors antithetical to anxiety. The patient begins by dealing with the least anxiety-producing situation in fantasy and progresses by steps to the greatest anxiety-producing situation. Medication, hypnosis, or special training in deep-muscle relaxation is sometimes used to help with the initial mastery of anxiety.

At the same time assertiveness training is used to help the patient express his or her sexual needs openly and without fear. Exercises in assertiveness are given in conjunction with sex therapy, and the patient is encouraged both to make sexual requests and to refuse to comply with requests perceived as unreasonable.

In one treatment variation, the sexual partner participates in the desensitization program. Instead of the therapist, the partner presents the hierarchy of situations to the patient. The therapist may also prescribe sexual exercises for the patient to perform at home, and, again, establish a hierarchy, starting with those activities that have proved most pleasurable and successful in the past. In all cases, a cooperative partner helps the patient to transport gains made during treatment sessions to sexual activity at home. Conversely, an obstructive or withdrawn partner can sabotage and slow down therapeutic progress.

INDIVIDUAL PSYCHOTHERAPY

Until the advent of sex therapy, clinicians treated sexual disorders as part of a more pervasive emotional disturbance, and treatment occurred during the course of general psychiatric treatment. Classic psychodynamic theory considers sexual inadequacy to have its roots in early developmental conflicts. One of the assumptions of psychotherapy is that the removal of the conflicts will allow the sexual impulse to become structurally acceptable to the patient's ego and thereby find appropriate means of satisfaction in the environment.

Individual psychotherapy is particularly useful for examining problems with intimacy, dependency, and closeness, problems which are so often accompanied by sexual dysfunction. In people whose capacity to trust is impaired, these problems prevent a mature, intimate relationship from developing. For them, sexual dysfunctions may serve a defensive purpose. Treatment focuses on the exploration of unconscious conflicts, motivation, fantasy, and various interpersonal difficulties. As these conflicts are resolved, the sexual functioning should improve, as should the patient's functioning in work and social spheres.

GROUP THERAPY

Group therapy is useful when a patient needs to examine both intrapsychic and interpersonal problems. In cases of sexual dysfunction, therapy group can be a strong support for the patient who feel ashamed, anxious, or guilty about a particular sexual problem. Th group is also a useful forum in which to counteract sexual myths and to educate patients regarding sexual anatomy, physiology, and varieties of behavior.

Groups organized specifically for the treatment of sexual disorder are often formed along homogeneous lines. Members may share the same problem, such as premature ejaculation or anorgasmia, or they may all be of the same sex with different sexual problems. Some groups are heterogeneous, composed of both men and women who are experiencing different sexual problems.

Groups may be psychodynamically oriented, behaviorally oriented or primarily educational. When the members in a group have a particular problem in common, therapy is usually behavioral in approach. For example, patients suffering from premature ejaculation may participate in a short-term, intensive group experience. In the group members share their sexual histories, feelings of inadequacy, and concerns about acceptance. They receive specific physiologic information, sometimes with the aid of audiovisual material. Away from the group members do homework assignments. For instance, they may be instructed to masturbate while employing a stop-start technique. combination of group support and group pressure helps some of the participants complete assignments they might otherwise want to avoid

As the short-term group process nears termination, members are encouraged to talk about their experiences with their partners at home.

Groups have also been effective when composed of sexually dysfunctional married couples. The group provides the opportunity to gather accurate information, provides consensual validation of individual preferences, and enhances self-esteem and self-acceptance. Techniques such as role playing and psychodrama may be used in treatment. Such groups are not indicated for couples when one partner is uncooperative, when a patient is suffering from a severe depression or psychosis, when the patient is repelled by explicit sexual audiovisual material, or when either partner has a strong fear of groups.

Intensive group psychotherapy can be effective when exploring the psychodynamic personality makeup. Psychodynamically oriented groups less often focus on a specific sexual dysfunction than do the behaviorally oriented groups. Patients with sexual anxieties frequently use denial and projection. With such patients, member-to-member and member-to-therapist transferences and interactions allow for the rapid emergence of sexual conflicts related to past experiences with siblings, parents, and other significant persons.

RESULTS

The reported effectiveness of various treatment methods for a problem of sexual dysfunction varies from study to study. Demonstrating the effectiveness of traditional outpatient psychotherapy is just as difficult when therapy is oriented to sexual problems as it is in general. So many factors are involved and in such complex interaction that efficacy eludes precise assessment. In some cases, the patient improves in all areas except the sexual area. We can unfortunately be confident that the more severe the psychopathology associated with a problem of long duration, the more adverse the outcome.

When behavioral approaches are used, empirical criteria which are supposed to predict outcome are more easily isolated. Using these criteria, for instance, it appears that couples who regularly practice assigned exercises have a much greater likelihood of successful outcome than do more resistant couples or than couples whose interaction involves mechanisms of blame or projection. Flexibility of attitude is also a positive prognostic factor. Overall, younger couples tend to complete sex therapy more often than do older couples.

Masters and Johnson (1970) have reported higher positive results for their dual-sex therapy approach. (See Table 1.) They have observed the failure rates of their clients, defining failure as the failure to initiate

TABLE 1. Data from 790 Couples*

Complaint	Overall Failure Rate
Primary impotence	40.6
Secondary impotence	30.9
Premature ejaculation	2.7
Ejaculatory incompetence	17.6
Primary orgasmic dysfunction	17.6
Situational orgasmic dysfunction	24.8

*Table prepared from Masters and Johnson (1970) data

reversal of the basic symptoms of the presenting sexual dysfunction. They compare initial failure rates with five-year follow-up findings for the same couples. Although some have criticized their definition of the percentage of presumed successes, other studies have confirmed the effectiveness of Masters and Johnson's approach (Marks, 1981). One therapist, however, seems to be nearly as effective as a dual-sex therapy team.

In general, methods that have proved effective singly or in combination include training in behavioral-sexual skills, systematic desensitization, directive marital counseling, traditional psychodynamic approaches, and group therapy. Although treating a couple for sexual disorders is the mode preferred by most workers, treatment of individuals has also been successful.

Chapter 4

Sex Therapy: The Problem Cases
by Alexander N. Levay, M.D.

INTRODUCTION

When Masters and Johnson first introduced sex therapy, it seemed extremely effective and almost universal in its applicability. In recent years, however, such universal efficacy has been questioned (Zilbergeld and Evans, 1980; Sobel, 1980; Brody, 1980; Levay and Kagle, 1977b). Experience indicates that Masters and Johnson's technique works well primarily with people whose anxieties center on issues of sexual performance and are not rooted in unconscious sexual or interpersonal conflicts. Consequently, changes in the basic technique have been gradually introduced. The treatment format has become open-ended and flexible in the rate and sequence of task assignments. When indicated, other psychotherapies, principally psychoanalytic psychotherapy and conjoint therapy, are either integrated or coordinated with the sex therapy (Levay and Kagle, 1977b).

Even with these modifications, however, some cases are refractory or very difficult to treat. Treatment for the presenting sexual dysfunction may be blocked, sabotaged, or even discontinued because of factors within the couple or factors within one or both individuals. In such cases, evidently, it is necessary to clear away interpersonal or intrapsychic difficulties so that the sex therapy may begin.

Since the problems encountered in sex therapy are of necessity dyadic, we shall focus first on the marital problems which cause treatment failure and then on the individual problems which interfere with couple therapy. Finally, a consideration of coping capacities and defensive styles is related both to the sexual dysfunction and to the need for continued growth in the techniques of treatment.

MARITAL PROBLEMS CAUSING TREATMENT FAILURE

Traditional sex therapy deals with some interpersonal or marital problems. But since the couples seen are often self-selected, highly motivated, and encouraged not to focus on past hurts during the two-week treatments, many aspects of marital distress are temporarily set aside. In more extended treatment, however, marital problems become quite obvious. Generally, they fall into three categories: marital disillusionment, marital mismatch, or marital conflict.

Marital disillusionment best describes the distress of those couples who seek sex therapy as a way of dealing with their sense of ennui or dissatisfaction with the state of being married. The cultural, social, and political movements of the 1960's and 1970's produced many new concepts of social role. Those issuing from the sexual revolution contribute to some people's dissatisfaction with their marriages.

Sometimes, caught in the throes of life-cycle crises, couples mistakenly believe sex is the paramount indicator of personal adequacy and interpersonal relatedness. Such couples use sex therapy consciously or unconsciously to test the viability of the marriage.

The couple's sex life often improves in the course of sex therapy when life-cycle or other questions are left unanswered, but their commitment to the marriage may worsen as they discover that a good sex life is not the panacea they had expected. Sex therapy could not, nor was it intended to, take the place of resolving the disillusionment of life-cycle questions for men and women.

Couples who seek sex therapy as a way of dealing with unresolved differences in their goals, values, and essential ways of relating may be suffering from a *marital mismatch* which sex therapy cannot correct. Their sexual difficulties often originate in basic differences of style and attitude. Neither member of the couple is "wrong" or "neurotic" in what he or she wants out of marriage, but their objectives are different, and the incongruence of attitudes can undermine their relationship.

Short-term sex therapy or even extended sex therapy which bypasses these marital problems may produce good results initially. However, when such differences are left unresolved, they will often recur. Only when these issues are adequately dealt with do the couple's long-term sex life and marital life improve.

The third form of marital distress, *marital conflict,* does not necessarily involve the type of schism or disengagement seen in mismatched couples. Rather, couples in conflict may agree on goals, attitudes, and values, and they are intensely involved with each other. These couples are caught in defeating patterns, including power struggles, reenacted parent-child relationships, or out-and-out hostility and destructiveness. The couple in conflict does not disagree out of principle (although they may claim to) but rather out of their need to fight or to goad the other partner into behaving in certain ways. Much of what goes wrong between such couples involves transference issues. Sometimes the partner is manipulated into acting in ways similar to those of the opposite sex parent, and the process is reciprocal. Sometimes the transference involves negative sibling behaviors. In couples in conflict, the major interactions tend to be negative.

Although these couples are frequently in crises which make treatment difficult, the stability of the relationships should not be underestimated. Marital conflict, because it represents a continuation of family patterns which are, if not pleasant, at least known, comfortable, and neurotically gratifying, often results in a fierce sense of loyalty and permanence.

Couples in marital conflict frequently have a difficult time in sex therapy. Often they are consumed by an effort to get the therapist to take sides, to make the partner look bad, or otherwise to maintain the status quo of the relationship. It is not uncommon for the therapy to be aborted as soon as significant change begins to occur. Couples in conflict, more than those who are disillusioned or mismatched, need extensive marital therapy before sex therapy can be effective (Levay and Kagle, 1978).

Gridlock Couples

In a particularly malignant form of marital conflict, a variety of individual and interpersonal factors combine to characterize what the author calls the *gridlock couple*. Factors characterizing the gridlock couple include (1) a difficulty in handling shared experiences which results in joint tasks being avoided or not succeeding; (2) a skewed distribution of affect, in which one partner appears significantly more gentle, caring, tender, and capable of positive affect than does the other; (3) a marked dependency of the first partner on the second partner for a sense of worth, esteem, and approval, especially in the area of sexual functioning; (4) a notable hostility or contempt or both in the second partner toward the first partner and unconsciously toward all people of the opposite sex; and (5) a profound dependency of the hostile or contemptuous second partner on his or her mate and their state of being married for emotional security. Any attempt by either partner to terminate the relationship is usually preemptively crushed by the other. In these cases, when symptoms are initially reversed, a continuous cycle of relapses and renewed symptom reversals begins, ultimately terminating in the treatment failure.

The history of these couples frequently is that the dependent partners had fiercely controlling mothers who had actively suppressed their aggression and autonomous strivings. Conditioned while young to secure love from their mothers by active compliance, they had performed only under the direction of and according to the specifications of their mothers, and they had catered to or even anticipated their mothers' emotional needs. The aggressive partners had not experienced love when young. Having known physical or emotional abuse instead of love, they developed maladaptive defense systems which warded off not only the repetition of past traumas in the here and now, but also the "threat" of love and tenderness as well.

Throughout treatment such couples need to maintain their familiar system. In their complicated relationship, the dependent partner's deficiencies are held responsible for the other's unhappiness, while the hostile partner can deny personal sexual difficulties, underlying hostility toward the spouse, and presumably comparable guilt. So overriding is the need to maintain this system that it completely cancels out the need to resolve the sexual problem. As the case illustrates, the complexities of treatment are considerable.

CASE 1 A handsome pilot, who was a premature ejaculator and infertile because of a postinfectious obliteration of both sperm ducts, was married to an aggressively seductive woman who was the victim of childhood maternal sadism. The wife was very limited in her capacity to show and receive love. She was habitually defensive, hostile, and distrustful of positive feelings.

Against her husband's wishes, but with his passive compliance, she adopted a handicapped child, once had herself artificially inseminated, and had an affair with his friend, resulting in a kept pregnancy. During therapy she heaped abuse on her husband because of his sexual difficulties. Only after considerable work did her attitude seemingly improve. As a result, her husband's premature ejaculation began to clear up rapidly, and he experienced an upsurge of warmth and affection towards her. This degree of tenderness and newly found sexual gratification stimulated great anxiety which the wife needed to ward off by resuming her vituperative, abusive behavior. Her behavior guaranteed cessation of the husband's newly found potency and ardor. Interpretations to her of the true meaning of her continuously disruptive and abrasive behavior fell on deaf ears, and therapy could only be started all over once again, never to be successfully completed.

INDIVIDUAL PROBLEMS CAUSING TREATMENT FAILURE

Good sexual functioning between adults is sexually gratifying and emotionally fulfilling, allowing both partners to give and receive while they remain individually autonomous. The result is a strengthened sense of well-being for both the individual and the couple. The personality problems of one partner or of both can cause considerable pathology in their sexual relationship. One or both may manifest impairments in specific ego functions, such as those reported in the areas of pleasure, intimacy, and cooperation (Levay and Kagle, 1977a). Such impairments can, in turn, impede gratification of sexual needs, the fulfillment of a need to feel cared about, close, and loved, or the ability to reciprocate.

Deficiencies of Ego Functions

People with pleasure disorders are blocked in their ability to identify, experience, or enjoy pleasurable sensations. They therefore cannot be gratified. Those with an excessive need state, on the other hand, have such overdetermined needs in the area of sexual gratification that no amount of sexual activity can fulfill them. They want "perpetual sex" as a substitute for the love and nurturing they lacked in childhood. Relationships with such dependent partners are draining because of the amount of sex and togetherness they require and because these partners tend to have difficulty reciprocating.

People who have difficulty with intimacy cannot enjoy closeness because it makes them overwhelmingly anxious. A subgroup of these patients harbor deep-seated hostility and choose to express their aggression when experiencing intimacy. While such hostile reactions can be defensive against the anxiety of intimacy, the primary intent here is not to love but to hurt. It could be said that such patients are not "in love" but "in hate." They inflict their hostility in intimate moments in order to distress or disable the partner and wreak havoc on the partner's sexuality. If dependent patients drain the partner, hostile patients tend to destroy the partner or at least his or her sense of intimacy, sexual performance, and pleasure. Needless to say, they do the same to themselves, but the consequences of their behavior to themselves are ego-syntonic and are not experienced as either pain or loss.

Pleasure and intimacy dysfunctions can be unilateral, but cooperative disorders almost invariably involve both spouses. The primary aspect of cooperative disorders is an inability to collaborate or to agree on common goals, priorities, or values. Viewed as an ego deficiency, however, a cooperative dysfunction involves an underlying need to compete with or to deprive the partner, a need usually accompanied by other manifestations of transferential rage and retaliation. Giving to the partner is experienced as a loss or defeat. The self-object axis, as it manifests itself in this group, runs from the narcissists, who are so self-involved that they are unable to relate to the needs of others, to the pathological altruists, who can give endlessly but are totally incapable of receiving. Not surprisingly, pathological narcissists are frequently paired with pathological altruists; they complement each other. At base, however, their relationship is essentially depriving, either of the self or of the other.

Nonerotized Aggression and Hostility

Cumulative clinical experience indicates that nonerotized aggression in a sexual setting plays an important role in producing and maintaining sexual dysfunction and merits special attention in a discussion of problem cases. At the outset any discussion of aggression and hostility in the sexual arena ought to emphasize the universal condition which creates hostility in all people. People do not learn appropriately about sex in childhood and may even be sexually deprived. In contrast to other areas, such as sports, health care, or academics, where parents lovingly, constantly, and consistently facilitate their children's growth and development, sex is neglected and even taboo. Parents consistently frustrate the child's sexual needs. At the same time, children are well aware that parents gratify each other sexually and experience the unique closeness that accompanies sexual intimacies. Children themselves are, out of hand and without appropriate explanation, excluded from participation. They feel confusion, jealousy, rejection, hurt and, particularly, aggressive feelings.

This universal condition of sexual deprivation may account in part for Stoller's assertion that sexual arousal has its roots in aggression (Stoller, 1976). In many people these factors will probably not generate serious problems. The predominantly positive input they have received throughout childhood will help them overcome the adverse influences on their sexual growth and development. But if these emotions re-emerge during adult sexual years, they affect the quality of intimacy, responsiveness, and pair-bonding in predictably negative ways.

For purposes of clarity, nonerotized aggression must be distinguished from erotized aggression, which, if experienced or entered into with a suitable matching partner, does not lead to sexual dysfunction but to an enhanced sexual experience. The erotized forms of aggression range from mild expressions of aggression, physical or psychological "love nibbles" so to speak, to outright physical or psychological hurt. It should be pointed out, however, that in such mutually gratifying sexual exchanges, often called sadomasochistic, people take care not to inflict any kind of real physical or emotional harm. Both partners need to maintain the primacy of pleasurable aspects of their exchanges and tend to ignore the implicit psychological harm involved in the perpetuation of their pathological pattern. If aggression gets out of hand between such couples, as it all too often does, it usually takes place outside the sexual arena.

Nonerotized aggression, while it is expressed during sex, is not part of either partner's sexual arousal system. This nonerotized aggression is best described as hostility because the conscious or unconscious intention is to distress the partner emotionally or to render him or her sexually disabled. A person chooses to express the aggression in the sexual arena since it arouses particularly hostile feelings in the susceptible partner. The partner is particularly vulnerable to aggressive behavior in this context if he or she experiences and expects tender or loving feelings.

The aggression involved in these exchanges can be primary or secondary. *Primary* aggression stems from impaired childhood development. If a child has experienced intense detachment or intense hostility on the part of one or both parents, accompanied by physical or emotional abuse, he or she may develop a maladaptive defense system which wards off not only a repetition of past hurts but any closeness, including love and tenderness, which is experienced as threatening.

A woman who has been physically abused and also excessively aroused or traumatized sexually by watching her parents in unbridled lovemaking may grow up with uniquely anxious associations to sexuality. In the marital transference she may defensively victimize her husband.

> **CASE 2** A woman equated sex with rape because of a mistaken childhood notion, derived from watching her parents in lovemaking, that sex is something a man does to a woman in violence. This notion was reinforced by her daytime experience of her father who was given to violent outbursts, often beating her with a strap. As a result, the woman had an acute anxiety attack when she went to buy bedroom furniture before her marriage to a gentle and kind man. She felt that she was selecting the furniture on which she was to be raped. After the marriage, she would consistently and preemptively strike so that her husband would lose his arousal. (It was only later, incidentally, that she discovered that her childhood impression of sex was a distortion. Through conversations she realized that her mother was orgasmic, loved sex, initiated it, and in general had a wholesome appetite for it.)

A more common form of nonerotized aggression which is treated in sex therapy is *secondary* aggression, anger which comes from frustration due to failed sexual experiences between couples. If one partner is particularly sensitive, misinterpreting the failed sexual experience as a sign of rejection or indifference on the other's part, the hostility of that partner can be intense, even sadistic. However, as soon as the couple is helped in therapy to have sexual experiences that are gratifying, the hostility evaporates almost instantly, a sure indication that the aggression has indeed been secondary. By contrast, if restoration to good sexual functioning makes the partner extremely anxious, this indicates that the aggression is of the primary type.

The course of nonerotized aggression can be influenced by the guilt it engenders during sexual contact. One partner may experience guilt over inflicting emotional pain and sexual dysfunction on the other and may also feel guilty about the other's counterreactions. Some of the developmental factors that led to pleasure in aggression can be counterbalanced by conscience mechanisms which deem such aggression unacceptable. Patients whose conscience mechanisms function well are easier to treat than others, because the conscience mechanisms supply motivation and make the aggressive behavior ego-dystonic.

The partner's reactions themselves have important implications for treatment outcome. The partner may be crushed by the hostility, become depressed and withdraw, or retaliate in the form of vituperative counterattack. In either case, the immediate outcome will be different. In all instances, the couples run a long-term risk of destroying their sexual life altogether. Only a very strong partner, who can withstand the aggression and not respond to it destructively, will be able to tolerate the relationship. He or she can handle the aggression as the partner's problem, seek treatment, and participate in the treatment constructively by helping the partner to identify the sources of aggression, enabling him or her to drop the aggressive behavior.

Other Individual Factors

A variety of other individual conflicts can disrupt a couple's ability to be sexual and can also interfere with the course of treatment. Space permits but brief mention of some of the most important. The pre-oedipal fears of separation and abandonment and of fusion, as well as oedipal issues, may be significant. Unconscious conflicts based on impaired dyadic relationships between mother and child, as well as on the triadic difficulties of the oedipal phase, have obvious implications for a person's relationships. The triad of the couple and the therapist may be especially significant and problematic for some people.

The quality of sibling relationships is also taken into serious account in sex therapy because sibling transferences to spouses tend to predominate over parental transferences. If couples have had good primary object relations with parents and have only unresolved difficulties with siblings, their problems in the marriage tend to be more benign and treatable. Where parental transferences as well as sibling transferences to spouses take place, and where these are complicated by unresolved preoedipal issues, the cases are extremely difficult to treat.

When other developmental factors involving childhood trauma are introduced, the problems are significantly compounded. Physical or emotional abuse, pathological punishment for childhood sexual behaviors, incest, and childhood deprivation, by themselves or in combination with those factors discussed previously, can cause considerable difficulty in sexual functioning and the treatment of sexual problems.

DEFENSIVE STYLES AND COPING CAPACITIES

Not only are the psychosexual disorders consequences of developmental factors, unconscious conflicts, and deficiencies in ego functions, they may also be strongly tied to defensive styles and capabilities. Some dysfunctions appear to be the result of breakdowns of coping mechanisms; premature ejaculation, impotence, or impulsive sexual acting out are examples. Others, such as the sexual phobias, desire disorders, nonorgasmic responses, and vaginismus, are defensive over-deployments of coping mechanisms and coping operations.

In general, premature ejaculation in men and orgasmic disorders in women are the easiest syndromes to treat because intrapsychic conflict is usually only minimally involved. Orgasmic difficulties in men tend to be more severe. Arousal disorders in men (impotence) can run the gamut from being mild performance issues to the severest form of defensive fear against aggression or abandonment. Sexual phobias can be effective defenses, in that phobics simply avoid the sexual situation. But since phobic patients often have rather weakened ego strength, treatment may be difficult. Even the perversions and homosexuality (which is no longer considered a perversion) are best seen as defensive operations that have become characterological or institutionalized.

The real difference in treatment outcome is not whether a person is suffering from a desire disorder or from premature ejaculation; rather, the degree and type of ego strength and coping capacity make the difference in treatment. The less a person has or the more over-deployed and misapplied the defenses are, the more difficult the treatment will be. The discussion which follows of necessity omits some of the more commonly observed syndromes, such as the sexual phobias and delusions, and focuses on desire and impulse disorders, homosexuality, and fetishism.

Desire Disorders

Lately it has been fashionable to think of desire disorders as a new syndrome. In fact, desire disorders have always existed. Now that the original sex therapy patient population with its relatively mild disorders has been depleted, patients with deeper disorders are coming for sex therapy.

People with desire disorders usually have good ego strength. Theirs is a misapplied defensive strength based on unconscious fears about sex which make them cut off desire at the pass. Like patients who use phobic avoidance, however, patients with desire disorders have sometimes had no sexual experiences in years, which means they have suffered an inordinate secondary loss of accumulated adult sexual experiences. The fact that a small group of people with desire disorders are virtually sexual innocents adds major problems to the therapeutic task.

Impulse Disorders

People who impulsively act out sexually not only do not avoid the situations that they should; they feel such sexual desire that they act on it before they consider the implications of their actions or their feelings for the particular person. These people usually come into sex therapy only after they have gotten into deep trouble. They have true and deep ambivalence, the two halves of the ambivalence being completely split apart. Suspending their defenses, they impulsively act on half of their ambivalence to bypass the other. Once they have acted, the other half strikes back, and they are likely to react impulsively again but, this time, in the opposite direction. At first they might plunge into an affair, feeling intense sexuality, love, and a sense of commitment. Then, when the other half of the ambivalence strikes, they feel no desire for the person and never want to see him or her again.

Homosexuality

The traditional way of viewing sexuality was to categorize it as homosexual, heterosexual, or perverse. Clinical evidence suggests a better way of viewing it, considering that people are sexual and that they can be sexual with members of the opposite sex and with members of their own sex. This does not mean that people are bisexual. Most people clearly have a heterosexual or homosexual preference, probably based in large measure on some form of biological loading. In some individuals, of course, neither form of sexuality is comfortable and pleasurable.

Our culture is, on the one hand, strongly in favor of heterosexuality and, on the other, opposed to homosexuality. Culturally speaking, fear of rejection and a sense of perversion attach to homosexuality. Because of the vicissitudes of childhood, some people use homosexuality as a defense against their feared heterosexuality. Conversely, some latent homosexuals use heterosexuality as a defense against their homosexuality (the Don Juan syndrome).

In therapy with those who wish to become heterosexual, the purpose is not to "cure" the homosexuality. Rather, when the patient has no biological reason to be homosexual, one uncovers the roots of the fears attaching to heterosexuality. Unconscious fears are made conscious, and their impact is reduced. Treatment is difficult because defensive homosexuality is likely to have been reinforced by homosexual experiences over many years, creating an embedded pleasure pattern that is exclusively homosexual. Patients may also benefit from corrective heterosexual experiences with a suitable partner in judiciously introduced sex therapy exercises. The exercises help to desensitize patients behaviorally to heterosexual fears and resensitize them to heterosexual pleasures. Gaining the partner's acceptance of the homosexuality is helpful unless the partner excessively condones or encourages the homosexual expression. This could lead to a regressive resistance to the therapy introduced by the partner.

Fetishes

Fetishes and related phenomena are best seen as quasi-characterological defenses in the sexual area against overwhelming and unbearable anxiety about involvement with persons of the opposite sex. Fetishes are seen almost exclusively in men, and severity varies in degree. In severe cases the fetishist prefers to have sex by himself with the fetish. In milder cases fetishists will have sex with other persons provided that the fetish is worn. Milder cases are more often seen in sex therapy, and results are remarkably good.

The fetish is best seen as a transitional object (Person and Ovesey, 1976). It protects against undue, unbearable, incestuous involvement with the mother and transfers the safety of the mother to the new and feared woman. Fetishes also protect against castration anxiety and other anxieties. Similar mechanisms are at work in transvestites who need a more extensive protection against overinvolvement with the mother. Dressing like the mother makes them feel safer with another person. The garter belt, for example, is a protective displacement mechanism. The sight of the mother's genitals is an overwhelming sexual stimulus, and the absence of the penis is a source of anxiety. Emotion can be displaced onto an article of clothing worn near the genitals. Masquerading as a substitute penis, the article reduces the castration anxiety occasioned by the sight of the mother's penisless genitals. The therapist helps the patient work through the roots of fear and anxiety and, in combination with appropriate sex therapy exercises, can help him to correct the disorder.

CONCLUSION

By and large the various sexual syndromes in both sexes fall into a hierarchy of treatment difficulty. All of the syndromes, however, are sometimes difficult to treat. The factors that determine the degree of difficulty in any given case are unconscious conflicts, ego deficiencies, and severely impaired developmental histories. When the dysfunctions appear as breakdowns of defenses, or as the products of a maladaptive deployment of excessive defense mechanisms, treatment may be further complicated. Patients with deficient coping mechanisms need to be helped to acquire better ways of coping with their sexual arousal, anxieties, dysphoric affects, and aggression. By contrast, overly defended patients have to be helped to reduce, move, or lay to rest some of their excessive and unnecessary defensive deployments so that sexual functioning can resume.

The therapist works in two ways (1) by making unconscious fears and conflicts conscious, thereby demonstrating their unrealistic basis, and (2) by the judicious assignment of behavioral tasks. In the process of therapy two factors that add to the difficulty of treating these complex patients (and partners) are negative transferences towards the therapist and the resistances which develop. Either may need to be dealt with analytically, although sometimes they can be successfully bypassed through the use of purely behavioral techniques (Weissberg and Levay, 1981; Levay, Kagle, and Weissberg, 1979a).

Sex therapy for the difficult cases has come full circle, and, once again, it is traditional individual psychoanalytic psychotherapy or conjoint therapy that is used to treat the problem. Masters and Johnson's sex therapy exercises are important adjuncts. As behavioral treatment modules, they are effective when introduced at suitable points. In some patients, however, the unconscious conflicts are so deeply entrenched and the traumatic childhood residues are so overriding that the problems remain very difficult to resolve. Thus sex therapy, to paraphrase Freud, has become "terminable and interminable."

Chapter 5

Medicine, Surgery, and Sexual Dysfunction
by Robert Dickes, M.D.

INTRODUCTION

Doctors are generally unaware of the extent of the emotional traumas patients suffer during acute and chronic illness. When patients are unable to deal emotionally with the problems stemming from a physical illness, many physicians are surprised. Especially in sexual matters, the doctors may overlook the initial signs of impending difficulty. Not only do most physicians overlook or avoid patients' sexual problems; sometimes the doctor actually causes problems by improper management of the patient's sexual anxieties. Unfortunately, the psychiatrist is usually consulted only when the patient requests help and after the patient's problems have escalated. When the patient with organic difficulties, past or present, does consult the psychiatrist about a sexual problem, the psychiatrist must consider carefully how the organic disease may be affecting the patient's sexual functioning.

MEDICINE

Cardiovascular Disorders

Patients suffering from an acute myocardial infarct are usually anxious and fearful of dying, not only during the acute phase, but also during convalescence and between bouts of infarction. Most patients recover sufficiently from the average infarct to return to home and work in a matter of weeks. These weeks are a time of great anxiety for the patient, who fears facing the workaday world. Although patients rarely express their concern, most are anxious about sexual activity. Recovery from cardiovascular injury is almost always sufficient to permit the patient to engage in a full range of sexual activity as soon as is practical (Soloff, 1977). Clearly, patients need physicians who know these facts and can help them deal with their fears and anxieties. Inappropriate management, on the other hand, can lead to a phobic avoidance of sex. Previously well-balanced, functioning marriages may suffer severe disruptions and eventual divorce, if not a sort of armed neutrality. Husband and wife rarely get psychiatric help until the marriage begins to suffer.

When the psychiatrist does get involved, he or she must deal with many specific issues. He or she must obtain from the patient's physician as much knowledge as possible of the patient's physical state and also establish a good working relationship with the physician. The psychiatrist should be aware that when the patient's illness is life threatening, the transference to the internist may be much more positive than to the psychiatrist. The psychiatrist then must also negotiate with the internist to insure his or her cooperation. When the internist is not cooperative, the psychiatrist must be very careful to avoid countertransference reactions. A noncontentious relationship with the internist is of great help at such a time and, with the patient's consent, discussion between the two specialists can be very helpful. Most physicians will be only too glad to share the responsibility and to allow the sexual difficulties and emotional stresses to be dealt with by the psychiatrist.

Most patients understand very little about anatomy and physiology. Usually the internist will have carefully explained the patient's condition. The psychiatrist should review the facts and their sexual implications with the patient. Often the psychiatrist will have to detail what has happened to the heart and how it was healed.

The patient's spouse must also be a partner in the therapeutic process. Unconsciously, spouses view becoming ill as a hostile act, which in turn makes them feel hostile. The illness also places great burdens on the spouse, leading to resentment and guilt feelings. Some partners may therefore require help in managing their concealed and overt hostilities. Support and instruction should supplement necessary interpretations of their emotional reactions to their partners' illness. The reduction of tensions helps the relationship and therefore the couple's sexual functioning. Sensate focus exercises also can help, both to direct sexual activity and to reduce anxiety, as well as to focus attention on the relationship.

In general, patients who have functioned well prior to acute illness return to normal sexual functioning without difficulty. If, however, a sexual dysfunction antedates the physical illness, the psychiatrist must necessarily deal with the entire premorbid state. A well-balanced patient will respond quickly to the rapid method of sex therapy that uses sensate focus exercises. Others may require a longer-term and more analytic approach.

Other circulatory disturbances, such as stroke, peripheral vascular diseases, emboli, and so forth, can occasion the development of sexual problems and impotence. Psychological treatment can use the basic approaches of brief sex therapy. The types of goals for sexual functioning must be responsive to the type and location of the lesions. If the man cannot achieve an erection for physiological reasons, nongenital contact and lovemaking short of intercourse may be sensible goals. Patients have reported much benefit and pleasure even when genital union is impossible. For people who have been together a long time, acceptance of the physical difficulty without guilt and frustration will come from a realistic acceptance and adjustment to the actualities.

Endocrine Disorders

Psychiatrists are often prone to label cases of impotence as psychogenic without seeking careful competent diagnostic screening to explore other causes. In a recent study of 105 consecutive patients with impotence, Spark, White and Connolly (1980) concentrated on the hypothalamic-pituitary-gonadal axis, and they discovered that 37 of these patients had organic dysfunctions which had been undiagnosed. To discover a year or so after treatment begins that the patient's difficulty is really of organic origin is embarrassing. Patients who complain of what seems to be a psychogenic sexual dysfunction should always receive a thorough examination, including an evaluation of possible endocrine disorders. Possibilities include the adreno-genital syndrome, which is noted for the masculinization of the female genitals and masculine behavior. Most youngsters with this syndrome do grow into normal womanhood. Other endocrine disorders which impair sexual function are acromegaly, Cushing's syndrome, and concealed Addison's disease.

Metabolic Diseases and Chronic Illness

Many chronic metabolic diseases affect sexual functioning. Diabetes mellitus is a prime example. The organic factors causing impotence in this illness have been demonstrated in several studies. Finding that 37 out of 45 impotent diabetics had neurogenic vesicular abnormalities, Ellenberg (1971) concluded that neuropathy of the automatic nervous system was involved. Faerman et al. (1974) confirmed these findings; they found lesions of the nerve fibers controlling erections. Vascular lesions of the pudendal arterial systems have also been reported. Psychiatrists should become aware that the first symptom a diabetic patient notices may be a developing impotence. Chronic illnesses, ranging from rheumatic arthritis to malignancy, also interfere with sexual function, but they are too numerous to discuss in detail.

A Word of Caution

Nocturnal Penile Tumescence (NPT) studies have been used to determine the presence of organic factors in impotence. If good erections, as measured by the NPT apparatus, do not occur for three nights successively, some researchers have claimed, organic disease is probable. Similarly, they presume, good erections indicate a psychic cause for the erective difficulty. A word of caution is necessary. Wasserman et al.

have pointed out, "The basic assumption that NPT measurements can distinguish psychogenic from organic impotence has never been demonstrated in patients shown to be psychogenically and organically impotent independent of the NPT measurements themselves" (1980, 575). Direct observations of the patient's fullest erections are necessary before any conclusion is made.

SURGERY

Most serious operations have a deleterious effect upon a person's basic body image and inflict a psychic trauma of greater or lesser extent. Those operations which mutilate, those designed to counteract cancerous disease, and those performed on the reproductive apparatus are especially prone to damage a person's basic self-image. The threat to the person's psychological balance can be considerable and may necessitate psychiatric intervention. The clinical picture, as it eventually emerges, has many facets, including the patient's previous mental health and basic character structure. Excessive dependency and the regressive effects of hospitalization may well produce temporary or prolonged psychic imbalance.

Unconsciously, many patients perceive surgical interventions as a form of punishment for misdeeds, usually sexual in nature. This is especially true for mutilating operations, which activate unconscious associations with castration fears. The fear and guilt such patients feel is sometimes so great that it is no wonder that they become anxious about their sexual performances. The anxiety itself can induce impotence or other sexual dysfunctions. Where anxiety is rooted in conscious conflicts, treatment will be most difficult, since problems stem from early childhood. When more superficial factors, such as ignorance, weakness, and so forth, are causing the sexual dysfunction, patients respond much more readily to treatment. Depression, commonplace after illness and surgery, requires the usual special attention.

The duration and type of care depends upon the patient's psychological state. Assessing the patient's state, the psychiatrist must be aware of the actual effects of the operation, whether the defect in functioning is permanent or temporary, and whether to expect a difficulty in the patient's social sphere or earning capacity. In some cases, a team, including the psychiatrist, should work to enable the individual to regain an appropriate place in society. When a disability remains, the psychiatrist must help the patient adjust to reality and to deal with his or her guilt about the disability.

Surgery on the Male

The kidneys, ureters, and bladder are not considered parts of the sexual apparatus, but rather of the excretory apparatus. Most patients, therefore, do not consider operations on these parts to be operations on their sexual organs. Following convalescence, the normal male generally has no problem in regaining sexual potency and leading an active sex life.

The situation is quite different for operations on the urethra, since it functions both as part of the sexual apparatus and as part of the excretory system. Urethral surgery can affect both urination and ejaculation and create considerable pain. Painful ejaculation obviously can inhibit sexual activity. If the dysfunction continues long past the period of healing, it is likely to be of psychological origin. The therapist, after assuring that the healing is complete and that the dysfunction is psychological, may institute the appropriate treatment.

Orchidectomy does not necessarily result in impotence, since the testes are not involved in producing an erection. Erection is due to the distribution of blood to the corpus cavernosum and corpus spongiosum. Many patients do not realize that a healthy, stable male can ordinarily achieve erections after an orchidectomy.

When testicular removal is due to carcinoma, however, the operation is often followed by either chemotherapy or radiation therapy or both. These are profoundly debilitating, and the patient will not return to his former state of sexual functioning unless and until the debilitation ceases. If sexual incompetence becomes the rule due to the extent of the operation and therapies, it may be of much lesser consequence than the patient's fear of losing his life. Appropriate discussion of these fears and the factual situation may help both the wife and the patient. Joint or separate sessions may be indicated. The emotional support provided by proper psychiatric help can make the difference in saving a marriage, and possibly in saving sexual competence.

Every surgical situation induces a depression, usually temporary. This universal depression may be deepened by a patient's loss of confidence, earning power, or sexual competence or by other factors. In such cases, couples therapy is almost always required in order to help the wife to deal with her own problems.

Vasectomy has become relatively commonplace. The operation is simple, and many now consider it the best means of contraception. The sterility, however, is usually permanent. A candidate for vasectomy should receive a careful psychiatric evaluation, so as to ascertain his stability and the likelihood of his adaptation to the irreversible consequences. Adequate previous sexual performance and a long-term, stable sexual pattern indicate the patient is suitable for this operation.

Prostatectomy is a common operation in older men. The retrograde ejaculation which frequently ensues should be explained to the patient before the operation so he can anticipate and adjust to it. This helps him avoid an anxious reaction to the effects of the operation.

Extensive pelvic dissection may lead to a resultant impotence, since the vascular supply to the penis may be disrupted. Men who require such operations for cancer should know about the resulting loss of potency and the other complications, such as urinary incompetence. In these cases, no amount of psychological help will enable the man to regain erectile ability. However, he and his wife can benefit from help with their emotional responses and learn to enjoy sexual pleasure without vaginal containment.

Surgery on the Female

In our culture female physical attractiveness and childbearing ability are highly valued. Because of this, these traits are fundamental to many women's self-esteem and social acceptance. Any operation on a woman's reproductive organs is therefore very likely to cause her severe emotional distress, and it can interfere with her ability to enjoy sexual relations.

Because of the internalization of their sexual organs, women are much more subject than men to sexual fantasies concerning the effects of any operation, and their external body images are less coherent.

Psychiatrists treating women should be aware of this and understand why genital operations can cause them such significant emotional consequences.

THE BREAST   Operated upon for carcinoma of the breast, a woman is already well aware of the dangers of dying. What we psychiatrists need to remember is that a woman's sense of her own value often rests upon her appearance, and that our society considers the breast a main part of her attractiveness. Women who have a mastectomy, therefore, are prone to feel unattractive and to fear a loss of love. The fear of rejection has led many a woman to act as though she were uninterested in sex or men, in effect quitting before being rejected. She is depressed about her general appearance and the scar and how they affect her partner. She may then suffer by initiating a rejection, which induces a counter-rejection. A vicious cycle is established which alienates her from people she loves.

Many men are unable to deal with the mastectomy's effects upon their partners. This may stem from a man's unconscious dependency on the breast. Moreover, when a woman loses her breast, it can stir up unconscious castration anxieties in the man, and he may develop an aversion at the very time the woman is most in need of his love, understanding, and support. In this way, depression can result for the man as well as for the woman.

Surgeons should be aware that if the man actively participates in the entire process leading to surgery, the postoperative course will be freer of difficulties and depression. Unfortunately, most surgeons do not undertake this involvement process, and we as psychiatrists see the end results.

Proper communication between the partners is essential. Mastering their fears requires exploring them, and, quite likely, exposing their unconscious roots. A modification of behavior technique can be helpful at the right time, step-by-step, looking at and touching the scar until it no longer produces adverse affects. After this, general sensate focus exercises may be instituted. Reconstructive surgery should be considered a viable rehabilitative approach, since a successful reconstruction can be of considerable value in reestablishing a woman's self-esteem.

THE UTERUS   Women's psychological responses to the removal of the uterus are quite variable. Generally, a malignancy produces greater psychological trauma than do fibromyomas. The patient's belief in the necessity of the operation is sometimes crucial in minimizing the emotional impact. Psychological maturity also favorably influences the outcome. Chronological age makes a difference, too. Since childbearing is of major importance to younger women, the removal of the uterus creates a much less favorable psychological climate for a young person than it does for an older one.

A partner's loving and accepting attitude also favorably influences the psychological outcome. Some men, however, are quite rejecting to their mates, whom they consider to have been surgically "mutilated." While they may offer many rational explanations for their rejecting attitudes, we must, of course, remember that psychological responses are not necessarily based upon logic. Primary-process thinking and deeply unconscious anxieties can influence a man's attitude, and the effects of such unconscious factors upon sexual performance can be enormous. It is a necessary part of the psychiatric task to render these hidden affects conscious and then to help alleviate the untoward effects of the emotions. As with other operations, depression follows and must be dealt with carefully. Again, we should remember that all operations may be viewed unconsciously as punishment and that this is especially true for operations on the sexual organs.

THE OVARIES   Bilateral oophorectomy causes sterility. Operations on the ovaries cause many of the same problems as operations on the breast and uterus. The same careful attention to the patient's and the partner's unconscious and conscious responses is necessary, as is care in working through deeply hidden affects and depression.

CONCLUSION
All illnesses and operations cause some psychological imbalance. The more serious illnesses and surgical operations are likely to produce serious psychological disturbances and to impair sexual functioning, as well as general psychological well-being.

A psychiatrist who intends to treat patients with the conditions discussed must be familiar with physical illnesses, treatments, and their general outcomes. Therapists must be careful not to initiate procedures which are beyond the patient's physical capacity. As a general rule, it is best to wait until convalescence is complete before dealing directly with sexual problems with sensate focus exercises. Once the patient's level of physical capacity has been established in cooperation with the medical or surgical caretaker, the psychiatrist can initiate a plan which is responsive to the patient's physical and organic capabilities and limitations and which addresses the psychological needs and capacities of both patient and spouse.

Chapter 6 # Sexual Behavior in the Separated, Divorced, Widowed, and the Aged
by Ira B. Pauly, M.D.

INTRODUCTION
When the sexual aspects of a relationship are good, most couples seem almost not to notice them and even to take them for granted. But when sex becomes problematic, it becomes a source of conflict, increasingly difficult to ignore. Sexual problems often spill over into other aspects of the relationship. Similarly, when other aspects are strained, secondary sexual problems can ensue. Whatever the origin, if sexual problems remain unresolved for long, the couple is at risk of divorce or separation.

Some couples do continue in their relationships without resolving the sexual problems. They make adjustments, such as having extramarital involvements. Or they attempt to ignore their sexual problems and hang in there "for the children." Just as sex therapy can help many couples with their primary sexual dysfunctions, relationship therapy can be successful in improving those secondary sexual problems which arise from continuing hostility and resentment. All too frequently, however, the couple is unable or unwilling to continue the relationship, and separation and divorce finally do ensue. Thus, as we help people to deal with both primary and secondary sexual problems, as well as with their relationships, we must consider the possible impact of divorce and separation on their sexual functioning.

This chapter deals with the postmarital sexual relations of people who are separated and divorced and touches upon the special case of those whose separations are caused by the spouse's death. While some of the issues related to separated and divorced couples are obviously quite different from those related to widowhood, similarities are sufficient to warrant some common discussion. Especially when separation by divorce or widowhood occurs relatively early in life, the groups have a number of sexual concerns in common.

The sexual adjustment of the aged is of growing importance to psychiatrists. In many ways their sexual adjustment is a very different matter from that of people who have separated through death or otherwise from their spouses. Because of this, the sexual adjustment of the aged is considered separately. But since so many older persons lose their spouses in the course of adjusting to the personal and sexual changes of aging, our knowledge of postmarital sexuality is frequently relevant.

POSTMARITAL SEXUALITY

The literature contains very little information on the sexual behavior of people who are divorced, widowed, or otherwise separated from their spouses. This omission is unfortunate, since such a large number of people must adjust to these separations. There is little question that the time of adjusting to the separation is so painful and agonizing that the term *crisis* is well applied to it. If the individual is fortunate, he or she may find another even more suitable partner. For many, however, divorce and widowhood represent an overwhelming stress which results in unhappiness and depression of some magnitude and duration. "Folklore and outmoded research findings tend to hold that the subsequent marriages of divorced people are precarious. Possibly at one time, but currently the 'formerly married' are a different breed from their historical antecedents. Their subsequent marital and sexual experiences constitute an improvement, as a rule, over former experience" (Cuber, 1975, 67).

It is difficult to draw generalizations regarding adjustment, sexual or otherwise, without understanding the particular dynamics or circumstances involved. Although we might expect the same characterological factors which may have been problematic in the first marriage to cause difficulty in later relationships, people do learn from experience and are capable of change, with or without therapy. The reasons for becoming involved with a new partner and the quality of that new relationship are also likely to influence a person's adjustment to a later relationship. Several studies do indicate that the second marriage is likely to be rated better than the first (Udry, 1971; Gebhard, 1970).

Most of those who divorce or are widowed when they are young do remarry, two-thirds of the women and three-quarters of the men.

Widowers and divorced men have a distinct advantage over women in finding new partners, probably because of their greater freedom and mobility. For those who remarry, the first marriage must not have been so traumatic as to prevent remarriage. Motivations for remarriage are many and include a need for social and sexual companionship, a desire for financial security, a need to provide a good environment for children, and, of course, the obvious desire to enhance and prolong a newly acquired relationship.

Reed estimated that between 1970 and 1980 there were ten million divorces, including all of the first, second, third, and subsequent divorces (Reed, 1976). Some 25 percent of first marriages are terminated by divorce, annulment, or desertion. Kinsey showed that separated or divorced men continue the same frequency and type of sexual activity as they practiced before marriage (Kinsey et al., 1953). Women, on the other hand, tend to have a greater frequency of sexual activity after divorce than before marriage (Gebhard, 1970). Although a period of sexual abstinence usually immediately follows the marriage termination, most divorced and widowed women do eventually resume sexual activity. Some two-thirds to three-quarters of divorced women have sexual activity, compared to one-third to one-half of widows (Gebhard, 1970).

According to Reed, "There is some statistical support for the stereotypes of the gay divorcee and the merry widow" (1976, 250). In the age group under 45, 12 percent of divorcees and 16 percent of widows have multiple sexual partners. These data from the Kinsey studies are now several decades removed from current times. But it would seem that just as premarital sexual activity has increased to over ninety percent since then, the frequency of postmarital sexual behavior in younger women and men must now approach the one hundred percent mark.

In order to understand postmarital sexuality more fully, we must appreciate the age of the individual when his or her marriage terminates and the individual's age when he or she reengages in sexual behavior. When most couples first marry, say in their middle twenties, the man is at or slightly past the peak of his sexual interest, while the woman is likely to achieve her peak of sexual responsiveness in her middle thirties (Reed, 1976). By this time, the husband may have reached a plateau of sexual need and may have begun to reduce the frequency of intercourse. His ability to achieve erection is not impaired at this age, but his refractory period has grown longer, and he is less inclined to try for more than one orgasm in a given lovemaking session. The woman, however, may have only begun to become consistently orgasmic or capable of multiple orgasms. In the past partners in their forties accommodated to the man's level of desire for sex and had intercourse once a week. Recently, however, women have come to assert themselves and to request sex more frequently. Sex therapists are now quite familiar with the tired husband syndrome, a presenting complaint of many couples.

The emotional adjustment immediately after the separation or divorce is very difficult for many. This stressful period usually includes anger, resentment, hostility, a sense of rejection with resulting loss of self-esteem, and, finally, depression. The sexual complications of this situation are obvious, and the following brief vignette is illustrative:

A young man in his middle thirties entered therapy within three weeks after his wife became involved with a considerably older and more experienced man. His wife was quite open about her desire to pursue this relationship, and the patient felt he could not prevent her from doing so. He had just accepted a new job in another city, and when he arrived at his new position, he was alone and depressed and had been impotent with his wife on several occasions. He gave a history of being passive and submissive to a somewhat dominant mother and older sister. He was a virgin prior to meeting his wife, in his early twenties. Once before he had sought therapy when he experienced erectile failure during the stress of completing his dissertation.

After treatment began he continued to feel depressed for two to three weeks, returning on the weekends to see his young daughter, while his wife pursued her relationship with her lover. He was fearful of confronting her, somehow hoping this affair would soon end. He became increasingly angry and impotent, as well as humiliated and depressed. Improvement occurred when he realized he related to women in a submissive and passive manner for fear they would abandon him if he were assertive. Finally, he decided to express his anger openly to his wife, quickly felt relieved, and began to improve. Shortly thereafter, he became involved in a relationship with a woman who was obviously attracted to him. His previous erectile difficulties and lack of sexual drive were resolved, and he was able to respond quite well in this new relationship.

Depression and secondary sexual dysfunction, such as this man experienced, are also common among women who separate and divorce. While the troubled couple is still together, the woman may experience orgasmic dysfunction of a secondary type. Subsequent to separation or divorce, her sexual drive may temporarily diminish, and she may have no interest either in outside involvement or in self-stimulation. The distressing period of crisis may last for several months, and the period of adjustment can last as long as a year or two. The hostility and antagonism which both of the former partners so often act out are both demeaning to them and damaging to their children. Psychotherapy for individuals in this type of crisis can be very effective in helping patients to work through their troubled feelings more quickly than would otherwise occur.

For relatively young divorced and widowed women, the rate of coital orgasm in subsequent marriages is greater than in their first marriages (Gebhard, 1970). For the divorced woman, the reason may be a release from irritation of the old, unhappy relationship, or simply a better relationship, sexual and otherwise, than she formerly had. For the widow, the same explanations may pertain, or perhaps as time has gone on, the woman has achieved more freedom, has become more self-confident, and has decreased her inhibitions. After an initial period of social and sexual withdrawal, young divorced and widowed men and women continue to engage in sexual relations with at least the same drive and interest as they did before and during their previous marriages. Depending on the circumstances, they may have a greater sexual interest and more satisfying sexual relationships with their later partners.

A final vignette underscores another sexual consequence of either divorce or widowhood:

A 40-year-old woman, divorced for two years after a 17-year marriage, came in complaining of periodic migraine headaches. She worked as a medical technician, missed time at work occasionally, and was under considerable stress to maintain employment and care for her teenaged children. She was moderately depressed with associated anxiety and tension. It was clear she had internalized much anger, which would periodically express itself as symptomatic migraine headaches whenever an interpersonal event occurred which increased her resentment and frustration.

Since the divorce was finalized, she had been going with an older married man with whom she felt a sense of security. However, he was intermittently troubled with erectile difficulty, and when she desired sex, she would become involved in a casual relationship about which she later felt guilt. As her self-concept improved, she was able to terminate her relationship with her older friend, since he had no intention of divorcing his wife. She had learned to engage in self-stimulation to relieve sexual tension. She felt this ability to achieve orgasm by herself allowed her to be more selective in her social and sexual interaction with men. Also she was able to face being alone for the first time in her life without having to rely on someone else.

The sexual behavior of divorced and widowed people, like sexual involvement for all people, is highly specific to the individual. How people act sexually depends on age, psychological adjustment, general attitude toward the opposite sex, and the degree to which sex has become important in the overall life style. Today, as the vignette suggests, postmarital sex may not correlate with remarriage as much as it did in the past. Although most individuals elect to remarry, the trend seems to indicate that more individuals will engage in postmarital relationships without entering into marriage again.

AGING AND SEXUAL BEHAVIOR

Couples who arrive together at the middle years may enjoy the opportunity to change their relationships. Children are out of the home, or nearly so, and either spouse or both may be thinking more about home and retirement than about the pressures of work. Some couples find these middle years to be a "new discovery of each other and of qualities in the relationship, sexual and otherwise, which have been neglected or ignored for a period of years" (Cuber, 1975, 63).

For others, the reverse may be true. With the common bond of raising children behind them, the partners may feel little in common and find that they are basically incompatible. This latter situation accounts, to some extent, for the sharp increase in the divorce rate among middle-aged people. Some of these unhappy couples may remain together, playing down sex and thus contributing to the sexual stereotype that sexual activity decreases as time goes on.

With age, changes in sexual responsiveness and functioning do occur in both men and women. In their fifties and sixties, however, a couple may reestablish a quality and quantity of sexual expression that they were unable to enjoy in their forties. As well as intercourse, this newfound sexuality may include an affection and tenderness that are intensified by the growing awareness of mortality (Cuber, 1975). In some cases, the sexual behavior remains unchanged. Some couples maintain an active and regular sexual relationship as long as ill health or death does not intervene.

The woman's natural ability to lubricate the vaginal barrel and introitus may be reduced, and, for women beyond the middle fifties, responsiveness may be slowed. The vaginal walls may thin, the length and diameter of the vagina may be reduced, and the major labia may shrink (Masters and Johnson, 1966). A woman who maintains regular sexual activity can minimize these atrophic changes. Women who continue to have sexual intercourse once or twice a week into their sixties and seventies are able to respond and function effectively despite physiological changes. (Some of these postmenopausal changes can, of course, be offset with cautious use of hormone replacement therapy.)

For men, erectile difficulty is the only sexual dysfunction which correlates with age (Frank et al., 1978). After age fifty, the frequency of impotence increases markedly and continues to increase with each decade (Masters and Johnson, 1966). Some of this erectile failure is psychogenic and therefore reversible. In other cases, neurological and vascular disease cause impotence which is organic in origin and irreversible.

The ability to measure nocturnal penile tumescence during REM sleep has been very helpful in distinguishing organic from psychogenic impotence (Fisher et al., 1979). Nocturnal penile tumescence is at its peak during puberty, occurring during 32 percent of sleep in the 13- to 15-year-old group, and declining to twenty percent between ages sixty and 69 (Karacan et al., 1972, 1975; Fisher et al., 1979). In the last decade it has been possible to take direct measurements of penile blood pressure, and to correct vasculogenic impotence surgically (DePalma et al., 1978). Although some methodological problems remain, these techniques are beginning to create a wider range of treatment possibilities for the appropriate candidates.

In addition to difficulty with erections, older men take longer to ejaculate, ejaculation is less forceful, refractory time is longer, and they require greater stimulation if they are to respond with an erection. Like his female counterpart, the man can mitigate the effects of aging by sustained sexual activity. According to Masters and Johnson, "If elevated levels of sexual activity are maintained from earlier years and neither acute nor chronic physical incapacity intervenes, aging males usually are able to continue some form of active sexual expression into the 70- or even 80-year age group" (1966, 263). Pfeiffer summarizes the situation succinctly: "With the exception of specific existing diseases, physiologic changes do not ring a mandatory curtain on sexuality in either aging men or aging women" (Pfeiffer, 1979, 133).

Other factors besides physiological ones may reduce sexual activity among older people. Prevailing stereotypes cause us to feel that sexual expression by older persons is taboo. The same attitudinal set causes us to feel that sexual activity is taboo when one has a serious illness. Because aging is often associated with either acute or chronic illness, our culture takes a doubly negative attitude toward sexual expression in the elderly. Perhaps not wishing to believe that our parents "do it," we have adopted numerous attitudes which limit approval of sexual activity in the aging population.

Fortunately, many elderly persons themselves do not subscribe to these cultural myths. At age 68 about seventy percent of men still regularly partake in sexual activity, and at age 78 about 25 percent are sexually active (Pfeiffer, 1974). The myth that men have a certain number of shots to fire during their lifetime or that it is possible to "wear it out" seems unfounded.

While the level of sexual activity continues for men in or out of marriage, marital status makes all the difference for women. Very few unmarried older women report regular sexual activity. "The availability of a sanctioned sexual partner is the chief determinant" (Pfeiffer, 1979, 131). Because women live longer than men, there is a marked disproportion of available partners, approaching four to one in many environments. Although biology may not limit the sexual capabilities of aging women, they are faced with restricted opportunities to find appropriate partners. In general, given the opportunities for expression, the likelihood of continued sexual expression in later years is greatest for people who have been interested and active in younger years. One's sexual life style, it appears, is a kind of characterological feature which endures with age.

Conclusion

Despite some physiological and social problems related to aging, group norms regarding sexual functioning do not predict individual response. The choice rests with the individual, and the primary care physician can present a range of options and strategies for adjusting to sexual changes and limitations. Paraplegic and other disabled individuals have taught us that sexuality is not confined to having intercourse or limited to men who can get erections. Older patients are not reluctant to talk about sex. More often, it is the physician who is uncomfortable or embarrassed and who rationalizes his or her reluctance to discuss sex on the basis that it is inappropriate.

Currently, ten percent of the U.S. population are over 65 years of age, and by the 21st century, this age group will represent 25 percent of our population. With the advances in health care, diet, exercise, and so forth, people can expect to live longer and also to enjoy good health during the later years. The senior citizen, however, has been portrayed very negatively, as slow-witted, self-centered, irritable, unproductive, feeble, and, finally, "senile." Yet only four percent of this population are institutionalized or in need of total care.

Between ten percent and twenty percent of the elderly actually increase their sexual activity. This age group should be regarded as potentially sexual and helped to achieve the optimum of sexual enjoyment. "Sexual therapy directed to helping elderly couples become sexually liberated not only has positive social value but has enabled elderly couples to open communication, increase intimacy and self-esteem, and enjoy without guilt sexual pleasures society accords as acceptable to its youth" (Sviland, 1978, 359).

Health care professionals are only beginning to address the physical, social, psychological, and sexual concerns of their elderly patients. Geriatric medicine has come of age, and we are now beginning to push forward in this much neglected arena. By inquiring and by offering information and advice, we may contribute significantly to older people's enjoyment and quality of life. Physicians should be more sensitive to the adverse sexual consequences of the drugs they prescribe and of the surgical procedures they recommend. At the very least, they should discuss in advance the possible negative sexual consequences of drugs, surgery, or other treatment. If we cannot all be sex therapists, at least we should not add unnecessary, iatrogenic sexual problems.

Chapter 7

Gender and Gender Disturbance: Childhood, Adolescence and Adulthood

by Jon K. Meyer, M.D.

INTRODUCTION

The many constituent elements of human sexuality, both biological and psychological, have more or less specific places within the epigenetic sequence of sexual development. Among the most important of these components is gender identity, the basic psychological sense of maleness or femaleness.

Independent lines of research demonstrate that gender takes shape within the second year of life. Developmentally, gender formation marks the incorporation of sexuality into early body image and self-concept. In many respects, gender identity is the psychological foundation for the course of development (Meyer, 1980b).

There is, as yet, no consensus on the necessary or sufficient precursors of gender sense. Although in lower mammals stereotypic mating behaviors are determined by perinatal hormonal influences, such clear-cut biological controls have not yet been demonstrated in humans. In humans, the weight of the evidence appears to be on the side of psychological, rather than biological, dominance in gender formation. While it seems likely that biological factors precondition gender sense, it also appears that they are insufficient to determine it (Gadpaille, 1980; Meyer, in press).

As would be predictable from the early age at which gender identity is acquired, gender disturbance may be manifest even in childhood. However, such etiological possibilities as biological mishap, imprinting, or nonconflictual identity formation during blissful symbiosis do not appear compatible with our clinical experience. Clinically, gender dysphoria appears to grow out of pathogenic fantasies and introjections which themselves arise in the context of disturbed family relationships. The emotional pain at the origin of gender dysphoria is eased by the fantasy that things would be better if only they were different. At the heart of the clinical disturbance is a denial of anatomical attributes, an idealization of opposite sex characteristics, and a fantasy that sex reversal would bring harmony and tranquility. As might be expected, a pathological resolution of such an early developmental crisis results in a gender dysphoria characterized by multiple signs of ego and personality impairment (Meyer, in press).

Psychotherapy with transsexuals is a difficult undertaking and should use a frame of reference appropriate to patients with severe borderline character disorders.* Surgical reassignment, which could be viewed as the ultimate in cosmetic surgery, apparently does offer subjective palliation of gender disturbance.

GENDER IDENTITY IN CONTEXT

Confusion is common among the terms *sex, gender, gender identity, sexual identity, masculinity,* and *femininity,* all of which refer to

*Editor's note: In Part V, chapter 31, Kernberg discusses techniques of treatment for patients with borderline personalities.

aspects of sexuality. *Sex* denotes the biology of maleness and female-ness, e.g., karyotype, gonads, and genitalia. *Gender* or *gender identity* is a psychological construct which connotes a basic sense of maleness or femaleness or a conviction that one is male or female. While gender is normally consonant with biology and appears to be a function of it, gender may be quite free from biological constraint. For example, in transsexualism, the sense "I am a female" may contrast starkly with a male habitus.

Similarly, the terms *gender identity* and *sexual identity* are at times considered synonymous, but properly they refer to different and de-velopmentally sequential facets of personality. *Gender identity* is the earlier and more fundamental acquisition, referring to a basic amalga-mation of anatomical givens and reproductive potential into the early sexual self-representation. Gender identity is a product of the separation-individuation phase and is very likely consolidated with the achievement of object constancy (Mahler et al., 1975, 110). The development of *sexual identity,* for which the oedipal phase and adolescence are the watersheds, is marked by the acquisition of the qualities of masculinity, femininity, and personal eroticism, as these are expressed in sexual fantasies, preferences, and object choices. Sexual identity is normally, but not necessarily, a refinement of basic gender sense. For example, a feminine sexual identity may coexist with a male gender sense, as in some male homosexuals.

The transition from biological sex to gender and from gender iden-tity to sexual identity is so smooth in the normal situation that the elements of the process are difficult to appreciate. Patients with gender disturbance, on the other hand, provide an extraordinary clinical laboratory in which the components of gender formation are more discernible.

CLINICAL EXAMPLES
The following three cases and accompanying discussion illustrate childhood, adolescent, and adult forms of gender dysphoria. While these vignettes do not, by any means, encompass the full clinical spectrum, they do illustrate common themes from among the more than five hundred cases we have seen in the last 12 years.

Childhood Gender Dysphoria
The first illustration is excerpted from an evaluation of a gender dysphoric boy and his family.

> Jay,[1] a five-and-a-half-year-old child referred because of "feminine" behavior, was accompanied by his father, mother, and his six-and-a-half-year-old adopted brother. The youngest child, a twenty-month-old boy, had been left at home.
> Mother was a plain, slim, 29-year-old who described a difficult child-hood with an alcoholic mother and a "cold and remote" father. She met her husband at 13, dated few other men, and married at twenty. She presented herself as an asymptomatic individual on the MMPI, but on projective testing her responses were poorly structured and frequently peculiar.[2] Generational boundaries seemed confused, and masculine and

[1]All names are pseudonyms.
[2]Natalia Chapanis, Ph.D., supervised and interpreted the psychological testing of the two boys and their family.

feminine figures were not clearly distinguished. Coldness, emptiness, and distance colored her description of parental images.

Father, a 31-year-old, white-collar worker with a "difficult" temper, related with obvious pride how well Jay could imitate females. Father presented himself as a normal individual on the MMPI but was defensive and guarded on projective testing. His stories suggested a wish for contact with other males but a fear of explosive violence, and they portrayed maternal figures as distant and uninvolved.

The parents had been married for three years when they adopted Jay's older brother. One month after the adoption, Jay was conceived. Because of a bloody vaginal discharge in the first trimester, it was feared that the pregnancy would abort, but gestation and delivery were otherwise uneventful. The parents recall Jay's first year of life as unremarkable. Specifically, there was no excessive body contact or emotional attachment between mother and son. If anything, mother may have been distant and preoccupied because of her own aloofness and because she had another infant in the household.

When Jay was a year old, his father was stationed overseas. During this interval, mother and the two boys lived next door to her parents, and mother became caught up once more in the difficult relationship with them. When father returned, Jay (age two) ignored him. Six months after father's return, mother again became pregnant, and it was then that Jay's feminine behavior was noticed. He wore a dish towel on his head to simulate long hair, showed a preference for playing with pots and pans rather than his brother's trucks, and began to dress in mother's clothes and accessories. At age three he proclaimed he was going to grow up to be a girl and a mommy. Jay's parents consulted a pediatrician who said the boy would "outgrow it."

At our consultation, Jay spoke in a high-pitched, laboriously cute voice. He aggressively manipulated his older brother through coquettish behavior. For example, to avoid being kissed by Jay, his brother would give up a toy. Jay cognitively recognized that he was a boy but wanted to be a "nurse" when he grew up. He had girls for best friends, and was always the "mommy" when playing house. Jay was preoccupied with superficial sexual characteristics like wigs, girdles, and dresses. The patient drew himself as female without either arms or legs. He also drew the female figure without legs. When asked about the legs on the drawing of himself, he said, "They were cut off," but as for the female, he indicated, "I cut them off." On projective testing, loosely knit stories were filled with violence: a man killed a woman "in" her exposed breasts, an embrace led to the death of both parties, and "a killer killed a girl" while her parents watched. Father was seen as powerful and evil. There was a blurring of sexual complementarity: father married his grandfather and mother married her daughter.

Jay's older brother at six-and-a-half dressed and behaved appropriately to his gender. He was, however, sad and downcast and readily verbalized thoughts of sickness and death. In his projective stories he told of mutual tail cutting, and of a "knife" and a "killer" who were threatening to the female. With the help of "magic," however, a female can kill a male with the "knife." He told of a story of a father killing his son with a sledge hammer and blocked on pictures of bedroom scenes.

Jay showed the usual characteristics of a "pretranssexual" child, including his effeminacy, his cross-gender wishes, his selection of girls' games, his choice of girls as playmates, and his preoccupation with female accoutrements. As has been the rule in our experience, there was no history of special physical or emotional symbiosis, although Jay, the natural child, was clearly preferred. Mother was depressed, isolated, and conflictually overinvolved with her alcoholic mother and cold, remote father. Jay's father was absent for a year early in the boy's separation-individuation phase. He was neither effeminate nor distant, but he did have great difficulty with explosive rage, and he was unwittingly supportive of his son's femininity. Father's absence, mother's reinvolvement in a highly conflicted relationship with her parents, and Jay's jealousy at mother's pregnancy formed the most obvious backdrop to his symptoms. The patient, like his brother, was preoccupied with violence and dismemberment.

Children, like Jay, who are gender disturbed disavow the significance of their anatomical endowment and have fantasies of growing up to be the opposite sex. Although there are similar elements in the fantasies of neurotic children, in gender-disturbed children the denial of anatomy and the cross-sexual fantasies are more overt, concrete, and persistent. These children (and the adolescents and adults they become) have serious flaws in their sense of self. Furthermore, in interviews and projective testing, their parents show a similar, but covert, gender confusion, blurring of generational boundaries, and conflict surrounding sex and reproduction. "Pretranssexual" children long for closeness with mother, feel empty and hollow, are anguished over what they sense as her disregard, and experience severe anxiety at separations. Often they manifest their sensitivity to loss or abandonment symptomatically, through night terrors, enuresis, school phobias, and social inhibition.

We cannot emphasize strongly enough to our pediatric and family practice colleagues that psychiatric consultation is indicated for children with these danger signs and that such fundamental problems will not be outgrown. Although the symptoms may temporarily go underground in latency and the preteen years, they do so only to emerge with greater force in adolescence.

Adolescent Gender Dysphoria

During latency gender disturbance may become relatively quiescent, and it is unusual for us to see a child in the nine to 12 age range. With the internal sexual pressures of puberty and adolescence, however, gender disturbance later resurfaces as homophilia and disturbing anomie, which may reach suicidal proportions. (Unfortunately, we do not know how many gender dysphoric youngsters are among the successful adolescent suicides.) The adolescent gender dysphoric tends to emerge from the crisis (suicidal or otherwise) created by sexual impulses with a "transsexual" resolution of his dilemma. The following case history illustrates these points.

In her associations over several hours, the patient, a biological male who had been reassigned as female, turned ultimately to memories of an adolescent suicide attempt:

"[What was the suicide attempt about?] I fell in love with a boy... I knew I was different because I liked having sex with boys. I didn't really know how I could classify myself. I knew that there was a similarity between myself and homosexuals because I had read in the dictionary that homosexuals were attracted to their sex... and this I definitely was... Well, this fellow had graduated from... junior high school and I was upset at the thought that I would never see him again. Suddenly I realized that I must be homosexual. I went downtown and bought myself a bottle of Nytol. I went home. I sat in the bathroom and slit my wrists and took the whole bottle of Nytol. Well, I sat there and expected something quick to happen although it didn't. So I went to bed and put some newspaper down . . . and put my wrist over it so that the blood could drip there . . . Some noise woke me up in the middle of the night . . . I couldn't easily get up . . . the room was spinning . . . literally spinning . . . I had to hold onto the bed . . . and getting up was like rolling off the bed and crawling on my all fours to the bathroom . . . All I could do was let the vomit come down the side of my face because I didn't even have strength enough to hold my head up. The next morning I felt like hell. I didn't tell anyone what I did. My mother noticed the bandage on my arm and I told her that I cut it climbing a fence . . . I had written a love letter to this boy. I cut school that day . . . I went to his home and stole the letter when it was delivered . . . Then, I realized that I was definitely different and I wanted to find others like myself so that I could learn about myself."

Finding others like herself marked the coalescence of the patient's belief that she was transsexual. Although there were no further suicide attempts, the patient as an adult showed self-destructive and sadistic trends. (See also Meyer, 1974, 539–540.)

Adult Gender Dysphoria

Late adolescent and adult gender dysphoria takes many forms. However, our experience has led to the conviction that transsexualism is almost universally linked with paraphilia and expressed in the context of a borderline character disorder. In general, the more commonly recognized signs and symptoms of borderline character and paraphilia alternate with the transsexual presentation.

The patient, a middle-aged male, was next to the youngest among five children. His father, who traveled extensively, was frequently absent. Furthermore, the family was polarized, with the children siding with mother against father to the point of physical threats against father. Many arguments stemmed from father's open complaints that mother was not sexually satisfying. Nonetheless, the patient recalled with sadness that his father was gentle and decent after his mother died, and he wondered if the children had been "set up" by their mother.

The patient recalled his mother as a stern, harsh, and "asexual" woman. He was considered to be "mother's child" and felt that he had been used to replace a little girl, his older sister, who had died at birth. When the patient was 18 months old, his mother moved from the parental bedroom to sleep with him. This arrangement lasted until he was seven or eight, when his continued bed-wetting brought it to an end. By this time, the patient was mother's helpmate around the house and was going into the closet just to touch her clothes. He began actual cross-dressing at about age ten.

In early adolescence his masturbation involved articles of clothing, and he had masturbatory fantasies that were typically transvestitic. He imagined he was taken away by women and made to live with them, often in female clothes, while they used him as a sexual plaything.

The patient dated for the first time in college. During his first marriage, at a time when he was ill and bedfast, he began cross-dressing again after a long hiatus. This first marriage ended in divorce after 18 years and two children. (Both children had required extensive psychiatric contact, and the patient suspected they were schizophrenic.) He cross-dressed a great deal during the separation but "calmed down" after meeting a new girlfriend. Around the time he remarried his cross-dressing increased immediately before and after the marriage. The second marriage was brief, but the patient eventually married a third time. His desire to cross-dress returned three years after this marriage began, when his wife was going through a "cancer scare."

In recent years his problems were compounded by retirement and difficulties in finding employment. "Careerwise it was a jolt to realize that I wasn't as good a man as I thought I was and wasn't acceptable as I thought I was." His request for sex reassignment came on the heels of this involutional problem, from which he took refuge in female clothes and in the fantasy of surgical sexual transformation. In the acutely malignant transformation of his transvestism, emptiness and depersonalization reached such a critical point that suicide was a risk. Our program temporized with his request for surgery, and we insisted he have psychotherapy. Over the space of a year his cross-dressing and desire for sex reassignment diminished to tolerable levels, and they almost vanished when he found a woman who was interested in him. (See also Meyer, 1974, 530, 533.)

As this case illustrates, the transsexual presentation may be viewed as a regressive solution of a developmental crisis. In most cases the transsexual reaction will be of greater duration, thereby fitting the two-year criterion of DSM-III. It is our impression, nonetheless, that transsexualism is a reaction which is precipitated by developmentally related stresses, which follows a fluctuating course, and which reappears dramatically at times of stress. The stresses which precipitate transsexual reactions are, in general, those involving separation, abandonment, or demands for independent assertiveness: for example, death of a parent, birth of a child, illness of a spouse, or pursuit of a career (Bernstein et al., 1981; Meyer, in press; Meyer, 1980a, 1980b). If the patient is not operated upon, there appears over time to be a reversion or readjustment to the pretranssexual state.

CONSULTATION AND CLINICAL EVALUATION

Transsexual patients rarely request psychiatric consultation. Commonly the patient's initial focus centers on the wish for cross-sexual hormones and sex reassignment. Before succumbing to the pressure toward such actions, physicians ought to recognize that the search for sex reassignment is the patient's symptom. Similarly, the patient's stated transsexualism should be viewed as a presenting complaint like any other. Our experience has been that, when evaluation proceeds in an unhurried fashion, the apparently solid transsexual presentation will unravel. Beneath it will appear vulnerability to stress, primitive defenses, affect intolerance, identity diffusion, and polymorphous perverse sexual trends.

TREATMENT

The treatment of transsexualism is sometimes viewed as the exclusive province of the surgical subspecialties. Despite the transsexual's apsychological stance and assertion of the right to self-determination through surgery, psychotherapy should always be considered as a treatment option. Among children and adolescents, of course, psychotherapy should be the only treatment considered. The transsexual's apparently recalcitrant stance is not unique in psychiatric practice. A suicidal patient may believe that death is the only solace and that psychiatric efforts rob him or her of the right to self-determination. Nevertheless, most of us would offer psychotherapy, recognizing that no suicide is totally preventable and that, in the final analysis, the patient's life is in his or her own hands.

Psychotherapy

The considerable pessimism about psychotherapy in the gender dysphoria syndromes is in part warranted because of the severe ego impairment in these syndromes. In part, though, the pessimism derives from an erroneous assumption that the gender reversal is non-conflictual. In our cases, we discovered that the seemingly non-conflictual gender reversal was a type of character defense not dissimilar from the perversions.

Psychotherapy with transsexuals is complicated by problems in achieving a therapeutic alliance, in dealing with primitive defenses (such as denial, projection, and splitting), in coping with oral-narcissistic transferences, and in sublimating countertransference rage and fear. Yet our notorious failures are probably attributable not only to the transsexual's recalcitrance, but also to our technical and human failures. Because of unrecognized and unresolved countertransference reactions, we frequently either attack the wish for sex reassignment or align ourselves with it. Colluding with the patient's wish, even when we rationalize our alignment as being in the service of rehabilitation, makes it impossible for us to see or hear the patient's conflicts. Attacking the wish for reassignment, on the other hand, is a direct assault on a central, highly defended portion of a fantasy complex. The result of attack is simply to strengthen the patient's defenses without therapeutic benefit and with no strategic advantage to the course of treatment.

The psychotherapist must approach the wish for sex reassignment as any other wish, empathically, in the spirit of inquiry, and from a position equidistant between collusion and rejection. It can be pointed out, in good faith and with absolute sincerity, that the decision regarding sex reassignment is ultimately the patient's alone but that the patient ought to explore the wish psychotherapeutically, *before* irreversible surgery. (See also Meyer, 1980c.)

Whenever feasible, twice-weekly sessions are ideal. The patient cannot tolerate analytic abstinence or the regression fostered by the couch, and the psychiatrist must be available as an encouraging, sympathetic, and concerned person. The therapist must anticipate no-shows, interrupted treatment, overdue accounts, self-destructiveness, and intercurrent need for hospitalization. These symptomatic eruptions are best handled by being interested in their timing and the accompanying thoughts and feelings. Almost without exception, impulsive outbursts follow a loss, separation, perceived slight, or demand made on the patient. To be effective, interpretations should be geared toward loss, emptiness, and rage, rather than toward the developmentally more advanced concerns of anxiety and guilt. Treatment may provide nothing more than a stable point in the patient's life, a place to return for support at times of stress. On the other hand, treatment may help to replace the gender disturbance with a stable paraphilia. With the passage of time, unreassigned patients tend to drift into paraphilic adjustments, reappearing with further demands for surgery at times of stress, separation, or loss.

Surgery

In the ablation of primary and secondary sexual characteristics and the creation of opposite sex facsimiles, surgery has made remarkable strides, both cosmetically and functionally, With rare exception, patients who self-select for surgery through a trial period are subjectively pleased and show objective improvement (Hastings, 1974; Meyer and Reter, 1979).

However, at Johns Hopkins, in the only study to date using an unoperated comparison group to control outcome, we found that both operated and unoperated transsexuals improved according to objective criteria and that both improved to the same degree (Meyer and Reter, 1979). All other studies have unfortunately used the permanently surgically modified patient as his own "control." While the results from any one study must be viewed as tentative until replicated, it appears that reassignment confers no objective advantage in terms of social rehabilitation, although it is subjectively satisfying.

The results of the Hopkins study, which suggest that an unoperated comparison group improves as much as the operated, and problems in the research designs of other studies, require that we withhold judgment on the degree of advantage conferred by surgery until there are other well controlled studies.

GENDER DEVELOPMENT AND GENDER DYSPHORIA

Research with intersex children first suggested that gender identity was an early acquisition of the developing child (summarized by Hampson and Hampson, 1961). Subsequent work with transsexuals (Stoller, 1975) and child observation (Mahler et al., 1975) refined the concepts of gender formation. Generally, although not universally, it is conceded that the critical locus of gender development is within the intimate relationships of the nuclear family. More particularly, the locus is in the relationship between mother and child, where mother functions as the child's emotional template. The mothers of transsexuals may be depressed and bisexual (as well as disturbed in other ways), have remarkably strong penis envy, and are inclined to deny the anatomical distinctions between the sexes (Stoller, 1975; Meyer, in press). As a product of their bisexuality and penis envy, these mothers are envious and rejecting of their sons and their anatomy, and contemptuous and rejecting of their daughters and their anatomy.

Galenson, Roiphe, and their associates (1971, 1975) have described a preoedipal phase of genital interest at approximately 18 months of age. During this phase a child first recognizes the anatomical distinctions between the sexes and at the same time integrates the genitalia into the body image as part of a more general object- and self-consolidation. Normally parents foster this process through their recognition, acceptance, and comfort with the child's anatomy and with their own. At this vulnerable stage, however, the future transsexual receives no such confirmation.

Male or female toddlers who find themselves and their sexual attributes at the focus of mother's ambivalence and conflict, and who have no remedial experience with father, repudiate their own anatomy through primitive denial and seek to become less offensive by becoming, in fantasy, the opposite of what they are. Through this repudiation, they hope to create a blissful symbiosis with mother. Transsexual males, in fantasy and in actuality, rid themselves of their penises to lessen mother's (or her introject's) envy and rejection; females acquire penises, which lessens mother's contempt and rejection (Meyer, in press).

Transsexualism can be seen not so much as a reversal in core gender identity as a consequence of a desperate effort to repair painful and disturbed relationships and confusing gaps in body image. This formulation differs from those of others. Stoller (1975), for instance, suggests that transsexualism is the product of imprinting in a blissful symbiotic phase, the transsexualism representing the individual's true identity. As conceptualized here, transsexualism is an outgrowth of separation-individuation phase rejection, compensated for through the use of primitive, phase-specific defenses and the reparative fantasy of sexual transformation. As such, transsexualism represents an "as if" identity.

CONCLUSION

The wish for sex reassignment occurs in both sexes. The wish may be put into action and come to medical attention at almost any age and marks a discordance between sense of self and the configuration of anatomy. Clinical experience has led to a conviction that the patient's description of a dissonance between sex and gender is a symptomatic condensation of remarkable proportions.

A clinically broad and diverse group of patients seek sex reassignment. Characteristically, gender dysphoria interdigitates with perversion, with a broad spectrum of character disorders, and, occasionally, with psychosis. Pursuit of sex reassignment surgery occurs most frequently at times of separation or loss or occasions requiring independent assertiveness. Transsexual patients' ego strengths are insufficient to withstand formal psychoanalysis, but they can be treated within the parameters used in treating patients with severe borderline character disorders. Issues of therapeutic alliance, defensive structure, transference, the level of interpretation, and countertransference are similar to those found in treating the perversions and other borderline characters. When sex reassignment surgery is done, it is positively valued subjectively, but its effects on the objective life situation may be no greater than have been observed in an unreassigned comparison group.

Transsexualism may be viewed in the same way as other major psychiatric syndromes. Transsexuals are not "a breed apart." Like patients suffering from other syndromes, transsexuals have a recognizable and comprehensible place in the scope of mental and emotional disturbance.

Chapter 8

Incest and Rape: Repercussions in Sexual Behavior
by Carol C. Nadelson, M.D.

INTRODUCTION

Rape and incest are both forms of sexual abuse and must both be conceptualized along a spectrum of sexual experiences in which the common theme is one person's nonconsent. Incest represents the special circumstance in which the individuals involved are closely tied by a familial relationship.

The clinician's perspective on these issues differs from that of the lawyer or the police officer. For example, sexual intercourse is not frequently part of the sexual experience of prepubescent children (Mohr et al., 1964). Thus, it is not legally incest when a father fondles his nine-year-old daughter, but the meaning of the event, psychologically, may be very similar to the child. Likewise, the threat of violence to someone who is fearful for her life may be as coercive as a violent act in forcing compliance (Nadelson and Rosenfeld, 1980).

This chapter focuses on the experiences of the victims of sexual abuse and specifically considers the repercussions of these experiences on sexual adaptation. Recognizing that legal and clinical descriptions and definitions may differ, it provides a clinical perspective on the limited available data and considers the treatment implications.

INCEST AND SEXUAL ABUSE OF CHILDREN

Incest is a special form of rape or coercive sexual interaction. Each year more than 60,000 children are victims of sexual abuse. Seventy-five percent of these children are abused by someone who is known to them, generally a close friend or a family member, often the father. Among incest victims, as many as 25 percent may be victimized again later in their lives, and female victims are likely to become battered wives or mothers of incest victims (Federal Organizations for Professional Women, 1980).

Incest is defined in a variety of different ways, depending upon which sexual acts are included and which relationships are considered incestuous. Definitions of what are potentially incestuous relationships vary. For example, is a sexual relationship between the live-in partner of a parent and the child of that parent incestuous? Some authors define incest in terms of actual intercourse (Sloane and Karpinski, 1942), and others include oral genital contact, fondling, and exposure (Weiner, 1962).

In a useful alternative formulation, Brant and Tisza conceive of and define *sexual misuse* as "exposure of a child within a given social-cultural context to sexual stimulation inappropriate for the child's age and level of development" (1976, 2). Their definition of sexual misuse thus includes a range of sexual experiences in childhood, from rape to overt seduction, and it places incest within this larger context. The concept and the definition are also helpful in that they address the issues of age and type of sexual encounter.

THE AFTERMATH OF INCEST

The many hypotheses about the reasons for incest focus primarily on family instability and deprivation, but available prevalence data are not representative of the general population. Most of the data derive from court-referred cases, usually people from lower socioeconomic groups who represent "disorganized" families. Most affluent and resourceful people seem to avoid legal or correctional involvement or, for some other reason, are not included in most studies of incest or its repercussions.

As to the effects of incest, Ferenczi believed that childhood seduction had dire consequences. He stated that the children "feel physically and morally helpless . . . for the overpowering force and authority of the adult makes them dumb and can rob them of their senses . . . . The most important change . . . is the introjection of the guilt feelings of the adult which makes hitherto harmless play appear as a 'punishable offense' " (Ferenczi, 1933, 228). Some writers on the subject of effects have not regarded the experience to be pathogenic. But these researchers have focused on relatively superficial variables, particularly whether incestuous activity leads to aberrant behavior. They have paid very little attention to intrapsychic consequences (Rasmussen, 1934; Bender and Grugett, 1952).

Studies of the effects of childhood sexual assault on the person's orgasmic capacity in adulthood have conflicting results. Gagnon (1956) and Landis (1956) found no difference in coital experience for sexually assaulted and nonassaulted women. Hamilton, on the other hand, reported contrary findings: there was a "lower proportion of women with adequate orgasm capacity among those with sex aggressions before puberty" (cited by Gagnon, 1956, 89; in Katz and Mazur, 1979, 243). Rascovsky and Rascovsky (1950) reviewed a case of sexual abuse from which they concluded that the consummation of the incestuous wishes protected a vulnerable daughter from a manic depressive psychosis. Glover (1932) presented a similar idea in his discussion of a fetish or perversion as a defense against psychosis. Kinsey et al. (1953) reported that a few victims felt that their earlier preadolescent experience contributed favorably to later sexual adjustment. In the incestuous relationship the child is provided with some caring, and these data suggest that for some people any relationship may be better than none.

On the other hand, Flugel (1926) reported that half of a group of women arrested for prostitution said their first sexual experience had occurred with their fathers. Of the twenty women with three or more illegitimate pregnancies whom Malmquist (1966) studied, five reported early incestuous relationships.

Halleck's (1962) study of promiscuous adolescent girls indicated that their behavior often began with a sexual seduction by an older boy or man and that 15 percent were victims of incest. Although the seduction usually took place when the girl was in late puberty, many girls had prepubertal sexual experiences. Halleck noted that if the seduction occurred at a time in the child's life when she was deprived, isolated, or upset, the promiscuous behavior seemed to appear as a "neurotic compulsion." Halleck believed that the molested child was not ready to integrate her sexual impulses with mature modes of interpersonal relationship, and thus could develop distorted emotional responses and fixed misconceptions. In the subsequent years, these developments could produce serious sexual problems, including frigidity, fear of intercourse, or promiscuity.

Some authors suggest that rape in childhood may be responsible for later prostitution (DeFrancis, 1969; Macdonald, 1971, 204; Halleck, 1962, 1965; Peters, cited in "News Report," 1971, 27; Brownmiller, 1975, 309N; Giaretto, cited in Summit and Kryso, 1978). Peters believed that promiscuity was the woman's effort to desensitize herself to a fear of sex and was also a way of expressing disillusionment, hatred, and contempt for men (cited in "News Report," 1971, 27).

Studies coming from psychiatric clinics provide another important source of data. Rosenfeld et al. (1977) reported on thirty patients with histories of incest during childhood. They found that frigidity, promiscuity, and depressions were frequent problems in adults, while they observed behavior and learning disorders in children. The adults reported that sex with other men was not as satisfying as it had been with the incestuous object, generally the father. These patients also manifested intense guilt related to the contribution their incestuous experience had made to family disruption and related to their enjoyment of the experience. These authors confirmed reports that many abusing parents had been sexually abused as children. As incest seems to impair the child's ability to achieve an adult sexual and parenting relationship, it can perpetuate the pattern in subsequent generations, and this patterning, the authors stated, may be tied as much to the family setting in which the incest occurs as to the event itself.

But these findings must be assessed in light of the constraints of the research. Separating the consequences of the sexual involvement from the effects of deprivation and disorganization in the sample families is difficult, and the repercussions of early sexual experiences are subtle and varied, manifesting themselves immediately after the event or considerably later in life. Careful long-term studies should attempt to differentiate between the effects of variables such as the ages and relatedness of the participants, the duration and frequency of the sexual activity, the family environment, and such psychological factors as ego organization and object relations.

> **CLINICAL CASE 1** Mrs. A. was a 41-year-old housewife who requested help for marital and sexual problems which had intensified during the previous year. Although she was never actively interested in sexual relations, she had participated until one year prior to treatment. At that time her oldest daughter reached menarche, and Mrs. A. abruptly refused to have any sexual contact with her husband.
>
> In the evaluation she revealed that she had had a sexual relationship, including intercourse, with her father during her 13th year. Her mother had been away for a period of a few months caring for her own mother, who was ill. During the time her mother was absent, Mrs. A. began to menstruate. She felt abandoned by her mother and was frightened. When she turned to her father for help and support, he seduced her.
>
> Mrs. A.'s withdrawal from her husband was precipitated by her daughter's menarche. She had never told her husband about her past history. Nor was she conscious of the relationship between her withdrawal from her husband and her mother's withdrawal from her father, and the repetition that represented.

Superficially, Mrs. A. would appear to fit the criteria of "adequate adjustment" so frequently reported in the literature. She was married, had children, and was not promiscuous or involved with the law. But her appearance in the clinic alerts us to other manifestations of response to early sexual trauma later in life and emphasizes the need for a careful history.

THERAPEUTIC IMPLICATIONS

As the sexual repercussions of childhood sexual abuse become manifest in adulthood, it is a critical issue to know about the earlier events. The clinician must be vigilant, though, since the patient may not connect a present sexual problem with earlier events. Either the patient is not conscious of the connection, or the sexual experiences may be accompanied by such shame and guilt that the patient is unable to reveal what has happened.

Treatment need not differ substantially from the treatment of any patient with sexual problems, except that the transference-countertransference issues take on special dimensions. The therapist may become the fantasized abusing parent, creating a therapeutic impasse, or the repressed anger may emerge in such a way as to disrupt therapy. On the other hand, the therapeutic relationship itself may be sexualized such that the underlying issues are not worked through.

Countertransference problems generally revolve around the therapist's own intense affect and a tendency to overidentify with the "victim." The therapist may be so angered by the events reported that he or she misses the complexity of the relationship which spawned the sexual event. When this happens, the therapist can easily forget the patient's attachment to the incestuous parent and the caring, nurturance, and other positive parts of the earlier relationship. Thus, the mobilization of affect can be perilous, if it compromises the objectivity of the therapist.

If the patient is married, the involvement of the spouse in treatment is often helpful. But the same caution about countertransference pertains. Often, the spouse has not previously known about the relationship because the patient may feel so damaged, guilty, or compromised that she fears her spouse would reject her if she revealed the truth. Most often, the spouse is supportive. Polarizing the events, however, some spouses see only the negative aspects and cannot understand the attachment to the abusing parent. A husband may not understand how his wife can be concerned about the health or well-being of her aging father when he was once the perpetrator of an incestuous relationship. These are among the issues which make therapy particularly difficult and complex.

    CLINICAL CASE 2   When Mrs. B. was three years old, her father abandoned the family. Subsequently her mother obtained a divorce and within three years remarried. When she was ten years old, Mrs. B. began to engage in sex play, including fellatio, with her stepfather.

In describing her experience, she stated that she felt it was her responsibility to please him. Thus, when he made sexual advances, she did not resist. In fact, she was pleased by his attention and recalled some pleasure in the experiences.

When she reached puberty at age 12, she became more aware of her sexual feelings, understood more about what was taking place between her and her stepfather, and became angry and guilty. She began to avoid him and even ran away from home on one occasion, but she was unable to tell her mother why she had done this. She was angry with her mother, because she felt abandoned and vulnerable. She stopped all sexual contact with her stepfather and, for a period of several years, did not have any social contact with men at all.

When she was 16, she met her future husband at a Sunday School picnic. They saw each other frequently and developed a close friendship. She told him that she did not believe in sexual contact prior to marriage, and he was understanding of her wishes. After they married, he expected her to be sexually responsive, but she found herself unable to become sexually involved. In fact, she developed vaginismus.

After two years Mrs. B. was referred by her gynecologist for "sexual therapy." She had become increasingly angry, provocative, and withdrawn. Her husband, unaware of her history, was disappointed and angry. They were both fearful that their marriage could not endure.

After a careful evaluation, couples psychotherapy, in conjunction with treatment of her vaginismus by her gynecologist, was recommended. In the initial conjoint psychotherapy sessions, Mrs. B. was encouraged to share her pain and her concerns with her husband. She was frightened and ashamed, but with the encouragement of the therapist she was able to do this. She found, to her surprise, that her husband was supportive and kind. As they talked, they began to evolve a more understanding and compassionate relationship. As Mrs. B. began to trust her husband more, she was also able to work on the vaginismus with him and the gynecologist. Slowly, over the course of the next year, their sexual relationship improved and she became orgasmic.

This case raises several important considerations. While we see how the interplay of psychiatric and gynecological approaches and the couples approach were effective in this case, it is important to emphasize that no one approach or modality will be effective in every case. More often, treatment must be flexible so that it can enable the participants to use available resources and develop trust and alliance.

SEXUAL REPERCUSSIONS OF RAPE

Crisis theory has often been applied to rape. The theory describes a number of symptoms which last for several months and posits a gradual return to a precrisis level of adjustment (Burgess and Holmstrom, 1974b; McCombie, 1976; Hoff and Williams, 1975). While this theory can help us understand the dynamics of the short-term effects of rape, it does not address the long-term repercussions.

The concept of a posttraumatic disorder, on the other hand, quite accurately reflects the experience of rape victims. It provides an avenue to consider disorders arising later in life or those which occur over a prolonged period of time. Unfortunately, there are few reported studies that follow rape victims beyond one year. Still, some extrapolations are possible from data on childhood sexual abuse.

Generally, it has been assumed that prolonged or intense responses to external trauma occur in those individuals who are vulnerable by virtue of prior psychopathology or developmental disturbances. Recent data lead us to challenge this view (Titchener and Kapp, 1976). These data suggest that responses to traumatic events are complex and that they are determined by the specific nature and meaning of an event, as well as by the past history and adaptive capacity of an individual (Notman and Nadelson, 1976; Payne et al., 1976). Thus, ego defects alone are not enough to explain responses.

Rape should be included in the group of traumatic life events which can have substantial impact because of the nature of the trauma itself (Notman and Nadelson, 1976). During the first days and months following a rape, nearly every aspect of the victim's life is affected. Behavioral symptoms include altered sleep patterns, nightmares, changes in appetite, and aversion to sexual activity. Somatic symptoms include headaches, nausea, exhaustion, and tension. The range of emotional responses is wide. Victims experience fears, general anxiety, difficulty concentrating, intrusive thoughts about the event, lethargy, irritability, anger, guilt, and self-blame. Functioning at work, at school, or in the home may be impaired, and social relationships are also affected. Victims frequently move, curtail their activities, or change employment, as they struggle to readapt (Burgess and Holmstrom, 1974b; Sutherland and Scherl, 1970; Notman and Nadelson, 1976; Peters, 1975; Kilpatrick et al., 1979). Katz and Mazur (1979) reviewed the empirical studies of the aftermath of rape and found that researchers generally agree that victims usually recover within a year.

Most data have suggested that sexual symptoms are present after rape but are not often long-standing. Burgess and Holmstrom (1974a) found that fear of sex was an important symptom, particularly if the rape was the victim's first sexual experience. They also noted that those who had been sexually active prior to being raped were often unable to resume normal sexual interactions. Almost a third (31 percent) of a group of women who had been raped experienced a change in sexual attitude and a decrease in sexual desire, which contrasted with their previous level of sexual interest. They were reluctant to initiate sexual activities with husbands and boyfriends, although they had previously done so (Burgess and Holmstrom, 1974b). They felt that sex was "dirty," or they were too tense to perform sexually. Moreover, the sexual problems of the rape victim were often intensified by the attitude of a sexual partner who had difficulty dealing with the rape (Burgess and Holmstrom, 1974b; Notman and Nadelson, 1976).

Peters (1975) indicated that rape precipitated the development of sexual conflicts in 21 percent of the adolescents he studied. Among the conflicts were doubts about their ability to function sexually in future marriages (Peters, 1975). Younger rape victims were also noted to feel less attractive to men (Peters et al., 1976).

Burgess and Holmstrom (1978) have published one of the few follow-up studies of the long-term impact of rape. When they interviewed 81 of their original group of women again, four to six years after the rape, they found that a large number of symptoms persisted. In fact, only one-third of the total sample reported feeling that they had "recovered" within a period of several months. McCahill, Meyer, and Fischman (1979) followed 213 victims. A year after the rape, they reported, at least one-third of the victims still had symptoms. They were still experiencing changes in eating and sleeping patterns, increased fear of being alone on the streets, negative feelings toward unknown men, decreased social activities, and decreased sexual functioning.

Nadelson, Notman, Zackson, and Gornick followed 41 rape victims for 15 to thirty months following the rape (unpublished). Their data also indicated that, in a population with no previous history of mental illness or treatment for emotional disturbance, a large number of symptoms which the victims attributed to the rape persisted. Most victims felt that the rape had caused them to be mistrustful of men and that it was detrimental to social interactions. Three-quarters of the sample felt suspicious of men, and more than half felt restricted in going out. Half reported sexual difficulties which had not been present prior to the rape.

The incidence of sexual trauma in general is difficult to ascertain. Fitz et al. (1981) recently reported that, among a college survey sample, 7.7 percent of the females and 4.8 percent of the males had experienced sexual molestation, both homosexual and heterosexual. (This figure differs slightly from the Kinsey et al. [1948] figure of 9.2 percent.) Further, 25 percent of those women who were molested and ten percent of the men reported subsequent problems with sexual adjustment. The most frequent sexual problem cited was difficulty in achieving orgasm with sexual intercourse. The authors observed that the guilt induced by succumbing to molestation without physical force was a major compounding factor and that it contributed to subsequent symptoms. Noting that the females were more likely to view the experiences negatively than were the males, the authors conjecture that males may view these contacts, particularly in the prepubescent period, as "initiation," whereas females view them as "violation." The authors emphasize that "molestation must be considered a central issue with a substantial portion of the female population seeking treatment" (Fitz et al., 1981, 57).

THERAPEUTIC CONSIDERATIONS

On the premise that successful adaptation will occur within the year following the trauma, most treatment has been short-term. Individual counseling, which may or may not involve the family of the victim, and groups, including self-help groups, are the basic resources provided in rape crisis centers. Behavioral approaches have been reported to be particularly effective with the phobic symptoms which may appear as the aftermath of rape (Kilpatrick et al., 1979).

Hilberman (1976) claims consensus for three basic precepts regarding counseling: (1) crisis intervention will facilitate working through the trauma and diminish the likelihood of long-term psychopathologic consequences; (2) emotional support from whomever the victim comes in contact with is important during the crisis period; and (3) rape is a significant crisis for others close to the rape victim. As noted, however, the response to rape is not simply a crisis response. Since the implications of rape differ for women at different stages of the life cycle and in different family and social contexts, therapists must be concerned with both contextual factors and with long-term implications (Notman and Nadelson, 1976). For example, the experience of rape for an adolescent, for whom the rape is the first sexual experience, may be very different from the experience for the middle-aged, married woman. Even in the initial crisis consultation, the meaning of the event must be understood in the context of a victim's life, remembering that positive adaptation is facilitated when the external world provides validation and support (Burgess, 1978; Notman and Nadelson, 1976).

The specific nature of the events is also important to the therapy. For example, the meaning of a betrayal by a trusted person, or the significance of a particular violent or degrading experience, will be different for each victim. Also important are the circumstances of the immediate aftermath of rape. The attitudes and behavior of those with whom the victim comes in contact, e.g., police, health care providers, family, and friends, have important therapeutic implications. Disapproval, skepticism, or any communication that can be seen as critical can intensify guilt. If the victim has experienced sexual stimulation or orgasm, she is even more likely to feel guilt and shame and to suffer later sexual repercussions (Notman and Nadelson, 1976).

Thus, while it does appear that many recover within a year, in view of the evolving evidence about the long-term consequences of rape, it is important to consider and to provide access to subsequent therapy, should symptoms continue, recur, or emerge. Recent authors have emphasized the need to incorporate psychodynamic and interpersonal understanding with the behavioral approach originally proposed by Masters and Johnson (Nadelson, 1979).

CLINICAL CASE 3 Mr. and Mrs. C. were evaluated for "sexual problems." They were both 43 years of age and had been married for ten years. Mrs. C. had never been very interested in sex, and since the birth of their daughter four years before, she had become sexually unresponsive.

The C.'s were interested in attempting a behavioral approach to the treatment of their sexual problem since they had read about it. They did not want a long period of psychotherapy because Mrs. C. had spent three years in psychotherapy in the past, and while she found it rewarding in many ways, there was no change in her sexual feelings. Mr. C. did not feel that he had a problem and did not want to be involved unless it was "sex therapy."

The therapist did not feel that a struggle about treatment approaches would be productive, and a modified behavioral sexual therapy program was begun. For the first two sessions progress was steady. The C.'s reported that their communication was good, and they were able to do the prescribed exercises. However, Mrs. C. noted that her feelings had not changed and that she continued to be uninterested in sex, despite the fact that she was performing. She presented a classical picture of the obsessive mechanism of "spectatoring," typified by her comment, "I often wonder what the fly on the ceiling thinks."

The therapist was not surprised when, suddenly, in the midst of the fourth session, Mrs. C. became teary. She abruptly changed the topic and refused to pursue the discussion of the sexual interaction of the last week. It was not clear what precipitated this change. Mrs. C. continued to become more agitated, and she finally related a story that Mr. C. had never heard.

Fifteen years before, Mrs. C. had been working as a nurse in a small community hospital in her home town. One night, when she left work, she was followed and raped by her supervisor, a man who had been extremely attentive and kind to her. He warned her not to tell anyone, threatening to cause her to lose both her job and her reputation if she did. Since her family lived in the town, she was frightened, and she complied. At work the next day he behaved as if he had no relationship with her at all.

When Mrs. C. met her husband, she was ashamed to tell him of this event because she believed that she had allowed herself to be raped. She feared that he would reject her if he knew. Since she cared about him a great deal, she pretended to have sexual feelings. She had, in fact, had none since the rape had occurred.

Mr. C. responded warmly and supportively upon hearing the story. Over the next few months they continued to talk about Mrs. C.'s experience. Slowly their sexual relationship began to improve. Mrs. C. felt loved and valued by her husband, particularly since he was able to understand her pain. He, on the other hand, was relieved of his feelings of failure. Behavioral techniques were of value in the therapy, although they did not become a major component because Mr. C. experienced them as too coercive.

A request for direct sex therapy can be a way to avoid a painful discussion or confrontation. From a treatment point of view, though, sex therapy can be the context for developing enough of an alliance so that other treatment can proceed. Sex therapy alone is unsuccessful unless underlying concerns about sexual trauma are confronted, and as indicated, an integration of approaches can be most successful.

Rape may intensify previous existing conflicts in relationships and strain the relationships at the very time when the victim needs the most support. When the victim feels isolated, helpless, and guilty, those who are close have a key role in reducing feelings of isolation and helplessness. The aim of therapy, including sexual therapy, should be to facilitate the reestablishment of a sense of control, competence, and self-esteem.

CLINICAL CASE 4 Mrs. D., a 31-year-old married mother of two children aged six and eight, was alone at home when an intruder entered her house through an opened back door. Just minutes before, her eight-year-old daughter had gone off to school through that door, and Mrs. D. had left it open because her six-year-old son was expected home for lunch.

The intruder surprised Mrs. D. while she was in her bedroom. She was frightened that her son would appear, and she complied. The man raped her and then spent several moments rummaging through the house for valuables. He left when he heard someone at the door. Mrs. D. immediately called her husband, who took her to see the family physician. Although both he and her husband were supportive, Mrs. D. suspected that they both wondered, "How come the door was opened? Why did she comply? Why didn't she struggle?"

Over the next few weeks, she felt increasingly distant from her husband. She was repulsed by his sexual advances and felt that he was disapproving of her. She worried about the impact of the turmoil on her children, who seemed sullen and uncommunicative. She felt that she had been damaged, and she found herself feeling angry with all men, including her husband.

She decided that she needed to talk with someone. She found a woman therapist, who requested that her husband come in also, after meeting with her individually for several weeks. In an individual session with Mr. D., he revealed that he was indeed suspicious that his wife had not attempted to fend off her assailant and that she had "allowed this to happen." He had difficulty getting close to her because of these feelings and because he did have a sense of her as damaged. He was embarrassed and ashamed of his feelings because he cared deeply for his wife. He acknowledged that his response was more negative than he expected it would be.

The therapist saw Mr. and Mrs. D. both separately and together over the course of six months. She worked with each toward acknowledging feelings, and she helped them to share these in order to reestablish some understanding and trust. They were each relieved by this openness, although initially pained. Mrs. D. commented, toward the end of therapy, that the closeness that had developed between them had resulted from their ability to be honest and caring and to acknowledge "human failings."

COUNTERTRANSFERENCE ISSUES

A multitude of countertransference issues emerge when treating a rape victim. Among them are anger at the victim for complying and identification with the spouse as a victim. Even more frequently, however, the therapist overidentifies with the patient, particularly if the experience is described as brutal or demeaning. Counselors who have themselves been raped may find it difficult to separate their own experience from that of the victim, and they may project their own feelings, fantasies, and fears. Their empathic ability may, however, be supportive and validating.

Both therapist and spouse may also find that the anger aroused promotes such a motivation for vengeance that the internal struggle of the rape victim is neglected. The rape victim in the emergency room often finds that staff spend more time "talking down" her spouse, boyfriend, or father than they do with her. In part such behavior relates to the guilt of the man, who was not "protective," but it may also reflect a view of the victim as damaged property. If a sexual problem results from rape, the sexual partner may become impatient or suspicious, or he may even feel that the woman had a better sexual experience when she was raped than with him. He may then feel sexually demeaned and defensively need to reject his partner.

In working with victims of sexual abuse, one of the most important and difficult issues is the problem of infantilizing the victim or turning her into a "patient." Even more damaging is the possibility of treating the person like a defendant. To the victim both of these views fail to capture the experience, and they may be damaging in the attempt to regain self-esteem and a sense of self-worth. For those dealing with the rape victim they may represent ways to cope with the counter-transference aspects of this powerful encounter. The support and respect demonstrated in a sensitive interaction can, however, turn a painful and tragic event into an experience which promotes growth.

Bibliography for the Introduction

American Psychiatric Association. *Diagnostic and Statistical Manual of Mental Disorders, 3d ed.* Washington, D.C.: American Psychiatric Association, 1980.

Briggs, M.A. "The Use of Audiovisual Materials." In *Sex Education for the Health Professional: A Curriculum Guide,* edited by N. Rosenzweig and F.P. Pearsall. New York: Grune & Stratton, 1978.

Broderick, C.B., and Bernard, J., eds. *The Individual, Sex, and Society: A SIECUS Hand Book for Teachers and Counselors.* Baltimore: Johns Hopkins University Press, 1969.

Cooper, A.J. "Factors in Male Sexual Inadequacy: A Review." *Journal of Nervous and Mental Disease* 149 (1969): 337–359.

Derogatis, L.R., Meyer, J.K., and King, K.M. "Psychopathology in Individuals with Sexual Dysfunction." *American Journal of Psychiatry* 138 (1981): 757–763.

Lief, H. "Introduction to Sexuality." In *The Sexual Experience,* edited by B.J. Sadock, H.I. Kaplan, and A.M. Freedman. Baltimore: Williams & Wilkins Co., 1976.

Masters, W.H., and Johnson, V.E. *Human Sexual Response.* Boston: Little, Brown and Co., 1966.

Masters, W.H., and Johnson, V.E. *Human Sexual Inadequacy.* Boston: Little, Brown and Co., 1970.

Maurice, W., and Guze, S. "Sexual Dysfunction and Associated Psychiatric Disorders." *Comprehensive Psychiatry* 111 (1970): 539–543.

Sadock, V.A. "Special Areas of Interest." In *The Comprehensive Textbook of Psychiatry,* edited by H.I. Kaplan, A.M. Freedman, and B.J. Sadock. Baltimore: Williams & Wilkins Co., 1980.

Small, J.G., and Small, I.F. "Psychosexual Dysfunctions." In *The Comprehensive Textbook of Psychiatry, 3d ed.,* edited by H.I. Kaplan, A.M. Freedman, and B.J. Sadock. Baltimore: Williams & Wilkins Co., 1980.

Sussman, N. "History of Sexuality." In *The Comprehensive Textbook of Psychiatry, 3d ed.,* edited by H.I. Kaplan, A.M. Freedman, and B.J. Sadock. Baltimore: Williams & Wilkins Co., 1980.

Audiovisual Resources on Sexual Function and Dysfunction

Dr. Edward A. Mason[1] has assembled the following list of audiovisual resources and distributors to help professionals fill specific needs for training or therapy. The films and videotapes listed have been useful in workshops, lectures, seminars and clinical settings. Of the distributors listed, the Multi-Media Resource Center and Focus International have a particularly wide selection.

Selected Audiovisuals

ACTIVE PARTNERS, 18 min., color, sound, 16 mm (also video and super 8), 1979, by Dr. Marvin Silverman and Robert Lenz. Rent: $40, Purchase: $300 from Multi-Media Resource Center.
A couple discuss their concerns and adjustments to the male's spinal cord injury; they demonstrate pleasuring techniques for a quadraplegic.

1. Associate Professor of Psychiatry; Harvard Medical School

COPING WITH SERIOUS ILLNESS: SEXUALITY, 30 min., color, sound, 16mm and video, 1980, by David Tapper. Rent: $60, Purchase: $600 16mm, $225 (videocassette) from Time-Life Video.
Part of a series using footage from "Joan Robinson: One Woman's Story," this one focusing on sexuality and the need for loving during illness.

FEELING GOOD, 25 min., color, sound, 16mm film (also video and super 8), 1975, by Laird Sutton. Rent: $55, Purchase: $360 from Multi-Media Resource Center.
A male masturbation film.

FEMALE ANORGASMIA AND ITS TREATMENT, 60 min., color, video, 1978, by Dr. Malcolm Freedman. Rent: $30, Purchase: $110 from Emory University. Discussion of the absence of orgasmic response and demonstration of Annon's therapy techniques.

GIVE TO GET, 11 min., color, sound, 16mm film (also video and Super 8), 1971, by Laird Sutton. Rent: $35, Purchase: $220 from Multi-Media Resource Center.
A couple moves from massage to intercourse.

INCEST: THE VICTIM NOBODY BELIEVES, 23 min., color, sound, 16mm film (and video), 1976, by J. Gary Mitchell. Rent: $60, Purchase: $385 from MTI Teleprograms.
Three young women candidly discuss their experiences and the impact on their lives.

MARGO, 11 min., color, sound, 16mm film (also video and super 8), 1972, by Laird Sutton. Rent: $35, Purchase: $220 from Multi-Media Resource Center.
A female masturbation film.

PHYSIOLOGICAL RESPONSES OF THE SEXUALLY STIMULATED FEMALE IN THE LABORATORY, 16 min., color, sound, 16mm film, 1974, by Dr. Gorm Wagner. Discussion guide included. Rent: $50, Purchase: $320 from Focus International.

PHYSIOLOGICAL RESPONSES OF THE SEXUALLY STIMULATED MALE IN THE LABORATORY, 16 min., color, sound, 16mm film, 1975, by Dr. Gorm Wagner. Discussion guide included. Rent: $50, Purchase: $320 from Focus International.
Both provide observations and have been widely used for students and patients because of their clinical tone.

PROBLEMS OF GENDER IDENTITY, 55 min., color, sound video. Rent: $35, Purchase: $200 from Blue Hill Educational Systems. One of a series dealing with concepts of gender role and illustrating the more common disturbances.

SQUEEZE TECHNIQUE, 10 min., color, sound, 16mm (also video and super 8), 1972, by Laird Sutton. Rent: $35, Purchase $215 from Multi-Media Resource Center.
A couple demonstrates the Semans technique for treatment of premature ejaculation.

TRYING TIMES: CRISIS IN FERTILITY, 33 min., color, 16mm film (and video), 1980, by Joan Finck. Rent: $50, Purchase: $480 from Fanlight Productions.
A film for professionals and involuntarily childless couples about causes, impact, investigation of, and clinical services for infertility.

Distributors

Barr Films
P.O. Box 5667
Pasadena, CA 91107

Benchmark Films, Inc.
145 Scarborough Road
Briarcliff Manor, NY 10510

Blue Hill Educational Systems, Inc.
52 S. Main Street
Spring Valley, NY 10977

Churchill Films
662 N. Robertson Blvd.
Los Angeles, CA 90069

Centron Educational Films
1621 W. 9th Street
P.O. Box 687
Lawrence, KS 66044

Cleveland Health Education Museum
8911 Euclid Avenue
Cleveland, OH 44106

Emory University
School of Medicine
69 Butler Street, S.E.
Atlanta, GA 30303

Extension Media Center
University of California
2223 Fulton Street
Berkeley, CA 94720

Fanlight Productions
P.O. Box 226
Cambridge, MA 02238

Focus International
1 East 53rd Street
New York, NY 10022

Guidance Associates
Communications Park
Box 3000
Mt. Kisco, NY 10549

Health and Education Multimedia, Inc.
50 E. 72nd Street, Suite 4B
New York, NY 10021

Health Sciences Consortium
200 Eastowne Drive, Suite 213
Chapel Hill, NC 27514

Indiana University
Audio-Visual Center
Bloomington, IN 47405

Learning Corp. of America
1350 Avenue of the Americas
New York, NY 10019

Medcom Products
1633 Broadway
New York, NY 10019

MTI Teleprograms, Inc.
4825 N. Scott Street, Suite 23
Schiller Park, IL 60176

Milner-Fenwick, Inc.
2125 Greenspring Drive
Timonium, MD 21093

Multi-Media Resource Center
1525 Franklin Street
San Francisco, CA 94109

New Day Films
P.O. Box 315
Franklin Lakes, NJ 07417

PBS Video
475 L'Enfant Plaza, S.W.
Washington, DC 20024

Perennial Education, Inc.
477 Roger Williams
P.O. Box 855 Ravinia
Highland Park, IL 60035

Polymorph Films
118 South Street
Boston, MA 02111

Spenco Medical Corporation
P.O. Box 8113
Waco, TX 76710

The Stanfield House
12381 Wilshire Blvd., Suite 203
Los Angeles, CA 90025

Texture Films, Inc.
1600 Broadway
New York, NY 10019

Time-Life Video
Box 666 Radio City Station
New York, NY 10019

Trainex Corporation
P.O. Box 116
Garden Grove, CA 92642.

Bibliography for Chapter 1

American Medical Association. *Human Sexuality.* Chicago: American Medical Association, 1972.

American Psychiatric Association. *Diagnostic and Statistical Manual of Mental Disorders, 3d ed.,* Washington, D.C.: American Psychiatric Association, 1980.

Brown, E., Brown, G.M., Kofman, O., and Quarrington, B. "Sexual Function and Affect in Parkinsonian Men Treated with L-Dopa." *American Journal of Psychiatry* 135 (1978): 1552–1555.

Gartrell, N.K., Loriaux, D.L., and Chase, T.N. "Plasma Testosterone in Homosexual and Heterosexual Women." *American Journal of Psychiatry* 134 (1977): 1117–1119.

Greenblatt, R.B., and McNamara, V.P. "Endocrinology of Human Sexuality." In *The Sexual Experience,* edited by B.J. Sadock, H.I. Kaplan, and A.M. Freedman. Baltimore: Williams & Wilkins Co., 1976.

Kinsey, A.C., Pomeroy, W.B., Martin, C.F., and Gebhard, P.H. *Sexual Behavior in the Human Female.* Philadelphia: W.B. Saunders. Co., 1953.

Langman, J. *Medical Embryology, 2d ed.* Baltimore: Williams & Wilkins Co., 1972.

Masters, W.H., and Johnson, V.E. *Human Sexual Response.* Boston: Little, Brown and Co., 1966.

Masters, W.H., and Johnson, V.E. *Human Sexual Inadequacy.* Boston: Little, Brown and Co., 1970.

McLean, P.D. "Brain Mechanisms of Elemental Sexual Functions." In *The Sexual Experience,* edited by B.J. Sadock, H.I. Kaplan, and A.M. Freedman. Baltimore: Williams & Wilkins Co., 1976.

Novak, E.R. *Textbook of Gynecology, 9th ed.* Baltimore: Williams & Wilkins Co., 1975.

Perry, J., and Whipple, B. "Pelvic Muscle Strength of Female Ejaculators: Evidence in Support of a New Theory of Orgasm." *Journal of Sex Research* 1 (1978): 22–39.

Sadock, V.A. "Sexual Anatomy, Endocrinology and Physiology." In *The Comprehensive Textbook of Psychiatry, 3d ed.,* edited by H.I. Kaplan, A.M. Freedman, and B.J. Sadock. Baltimore: Williams & Wilkins Co., 1980.

Sherfey, M.J. *The Nature of Evolution of Female Sexuality.* New York: Random House, 1972.

Bibliography for Chapter 2

American Psychiatric Association. *Diagnostic and Statistical Manual of Mental Disorders, 2d ed.* Washington, D.C.: American Psychiatric Association, 1968.

American Psychiatric Association. *Diagnostic and Statistical Manual of Mental Disorders, 3d ed.* Washington, D.C.: American Psychiatric Association, 1980.

World Health Organization. *Manual of the International Classification of Diseases, Injuries, and Causes of Death, 9th rev.* Geneva: World Health Organization, 1978.

Bibliography for Chapter 3

American Psychiatric Association. "Psychosexual Dysfunction." In *Syllabus: Psychiatric Knowledge and Skills Self-Assessment Program.* Washington, D.C.: American Psychiatric Association, 1979.

Barbach, O.G. *For Yourself: The Fulfillment of Female Sexuality.* New York: Doubleday & Co., 1975.

Brady, J.P. "Behavior Therapy and Sex Therapy." *American Journal of Psychiatry* 133 (1976): 896–899.

Cooper, A. "Hostility and Disorders of Sexual Potency." *Comprehensive Psychiatry* 9 (1968): 621–626.

Derogatis, L.R., Meyer, J.K., and King, K.M. "Psychopathology in Individuals with Sexual Dysfunction." *American Journal of Psychiatry* 138 (1981): 757–763.

Kinsey, A.C., Pomeroy, W.B., and Martin, C.E. *Sexual Behavior in the Human Male.* Philadelphia: W.B. Saunders Co., 1948.

Lansky, M.R., and Davenport, A.E. "Difficulties in Brief Conjoint Treatment of Sexual Dysfunction." *American Journal of Psychiatry* 132 (1975): 177–179.

Lobitz, W.C., and Baker, E.L. "Group Treatment of Single Males with Erectile Dysfunction." *Archives of Sexual Behavior* 8 (1979): 127–129.

LoPiccolo, J. "Sexual Dysfunction." In *Behavioral Medicine: Theory and Practice,* edited by O.F. Pomerleau and J.P. Brady. Baltimore: Williams & Wilkins Co., 1979.

LoPiccolo, J., and Lobitz, W.C. "The Role of Masturbation in the Treatment of Sexual Dysfunction." *Archives of Sexual Behavior* 2 (1972): 163–171.

Marks, I.M. "Review of Behavioral Psychotherapy, II: Sexual Disorders." *American Journal of Psychiatry* 138 (1981): 750–756.

Masters, W.E., and Johnson, V.E. *Human Sexual Response.* Boston: Little, Brown and Co., 1966.

Masters, W.E., and Johnson, V.E. *Human Sexual Inadequacy.* Boston: Little, Brown and Co., 1970.

Maurice, W., and Guze, S. "Sexual Dysfunction and Associated Psychiatric Disorders." *Comprehensive Psychiatry* 11 (1970): 539–543.

Meyer, J.K. "Individual Psychotherapy of Sexual Disorders." In *The Sexual Experience,* edited by B.J. Sadock, H.I. Kaplan, and A.M. Freedman. Baltimore: Williams & Wilkins Co., 1976.

O'Connor, J., and Stern, L.O. "Results of Treatment in Functional Sexual Disorders." *New York State Journal of Medicine* 72 (1977): 1927–1934.

Sadock, B.J., and Spitz, H.I. "Group Psychotherapy of Sexual Disorders." In *The Comprehensive Textbook of Psychiatry, 2d ed.,* edited by A.M. Freedman, H.I. Kaplan, and B.J. Sadock. Baltimore: Williams & Wilkins Co., 1975.

Sadock, V.A., Sadock, B.J., and Kaplan, H.I. "Comprehensive Sex Therapy Training: A New Approach." *American Journal of Psychiatry* 132 (1975): 858–860.

Sadock, V.A., and Sadock, B.J. "Dual-Sex Therapy." In *The Sexual Experience,* edited by B.J. Sadock, H.I. Kaplan, and A.M. Freedman. Baltimore: Williams & Wilkins Co., 1976.

Sadock, V.A. "Treatment of Psychosexual Dysfunctions." In *The Comprehensive Textbook of Psychiatry, 3d ed.,* edited by H.I. Kaplan, A.M. Freedman, and B.J. Sadock. Baltimore: Williams & Wilkins Co., 1980.

Bibliography for Chapter 4

Brody, J.E. "Success and Failure in Sex Therapy: Four Case Histories." *The New York Times,* November 11, 1980, p. c 1–2.

Kaplan, H. *The New Sex Therapy.* New York: Brunner/Mazel, 1974.

Kaplan, H. *Disorders of Sexual Desires.* New York: Brunner/Mazel, 1979.

Levay, A. "Ethical Issues in Sex Therapy and Research: A Review." *Values and Ethics in Health Care* 6 (1981): 61–64.

Levay A., Weissberg, J., and Blaustein, A. "Concurrent Sex Therapy and Psychoanalytic Psychotherapy by Separate Therapists: Effectiveness and Implications." *Psychiatry* 39 (1976): 355–363.

Levay A.N. and Kagle, A. "Ego Deficiencies in the Areas of Pleasure, Intimacy, and Cooperation: Guidelines in the Diagnosis and Treatment of Sexual Dysfunctions." *Journal of Sex and Marital Therapy* 3 (1977a): 10–18.

Levay A.N., and Kagle, A. "A Study of Treatment Needs Following Sex Therapy." *American Journal of Psychiatry* 134 (1977b): 970–973.

Levay A.N., and Kagle, A. "Recent Advances in Sex Therapy: Integration with the Dynamic Therapies." *Psychiatric Quarterly* 50 (1978): 5–16.

Levay A.N., Kagle, A., and Weissberg, J.H. "Issues of Transference in Sex Therapy." *Journal of Sex and Marital Therapy* 5 (1979a): 15–21.

Levay A.N., and Weissberg, J.H. "The Role of Dreams in Sex Therapy." *Journal of Sex and Marital Therapy* 5 (1979b): 334–339.

Magee, M. "Psychogenic Impotence: A Critical Review." *Urology* 5 (1980): 435.

Masters, W., and Johnson, V. *Human Sexual Inadequacy.* Boston: Little, Brown and Co., 1970.

Marmor, J., and Woods, S.M. *The Interface Between the Psychodynamic and Behavioral Therapies.* New York: Plenum Medical Book Co., 1980.

Michal V., and Pospichal, J. "Phalloarteriography in the Diagnosis of Erectile Impotence." *World Journal of Surgery* 2 (1978): 239–248.

Person, E., and Ovesey, L. "Transvestism, a Disorder of the Sense of Self." *International Journal of Psychoanalytic Psychotherapy* 5 (1976): 219–236.

Sobel, D. "Sex Therapy: As Popularity Grows, Critics Question Whether It Works." *The New York Times,* November 4, 1980, p. c 1–3.

Spark, R.F., White, R.A., and Connolly, P.B. "Impotence Is not Always Psychogenic: Newer Insights Into Hypothalamic-Pituitary-Gonadal Dysfunction." *JAMA* 243 (1980): 750–755.

Stoller, R. "Sexual Excitement," *Archives of General Psychiatry* 33 (1976): 899–909.

Weissberg, J.H., and Levay, A.N. "The Role of Resistance in Sex Therapy." *Journal of Sex and Marital Therapy* 7 (1981): [sic]

Zilbergeld, B., and Evans, M. "The Inadequacy of Masters and Johnson." *Psychology Today,* August 1980, pp. 28–43.

Bibliography for Chapter 5

Belt, B.G. "Some Organic Causes of Impotence." *Medical Aspects of Human Sexuality* 7 (1973): 152–162.

Cole, T.M. "Sexuality and Physical Disabilities." *Archives of Sexual Behavior* 4 (1975): 389–405.

Dickes, R. "Surgery, Medicine, Drugs, and Sexuality and the Physician's Role in Sex Education." In *The Comprehensive Textbook of Psychiatry, 3d ed.,* edited by H.I. Kaplan, A.M. Freedman, and B.J. Sadock. Baltimore: Williams & Wilkins Co., 1980.

Ellenberg, M. "Impotence in Diabetes: The Neurologic Factor." *Annals of Internal Medicine* 75 (1971): 213–229.

Faerman, I., Glocer, L., Fox, D., Jadzinsky, N., and Rapaport, M. "Impotence and Diabetes: Histological Studies of the Autonomic Nervous Fibers of the Corpora Cavernosa in Impotent Diabetic Males." *Diabetes* 23 (1974): 971–976.

Hollander, M.A. "Hysterectomy and Feelings of Femininity." *Medical Aspects of Human Sexuality* 3 (1969): 6–19.

Karacan, I., Salis, P.J., Ware, J.C., Dervent, B., Williams, R.L., Scott, F.B., Attia S.L., and Beutler, L.E. "Nocturnal Penile Tumescence and Diagnoses in Diabetic Impotence." *American Journal of Psychiatry* 135 (1978): 191–197.

Rodgers, D.A., Ziegler, F.J., and Levy, N. "Prevailing Cultural Attitudes About Vasectomy: A Possible Explanation of Postoperative Psychological Response." *Psychosomatic Medicine* 29 (1967): 367–375.

Rosen, J.S., Nanninga, J.B., and O'Connor, V.J. "External Sphincterotomy: Effect on Penile Erection." *Archives of Physical Medical Rehabilitation* 57 (1976): 511–513.

Scully, J.H., Dickes, R., and Bernstein, W.E. "The Difficult Surgical Patient." In *Understanding Human Behavior in Health and Disease, 2d ed.,* edited by R.C. Simons and H. Pardes. Baltimore: Williams & Wilkins Co., 1981.

Segraves, R.T. "Pharmacological Agents Causing Sexual Dysfunction." *Journal of Sex and Marital Therapy* 3 (1977): 157–177.

Sparks, R.F., White, R.A., and Connolly, P.B. "Impotence Is not Always Psychogenic: Newer Insights Into Hypothalamic-Pituitary-Gonadal Dysfunction." *JAMA* 243 (1980): 750–755.

Titchener, J.L. "Psychiatry in the Practice of Surgery and the Specialties: Somatopsychic Sequences." In *Textbook of Psychiatry for Medical Practice,* edited by C.K. Hofling. Philadelphia: J.B. Lippincott Co., 1975.

Wabrek, A.J., and Wabrek, C.J. "Mastectomy: Sexual Complications." *Primary Care* 4 (1978): 803–810.

Wasserman, M.D., Pollack, C.P., Speilman, A.J., and Weitzman, E.D. "Theoretical and Technical Problems in the Measurement of Nocturnal Penile Tumescence for the Differential Diagnosis of Impotence." *Psychosomatic Medicine* 42 (1980): 575–585.

Bibliography for Chapter 6

Abram, H.S., Hester, L.R., Sheridan, W.F., and Epstein, G.M. "Sexual Functioning in Patients with Chronic Renal Failure." In *Handbook of Sex Therapy,* edited by J. LoPiccolo and L. LoPiccolo. New York: Plenum Press, 1978.

Cuber, J.F. "The Natural History of Sex in Marriage." *Medical Aspects of Human Sexuality* 9 (1975): 51–75.

DePalma, R.G., Levine, S.B., and Feldman, S. "Preservation of Erectile Function After Aortoiliac Reconstruction." *Archives of Surgery* 113 (1978): 958–962.

Ellenberg M. "Impotence in Diabetes: The Neurologic Factors." In *Handbook of Sex Therapy,* edited by J. LoPiccolo and L. LoPiccolo. New York: Plenum Press, 1978.

Fisher, C., Schiavi, R.C., Edwards, A., Davis, D.M., Reitman, M., and Fine, J. "Evaluation of Nocturnal Penile Tumescence in the Differential Diagnosis of Sexual Impotence: A Quantitative Study." *Archives of General Psychiatry* 36 (1979): 431–437.

Frank, E., Anderson, C., and Rubinstein, D. "Frequence of Sexual Dysfunction in 'Normal' Couples." *New England Journal of Medicine* 299 (1978): 111–115.

Friedman, J.M. "Sexual Adjustment of the Postcoronary Male." In *Handbook of Sex Therapy,* edited by J. LoPiccolo and L. LoPiccolo. New York: Plenum Press, 1978.

Gebhard, P.H. "Postmarital Coitus Among Widows and Divorcees." In *Divorce and After,* edited by P. Bohannan. New York: Doubleday & Co., 1970.

Golden, J.S. "How You Can Help Patients with Physical Ailments to a Better Sex Life." *Medical Times* 104 (1976): 83–91.

Hellerstein, H.K., and Friedman, E.H. "Sexual Activity and the Post Coronary Patient." *Scandinavian Journal of Rehabilitation Medicine* 2 (1970): 109.

Higgins, G.E. "Aspects of Sexual Response in Adults with Spinal-Cord Injury: A Review of the Literature." In *Handbook of Sex Therapy,* edited by J. LoPiccolo and L. LoPiccolo. New York: Plenum Press, 1978.

Karacan, I., Hursch, C.J., and Williams, R.L. "Some Characteristics of Nocturnal Penile Tumescence in Elderly Males." *Journal of Gerontology* 27 (1972): 39–45.

Karacan, I., Williams, R.L., Thornby, J.I., and Salis, P.J. "Sleep-Related Penile Tumescence as a Function of Age." *American Journal of Psychiatry* 132 (1975): 932–937.

Kinsey, A.C., Pomeroy, W.B., Martin, C.E., and Gebhard, P.H. *Sexual Behavior in the Human Female.* Philadelphia: W.B. Saunders Co., 1953.

Levay, A., Weissberg, J., and Blaustein, A. "Concurrent Sex Therapy and Psychoanalytic Psychotherapy by Separate Therapists: Effectiveness and Implications." *Psychiatry* 39 (1976): 355–363.

LoPiccolo J., and LoPiccolo L., eds. *Handbook of Sex Therapy.* New York: Plenum Press, 1978.

Masters, W.H., and Johnson, V.E. *Human Sexual Response.* Boston: Little, Brown and Co., 1966.

May, J., and Pauly, I.B. "Sexual Activity in the Cardiac Patient." *Seminars in Family Medicine* 1 (1980): 73–86.

Pauly, I.B. "Sex and the Life Cycle." In *The Comprehensive Textbook of Psychiatry, 3d ed.,* edited by H.I. Kaplan, A.M. Freedman, and B.J. Sadock. Baltimore: Williams & Wilkins Co., 1980.

Pauly, I.B., and Goldstein, S.G. "Physicians' Perception of Their Education in Human Sexuality." *Journal of Medical Education* 45 (1970): 745–753.

Pfeiffer, E. "Sexuality in the Aging Individual." *Journal of the American Geriatric Society* 22 (1974): 481–484.

Pfeiffer, E. "Sexuality and the Aging Patient." In *Human Sexuality,* edited by R. Green. Baltimore: Williams & Wilkins Co., 1979.

Reed, D.M. "Sexual Behavior in the Separated, Divorced, and Widowed." In *The Sexual Experience,* edited by B.J. Sadock, H.I. Kaplan, and A.M. Freedman. Baltimore: Williams & Wilkins Co., 1976.

Regestein, Q., and Horn, H. "Coitus in Patients with Cardiac Arrythmias." *Medical Aspects of Human Sexuality* 12 (1978): 108–125.

Renshaw, D. "Impotence in Diabetes." In *Handbook of Sex Therapy,* edited by J. LoPiccolo and L. LoPiccolo. New York: Plenum Press, 1978.

Scalzi, C., Loya, F., and Golden, J.S. "Sexual Therapy of Patients with Cardiovascular Disease." *Western Journal of Medicine* 126 (1977): 237–244.

Sviland, M.A. "Helping Elderly Couples Become Sexually Liberated: Psychosocial Issues." In *Handbook of Sex Therapy,* edited by J. LoPiccolo and L. LoPiccolo. New York: Plenum Press, 1978.

Udry, J.R. *The Social Context of Marriage, 2d ed.* Philadelphia: J.B. Lippincott Co., 1971.

Wabrek, A., Wabrek, C., and Burchell, R. "Marital and Sexual Counseling After Mastectomy." In *Human Sexuality,* edited by R. Green. Baltimore: Williams & Wilkins Co., 1979.

Bibliography for Chapter 7

Bernstein, S.M., Steiner, B.W., Glaister, J.T.D., and Muir, C.F. "Changes in Patients with Gender-Identity Problems After Parental Death." *American Journal of Psychiatry* 138 (1981): 41–45.

Gadpaille, W. "Biological Factors in the Development of Human Sexual Identity." *Psychiatric Clinics of North America* 3 (1980): 3–20.

Galenson, E., and Roiphe, H. "The Impact of Early Sexual Discovery on Mood, Defensive Organization, and Symbolization." *Psychoanalytic Study of the Child* 26 (1971): 195–216.

Galenson, E., Vogel, S., Blau, S., and Roiphe, H. "Disturbance in Sexual Identity Beginning at 18 Months of Age." *International Review of Psychoanalysis* 2 (1975): 389–397.

Hampson, J.L., and Hampson, J.G. "The Ontogenesis of Sexual Behavior in Man." In *Sex and Internal Secretions,* Vol. 2, edited by W. Young. Baltimore: Williams & Wilkins, Co., 1961.

Hastings, D. "Postsurgical Adjustment of Male Transsexual Patients." *Clinics in Plastic Surgery* 1 (1974): 335–344.

Mahler, M., Pine, F., and Bergman, A. *The Psychological Birth of the Human Infant.* New York: Basic Books, 1975.

Meyer, J. "Clinical Variants Among Applicants for Sex Reassignment." *Archives of Sexual Behavior* 3 (1974): 527–558.

Meyer, J. "Paraphilia." In *The Comprehensive Textbook of Psychiatry, 3d ed.,* edited by H.I. Kaplan, A.M. Freedman, and B.J. Sadock. Baltimore: Williams & Wilkins Co., 1980a.

Meyer, J. "Body Ego, Selfness, and Gender Sense." *Psychiatric Clinics of North America* 3 (1980b): 21–36.

Meyer, J. "Psychotherapy in Sexual Dysfunctions." In *Specialized Techniques in Individual Psychotherapy,* edited by T. Karasu and L. Bellak, New York: Brunner/Mazel, 1980c.

Meyer, J. "The Theory of the Gender Identity Disorders." *Journal of the American Psychoanalytic Association* (in press).

Meyer, J., and Reter, D. "Sex Reassignment." *Archives of General Psychiatry* 36 (1979): 1010–1015.

Stoller, R. *Sex and Gender, Vol. II: The Transsexual Experiment.* New York: Jason Aronson, 1975.

Bibliography for Chapter 8

Bauer, R., and Stein, J. "Sex Counseling on Campus: Short-Term Treatment Techniques." *American Journal of Orthopsychiatry* 43 (1973): 824–839.

Bender, L., and Grugett, A. "A Follow-up Report on Children Who Had Atypical Sexual Experience." *American Journal of Orthopsychiatry* 22 (1952): 825–837.

Brant, R., and Tisza, V. "Sexual Misuse of Children." Unpublished manuscript, 1976.

Brownmiller, S. *Against Our Will: Men, Women and Rape.* New York: Bantam Books, 1975.

Burgess, A.W., and Holmstrom, L.L. "Rape Trauma Syndrome." American Journal of Psychiatry 131 (1974a): 981–986.

Burgess, A.W., and Holmstrom, L.L. *Rape: Victims of Crisis.* Bowie, Md.: Robert J. Brady Co., 1974b.

Burgess, A.W., and Holmstrom, L.L. "Recovery from Rape and Prior Life Stress." *Research in Nursing and Health* 1 (1978): 165–174.

Capraro, V.J. "Sexual Assault of Female Children."

Annals of the New York Academy of Sciences 142 (1967): 817–819.

DeFrancis, V. *Protecting the Child Victim of Sex Crimes Committed by Adults, Final Report.* Denver: The American Humane Association, Children's Division, 1969.

Federal Organizations for Professional Women. *Women and Health Roundtable Report,* Vol. 4. Washington, D.C.: Federal Organization for Professional Women, 1980.

Ferenczi, S. "Confusion of Tongues Between Adults and the Child" (1933). *International Journal of Psychoanalysis* 30 (1949): 225–230.

Finch, S.M. "Sexual Activities of Children with Other Children and Adults." *Clinical Pediatrics* 6 (1967): 1–2.

Finch, S.M. "Adult Seduction of the Child: Effects on the Child." *Medical Aspects of Human Sexuality* 7 (1973): 170–193.

Fitz, G., Stoll, K., and Wagner, N. "A Comparison of Males and Females Who were Sexually Molested as Children." *Journal of Marital and Sexual Therapy* 7 (1981): 54–59.

Flugel, J. *The Psychoanalytic Study of the Family.* London: Hogarth Press, 1926.

Gagnon, J.H. "Female Child Victims of Sex Offenses." *Social Problems* 13 (1956): 176–192.

Glover, E. "Common Problems in Psychoanalysis and Anthropology." *British Journal of Medical Psychology* 12 (1932): 109–133.

Gordon, L. "Incest as Revenge Against the Pre-Oedipal Mother." *Psychoanalytic Review* 42 (1955): 284–292.

Halleck, S.L. "The Physician's Role in Management of Victims of Sex Offenders." *JAMA* 180 (1962): 273–278.

Halleck, S.L. "Emotional Effects of Victimizations." In *Sexual Behavior and the Law,* edited by R. Slovenko. Springfield, Ill.: Charles C. Thomas, 1965.

Hilberman, E. *The Rape Victim,* New York: Basic Books, 1976.

Hoff, L.A., and Williams, T. "Counseling the Rape Victim and Her Family." *Crisis Intervention* 6 (1975): 2–13.

Katz, S., and Mazur, M.A. *Understanding the Rape Victim: A Synthesis of Research Findings.* New York: John Wiley & Sons, 1979.

Kilpatrick, D.M., Veronen, L.J., and Resnick, P.A. "The Aftermath of Rape: Recent Empirical Findings." *American Journal of Orthopsychiatry* 49 (1979): 658–669.

Kinsey, A.C., Pomeroy, W.B., and Martin, C.E. *Sexual Behavior in the Human Male.* Philadelphia: W.B. Saunders Co., 1948.

Kinsey, A.C., Pomeroy, W.B., Martin, C.E., and Gebhard, P.H. *Sexual Behavior in the Human Female.* Philadelphia: W.B. Saunders Co., 1953.

Landis, J.T. "Experiences of 500 Children with Adult Sexual Deviation." *Psychiatric Quarterly Supplement, Part 1,* 30 (1956): 91–109.

Lewis, M., and Sarrel, M. "Some Psychological Aspects of Seduction, Incest, and Rape in Childhood." *Journal of the American Academy of Child Psychiatry* 8 (1969): 606–619.

Lukianowicz, N. "Incest." *British Journal of Psychiatry* 120 (1972): 301–313.

Macdonald, J.M. *Rape Offenders and Their Victims.* Springfield, Ill.: Charles C. Thomas, 1971.

Malmquist, C. "Report on Females with Three or More Illegitimate Pregnancies." *American Journal of Orthopsychiatry* 36 (1966): 476–484.

Massey, J.B., Garcia, C.R., and Emich, J.P., Jr. "Management of Sexually Assaulted Females." *Obstetrics and Gynecology* 38 (1971): 29–36.

McCahill, T.W., Meyer, L.C., and Fischman, A.M. *The Aftermath of Rape,* Lexington, Mass.: Lexington Books, 1979.

McCauldron, R.J. "Rape." *Canadian Journal of Corrections* 9 (1967): 37–57.

McCombie, S.L. "Characteristics of Rape Victims Seen in Crisis Intervention." *Smith College Studies in Social Work* 46 (1976): 137–158.

Mohr, J., Turner, R., and Jerry, N. *Pedophilia and Exhibitionism.* Toronto: University of Toronto Press, 1964.

Nadelson, C. "Treatment of Sexual Dysfunction." In *Outpatient Psychiatry,* edited by A. Lazare. Baltimore: Williams & Wilkins Co., 1979.

Nadelson, C., Notman, M., Zackson, H., and Gornick, J. "The Long-term Impact of Rape: A Follow-up Study." Unpublished manuscript.

Nadelson, C. and Rosenfeld, A. "Sexual Misuse of Children." In *Child Psychiatry and the Law,* edited by D. Schetsky and E. Benedek. New York: Brunner/Mazel, 1980.

Nadelson, C. and Rosenfeld, A. "News Report: Rape Is an Ugly Word." *Emergency Medicine,* October 1971, pp. 23–27.

Notman, M.T., and Nadelson, C. "The Rape Victim: Psychodynamic Considerations." *American Journal of Psychiatry* 133 (1976): 408–413.

Parsons, T. "The Incest Taboo in Relation to Social Structure and the Socialization of the Child." *British Journal of Sociology* 2 (1954): 101–117.

Payne, E.C., Kravitz, A.R., Notman, M.T., and Anderson, J.V. "Outcome Following Therapeutic Abortion." *Archives of General Psychiatry* 33 (1976): 725–733.

Peters, J.J. "Child Rape: Defusing a Psychological Time Bomb." *Hospital Physician,* February 1973, pp. 46–49.

Peters, J.J. "The Psychological Effects of Childhood Rape." *World Journal of Psychosynthesis* 6 (1974): 11–14.

Peters, J.J. "Social Psychiatric Study of Victims Reporting Rape." Presented at the 128th Annual Meeting of the American Psychiatric Association, Anaheim, Calif., May 5–9, 1975.

Peters, J.J., Meyer L., and Carroll, N. "The Philadelphia Assault Victim Study; Final Report from the Institute of Mental Health." Bethesda, Md.: NIMH, June 30, 1976.

Price, V. "Rape Victims—The Invisible Patients." *The Canadian Nurse* 71 (1975): 29–34.

Rascovsky, M., and Rascovsky, A. "On Consummated Incest." *International Journal of Psychoanalysis* 31 (1950): 42–47.

Rasmussen, A. "The Importance of Sexual Attacks on Children Less than 14 Years of Age for the Development of Mental Disease and Character Anomalies." *Acta Neurologica et Psychiatrica Belgica* 9 (1934): 351–434.

Renshaw, D.C., and Renshaw, R.H. "Incest." *Journal of Sex Education and Therapy* 3 (1977): 1–7.

Rosenfeld, A., Nadelson, C., Krieger, M., and Backman, J.H. "Incest and Sexual Abuse of Children." *Journal of the American Academy of Child Psychiatry* 16 (1977): 327–339.

Sloane, P., and Karpinski, E. "Effects of Incest on the Participants." *American Journal of Orthopsychiatry* 12 (1942): 666–673.

Summit, R., and Kryso, J. "Sexual Abuse of Children: A Clinical Spectrum" *American Journal of Orthopsychiatry* 48 (1978): 237–251.

Sutherland, S., and Scherl, D.S. "Patterns of Response Among Victims of Rape." *American Journal of Orthopsychiatry* 40 (1970): 503–511.

Titchener, J.L., and Kapp, F.T. "Family and Character Change at Buffalo Creek." *American Journal of Psychiatry* 133 (1976): 295–299.

Weber, E. "Sexual Abuse Begins at Home." *Ms,* April 1977, pp. 64–67.

Weiner, I. "Father-Daughter Incest." *Psychiatric Quarterly* 36 (1962): 607–632.

II

The Schizophrenic Disorders

Part II

The Schizophrenic Disorders

Authors for Part II

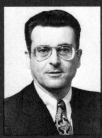

Robert Cancro, M.D., Med.D.Sc., Preceptor

Professor and Chairman
Department of Psychiatry
New York University Medical
   Center

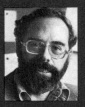

John S. Strauss, M.D.
Professor of Psychiatry
Yale University School of Medicine

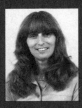

Lynn E. DeLisi, M.D.
Adult Psychiatry Branch
Division of Special Mental Health
   Research
Intramural Research Program
National Institute of Mental Health
Saint Elizabeths Hospital

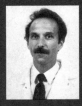

Steven G. Potkin, M.D.
Adult Psychiatry Branch
Division of Special Mental Health
   Research
Intramural Research Program
National Institute of Mental Health
Saint Elizabeths Hospital

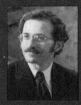

Robert Paul Liberman, M.D.
Professor of Psychiatry
UCLA School of Medicine
Director, Mental Health Clinical
   Research Center and
   Rehabilitation Research and
   Training Center
Chief, Rehabilitation Medicine
   Service at the Brentwood
   VA Medical Center

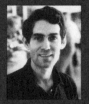

Richard Jed Wyatt, M.D.
Adult Psychiatry Branch
Division of Special Mental Health
   Research
Intramural Research Program
National Institute of Mental Health
Saint Elizabeths Hospital

Neal R. Cutler, M.D.
Adult Psychiatry Branch
Division of Special Mental Health
   Research
Intramural Research Program
National Institute of Mental Health
Saint Elizabeths Hospital

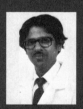

Dilip V. Jeste, M.D.
Adult Psychiatry Branch
Division of Special Mental Health
   Research
Intramural Research Program
National Institute of Mental Health
Saint Elizabeths Hospital

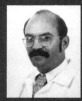

Joel E. Kleinman, M.D.,Ph.D.
Adult Psychiatry Branch
Division of Special Mental Health
   Research
Intramural Research Program
National Institute of Mental Health
Saint Elizabeths Hospital

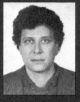

Daniel J. Luchins, M.D.
Adult Psychiatry Branch
Division of Special Mental Health
   Research
Intramural Research Program
National Institute of Mental Health
Saint Elizabeths Hospital

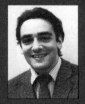

Daniel R. Weinberger, M.D.
Adult Psychiatry Branch
Division of Special Mental Health
   Research
Intramural Research Program
National Institute of Mental Health
Saint Elizabeths Hospital

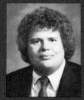

Douglas W. Heinrichs, M.D.
Chief of Outpatient Research
   Programs
Maryland Psychiatric Research
   Center
Assistant Professor of Psychiatry
University of Maryland

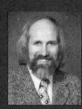

**William T. Carpenter,
Jr., M.D.**
Director
Maryland Psychiatric Research
   Center
Professor of Psychiatry
University of Maryland

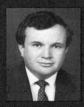

Samuel J. Keith M.D.
Chief
Center for Studies of Schizophrenia
Clinical Research Branch
National Institute of Mental Health

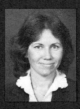

Susan M. Matthews
Research Analyst
Center for Studies of Schizophrenia
Clinical Research Branch
National Institute of Mental Health

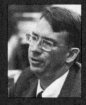

John M. Davis, M.D.
Director of Research
Illinois State Psychiatric
  Institute
Gilman Professor of Psychiatry
University of Illinois School of
  Medicine

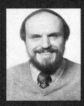

Philip Janicak, M.D.
Illinois State Psychiatric Institute

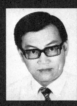

Sidney Chang, M.D.
Illinois State Psychiatric Institute

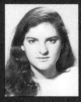

Karen Klerman
Illinois State Psychiatric
  Institute

Introduction
by Robert Cancro, M.D. Med. D.Sc.

Excellent descriptions of people who manifested symptoms which today would be diagnosed as schizophrenic illnesses have been available for well over two hundred years. Such people have most certainly always been with us, but they have not been observed and described with equal interest at all times. Useful though the descriptions may be for some purposes, they do not in the aggregate automatically yield a valid classification of mental disorders. Expecting them to do so would be like creating a nosology of rashes based entirely on their appearance. Maculopapular rashes obviously do not share a single etiology, respond to a single treatment, and have a uniform outcome over time. So it is with the schizophrenic disorders. Their manifestations are multi-determined as to etiology, pathogenesis, course, and outcome. Even clinically useful diagnostic groupings do not necessarily constitute a scientific classification of illness. To be scientific the nosology must be based on etiology and pathogenesis. The Schizophrenic Disorders are a classical example. While the grouping has some clinical utility, it is not a scientific classification.

Any attempt to present the history of the concept of the schizophrenic disorders is inherently arbitrary. Nevertheless, many would agree on beginning with the introduction of the term *démence précoce.* Morel (1852–1853) used the term to describe a 14-year-old boy whose symptoms included disorganization of thought. Although Morel did not himself use the term to represent a category of disease but to describe a particular finding in an individual patient, the term was subsequently borrowed, rephrased into the Latin-like term *dementia praecox,* and used to label a disease entity.

During the fifty years following the publication of Morel's treatise, the influence of German psychiatry on nosology became dominant. German psychiatry attempted to identify real disease entities rather than to restrict itself merely to a description of symptoms. The search for disease entities was profoundly stimulated by the work of Koch on the bacterial transmission of tuberculosis. He demonstrated that very different clinical pictures could be presented by the same disease entity, thereby offering a solution to the problems posed by the limitations of diagnosis based exclusively on clinical features.

Kraepelin saw the importance of Koch's work for general medicine and its implications for psychiatry. In an effort to apply some of Koch's postulates to mental disorders, he separated patients with thinking disturbances into two groups—those who tended to deteriorate and those who tended to improve. Thus, having subdivided the patients on the basis of outcome, Kraepelin (1899) called the two categories dementia praecox and manic-depressive psychoses, respectively. While he did recognize that his prognosis-based classification was not internally consistent, his effort was to create a nosology which would yield disease entities.

Bleuler (1911) moved away from the disease-entity model and introduced the concept of a syndrome into psychiatric nosology.

Bleuler saw the core defect of this syndrome as a splitting of or a loss of harmony amongst the different kinds of mental functions which are normally integrated. More importantly, he spoke of "the group of the schizophrenias," recognizing that the group included at least several diseases. These diseases shared the common feature of splitting of mental functions but differed as to etiology, pathogenesis, course, and outcome.

The continuation and detail of this history of the concept of the schizophrenic disorders are available elsewhere (Cancro and Pruyser, 1970).

The purpose here is to emphasize a fundamental conflict between the disease-entity approach and the syndrome approach. The disease-entity approach assumes that there are real, specific, and actual diseases in existence, diseases whose presence can be recognized by their clinical manifestations. The syndrome approach aims to reduce population heterogeneity by creating groups which tend to share certain signs and symptoms. The approaches to nosology differ in their ambitiousness and presumed validity. The need to classify is ever present, since the data of observation must be organized in some fashion. Yet any classification entails an artificial imposition on the data of a particular view point. At the very least, data must be organized in a manner consistent with our ways of thinking. Classifications need not be Platonic in nature, but they must be useful. If classifications are helpful in producing new hypotheses or new insights into the data, then they are of value. If they are merely receptacles into which observations can be placed, and if they do not stimulate new knowledge, then they are of little value.

At the present time all of the efforts to diagnose and classify the schizophrenic disorders are based on clinical features. These features may be symptoms, premorbid personality, course, response to a particular treatment, and so forth, but they remain clinical phenomena. And any classification based on such phenomena must be arbitrary. Every clinical feature is multidetermined and therefore cannot yield a group which is homogeneous as to the etiology or pathogenesis of that feature. A truly scientific classification must await a knowledge of etiology and pathogenesis. Until then the categories will depend on clinical features and therefore will remain arbitrary but hopefully not capricious. In the interim every student of the schizophrenias will fall into the error of reifying the concept and treating it as a real entity. This will be manifested, for example, by references to people having *it* or that *it* does not necessarily lead to deterioration. Obviously, the autistic use of language is not restricted to the members of the group of the schizophrenias.

In the chapter which follows Dr. John Strauss reviews the clinical features of the schizophrenic disorders and discusses the implications of DSM-III for the development of our understanding and management of these complex conditions.

Chapter 9

The Clinical Pictures and Diagnoses of the Schizophrenic Disorders†
by John S. Strauss, M.D.

INTRODUCTION

Whether one has worked in the field for years or is just beginning, one can very easily construct a picture of schizophrenia that is stereotyped—and misleading. Such a picture tends to perpetuate itself. By limiting the types of contact made and the assessment approaches used with patients, it promotes stereotyped treatment methods and stereotyped patient responses.

Is a person with "true" schizophrenia someone who hears certain voices, has severely disordered communication, relates minimally, is incapable of working, and will always be that way? Or does "true" schizophrenia also include people who function well in work and social situations, respond to psychosocial treatments, and perhaps recover totally? These issues, the center of controversy since Kraepelin first defined the concept of dementia praecox, need to be continuously reappraised. Most recently a reappraisal became important as the same issues influence and are influenced by the new rules for diagnosing the Schizophrenic Disorders.

Two dominant views about schizophrenia reflect polar opposites on these issues and their ramifications. The view originated by Kraepelin and reflected by those who have since followed his orientation is that schizophrenia is a disorder, probably of organic origin, marked by a particular age of onset and symptom picture and by a deteriorating course.

The contrasting view is most commonly associated with psychodynamic thinking. In this view, schizophrenia is seen more as a point in the course of a developmental trajectory. At that point, the eruption of particular symptoms arises from vulnerabilities which are developmentally, and perhaps constitutionally, determined. This view focuses not so much on the symptoms themselves, or even on diagnostic questions, but rather highlights assumed underlying processes, such as problems with interpersonal relations and distortions in the meanings drawn from experiences and perceptions.

The first view tends to focus especially on symptoms and prognosis with the hope that an underlying organic etiology can be discovered. The second view focuses primarily on the underlying psychological processes that generate distortion of social relationships and meaning and that are determined by developmental precursors. These two views, here somewhat overdrawn, have often been proposed and disputed as though they were mutually incompatible. But it is possible that they are like two halves of a jigsaw puzzle that have been put together independently. The final picture may not be clear until they have been joined.

Eugen Bleuler pioneered such an effort. In the process of changing the name of the disorder from dementia praecox to schizophrenia,

†This chapter is based in part on work supported by the National Institute of Mental Health Grant No. MH 00340.

Bleuler struggled repeatedly with the basic conceptualization of the disorder. Throughout his career, he struggled to balance a focus on symptom description with considerations of underlying psychopathological process. He also attempted to balance the view that etiology may be organic, precluding full recovery, with the view that symptoms have important psychological meanings and are influenced by psychosocial factors. In this struggle, Bleuler generated a series of writings which have often been seen as confusing (Stierlin, 1967). Perhaps this apparent confusion reflects the difficulty that the field more generally experiences as it tries to reconcile or even cope with two parts of the puzzle.

The clinical picture of schizophrenia has become clearer as a result of careful descriptive studies emphasizing reliability of assessment, careful sampling, and follow-up, and this has made it increasingly difficult to ignore either of the two parts. The current Diagnostic Manual of the American Psychiatric Association, DSM-III, focuses essentially on descriptive characteristics in defining schizophrenia. The manual can serve either as a definitive statement that there is a disease, schizophrenia, that is essentially static in nature, or it can serve as a tentative basis for a bootstrap approach to treatment and research, not only at a descriptive level, but also in regard to biological and psychodynamic phenomena. Such a bootstrap approach would, for instance, evaluate enzymes as well as development, or genetics as well as meaning, to see how these factors validate or modify the diagnostic concept. This second approach to DSM-III would promote recognition of the many characteristics and considerable variability in the clinical pictures of schizophrenia and would enable incorporating this variability into the diagnosis, understanding, and treatment of the disorder and the people who have it. The bases for these views become apparent in the following discussion of the cross-sectional and longitudinal aspects of the clinical pictures of the schizophrenic disorders and of the people affected by them.

THE CROSS-SECTIONAL CLINICAL PICTURE

In the past, the most widely accepted cross-sectional definitions of schizophrenia were far narrower than those commonly used in the United States. The original description by Kraepelin involved clinical pictures that included certain types of delusions and hallucinations, severe disorders of thinking, incongruous or flattened affect, disorders of the will, and bizarre behavior. In this widely accepted view of schizophrenia, patients with significant degrees of depression or elation were often considered as not having schizophrenia, and certain kinds of hallucinations and delusions, such as delusions of grandeur or persecution, were considered nonspecific and equally likely to indicate other kinds of psychoses. Schneider (1959), Langfeldt (1969), and others, for example, believed that delusions and hallucinations of many types were of limited diagnostic value. Certain delusions, however, such as being controlled by an outside force, and auditory hallucinations involving hearing voices talking about one's actions or thoughts, rather than criticizing the person, they deemed to be highly relevant, or even pathognomonic, for schizophrenia (Carpenter and Strauss, 1979).

American psychiatry, on the other hand, was influenced by the social as well as psychobiological views of Adolf Meyer and the modified psychodynamic and psychosocial views of Harry Stack Sullivan and others. Psychiatry in the United States therefore had focused more on a person's ability to relate interpersonally and to function generally and on broadly defined concepts of thought disorder. Thus, while most patients that clinicians outside the United States would consider schizophrenic were also diagnosed as schizophrenic in this country, a broad group of patients in addition to this central core also received the diagnosis of schizophrenia in the United States (Cooper et al., 1972; Kuriansky et al., 1977). This group often included persons with a considerable affective component to their hallucinations or delusions and, in some centers, practically anyone who related strangely with other people.

DSM-III considerably narrows the American cross-sectional view of schizophrenia. This has brought the American concept of schizophrenia much more into harmony with the view common to other parts of the world. Thus, Axis I of DSM-III defines schizophrenia symptomatically in terms of the presence of a rather narrow range of psychotic symptoms, such as limited kinds of delusions, hallucinations, or specific types of thought disorder. DSM-III also adds to Axis I the criteria of a six-month or greater duration, nonorganic etiology, age of onset before 45, and diminished social function. Since these criteria do not relate to symptom type, they are not really part of the syndrome, and some would have fit more logically into the other DSM-III axes.

The current American concept of schizophrenia is narrower, and the criterion of dysfunction in personal relationships is no longer central. The subtypes currently defined within the Schizophrenic Disorders are generally only minor modifications of Kraepelin's original subtypes. The Disorganized Type is essentially what was called hebephrenic in the past, and the Catatonic and Paranoid Types are generally unchanged from previous usage. In DSM-III the less traditional categories of Undifferentiated and Residual Types are also included. At the same time, schizophrenia-like disorders lasting less than six months, those with a marked affective component, and the categories previously labeled as borderline and latent schizophrenia are now no longer classified under the category of Schizophrenic Disorders.

This represents a return to what we might now consider psychiatric classicism, although these concepts were once considered quite radical. The return to classicism has several advantages. First, it brings American terminology into line with that commonly used in other parts of the world. Second, the operational diagnostic criteria provided by DSM-III contribute to the enhanced reliability of a concept whose use in this country in the past may have been so vague that communication was greatly hindered. The more reliable communication made possible by DSM-III is invaluable both for clinical and research purposes. Despite these advantages, the new scheme raises some important questions. What has become of the interpersonal and psychodynamic aspects of schizophrenia? Were they too unimportant to be of value? Or, in our grasping for clarity, have we sacrificed something crucial?

If, for example, schizophrenia is a set of disorders in which the basic processes are manifest in many different symptoms and syndromes, such as in tuberculosis, an excessive focus on specific syndromes themselves would obscure a major feature of the disorder. If, moreover, the basic processes have different manifestations over time, as in syphilis, a heavily weighted focus on syndromes could be seriously incomplete. And what if schizophrenia is primarily a pathological process that deviates on a continuum from normal functioning, as might be suggested by the concept of schizophrenia spectrum disorders (Rosenthal et al., 1971)? If this is so, then a careful isolation of only that type of schizophrenia with psychotic symptoms, or only that type which lasts for six months or longer, might prove to generate a rather artificial focus on only one segment of an entire process, a process which would be more accurately viewed in terms of degrees of deviation from a standard. If schizophrenia is an interactive developmental process, in which some characteristics are generated by a progressive interaction between an individual's biology, psychology, and environment and in which abnormality is exaggerated over time, the essence of this process might be lost by focusing primarily on symptomatology.

Thus, Bleuler's view that certain symptoms of schizophrenia, such as particular hallucinations and delusions, are essentially secondary to a more basic process is not merely an historical curiosity. Rather his view reflects the altogether current concern that emphasizing symptoms such as certain delusions and hallucinations as diagnostic criteria may distract treatment and research attention from the basic aspects of the clinical picture. With all the value that the current focus on the symptoms of schizophrenia has for reliable diagnosis, this focus is still but a convention, and it may already need to be tempered in the light of evidence from clinical experience and research (Strauss and Carpenter, 1981).

We can and should use DSM-III as the guide to diagnosing schizophrenia, but we must not act as though it automatically provides a sufficient recipe for defining the basic processes involved in etiology, treatment, and prognosis. Rather, we must go on to a broad-based assessment of other characteristics of the person, including his or her social functioning, distortions of meaning, psychological conflicts, and coping mechanisms (Strauss and Carpenter, 1981).

Although Axes II through V of DSM-III assist considerably in such a broad-based effort, the symptoms of schizophrenia tend to be so impressive, and are so central for Axis I classification, that all attention may be drawn to these bizarre manifestations. The multiaxial structure of DSM-III, even when axes are considered optional, should be used to focus on other aspects of the person as well. Environmental characteristics such as life events and the person's competence can be reflected in Axes IV and V. Attention to these axes increases diagnostic validity for prognosis and probably for treatment (Strauss and Carpenter, 1981). On the other hand, ignoring areas of competence, for example, whether in work or in interpersonal functioning, or even in mothering (Rodnick, 1974), generates a false view. Treatment decisions based on such a view may be faulty, and research efforts, too, may be distorted.

But even when all the present axes of DSM-III are used, an intensive focus on personal relationships and psychodynamics is not fostered (Karasu and Skodol, 1980). These areas, which many have considered basic to schizophrenia, are de-emphasized, but a longitudinal perspective may help to restore the proper emphasis.

THE LONGITUDINAL CLINICAL PICTURE

Prognosis, the likely outcome of disorder, is an important basis for defining the disorder. It also lets the patient, the patient's family, the clinician, and others know the probable evolutions and provides a baseline for research on treatment effectiveness. But a static view of prognosis, as exemplified in the concept of an outcome of schizophrenia, can be extremely misleading. Kraepelin's original view that schizophrenic patients have a deteriorating course with several possible end states, and even Bleuler's view that schizophrenic patients never completely recover, have been increasingly challenged.

More recent data indicate that as many as one-third of patients diagnosed schizophrenic recover completely. The percentage varies from study to study, depending on the diagnostic criteria used, the premorbid adjustment status of the individuals, and probably on environmental conditions and treatment received as well. There is evidence to suggest that the best way to estimate prognosis in schizophrenia is to consider symptom type, previous duration of disorder, previous level of social relationships, and previous level of work functioning. Each of these may be the best indicator of a person's likely functioning on that particular characteristic in the future (Strauss and Carpenter, 1978), and considering all of them together may be the most effective way to anticipate the patient's overall prognosis.

Still, as noted above, the concept of an outcome, or even of a prognosis, may be misleading. A growing body of studies indicates that a significant number of patients may improve or recover even after a period of severe illness that has lasted 15 years or more (Bleuler, 1974; Ciompi, 1980; Huber et al., 1975). Preliminary findings from another study suggest that such a recovery may occur at any one of several points following discharge from the hospital, even with patients who have previously had a chronic course (Harding and Brooks, 1980).

But not only may the longitudinal picture have complex patterns of downs or ups, it may also change qualitatively. The findings of postpsychotic depression (McGlashan and Carpenter, 1976) and of changing symptom pictures from subtype to subtype (Sneznevsky, 1968), even in patients diagnosed as schizophrenic by the strictest criteria, are evidence for such qualitative shifts. Some recent research focused intensively on the evolution of schizophrenia just prior to and following an episode suggests that certain other sequences of symptoms commonly occur (Herz, 1980; Docherty et al., 1978; Harrow et al., 1978). For example, before a psychotic exacerbation in schizophrenia, a series of symptoms such as anxiety, sleep loss, irritability, and sometimes depression occurs, suggesting that the psychotic episode itself may be the end point of an evolving process. Such findings are particularly important, because they may throw light on the nature of the disorder itself, and because they suggest that more sensitivity to these earlier stages of decompensation can enable more timely and perhaps more effective treatment intervention.

Several other findings suggest that, as well as being more variable and evolutionary than is often realized, the process of schizophrenia may be more flexible and dynamic than we have recognized. Environmental factors, such as institutional living, family conditions, and pharmacologic and psychosocial treatments may affect the course of disorder considerably (Barton, 1959; Brown et al., 1962; Gunderson, 1980; Hogarty et al., 1974; Leff, 1976; Wing, 1970). A pitfall of this view of the process is a tendency to view a person with a schizophrenic disorder as passively impacted upon by family, institutional, or other factors. But there is some evidence that people with schizophrenia, like people in general, use a range of coping mechanisms to deal with their symptoms and their environments. Thus, a chain of interactions between the individual and the environment may further determine the individual's prognosis (Strauss et al., 1981).

A brief review of what recent findings suggest about the salient characteristics of the prognosis and evolution of schizophrenic disorders may help to put these complications in perspective. (1) Prognosis is somewhat more guarded than in many types of functional psychiatric disorder, and a significant number of patients appear to become chronic. (2) In general, symptomatology is repeated in subsequent or continuing episodes, although shifts in symptomatology over time are not rare. (3) Premorbid functioning in social relations and work is an important predictor of later functioning in those same areas and of the person's course of disorder more generally. (4) The notion of outcome in schizophrenia may be misleading. Patients' clinical pictures may change, and recovery may occur at any time in their lives, even after an extended course of severe disorder. (5) Environmental factors, such as the living setting (institutions or certain family environments) and perhaps other factors such as work settings, may have considerable impact on determining the course of disorder. (6) The person with schizophrenia is probably not a passive recipient of factors that will determine the course of disorder. More likely, many characteristics of the individual, from willingness to participate in treatment to skills and motivation for more effective functioning, interact with environmental and treatment factors to influence prognosis over both the short and the long term.

But the longitudinal picture of schizophrenia cannot be entirely conveyed by a description of factors influencing the evolution of disorder following its onset. The period preceding onset is also important. At least some schizophrenic patients manifest characteristics of disorder before identifiable symptoms occur. Poor social relationships and antisocial behavior during adolescence are commonly found to have been present in persons who later become schizophrenic (Watt, 1978). According to psychodynamic theories, behavioral and psychological precursors may even be found to have existed during the childhoods of persons who later become schizophrenic (see, for example, Chodoff and Carpenter, 1975). Early problems with personal relationships have been a particular focus of such theories. Finally, genetic studies suggest that childhood withdrawal may be linked genetically to schizophrenia in the parent, and that this withdrawal may be an early sign of the child's vulnerability to adult schizophrenia (Heston, 1970; Kendler et al., 1981). Thus, the considerable evidence from genetic and descriptive studies combines with psychodynamic concepts to suggest that a child or an adolescent may have manifested characteristics of the disorder long before the onset of an adult schizophrenic disorder.

Current knowledge about the longitudinal perspective of schizophrenia thus ties together, although not very neatly, the social relations and symptom aspects of schizophrenia. From this perspective, it seems even less reasonable to neglect these aspects in diagnosis, patient assessment, treatment, or research.

CONCLUSIONS

How do the diagnostic criteria of DSM-III reflect these cross-sectional and longitudinal perspectives on the clinical picture of schizophrenia?

Although de-emphasizing the role of personal relationships, the DSM-III criteria do have the advantage of outlining conditions that most would agree are likely to be useful for description, prognosis, treatment indications, and etiology. However, even if the criteria do represent a current best estimate of the domain and boundaries of schizophrenia, DSM-III's clear rules for diagnosis suggest that its criteria are much more complete and definitive than the data would support.

The clarity of DSM-III tends to suggest that its categories, such as that of the Schizophrenic Disorders, provide a definitive description of a real disease entity. In spite of the advantages of DSM-III, there is a real danger that this clarity will promote incorrect and even dangerous beliefs about clinical pictures, etiology, and treatment. The danger lies in the potential for narrowing excessively the range of assessment, treatment, and research considerations. In all fairness, this danger may not ensue so much from DSM-III as from the human tendency to take something that is clearly and narrowly stated and then to lean too heavily on it for explaining and dictating a broad range of beliefs and actions.

Another problem with the DSM-III definition of the Schizophrenic Disorders is that it assists only minimally in providing a longitudinal view of disorder. The six-month duration criterion does not suffice as a way of addressing the long-term picture. The shifts over time that might reflect important longitudinal processes are essentially lost in the particular kind of disease concept implied by DSM-III.

The clinical picture of schizophrenia can be considered from both cross-sectional and longitudinal perspectives. Viewed from a cross-sectional perspective, schizophrenia may incorporate either a broad or a narrow range of individuals. Recently, as exemplified in DSM-III, there has been a tendency to narrow the range of symptoms that serve to identify the disorder. This has provided increased reliability, demonstrating the invaluable contribution that DSM-III has made to communication. But such a narrow device risks our missing other important factors. Especially for schizophrenia, the evidence for abnormalities in social relationships prior to onset of symptomatology, as well as during and after an episode, makes a failure to include characteristics of social relationships in a cross-sectional diagnosis a serious shortcoming. Despite the potential importance of these areas, there are admittedly serious problems in defining them specifically and reliably enough to have them serve as major bases for diagnostic decision making. The solution lies in between the current de-emphasis of these areas in DSM-III and the previous tendency to depend too heavily on them.

Longitudinally, the old concept that schizophrenia is a disorder that inevitably leads to deterioration or that never permits complete recovery seems to have been an oversimplification. The course of disorder is complex and variable, involving many independent areas of function and possibilities for exacerbation or recovery at many points during a person's lifetime, and the longitudinal aspect may also extend back before the onset of disorder. Whether this is developmental in the psychodynamic sense of the term or an early behavioral manifestation of some disordered process is not clear. In any case, the tendency in the past to equate childhood abnormalities and problems in social relationships entirely with psychodynamic orientations is no longer tenable. Genetic and descriptive studies as well have indicated the importance of these phenomena. In fact, this is a major potential meeting area between the biologic and the psychosocial approaches.

The diversity in the clinical picture of schizophrenia is considerable, both cross-sectionally and longitudinally. DSM-III provides important steps forward in its emphasis on reliability. DSM-III does provide an excellent, abbreviated guide for diagnosis, but to understand and treat schizophrenia we must know far more about the patients with whom we are working and about their environments than DSM-III requires of us. In the treatment and study of real patients, such abbreviated and stereotyped assessment procedures automatically discount too high a percentage of reality, disregard the reality of individual variation, neglect many areas of strength and weakness, and fail to consider important environmental and biological factors. Overlooking these realities could seriously jeopardize the scientific and humanitarian aspects of our work.

Introduction to Etiologic Studies of the Schizophrenic Disorders
by Robert Cancro, M.D., Med.D.Sc.

The previous chapter illustrates the central role that diagnosis plays in all research on the schizophrenic disorders. Clinical diagnosis defines the patient population to be studied. Because of this simple fact no study on etiology, treatment, or any other aspect of the schizophrenic syndrome can be independent of the problems of the validity and reliability of the diagnosis.

There is no independent test to confirm or to reject the diagnosis of schizophrenia. There is no tissue or body fluid which can be sent to the laboratory to ascertain which individuals are false positives or false negatives. Diagnosis remains a clinical activity based on arbitrarily selected clinical phenomena. This limitation of the diagnostic method guarantees heterogeneity in the sample and in part accounts for the fact that all studies of the schizophrenic syndrome are less reliable than is desirable. Moreover, some of the variability in the results of the different studies can be attributed to the problem of exclusively clinical diagnosis.

In addition to the heterogeneity that diagnosis causes, the heterogeneity inherent in the syndrome nature of the category of schizophrenic disorders causes difficulties for research. Since the category is defined by phenomena which are multidetermined, the nosologic use of the phenomena does not create a homogeneous group of patients. Patients are homogeneous only as to the presence of phenomena at a moment in time, not as to the origin or the prior or future presence of phenomena. This source of heterogeneity means that the results of studies on etiology can only be statistically significant, and the revealed etiologic factor will not be uniform throughout the sample. A factor which can be demonstrated as an etiologic agent in some people diagnosed as schizophrenic cannot be demonstrated to be an agent in others so diagnosed. Furthermore, the failure to demonstrate the presence of a particular factor is obviously not equivalent to demonstrating its absence. The confounding of negative findings with the demonstration that the factors are truly not present has led to much confusion in thinking about this disorder. It is also important to remember that statistical significance is not the same as clinical significance. A finding which holds true for ten percent of the schizophrenic population may be statistically significant, but it may also be clinically useless.

The following chapters review genetic, biochemical, and social factors in the etiology of the schizophrenic syndrome. The genetic data are presented first because they will help the reader to integrate biologic and environmental determinism into a more holistic model. This chapter, by the Preceptor, covers the most important research without going into fine detail because of the ready availability of a number of recent excellent reviews. The chapter on biochemical and morphological factors, by Dr. Richard Wyatt and his colleagues, is the most extensive of the three chapters in this section and, indeed, in this Part. This does not reflect its relative importance, but rather the need for an up-to-date review of a complex literature which is of broad interest to psychiatrists and other mental health professionals. Dr. Robert Liberman's chapter on social etiology presents the relevant studies in a manner more consistent with the chapter on genetics. The major works are cited, and a bibliography is given for more extensive reading.

Chapter 10

The Role of Genetic Factors in the Etiology of the Schizophrenic Disorders

by Robert Cancro, M.D., Med.D.Sc.

In the past, a reluctance to recognize the role of genetic factors in the etiology of the schizophrenic syndrome stemmed from the fear that recognizing the genetic factors would lead to therapeutic nihilism. Anything determined by a gene, it was thought, was immutable and inevitable. Only in recent years has neuroscience revealed the enormous plasticity inherent in the genotype. Indeed, the determinants of biology are in many ways more plastic and forgiving than are the determinants of social experience. With the increasing recognition that genotypes do not doom the bearer to an inevitable outcome, investigators have become more optimistic about the implications of the genetic studies for people with a schizophrenic illness. This chapter aims to clarify the bases of this informed optimism.

GENETIC STUDIES 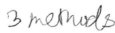 3 methods

Consanguinity Method

The rationale for the consanguinity method is deceptively simple. If a genetic factor is operating in the transmission of a disorder, the prevalence rate for that disorder will be higher in the family members of an afflicted individual as compared to the prevalence rate in the general population. Furthermore, the greater the degree of consanguinity, the higher the prevalence rate will be if a genetic factor is responsible.

There are obvious limitations to the power of the consanguinity method. It can only show that the prevalence rate in the families of schizophrenic index cases is or is not increased, and that the increase, if present, does or does not vary directly with the degree of consanguinity. Positive findings in a mental illness can easily be interpreted in social or environmental terms. Many things that run in families are not determined genetically but are determined by the shared psychological experiences of the family. Environmental factors could also explain why relatives who are closer in terms of consanguinity are more alike in their behaviors. The closer they are the more likely it is that their environmental experiences are similar. The consanguinity method is, therefore, not powerful in terms of supporting a genetic etiology, but it is a necessary first step in establishing the possibility of a genetic explanation.

In the first published study on the genetics of schizophrenia, Rüdin (1916) reported a significant increase in the prevalence rate of schizophrenia in the biologic relatives of his index cases. Later European studies by Schultz (1932) and Kallmann (1938) also reported increased prevalence rates in the families of index cases. Slater (1968) reviewed a number of the early studies and found a significantly higher prevalence rate in the biologic relatives of schizophrenics than in the general population. These studies also showed the positive relationship between the degree of consanguinity and the prevalence rate. The closer the blood relative, the more likely was there to be a schizophrenic illness. He reported that these findings were present in studies which had been conducted by investigators who had an environmental bias, as well as in those conducted by investigators who had a genetic bias.

The early consanguinity studies revealed the prevalence rate in first-degree relatives of schizophrenic patients to be between ten percent and fifteen percent, compared to a rate of approximately one percent in the general population. These studies also showed that the second-degree relatives were at a significantly greater risk than the general population, but less so than the first-degree relatives. More recent consanguinity studies by Lindelius (1970), Tsuang et al. (1974), and Stephens et al. (1975) are quite consistent in finding about a ten percent age-corrected risk for the disorder in siblings of index cases. These more recent studies are in good harmony with the earlier ones and involve different gene pools not examined in the initial reports.

Twin Method

The twin method of genetic research is more powerful than the consanguinity method. The rationale for the twin method is also quite simple. If genetic factors operate in the transmission of an illness, then monozygotic twins will show significantly greater concordance rates than dizygotic twins. Obviously, the term *concordance* means the occurrence of the same or clinically very similar conditions in both twins. In the case of a clinical illness, the determination of concordance is made on the basis of diagnosis and is no more reliable than the diagnostic technique. Cases of uncertain or probable schizophrenia must be assigned as either schizophrenic or not schizophrenic, and this assignment can reduce reliability. There are also different ways of determining concordance, and each will give different results on the same data. Pairwise concordance rates will be lower than the casewise concordance rates, given the same data. In comparing different studies, it is essential to know the method used for determining concordance and to make certain that the same method is applied before making any conclusions.

The concordance rate of schizophrenia in monozygotic twins has been consistently reported to be significantly higher than it is in dizygotic twins. The first report by Kallmann (1946) found striking differences in the concordance rates. The subsequent report by Slater and Shields (1953) on a different gene pool reported a significant difference between monozygotic and dizygotic twins. Methodological difficulties limited the generalizability of both of these early studies.

The more recent studies are methodologically much stronger and have been extended to larger populations of twins, thereby including index cases who were less severely ill and not necessarily chronically hospitalized. The five best include three done in Scandinavia, each done in a different Scandinavian country, representing a somewhat different gene pool (Tienari, 1963; 1968; Kringlen, 1967; and Fischer, 1973). The other two studies were done in English-speaking countries by Gottesman and Shields (1966) in England and by Pollin et al. (1969) in the United States. These five studies reported concordance rates for monozygotic twins in the range of six to forty percent, found that monozygotic concordance was significantly higher than dizygotic, and reported that the dizygotic rates were no higher than those found in ordinary siblings.

In 1963, Tienari initially reported a zero percent concordance rate in the monozygotic twins he studied. He had raised this figure to six percent by the time of his 1968 publication. In 1976, Gottesman and Shields reported that Tienari's monozygotic rate had now risen to 16 percent, even if all of the probable schizophrenics were treated as discordant. Utilizing the proband method and including some of the probable schizophrenics as concordant would raise the rate to 35 percent (Gottesman and Shields, 1976). The Tienari study was known for its initial failure to find a monozygotic-dizygotic difference, but over time, as more individuals became ill, the concordance rate for the monozygotes was significantly higher.

Kringlen (1967) found a significant monozygotic-dizygotic difference in his sample. A number of important negative findings also resulted from the Kringlen study. There were no significant differences between the concordance rate of dizygotes and the prevalence rate among regular siblings. Male and female twin pairs did not show significant differences. Finally, there was no significant difference between same sex and different sex dizygotes. All of these negative findings support a genetic etiology rather than a psychological explanation based on identity blurring.

The Fischer study (1973) was very powerful. Fischer followed the subjects of her study past the age of risk, and, therefore, virtually no age correction was necessary in her data. She found a monozygotic concordance rate of 56 percent (arrived at with the proband method). This is the best estimate of the true concordance rate because it involves almost no statistical age correction. This monozygotic concordance rate was significantly higher than the dizygotic rate. Fischer also studied the offspring of her population and found that the twins who were discordant for schizophrenia had the same percentage of schizophrenic offspring as did the twins who were concordant for the disorder. She also studied the twins as individuals and found that the twin who was free of schizophrenia was just as likely to produce a schizophrenic child as was the schizophrenic member of the twin pair. Actually, the 12.9 percent rate of schizophrenic offspring produced by nonschizophrenic twins was higher than the 9.6 percent of schizophrenic offspring produced by the schizophrenic twins, but the difference was not significant for a sample of that size. The conclusion, which is one of the most compelling in the genetic literature, is that the offspring of discordant twin members are as vulnerable to the schizophrenic illness as are the offspring of schizophrenic probands.

Pollin et al. (1969) reported on almost 16,000 twin pairs, a sample they derived from United States draft records. The size of the sample dwarfs the samples of all previous and subsequent studies. The sample was biased towards health, because both members of the twin pair had to pass the induction physical before they could be entered into the study. The early onset cases, who have the worst prognosis and most likely the highest concordance rates were therefore excluded. Despite this bias, the results showed that the concordance rate for the monozygotes was three times greater than the rate for the dizygotes. Parenthetically, the Pollin and Tienari studies were restricted to male twins. Because the Kringlen study found no sex differences, however, the Tienari and Pollin results can be generalized to all schizophrenics.

Taking these five twin studies as a group, Gottesman and Shields (1976) recalculated the concordance rate using the proband method. They found that the monozygotic concordance rate ranged between 35 percent and 58 percent, while the dizygotic concordance rate varied between nine percent and 26 percent. The author averaged the concordance rates of these five studies and found them to be 47 percent for monozygotes and 15 percent for dizygotes (Cancro, 1980). This threefold difference in average concordance rates is highly significant.

Adoptive Method

In the first published adoptive study on schizophrenics, Heston (1966) examined the prevalence rate of schizophrenia in the offspring of schizophrenic women. The offspring had been put up for adoption early in life and reared by their adoptive rather than their natural parents. He found that the prevalence rate for these children was not significantly lower than would have been expected if they had been raised by their biologic mothers. The offspring of his control group of nonschizophrenic women showed a prevalence rate which did not differ significantly from the general population rate. These data suggest that what matters in the prevalence of schizophrenia is who bears the child, not who rears it. But Heston's study had a number of methodological problems.

Many of these problems were addressed by the Danish adoption studies (Kety et al., 1968; Kety et al., 1975; Rosenthal et al., 1968; Wender et al., 1974). Under the leadership of Kety and Rosenthal a large population of children adopted in Copenhagen during a 24-year period were studied. More recently, they have conducted extensive psychiatric interviews with the biologic and adoptive relatives. The research team identified those adoptees who developed a schizophrenia-spectrum illness and those who did not. They then ascertained the prevalence rate for schizophrenia-spectrum illnesses in the biologic and adoptive relatives of the children. They found that the biologic relatives of the schizophrenic index cases, not the adoptive relatives, showed schizophrenia. The majority of the parents whose children subsequently became ill with a schizophrenic disorder did not develop their own schizophrenic illness until after the child was adopted. Parents who adopted a child whose biologic parents were free of schizophrenia, and who themselves developed a schizophrenic illness, did not produce schizophrenic offspring. Being reared by a schizophrenic parent is not in and of itself enough to produce a schizophrenic illness in an adopted child. Finally, there was no relationship between which biologic parent had the illness and the prevalence rate of the disorder in the offspring. The child of a schizophrenic father was as likely to be schizophrenic as was the child of a schizophrenic mother.

A behavioral scientist cannot speak of proof in the sense that a mathematician can. Behavioral science relies on evidence rather than proof. The total weight of the evidence from the genetic studies is impressive. A genetic factor does operate in the transmission of the disorder. This genetic factor is sufficiently powerful to override a number of environmental variables at the group, if not at the individual, level.

VULNERABILITY

It is obvious that a complex illness such as a schizophrenic disorder cannot be directly transmitted genetically. What is transmitted is a diathesis, or a vulnerability, which allows the individual to develop the syndrome in the face of certain environmental triggers. The genetic diathesis is viewed as necessary but not sufficient for the disorder, because not everyone with the diathesis will become ill. Perhaps it is best to think of the individual who has inherited the trait not as having the potential for an illness, but rather as having the capacity to develop certain signs and symptoms should he or she become mentally ill. The transmitted phenotype may be nothing more than a statistical variation of the degree of expression of that trait in the general population. Individuals with that variation have the capacity for a schizophrenic form of illness if they become psychotic. People with different variations of that same trait can also become psychotic, but would show different signs and symptoms and would be labeled as having an illness other than a schizophrenic disorder. This way of thinking about the transmitted trait merely means that some people have a variation on the trait which underlies the capacity for the form of a schizophrenic illness and that these people are statistically unusual both in health and illness. They are unusual in a statistical rather than in a moral sense. The rationale behind this formulation holds equally well for multiple traits, but is presented in terms of a single trait for purposes of clarity.

It is important to remember that genes are nothing more than encoded information. Genes represent instructions which may or may not be activated by environmental factors. Since environmental factors activate the structural and regulatory genes, they ultimately determine the active genetic makeup of the individual. In this sense, it can be said that the environment determines which of the many genetic potentials inherent in a given individual will actually be activated. Environment, technically, is the biochemical bath in which the gene sits. This bath is influenced by social and psychological events through physiologic pathways. The manner in which social experiences are translated into physiologic events is poorly understood. Nevertheless, it is this inter-action of genetic and nongenetic factors which produces the final phenotypes which characterize a given individual.

Any phenotype of interest can be arrived at from different genotypes. The identical trait in different individuals can be derived from different genes. Being phenotypically identical does not make individuals gen-etically identical. Furthermore, the same gene activated by different environments will produce different phenotypes. The difference in phenotype can be quantitative, e.g., taller or shorter, or qualitative, e.g., presence or absence of audiogenic seizure susceptibility. Obviously, the range of phenotypic outcomes inherent in any given genotype is not infinite, but neither is it fixed or predetermined. The richness of biologic diversity and the plasticity in the biologic system are so great that it is tempting to conclude that no single gene or environment will inevitably produce a schizophrenic disorder.

CONCLUSIONS

Because different gene-environment combinations can produce the phenotype or phenotypes which are necessary but not sufficient for the schizophrenic syndrome, there must be multiple etiologic pathways through which the syndrome can develop. This etiologic diversity is based on the insights of biology and not on the inadequacies of diagnosis. A valid classification of the schizophrenic disorders must be based on the nature and timing of the gene-environment interactions which would produce particular subtypes of the disorders.

The genetic studies also tell the informed observer that a particular symptom which is used for diagnostic purposes may evolve through different mechanisms at different times. Its presence, therefore, at a particular moment in the course of the illness would prevent neither its absence at other moments nor its recurrence at a later date on a different etiopathogenic basis. The clinical symptoms of the disorder are disjunctive within the individual as well as between individuals.

The genetic heterogeneity which is inherent in the schizophrenic disorders leads to variability in every clinical manifestation of the illness. This variability manifests itself in etiology, pathogenesis, pre-senting picture, recurrences, and outcome. Obviously, there can be no correct treatment, let alone a single treatment for such a heterogeneous group of disorders. Any treatment which is useful for certain patients will be useless for others and harmful to the remainder. There can be no treatment which will be good for all schizophrenic patients. The challenge of treatment remains in informed and honest trial and error.

Chapter 11

Social Factors in the Etiology of the Schizophrenic Disorders
by Robert Paul Liberman, M.D.

Current conceptualizations of schizophrenia still revolve around speci-fic and operational descriptions of its symptom states, which are viewed as the multidetermined outcomes of organismic, environmental, and social conditions. Despite considerable recent advances in the neurosciences, schizophrenia remains a clinical entity. It is still recognized and diagnosed phenomenologically, by observing characteristic subjective experiences and overt behavioral signs. The phenomenology of schizophrenia is fluid and dynamic, but the onset, continuance, exacerbation, relapse, remission, and adaptation of schizophrenic symptoms and behaviors are presumed to be in some kind of homeostatic balance with biological, social, and environmental events. This conceptualization of schizophrenia is the currently popular *stress-diathesis* model (Zubin and Spring, 1977; Marsella and Snyder, 1981). Under this model, the signs and symptoms that DSM-III identifies as pathognomonic of schizophrenia would be viewed as flimsy and changing barometers of interacting determinants which themselves stem from underlying biological and external social processes.

While research is advancing toward a better appreciation of the specific biological and environmental variables, a knowledge of the social and environmental factors warrants review. This chapter reviews that knowledge. In particular, the chapter discusses social and cultural variables which influence the symptom states of schizophrenia, highlights the social factors which affect its prognosis, reviews the social outcomes or consequences of schizophrenia, and, finally, considers the social variables which can assist in the management of schizophrenia.

SOCIOECONOMIC FACTORS

One of the most robust findings in schizophrenia research has been the discovery of disproportionately large numbers of schizophrenic persons in the lower social classes. Over fifty epidemiological studies have been conducted during a forty-year period in Denmark, the United States, Great Britain, Norway, Sweden, Taiwan, Finland, and Canada, among others. These studies have established a higher-than-expected rate of schizophrenia among the lowest social class levels (Kohn, 1976). But these findings are for urban areas, and a few studies in rural areas report contrary results. In the villages of India, six studies have indicated that schizophrenia occurs more often in higher-order castes, such as the brahmin (the aristocracy), the bania (the traders), the rajputs (the landowners), and the kayasthas (the civil servants).

Earlier theorists speculated that the generally higher prevalence of schizophrenia in the lower social classes was evidence for the etiological roles of social stressors, social isolation, and social deprivation. More recent research, however, casts doubt upon such causal links, suggesting, rather, that the greater number of schizophrenics found in the lower social classes is due to selection, drift, and sociomedical variables.

Selection is the process by which the poor premorbid characteristics and insidious onset of schizophrenia handicap an individual's upward progression on the social class ladder. The genetic vulnerability for schizophrenia, with its phenotypical cognitive and behavioral premonitory deficits in the growing-up years, can impair the young person's educational and occupational attainment. Achievements in these areas, of course, determine social class. Once the actual schizophrenic illness begins, the person's progress in school and jobs may be further

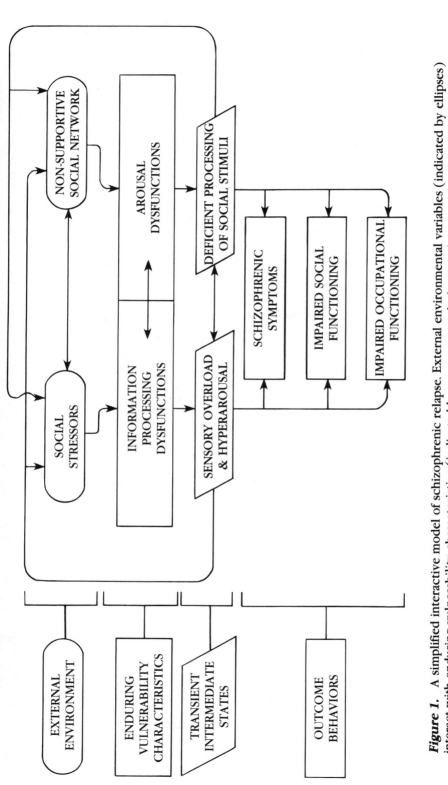

Figure 1. A simplified interactive model of schizophrenic relapse. External environmental variables (indicated by ellipses) interact with enduring vulnerability characteristics (indicated by upper rectangles) to produce transient intermediate states (indicated by parallelograms). The transient intermediate states create a vicious cycle by feedback to the environmental variables. The end results of the vicious cycle are the outcome behaviors (indicated by lower rectangles).

disrupted, causing an even greater drift downward in the social class structure.

In support of this explanation for the class bias in schizophrenia, the seven most methodologically rigorous of eleven studies of social mobility and schizophrenia have shown either downward mobility or lower-than-expected upward mobility among schizophrenics (Eaton and Larry, 1978; Bland and Orn, 1981). A quantitative model of the process of selection and drift suggests that class differentials in schizophrenia can be completely explained by the selection-drift hypothesis and that the most important stressors related to the onset of schizophrenia are probably classless (Eaton, 1980). The tendency of schizophrenics to be occupationally disadvantaged in urban society has major implications for treatment and rehabilitation.

The confirmation of the selection-drift explanation for the accumulation of schizophrenics in the lower urban classes does not diminish the etiologic importance of social factors in the development and course of schizophrenia. In fact, social variables are thereby highlighted and better specified as to the part they play in the pathogenesis and course of schizophrenia. For example, the premorbid social deficits of individuals destined to become schizophrenic impair their social mobility and predict poor outcome in the illness. Other important social factors that may interact with genetic vulnerability are attitudes and behavior in relation to health and differential access to quality health care. Lower class individuals know less about symptoms and their meaning, are less likely to seek medical and psychiatric care when symptoms develop, are less likely to attempt remediation of premorbid problems, and are less likely to receive the best psychiatric care (Karno and Edgerton, 1969; Weaver, 1973; Rushing and Ortega, 1979). Working class and unskilled individuals with schizophrenia in remission are at greater risk for unemployment and financial losses when the economy is depressed, and, hence, they are more likely to experience stress leading to decompensation and rehospitalization (Brenner, 1973).

CULTURAL FACTORS

Is schizophrenia universal? Do cultures and ethnic patterns have an impact on the incidence, severity, content, and outcome of the disorder? These questions were raised by the International Study of Schizophrenia sponsored by the World Health Organization (WHO) during the past 15 years. Using a standard and reliable mental status interview, the Present State Examination (PSE) (Wing et al., 1974), psychiatrists elicited characteristic symptoms of schizophrenia and other disorders in over 1,000 patients who presented for treatment at nine international centers. A computer program, based on Schneiderian first-rank symptoms of schizophrenia, was used to make the diagnosis of schizophrenia in a common, unitary fashion. An early phase of the WHO study had indicated that the incidence of schizophrenia was similar between New York and London. When the PSE was used to elicit symptoms in a standard way, the WHO study found a high degree of similarity among all nine centers.

A follow-up study on the original patients was conducted in all nine centers two years after the initial evaluations (Sartorius et al., 1977). Averaged over the nine countries, about one-third of the patients were totally free of symptoms, while about a quarter were still seriously ill. When the two-year outcome was examined in each country separately, unexpected and striking differences were found. Patients from Ibadan in Nigeria and Agra in India had made the best progress (58 percent symptom free in Ibadan), and those from Aarhus in Denmark had fared the worst (eight percent symptom free). Across all of the outcome measures, the schizophrenic patients from the developing countries (India, Nigeria, Colombia) did better than their counterparts from the more advanced, industrialized countries.

One explanation for this finding is that schizophrenia represents a group of disorders, with different biological and genetic bases, whose distribution varies in different ethnic groups. An alternate hypothesis is social: differences in the cultures of the participating countries account for differences in prognosis. For example, a schizophrenic returning to an undemanding rural life might function better and have less stress and symptoms than a schizophrenic returning to an overstimulating urban environment in an industrial society. Another important element helping to explain these findings is cultural: the differences in course of illness might be explained by more supportive family and neighborhood relationships in the developing countries.

The longitudinal WHO study sheds light on earlier studies which were conducted less rigorously and more cross-sectionally. These studies found differences in the prevalence of schizophrenia among various ethnic groups. More insidious courses of illness, rather than increased incidence, might account for the variations in prevalence these studies found. The differential prevalence of schizophrenia among various ethnic groups may thus be accounted for on the basis of cultural and familial elements that affect the prognosis and course of already established schizophrenic disorders. More detailed longitudinal follow-up studies of various ethnic groups, using standardized interview and diagnostic methods, may provide additional clues regarding pathogenic factors in the social environment.

A recently published longitudinal study of this type was based upon five-year follow-up data collected on a sample of 66 first-admission schizophrenic patients from Sri Lanka (Waxler, 1979). Social adjustment and clinical status of the patients were remarkably good at the five-year follow-up point. Mirroring the results from the WHO study of Nigeria and India, 66 percent of the schizophrenics had little or no symptoms, and 58 percent were playing normal social roles at home. These good outcomes could not be explained by any artifacts of sampling or diagnostic methods, by type of treatment, or by the family's willingness to tolerate deviance. Rather, it was conjectured, the good outcomes could be attributed to the nonindustrial society's beliefs and practices encouraging rapid return to functioning after a brief illness.

Migration and Misdiagnosis of Schizophrenia

A frequent sociocultural finding has been an increased incidence and prevalence of schizophrenic disorders among people who migrate from one culture to another (Torrey, 1979). Recently, however, studies using more careful diagnostic practices, standardized mental status interviews, and DSM-III have challenged the validity of these findings. Studies from South Africa and Britain, for example, suggest that the previously reported high incidence of schizophrenia among immigrants is attributable to the misdiagnosis of transient, brief, reactive psychoses (Littlewood and Lipsedge, 1981; Carpenter and Brockington, 1980; Cheetham and Griffiths, 1981).

In a United States example of misdiagnosis, evidence now points to an artifactual overdiagnosing of blacks as schizophrenic because of white psychiatrists' ignorance of black values, culture, and personality trends (Adebimpe, 1981). One study has reported that paranoid schizophrenia was diagnosed twice as often among blacks as among whites (Adebimpe, 1981). The gradual adoption of more stringent diagnostic criteria from DSM-III should help clinicians avoid the errors of stereotyping and false-positive symptoms. Reducing these errors will in turn reduce the stress, stigma, and iatrogenic illness caused by labeling individuals as more pathological than they really are.

STRESSORS

In the stress-diathesis view of schizophrenia, any event that requires adaptation is characterized as a stressor, whether the event is positively or negatively perceived and valued. Recent research has indicated that perception does make a difference in the outcome. A person's perception of the nature of the life change in large part determines whether the adaptation will lead to strain and stress. Furthermore, the negatively valued and perceived life events—undesirable, uncontrolled, and unanticipated events—appear to explain the bulk of the psychological, physical, and subjective distress and strain that individuals experience (Streiner et al., 1981).

Life events have been implicated in the process of relapse in schizophrenia. In a landmark study in England, Brown and Birley (1968) found a piling up of such events in the three weeks prior to hospitalization, and they did not find such an accumulation in the normal control group. The researchers drew distinctions between events that could be consequences of the insidious development of the schizophrenic symptoms and those that occurred totally outside the control of the individual. Only the latter were included in the calculations of differential rates of life changes between schizophrenics and normals.

To determine life events, both agreeable and noxious, researchers had the patient and a significant other describe disappointments, losses, damages, and fulfillments that could be specifically dated during the three-month period preceding the psychotic episode that required hospitalization. Of the schizophrenic sample sixty percent experienced abrupt changes in their social environments during the three-week period before hospitalization, compared to only 14 percent of the normal controls. Birley and Brown (1970) found that this concentration of life events occurred just prior to the first psychotic episode in young schizophrenics and prior to exacerbations and repeated relapses in more chronic schizophrenics.

In another investigation of the relationship of life events to relapse, the researchers found that patients who relapsed while taking neuroleptic medication were more likely to have experienced major life events in the period immediately preceding the flare-up of symptoms than were schizophrenics who relapsed without medication (Leff and Wing, 1971; Leff et al., 1973). These investigators concluded that the medication may protect vulnerable schizophrenic patients from the routine demands of daily living but not from large changes in their environments.

In the only other methodologically adequate study of life events and schizophrenia, researchers in New Haven interviewed first-admission schizophrenics and controls on the frequency of life events during the one-year period prior to the onset of their symptoms (Jacobs and Myers, 1976). Like other studies, this study also found a higher rate of life events for the schizophrenic patients than for the controls. One recently published study, which used a prospective design, found that problematic life events had significant associations with depression, but not with schizophrenia (Robin et al., 1980). Indeed, while the preponderance of evidence suggests a linkage between life events and onset and exacerbation of schizophrenia, most studies do indicate a greater correlation between life events and depression (Spring, 1981).

In a macroeconomic analysis of antecedents to schizophrenic psychopathology, Brenner (1973) studied the relationship between the unemployment rate and admissions to New York State public and private mental hospitals from 1914 to 1967. There was a substantial correlation between poor economic conditions and hospital admissions, and many of the admissions were schizophrenics. Although this correlation may be explained in a number of ways, it is possible that poor economic conditions precipitate the onset of symptoms or exacerbate them by increasing the number of noxious life events to which an individual must adapt.

Because of their perceptual and cognitive impairments and their psychological vulnerability, schizophrenics may be stressed by small-scale and everyday life events that would not be upsetting to others. The accumulation of minor but unexpected or confusing changes could conceivably tip the balance toward decompensation. Before the nature of the effect of stress on schizophrenia can be clearly determined, the concept of *onset* will need to be clarified so that the occurrence of stressors can be temporally related to the onset of symptoms. Onset can be defined as the first signs of prodromal symptoms and behaviors, or it can be defined as the appearance of the first-rank, characteristic symptoms of schizophrenia. Further research into the stressful factors which may trigger psychotic episodes should also conceive of a broader context made up of more remote stressors that influence the vulnerability to schizophrenia.

FAMILY FACTORS

A series of family studies began over the past two decades at the Medical Research Council's Social Psychiatry Unit at the Institute of Psychiatry in London and have continued in studies located in Denmark, India, and the United States. These studies have highlighted how the emotional climate in the family can influence the course of schizophrenic illness in a family member. Accumulated evidence points to interpersonal processes within the family as the most powerful predictors of relapse in a person having an established schizophrenic illness. Confirming results from three separate studies conducted in London over a 15-year period have revealed that patients returning to families that are high on expressing criticism and emotional overinvolvement relapse four times as often as patients returning to families that are low in these categories of expressed emotion (EE). Of patients who returned to homes where a family member was high on EE, 51 percent relapsed during the nine months after discharge, whereas only 13 percent relapsed who returned to low EE families (Vaughn and Leff, 1976). The diagnosis of schizophrenia and clinical determinations of relapse were made on the basis of the appearance of schizophrenic symptoms elicited by interviews using the PSE, not simply on the basis of rehospitalization or social functioning.

Since high EE did not explain all of the variance (nearly half of the patients from high EE homes did not relapse), the investigators conducted secondary analyses to identify other contributing factors. The two factors that did correlate with relapse were maintenance on antipsychotic drugs and amount of face-to-face contact between the patient and relative during the postdischarge period. Figure 2 shows how the use of antipsychotic medication and less than 35 hours per week of face-to-face contact protected schizophrenic individuals from relapse in high EE families, but not those in low EE families. Patients who lived with family members high on EE, who spent much time with their relatives, and who were not protected by maintenance drug therapy had a very poor outcome, with 92 percent of them relapsing. Relapse rates dropped if one of the two protective factors was operating. Outcome was best of all, equivalent to that of patients returning to low EE households, for those who had both protective factors operating.

In an American replication of these English studies the author and his colleagues at UCLA and the Mental Health Clinical Research Center for the Study of Schizophrenia at Camarillo State Hospital have found an uncanny duplication of the English results, with 57 percent of the high EE cases but only 17 percent of the low ones relapsing within nine months of discharge from the hospital (Vaughn et al., in press).

A much greater proportion of the families in California were high on EE than in England. In London, 45 percent of the families were high on EE, but in California almost seventy percent of the families were high on EE. Disproportionately larger numbers of high EE families of schizophrenics are also being found in replications of the EE studies in Rochester, Pittsburgh, and Chicago, while in India almost all the families are low on EE. In a replication of the EE work with Spanish-speaking, Mexican-American families containing a schizophrenic member, preliminary results suggest that the proportion of high EE families is midway between the Indian and English rates. These international and cross-cultural studies suggest that cultural factors may determine the proportion of families high on EE, but that once present, high EE predisposes toward schizophrenic relapse regardless of culture. The studies may also explain why schizophrenic illnesses run a more benign course in underdeveloped countries. Families in these countries are less critical and more tolerant and supportive of their schizophrenic members.

Interesting relationships have also emerged from a study that measured both EE and life events in the three months before development of schizophrenic symptoms. Exacerbations in patients living with high EE relatives were not associated with an increase in life events, but life events did occur in excess among relapsing schizophrenics who lived with low EE relatives. The maximum difference occurred in the three weeks before onset of the relapse (Leff and Vaughn, 1980).

The findings on the strong effects exerted by family factors on

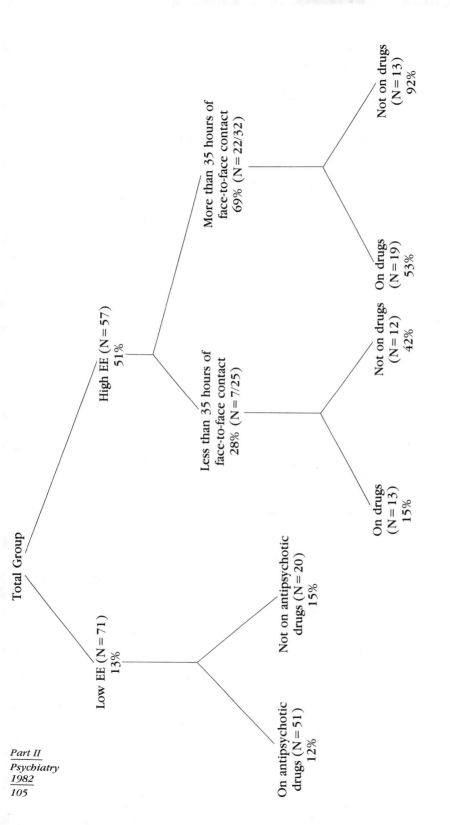

Figure 2. Nine-month relapse rates of 128 schizophrenic patients who were living with relatives rated high and low on EE. Data are drawn from two separate studies carried out a decade apart in London (Brown et al., 1972; Vaughn and Leff, 1976).

schizophrenic relapse point the way to more specific forms and goals of family therapy in the treatment of schizophrenia.*

SOCIAL SUPPORT NETWORKS

Only recently have social psychiatry investigators begun to shift attention from social stressors and noxious family and environmental conditions to the supportive and positive events and relationships that might attenuate the onset or course of schizophrenia. In one such attenuating circumstance is the child who begins life at risk for psychopathology or deviance but, because of favorable social learning environments, proves invulnerable to the stressors that provoke decompensation (Garmezy, 1974). In some instances, a socially competent and caring person, possibly a parent or parent-surrogate, may provide compensatory, emotionally supportive experiences and clear communication to the genetically vulnerable child. This may offer some explanation for the fact that not all vulnerable children go on to develop schizophrenia. Similarly, the availability of special help and support during stressful periods, e.g., adolescence, leaving home, supporting self, death of parent, may preempt the onset of schizophrenia in a vulnerable person.

Within the past twenty years, the concept of social support networks has arisen among sociologists, anthropologists, and social psychiatrists. Of the 1,000 to 1,500 people known to the average person, there appears to be a remarkably stable network of twenty to thirty persons with whom social contact is the most frequent and meaningful. People have network ties with relatives from nuclear and extended families and with friends, neighbors, social agency officials, and work associates. Characteristics of adult network relationships include frequency of contact, emotional quality (positive vs. negative), instrumental or affectional purpose, diversity of interactions, degree of reciprocity, and mutual interdependency vs. unidirectional dependency. While many methodological dilemmas still confront the researcher who attempts to ascertain valid and reliable features of social networks, the significant importance of these everyday social relations in the course, management, and quality of the schizophrenic experience is increasingly evident.

The individual's social support network can be considered an extension of his or her social competence. Socially supportive relationships can serve as a supplementary mechanism for effective coping and problem solving with the stressors of everyday life. Most of the work done in the area of social support has focused on its impact on already established, usually chronic schizophrenic disorders. Social support and associated networks are usually defined as relationships accessible to the vulnerable or schizophrenic individual, generally kinfolk or close friends and neighbors. The study of social support networks represents an important shift in interest from analysis of the relationship between static social categories such as socioeconomic status and schizophrenia to analysis of more dynamic social processes as they directly affect schizophrenia. Social support should be discriminated from social network. The former connotes relationships that contribute positively to the individual, while the latter is a more neutral concept that

*Preceptor's note: Keith and Matthews discuss the therapeutic implications of this family research in their chapter.

describes the frequency, number, and type of connections between people without regard to their positive or negative impacts.

They shrink after onset of schiz.

Studies comparing the social networks of established schizophrenics with those of normal or other deviant populations have led to a general consensus that schizophrenics' networks are smaller and that the constituent relationships are simpler and marked by more dependent ties (Lipton et al., 1981). Schizophrenic individuals have fewer intimate relationships with their network members, and their networks consist disproportionately of family members. Structurally, the social support networks of first-admission schizophrenics are larger and more interconnected than those of patients with multiple admissions. The social contacts of the chronic schizophrenics are characterized by more limited types of exchanges as well as by greater dependency (Lipton et al., 1981). Together with data from a retrospective study of hospitalized schizophrenics, which revealed that only one-sixth of the patients had been severely socially isolated during adolescence (Kohn and Clausen, 1955), these findings suggest that the most dramatic changes in social networks develop after the patient's first hospitalization.

Several researchers have focused on social network clusters outside of the family, most notably on relationships within the single-room occupancy hotels which house many exhospitalized chronic schizophrenics in New York and other large cities. In a series of investigations in such hotels, investigators found that the expatients' reports of satisfaction with life and favorable social functioning correlated with casual rather than intimate or nurturing relationships with other residents of the hotel (Lehmann, 1980; Lipton et al., 1981). More intense affiliative relationships in the hotel, as well as contacts with relatives outside the hotel, were associated with lower levels of life satisfaction and well-being. It appears from these studies that a quiet, undemanding, somewhat isolated social experience may be actually supportive and contribute to positive outcomes in schizophrenics. The studies await replication in nonfamily residential settings other than the somewhat unique hotels.

Findings from both family and nonfamily social network clusters, thus, suggest that intrusiveness, demands to perform normally, and intimacy may have harmful effects on the course of established schizophrenia. These data amplify the understanding of the long-known relationship between social stimulation and psychopathology in schizophrenia. Studies in both England and the United States have documented that florid schizophrenic symptoms reemerge in long-stay, hospitalized patients when they are exposed to a demanding, total-push rehabilitation effort (Wing, 1978). Social pressure, whether it comes from families, friends, or professionals, can have harmful effects on schizophrenics regardless of its positive intentions. A caveat should be noted, however. The harmful effects of social pressure and expectations can be ameliorated or eliminated by structuring expectations with clear and specific goals, by requesting small changes gradually over a period of time, and by providing abundant amounts of positive reinforcement or feedback for progress (Liberman et al., 1976; Liberman et al., 1980).

SOCIAL COMPETENCE

In conceptualizing the interaction between genetic vulnerability and environmental stressors leading to schizophrenic symptomatology, an intervening variable requiring attention is the socially learned competence and problem-solving skill of the vulnerable individual. Since the time of Kraepelin, clinical lore has suggested that schizoid traits in childhood and adolescence predisposed individuals to developing schizophrenia. In a longitudinal study of adolescent children of severely schizophrenic vs. healthy mothers, Mednick and Schulsinger (1970) found that more of the offspring of schizophrenics were rated by their teachers as passive, withdrawn loners with idiosyncratic thinking. In a ten-year follow-up of these youngsters, Schulsinger (1976) found that the offspring of schizophrenics had an excess of schizophrenic illness. Other investigators have described young schizophrenic patients with "premorbid asociality." From early childhood the patients were friendless, scapegoated, and socially incompetent, and they had academic difficulties and a limited range of interests (Quitkin et al., 1973; Kasanin and Rosen, 1933). While it appears clear that some proportion of schizophrenic patients do show schizoid traits before the onset of their illness, it is not clear how many persons with schizoid traits later go on to become schizophrenic.

Premorbid Social Adjustment and Outcome

Pre-morbid schizoid pers. more related to prognosis than onset

Although not much direct evidence exists to suggest that poor social skills development or a schizoid personality is etiologically linked to schizophrenia, considerable evidence points to the influence of poor premorbid social adjustment on the subsequent course of schizophrenia. Investigators have for many years recognized correlations between premorbid social inadequacy and symptomatic outcome and rehospitalization (Zigler and Phillips, 1961; Levine and Zigler, 1973; Strauss and Carpenter, 1974). Many studies have shown that the higher the person's level of social adjustment prior to developing schizophrenic symptoms and requiring hospitalization, the better will be his or her posthospital outcome (Hersen and Bellack, 1976b). The Phillips Premorbid Scale and its many derivatives generally measure education, occupation, heterosexual adjustment, and the range and depth of personal relationships from childhood to the present. Studies utilizing premorbid adjustment ratings show associations with global ratings of improvement and indices of rehospitalization (Kokes et al., 1977).

Gittelman-Klein and Klein (1969) investigated how childhood and adolescent social adjustment correlated with the two-year outcomes of 86 schizophrenics. Each of their items reflecting premorbid adjustment significantly correlated with the three measures of outcome (correlation coefficients ranged from 0.27 to 0.55).

Poor development of social skills as a prognostic feature in the course of schizophrenia is compounded in males, whose peak age for onset of schizophrenia is 20 to 22, approximately five years earlier than for females (Watt and Szulecka, 1979). This may account for the generally observed better outcome of schizophrenia in women (Shepherd, 1957).

Specific Social Skill Deficits

While the data from studies using premorbid social adjustment scales are based on retrospective and global ratings of interpersonal competence, a body of more direct and prospective evidence has recently developed showing that schizophrenic persons have major deficiencies in discrete social skills. In unmarried schizophrenics, lack of conversational skills and impaired confidence to form relationships with the opposite sex have been identified (Falloon et al., 1978). Spivack and his colleagues have identified six cognitive problem-solving skills related to social effectiveness: problem recognition, means-ends thinking, alternative generating, causal thinking, perspective taking, and consequential thinking (Spivack et al., 1976). In a series of studies these investigators have found that in comparison with normals, psychiatric patients generate fewer response alternatives to interpersonal problems, fewer means to achieve a goal, and fewer means that are relevant (Platt et al., 1975; Spivack et al., 1976; Platt and Siegel, 1976).

Social performance spontaneously enacted with confederates in natural situations or in role-play situations has been measured by directly recording discrete behaviors presumed to be important elements of social skill. Schizophrenic individuals, as compared to normal controls, have been found to exhibit less eye contact, greater response latency, more dysfluencies, and less self-assertion (Hersen and Bellack, 1976a).

Work and Schizophrenia

In a thirty- to forty-year follow-up study of 200 schizophrenics, Tsuang (1980) and colleagues at the University of Iowa have found that continuation of symptoms is associated with poor occupational outcome. Those twenty percent of schizophrenics who were symptom free during most of the follow-up period actually demonstrated an increase in their occupational status from the time of their illness episode.

While the severity and chronicity of symptoms and the number and duration of hospitalizations are inversely correlated with subsequent work adjustment, the most powerful predictor of posthospitalization work pattern is the patient's premorbid occupational history. If a patient has, prior to the onset of illness, worked effectively and stably, the chances for continued success at work are high (Huffine and Clausen, 1979). On the other hand, if the patient did not develop work habits prior to the schizophrenic disorder, vocational adjustment is unlikely to occur (Strauss and Carpenter, 1974; Brown et al., 1966; Simmons, 1965).

The disability compensation mechanisms contain disincentives that reduce job and work success in schizophrenic individuals. Social Security Disability, Supplemental Security Income, and Veterans Benefits are all contingent upon the maintenance of disability. An individual who receives these benefits must surrender them as soon as a job is obtained. This is obviously threatening to the many individuals who are well aware of the fragility of their recovery. Rather than risk losing a secure income base, they are frightened away from seeking a job (Ludwig, 1981).

A recent study of disincentives to vocational rehabilitation among disabled patients found that the number of sources of disability benefits and family income were the most potent predictors of rehabilitation outcome (West Virginia Rehabilitation Research and Training Center, 1980). The more sources of benefits, the less likely was placement in competitive employment, and patients who received benefits from three or more sources had a zero employment rate. If the patient's family was below the poverty level, successful rehabilitation was less likely. Furthermore, the patient was less likely to cooperate with the vocational rehabilitation agency or to seek a job if he or she could make more money from benefits than from working.

In a Madison, Wisconsin program chronic psychiatric patients were provided round-the-clock support by a team of professionals who aimed to teach daily living skills. Patients were placed in sheltered workshops, in jobs, and in transitional volunteer jobs with charitable agencies. This comprehensive social rehabilitation approach was effective in maintaining patients in the community at a reasonable quality of life and in keeping them relatively free of symptoms (Stein and Test, 1978). From the point of view of work, this community-based program produced twice as much work capacity, as gauged by earnings, as did a standard state hospital treatment. In addition, those patients who were actively involved in sheltered or competitive employment were the least likely to relapse and return to the hospital (Greco and Stein, 1980). Other studies have confirmed the relationship between involvement in work activities, patients' occupational and social skills, and rehabilitation outcome (Anthony et al., 1978).

SOCIAL INTERVENTIONS AND REHABILITATION

Enough is now known of the social and family factors which influence the course of schizophrenia to prescribe psychosocial interventions as well as pharmacological agents for schizophrenics. For the acutely ill schizophrenic with florid symptoms, drugs are unquestionably indicated. Social interventions during the acute stage should aim to reduce levels of stimulation and arousal, should provide clear expectations with low performance requirements, and should offer accepting, tolerant, and nondemanding supportive relationships. Psychosocial treatment can play a key role in maintaining remission and community tenure, and maintenance medication also seems essential for many schizophrenics, but not for all.

Social Learning in the Psychiatric Milieu

Using highly trained paraprofessional therapists for remediating the bizarre symptomatic behaviors and the social and self-care deficits of the most chronic, institutionalized schizophrenics, Paul and his colleagues have tested a token economy program based on social learning principles (Paul and Lentz, 1977). Comparing the social learning approach with equally intensive therapeutic community methods and conventional custodial care, they had impressive and clear-cut results favoring the social learning approach. The social learning program emerged as effective on an absolute level, in that over a third of the patients were functioning at a level indistinguishable from normals, and it was also significantly more effective relative to both the traditional hospital program and the milieu therapy program.

Family Interventions

Early controlled studies of family intervention had the promising results of reduced hospitalization and symptomatology rates among schizophrenics (Mosher and Keith, 1979). Several teams are now refining family therapy methods to reduce more specifically those noxious family interactions that have been associated with high relapse rates. Liberman, Falloon, and their associates have established two formats aimed at reducing high levels of EE among patients and their relatives: a multiple family group therapy and an in-home family intervention. The multiple family group met in a storefront in a shopping center for nine weekly sessions while the patients were receiving hospital care. Patients and relatives together attended sessions that included education on schizophrenia and its treatments, as well as intensive training in family communication skills. Although the total sample was small, comparisons with patients and families receiving no family therapy or those receiving an insight-oriented therapy suggested a lower relapse rate for those attending the group meetings (Liberman, et al., submitted; Falloon et al., 1981).

Falloon (1981) has adapted this model for a controlled clinical trial comparing in-home family therapy with individual supportive therapy, both in conjunction with optimal provision of neuroleptic medication. Patients from families high on EE were randomly assigned to each treatment condition. At the one-year follow-up point, approximately fifty percent of the patients in the conventional, individual aftercare program had relapsed, while only nine percent of the family therapy patients had relapsed.

Social Skills Training

Social skills training is a behavior therapy approach which attempts to improve patients' performance in critical life situations. It assumes that each individual always does the best that he or she can, given the person's biological endowment, cognitive limitations, and previous social learning experiences. When an individual's "best effort" fails to meet interpersonal needs and goals, it is an indication of a situation-specific deficit in the individual's repertoire. Whatever the source of the person's deficit of skills, systematic training in more effective response alternatives should be able to help the person overcome or partially compensate for the deficits. The training can take place *in vivo* with the people actually involved with the patient's real-life problems, or it can take place via role playing (Liberman et al., 1975; Goldstein, 1973; Trower et al., 1978).

While social skills training appears to be an encouraging new approach to the rehabilitation of chronic schizophrenics, training effects have been primarily demonstrated during periods of active therapy. The generalized and durable impacts of training have yet to be documented and replicated. More research must also be done to clarify whether improvements in social skills lead to improvements in other domains, such as psychopathology, social adjustment, self-care skills, cognitive capacities, motivation, and affect. While most of the brief treatment studies to date suggest that social skills training starts patients on a trajectory of change, only long-term studies can assess truly durable improvements in functioning and quality of life.

SUMMARY

Based on the discovery of social factors which affect the course of schizophrenia, an empirically based foundation for the psychosocial treatment of schizophrenia has been laid. New methods for both acute and maintenance treatment are focused on specific behavioral, social, and family problems of the schizophrenic and have improved the coping and adjustment of schizophrenics in hospital, family, and community milieus. No longer in competition with each other, drug and psychosocial therapies have been combined to potentiate favorable outcomes, thereby giving powerful encouragement to the eclectic therapist.

Social factors exert direct effects on the etiology and course of schizophrenia and also moderate its etiology and course through interaction with genetic and biological factors. The development or exacerbation of schizophrenic symptoms in biologically vulnerable individuals emerges from the homeostasis between the intensity of the individual's social stressors and their interpersonal problem-solving skills and support networks.

While problem-solving skills and social support are in scarce supply in the lower socioeconomic strata, the disproportionately large numbers of schizophrenics in the lower classes appear to be a function of drift downward rather than being directly linked to causal class factors. Characteristic schizophrenic symptoms are found universally, but the course of the disorder is much less severe in undeveloped countries, possibly because of the more benign social environments found in preindustrial societies.

Social stressors and life events have been implicated in the onset and exacerbation of schizophrenia, but aside from family stressors, no specificity between environmental precipitants and symptoms has been established. Excessive criticism or emotional overinvolvement by family members appears to provoke relapse in schizophrenics. As a consequence of the impairments produced by the disorder, the social networks of schizophrenics are smaller, burdened by dependency ties, and less intimate than those held by normals. It is thus evident that social factors function both as influences on schizophrenia and as consequences of the disorder.

Beginning with the optimistic assumptions that our schizophrenic patients have the capacity to learn and that their relatives' attitudes and feelings can become more positive, we can go on to design conducive and supportive environments both in and out of hospitals to override the biologically mediated diathesis toward schizophrenia. We can thereby continue to make important progress in helping our schizophrenic patients live more rewarding lives.

Chapter 12

Biochemical and Morphological Factors In The Etiology Of The Schizophrenic Disorders

*by Richard Jed Wyatt, M.D., Neal R. Cutler, M.D.,
Lynn E. DeLisi, M.D., Dilip V. Jeste, M.D.,
Joel E. Kleinman, M.D., Ph.D., Daniel J. Luchins, M.D.,
Steven G. Potkin, M.D., Daniel R. Weinberger, M.D.*

INTRODUCTION

The psychiatric nosologist interested in schizophrenia must work first to distinguish schizophrenia sharply from other disorders and second to divide schizophrenia into meaningful subgroups. These centrifugal and centripetal efforts are no more clearly seen than in the contrasting efforts of Kraepelin and Bleuler. Kraepelin (1971) brought together what generally appeared to be a diverse group of disorders under the name of dementia praecox, distinguishing it from other types of disorders. And Bleuler (1950), while slightly expanding the boundaries around dementia praecox, emphasized that schizophrenia is a group of disorders by titling his famous monograph *Dementia Praecox or the Group of Schizophrenias.*

Prior to and since Kraepelin's and Bleuler's achievements and with ever-increasing intensity, psychologists and psychiatrists have tried to distinguish schizophrenia externally from the rest of psychosis and to draw boundaries internally between subtypes of schizophrenia. Our primary tools during most of this time have been phenomenological. Now, with careful clinical observations, we can usually distinguish schizophrenia from other disorders with good reliability.

The high reliability of the phenomenological approach has been largely due to the willingness of experienced clinicians to agree on what appear to be relatively arbitrary and intuitively derived diagnostic thresholds. For example, DSM-III requires that there have been six months of continuous disability before a patient may be diagnosed schizophrenic. This demarcation, based upon the patient's past, undoubtedly has a predictive value. But using this time-dependent phenomenological threshold, particularly if schizophrenia is a progressive disorder, risks the loss of important time as the patient, physician, and family wait for six months to elapse. During this time they may develop a false sense of security and fail to make realistic plans for the future. Furthermore, when the etiologies of the disorder are uncovered, we may well find that the time criterion should be varied across different forms of the disorder. A single primary cause could be responsible for an acute, a remitting, or a chronic illness. And either the severity of the primary cause or the biological and psychological environment or both could determine the time-dependent severity of the individual's illness. Thus, while the phenomenological approach has improved in recent years, developing tests related to the biological or other etiology would greatly improve the accuracy and timeliness of diagnosis.

This chapter reviews many of the current biologic and biochemical themes in schizophrenia research. It focuses particularly on those findings that seem to cluster together in a group of patients. Some of the clustering appears both to make sense physiologically and also to further the definition of dimensions[1] within schizophrenia. The authors discuss these dimensions at the end of the chapter. The dimensions, which require using both biological and phenomenological distinctions, greatly overlap and are not synonymous with subtypes. The subtype concept implies distinct nonoverlapping groups. The dimensions, on the other hand, are a different kind of organizational schema and are of heuristic value. The following review of the current state of selected biochemical and morphological research into schizophrenia is intended both as a foundation for the discussion of the dimensions and also as a summary of the findings themselves.

[1]*Dimension* is defined by Webster's Third New World International Dictionary (1978) as "the particular set of circumstances or environmental factors within which someone or something exists or with reference to which something is viewed."

ABNORMAL IMMUNE MECHANISMS, PLASMA FACTORS, AND VIRUSES

The Immune System

A primary function of the immune system is to distinguish self from nonself, thus protecting the body's internal environment from external environmental changes. This function is accomplished by a complex network of cellular and extracellular interactions.

Lymphocytes, the main cellular component of the immune system, are either bone marrow (B-cells) or thymus-dependent (T-cells) in origin. B-cells, when stimulated by antigens, proliferate and differentiate forming clones of plasma cells producing specific antibodies. T-cells, while predominantly responsible for the so-called cellular immune responses, also may be either "helpers" or "suppressors" of the B-cell system; thus, T-cells play a role in the regulation of humoral immune response (see Figure 1).

IMMUNOLOGY, BRAIN, AND SCHIZOPHRENIA An association between the central nervous system and immunity is well recognized. Even before much of the field of immunology was known, the central nervous system was considered to be involved in the development of immunity, and the brain thought to be the organ initiating the anaphylactic reaction. For the last thirty years, the status of the immune system in schizophrenic patients has been studied extensively.

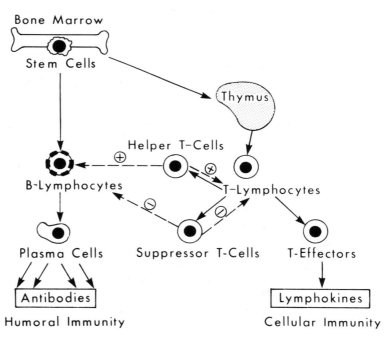

Figure 1. Schematic model of the functions and interrelationships of the main components of the immune system. Solid arrows indicate direction of derivation, broken arrows indicate influence (−) inhibition; (+) enhancement.

LYMPHOCYTE HISTOLOGY Early researchers reported histological changes in lymphocytes of schizophrenic patients. Kamp (1962) demonstrated abnormal nuclear staining and increased cytoplasmic glycoprotein in the lymphocytes of schizophrenic patients, while Fessel (1963) found an increase in lymphocytic lobular structure.

IMMUNITY, PHYSICAL ILLNESS, AND SCHIZOPHRENIA Asthma, an allergic or hyperimmune response, has been notably absent among psychotic patients (Funkenstein, 1950). Cancer, which may reflect abnormal immune mechanisms, has also been found to be less frequent among schizophrenic populations, although not all epidemiological studies are in agreement (Torrey, 1980). Finally, response to infection in schizophrenic patients, an indication of immune competence, appears to vary. While early studies showed an elevation in the rate of tuberculosis infection among psychiatric populations, later ones find no evidence of increased incidence of infection (Doust, 1952; Baldwin, 1979).

IMMUNOGLOBULINS Immunoglobulins A, G, and M (IgA, IgG, and IgM) have been studied in plasma and cerebrospinal fluid (CSF) of chronic schizophrenic patients (see Table 1). While some studies report significant elevations of immunoglobulins in schizophrenic patients compared with controls (Strahilevitz, 1976; Torrey, 1978; Gowdy, 1980), others find no differences (Solomon et al., 1969; DeLisi et al., in press). Domino (1975) found low levels of IgA in acute schizophrenics and found IgA elevations in chronic schizophrenic patients. Amkraut et al. (1973) found that patients with low amounts of IgA and IgG were more likely to recover during treatment than those with high IgA and IgG. Pulkkinen (1977) reported that the severity of the psychotic illness, as well as prognosis and recovery, was negatively correlated with the concentration of total IgG and also found that withdrawn patients had high IgM concentrations, while paranoid patients had low concentrations.

The lack of consistency in these reports may be due to the diagnostic heterogeneity, as well as the age, gender, and racial characteristics of populations sampled. The significance of altered immunoglobulin levels for schizophrenia is not well understood, although high levels of immunoglobulins have been proposed to be a reaction to a viruslike substance (Torrey et al., 1978; Crow et al., 1979) or a manifestation of an autoimmune disease (Heath and Krupp, 1967a).

CELLULAR IMMUNITY Early reports of cellular immunity, particularly delayed hypersensitivity, in schizophrenic patients noted various changes in antibody response to intradermally administered antigens. Vaughn et al. (1949) and Molholm (1942) found diminished skin responses to pertussis and guinea pig serum respectively, but Friedman et al. (1967) found an accelerated response to cholera vaccine, and Solomon et al. (1970) found that the response of schizophrenic patients to tetanus toxoid was no different from that of controls.

Recently developed techniques for separating lymphocytes into B- and T-cell populations have enabled investigators to explore other aspects of the cellular immune system in schizophrenic patients in comparison with controls. Vartanian et al. (1978) reported an elevation

TABLE 1. IMMUNOGLOBULIN CLASSES

	IgG	*IgM*	*IgA*	*IgE*	*IgD*
CON-CENTRATIONS IN SERUM AND CSF	Normally 8-16 mg/ml serum, .028-.106 % total CSF protein	Normally .5-1.0 mg/ml serum, Trace amounts in CSF	Normally 1.4-4.2 mg/ml serum, 0-.02% total CSF protein (Major Ig in secretory fluids)	Trace-.006 mg/ml serum, ? in CSF	.003-.4 mg/ml serum, ? in CSF
FUNCTION	Antibodies against viruses, toxins, and Gram positive bacteria. Appears after an initial IgM response and lasts longer	Typically against Gram negative bacteria. Appears rapidly in response to antigen	First line of defense against bacteria and viruses in respiratory, intestinal, and reproduction systems	Allergic, anaphylactic reactions, and parasitic infections	Unknown

in percentage of B-cells and a low percentage of T-cells in schizophrenic patients compared with controls. Nyland et al. (1980), while confirming the T-cell finding in acute schizophrenic patients, failed to find any T- or B-cell differences in chronic schizophrenics. Nevertheless, the higher proportion of B-cells supports the above reports of higher circulating immunoglobulin concentrations, while the lower percentage of T-cells may indicate an alteration in cellular immunity as well. Vartanian and colleagues (1978) and Liedeman and Prilipko (1978) additionally found the level of *in vitro* physiological activity of peripheral T-lymphocytes from chronic schizophrenic patients reduced and have attributed this to the presence of factors in the serum of schizophrenic patients.

AUTOIMMUNITY One mechanism for self-injury by the immune system involves the formation of antibodies directed against the body's own tissues. Examples are the antinuclear antibodies and the rheumatoid factors that are present in high concentrations in the serum of patients with systemic lupus erythematosus and rheumatoid arthritis. Elevated serum antinuclear antibody titres are present in approximately twenty percent of chronically hospitalized psychiatric patients while present in only one percent of the general population. The higher titres of antinuclear antibodies in hospitalized psychiatric patients, however, appear not to be specific to schizophrenia. Furthermore, chronic neuroleptic treatment seems to be associated with the higher titres (Johnstone and Whaley, 1975). Rheumatoid factors also appear to be elevated in populations of schizophrenic patients (Wertheimer, 1961), despite the paucity of rheumatoid arthritis among schizophrenic populations (Gregg, 1939). Systemic lupus erythematosus, on the other hand, is found frequently in mental hospitals. Patients diagnosed for several years as schizophrenic are later found to have systemic lupus erythematosus, and conversely patients with a primary diagnosis of lupus also develop neurological signs and schizophrenic-like symptoms. It is not certain whether some lupus patients are initially misdiagnosed as schizophrenic or whether there is an association between these two illnesses (Fessel and Solomon, 1960).

In addition, some isolated reports suggest increased autoantibody production in schizophrenic patients. Jankovic et al. (1979) found a high incidence of delayed skin hypersensitivity (a T-cell function) to human brain protein in psychiatric patients, particularly those patients known to have cerebral atrophy. Finally, antibodies against human lymphocytes (antithymic antibodies) have been found in elevated levels in schizophrenic populations (Koliaskina et al., 1980).

NEUROLEPTICS AND IMMUNITY All the above data are inconclusive. We do not know if any of these findings predate the development of the illness, coincide with it, or are associated with illness chronicity. Nor do we know how each isolated finding might be correlated with the others. Moreover, these problems are complicated by the fact that neuroleptics have been associated with several immunological abnormalities in psychiatric patients.

Patients who have been on neuroleptics for a long time are reported to have a high incidence of splenic enlargement (Zarrabi et al., 1979). Neuroleptics have also been associated with abnormal lymphocyte morphology (Fieve et al., 1966), with a decreased response to lymphocyte mitogens, and with other inhibitory effects on indices of cellular immunity (Ferguson et al., 1978). Zarrabi et al. (1979) found that the percentage of T-lymphocytes was below normal in 13 of 41 chronic schizophrenic patients on long-term chlorpromazine treatment, but Ferguson et al. (1978) found no difference in T-cell percentages in chlorpromazine-treated patients. Antinuclear antibodies are increased in chronic medicated schizophrenic patients, and chlorpromazine has been linked to the development of lupus erythematosus (Ananth and Minn, 1973). In one study chlorpromazine inhibited the antibody response to oral polio vaccine virus when daily treatment was started four weeks prior to vaccination but not when the chlorpromazine was started on the day of immunization (Saunders and Muchmore, 1964).

In addition, neuroleptic treatment may decrease immunoglobulin production. Although this is suggested by both *in vivo* (Gowdy, 1980) and *in vitro* (Lovett et al., 1978) observations, some investigators have found enhanced antibody response in laboratory animals after phenothiazine treatment (Kerbikov, 1961).

Despite the strong evidence for neuroleptic suppression of both cellular and humoral immunity, there remain some indirect indications that alterations in the immune status of schizophrenic patients precede neuroleptic treatment. Decreased prevalence of rheumatoid arthritis, decreased prevalence of allergy, and decreased cellular immune responses have been noted prior to the advent of neuroleptic treatment.

Plasma Factors

The search for a biochemical etiology of schizophrenia has led some investigators to search for substances that are present in the blood of schizophrenic patients but not in the blood of controls, substances that are able to alter behavior in normal subjects or animal models. Two such substances have been heavily studied. One, taraxein, appears to be an immunoglobulin, the other, the Frohman factor, an α-2-globulin.

TARAXEIN Heath and co-workers (1957) first reported the presence of a substance they named taraxein in the blood of schizophrenic patients. When injected into healthy subjects, taraxein produced schizophrenic-like symptoms. They later reported the ability of taraxein to produce abnormal EEG spiking in the-septal region of the brains of monkeys, an abnormality similar to those they had seen in the EEG's of schizophrenic patients (Heath et al., 1970). Since taraxein was then found to be a particular subfraction of IgG, Heath and co-workers proposed an autoimmune hypothesis for the genesis of schizophrenia (Heath and Krupp, 1967a). Specifically they theorized that schizophrenic symptomatology results from the formation of autoantibodies to brain tissue, particularly of the limbic system. The resultant antibody, deposited on brain tissue, might then interfere with certain aspects of brain function, ultimately resulting in schizophrenic symptoms. In further support of their hypothesis, Heath and Krupp (1967b) demonstrated antibody deposition on neural cell nuclei of post-mortem schizophrenic brain tissue, particularly from the septal region and basal caudate nucleus. Several subsequent investigators have been unable to confirm the presence or specificity of taraxein, while others have supported Heath's work (reviewed by Wyatt et al., 1971).

While they did confirm Heath's basic findings in monkeys, Bergen et al. (1980) have alternatively proposed that the biological activity observed with taraxein and other plasma factors may be the manifest activity of a small molecule attached to the protein. The function of the protein might be to serve as a carrier for the biologically active small molecule. While these hypotheses are intriguing models for the production of psychoses, taraxein remains a controversial substance. Further confirmation and correlation with other immunologic findings in schizophrenia are still wanting.

FROHMAN FACTOR   The Frohman factor, Bergen's plasma fraction (Bergen et al., 1968), and a factor isolated by Russian workers (Koliaskina et al., 1967) all appear to be α-2-globulins and probably identical substances. While the Russian workers feel there is an association between their factor and immunologic abnormalities, Frohman and colleagues have associated their protein with abnormal tryptophan metabolism.

Approximately twenty years ago, Frohman and colleagues (1960) reported the isolation of a protein factor that altered the anaerobic metabolism of chicken red blood cells, producing lower pyruvate and higher lactate concentrations. From this ensued studies of lactate/pyruvate (L/P) ratios in schizophrenic patients' sera compared with those of controls, using L/P ratios as predictors of the illness. Schizophrenic sera could be differentiated from controls, by this method in some laboratories though not in others (reviewed by Wyatt et al., 1971).

Frohman et al. (1971) subsequently renamed their factor the S-protein and characterized it as an α-2-globulin having a molecular weight of 263,500 and containing approximately eighty percent lipid. When isolated from plasma of schizophrenic patients, they hypothesized, the protein is in an active form or an α-helical configuration and causes more tryptophan to accumulate in cells than the inactive form or β-helix isolated from controls causes in them. They emphasize that the active S-protein may be connected to other reports of abnormal indole metabolism and the accumulation of dimethyltryptamine (DMT) in schizophrenic patients. This structural alteration, however, may not be specific to schizophrenia. They also found a high percentage of the α-helical molecule in plasma from normal individuals under psychological stress.

More recently, Frohman et al. (1973) postulated the presence of a second protein, the anti-S-protein, which counteracts the action of the S-protein, shifting its equilibrium towards the inactive form. They have further characterized the active site of the anti-S-protein as a tripeptide, threonyl-valyl-leucine, and have synthesized this compound in their laboratory. Since Frohman and colleagues hypothesize that a deficiency in the anti-S-protein may be relevant to the pathogenesis of schizophrenia, their plans include clinical trials of threonyl-valyl-leucine in patients. The hypotheses of Frohman and other propositions concerning a blood-borne mechanism for schizophrenia await further clarification and confirmation from other laboratories.

Viruses

SLOW VIRUS   During the 1950's several reports from the Soviet Union associated viruses or viruslike particles with schizophrenia

(Rimon et al., 1979). Western interest in this field is of later origin and relates to the discovery of slow virus infections. Such viruses include (1) the conventional viruses that are responsible for illnesses such as measles, but can also produce a disease such as subacute sclerosing panencephalitis many years after the initial contact and (2) the newly discovered so-called slow viruses that have now been shown to cause Kuro and other dementing disorders including Creutzfeldt-Jakob disease. Since these slow viral infections may be acquired years before they produce any clinical effects, and since they may produce degenerative changes of the CNS without apparent inflammation, it has been suggested that they are relevant to schizophrenia (Torrey and Peterson, 1976). This viral hypothesis has gained increased attention with recent computed tomography (CT) findings, suggesting brain atrophy in schizophrenia, and with neuropathologic studies revealing gliosis (Stevens, 1981) or degeneration (Averback, 1981) in midbrain and limbic structures. The three main lines of evidence that support albeit circumstantially, this viral hypothesis are clinical, epidemiological, and immunological.

CLINICAL STUDIES   Clinically, it is known that many neurological disorders can mimic schizophrenia (Davison and Bagley, 1969) and that the viral encephalitides may frequently present such a picture. Both during the 1918 influenza epidemic and during the epidemic of encephalitis lethargica, a schizophrenic presentation was not unusual. Even today, herpes encephalitis must be considered in the differential diagnosis of acute schizophrenia (Raskin and Frank, 1974). In this regard, it is of interest that in a neuropathological study of schizophrenic brains, seven of the eight had lesions that mimicked encephalitis and that were concentrated in the area of the trigeminal nucleus, for which the herpes virus shows a predilection (Fisman 1975). A more exotic disorder, Vilyuisk encephalitis, found in the Yakut Republic of the USSR, is believed to be due to a slow virus and can be clinically indistinguishable from schizophrenia. Another clinical phenomenon that may be relevant to the viral hypothesis is the high frequency of abnormal dermatoglyphics in schizophrenia. The finding that such abnormalities can be produced by fetal infections with either rubella or cytomegalovirus has been offered as additional evidence for this hypothesis (Torrey and Peterson, 1976).

EPIDEMIOLOGICAL STUDIES   The epidemiology of schizophrenia is controversial. Although conventional wisdom teaches that the incidence does not vary over time or place, Torrey (1980) has accumulated contrary evidence. He emphasizes that the first descriptions of the disorder occurred early in the nineteenth century. Also schizophrenia appears to be extremely rare in certain areas that have limited contact with the West, e.g., New Guinea and the highlands of Papua. When schizophrenia does occur, it appears to have a more benign course in relatively underdeveloped areas (Murphy and Raman, 1971). Furthermore, in some areas in the West, e.g., Croatia and Ireland, the prevalence of schizophrenia is markedly elevated. Although these findings could be interpreted as supporting the role of culture in schizophrenia, they are also compatible with a viral etiology. Several viral diseases which were rare in primitive cultures became more prevalent with the concentration of the population in urban areas

Moreover, viral infections are not uncommonly concentrated in specific endemic areas, often related to the presence of vectors, e.g., the equine encephalitides.

Another unusual feature of the epidemiology of schizophrenia is that a disproportionate number of schizophrenics were born in the late winter and early spring. This has been confirmed in several locales (see Torrey et al., 1977). Some viral infections, e.g., measles and rubella, also show a peak incidence during these months. To relate the viral hypothesis of schizophrenia to genetic studies, it is of interest that reanalysis of data from the Danish cross-fostering studies did show the expected season of birth effect among schizophrenics without a family history of the illness, but not among those with a family history (Kinney and Jacobsen, 1978).

IMMUNOLOGICAL STUDIES Laboratory studies to support the viral hypothesis are in an early stage. One nonspecific approach has been to study the levels of either serum or CSF immunoglobulins in schizophrenics, since these are often elevated in viral diseases. Several reports have noted an elevation in specific immunoglobulin fractions, usually IgA, in the serum of schizophrenics, although others have failed to replicate these findings (see DeLisi et al., in press). Researchers have also attempted to study immune responsiveness to specific viral agents. Reports of elevated serum antibody titres in response to herpes simplex type 1 virus (Halonen et al., 1974) have not subsequently been confirmed (Rimon et al., 1979). Skin testing with antigen from this virus has produced a high frequency of positive responses in schizophrenics and in many other psychiatric patients (Libíková et al., 1980). An elevation of the ratio of CSF to serum antibody titres has been reported for both measles (Torrey et al., 1978) and cytomegalovirus (Albrecht et al., 1980). At least in the case of the cytomegalovirus, however, the deviation from normal was not an elevation of the CSF titres but a decrease in the serum titres.

These studies are somewhat problematic because both chronic hospitalization and the long-term use of neuroleptic medications may alter the immune system. Furthermore, levels of antibodies to specific viruses may vary in populations depending on their HLA type. This has been a problem in research on multiple sclerosis. Although there have been reports of an increase of measles antibody titres in multiple sclerosis, it appears that it is only those multiple sclerosis patients with specific HLA antigens who have increased antibody titres. Multiple sclerosis patients with other HLA types do not have such increases (see Carp, 1978). Since specific HLA antigens may be associated with schizophrenia (McGuffin, 1980), the HLA type of patients may be important for future studies.

There have been attempts to isolate and propagate viruses from tissue or body fluids of schizophrenics. Tyrrell et al. (1979) were able to demonstrate a cytopathic effect of CSF from 13 of 38 schizophrenics. They were not able to propagate the responsible agent, and a similar effect was noted in the CSF of eight of 11 patients with various neurological disorders not believed to be due to a viral agent, i.e., Huntington's chorea.

Although these recent laboratory studies aimed at supporting the viral hypothesis of schizophrenia are subject to criticism and in need of replication, new and more powerful techniques for studying the viral hypothesis do exist. In particular, study of post-mortem materials for evidence of viral infection, using either immunologic techniques or recombinant RNA probes, may provide more definitive answers (Haase et al., 1981).

MORPHOLOGICAL CHANGES

Computed Tomography Scans

Recent investigations with computed tomography (CT) have reopened a question raised earlier in this century with pneumoencephalography, namely, whether some chronic schizophrenic patients have cerebral atrophy. The CT studies suggest that as a group chronic schizophrenic patients differ from normal control subjects in the following ways. (1) They have significantly larger lateral cerebral ventricles. (2) They are more likely to have dilated cortical fissures and sulci. (3) They have a greater prevalence of apparent atrophy of the anterior cerebellar vermis (for review see Weinberger and Wyatt, in press[a]). In addition to these group differences, at least one patient has been observed with atrophic pons and cerebellum (Weinberger and Wyatt, in press[b]). Together these findings indicate that CT abnormalities suggest a structural brain disorder, probably atrophy or a dysplastic process, occurring in some individuals diagnosed as schizophrenic. It is unclear, however, whether these findings are relevant to the pathogenesis of a form of schizophrenia or whether they develop secondarily. The possi-

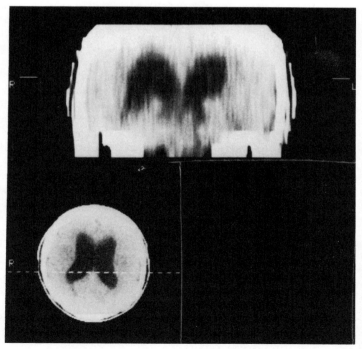

Figure 2.   CT scan of schizophrenic patients in horizontal (top) and coronal sections showing enlarged ventricles. Normal ventricles are slit-like in nature. Dashed line is level of coronal section.

bility that they are the result of somatic treatment or of institutionalization, although difficult to rule out, does not appear probable (Weinberger and Wyatt, in press[b]).

CLINICAL RELEVANCE   Several reports have suggested that one of the CT findings, ventricular enlargement, may have clinical relevance. Johnstone et al. (1978) found enlarged ventricles to be associated with the so-called negative schizophrenic symptoms, i.e., affective flattening, retardation, and poverty of speech. Five studies of schizophrenic patients found poorer performance on neuropsychological testing in patients with enlarged ventricles (Weinberger and Wyatt, in press[a]). Enlarged ventricles have also been associated with neurological signs of diffuse cerebral dysfunction ("soft signs") and with poor smooth-pursuit eye tracking (Weinberger and Wyatt, in press[b]).

In a retrospective study of premorbid adjustment, Weinberger et al. (1980b) reported that the 19 large-ventricle patients had poorer adjustment than did the 32 normal-ventricle patients, particularly during childhood. Furthermore, despite the fact that the study sample was biased towards poor premorbid adjustment, they found that the nine patients with the poorest adjustment scores during childhood all had enlarged ventricles, as compared with only three of the 14 with the best adjustment. The results of the study suggest that either poor premorbid schizophrenic patients are somehow at greater risk for developing enlarged ventricles, or that ventricular enlargement in such patients is an indication of an early developmental brain disorder that interferes with normal social maturation.

Perhaps the most intriguing of the clinical studies of ventricular enlargement in schizophrenic patients is a National Institute of Mental Health (NIMH) study of response to neuroleptic drug therapy (Weinberger et al., 1980a). The NIMH group found that after eight weeks of standard drug treatment the patients with enlarged ventricles (N = 10) had a significantly poorer response than did the other patients (N = 10). The difference could not be explained by differences in drug dose or serum drug concentrations. This finding has implications for the dopamine hypothesis of schizophrenia (see also later discussion of this hypothesis). It suggests that the dopamine hypothesis is less relevant for patients with enlarged ventricles. The NIMH group has pursued this further in a series of studies of dopamine-related clinical phenomena, e.g., prolactin concentrations, apomorphine response, and eye blink rates, and the results are consistent with the notion that patients with large ventricles do not fit the dopamine hypothesis as well as other patients (Weinberger and Wyatt, in press[b]).

These studies seem to suggest that structural brain abnormalities as seen on CT scans, in particular ventricular enlargement, are clinically, if not pathogenically, meaningful. But some words of caution are necessary. The number of CT studies are relatively few, and studies reporting clinical correlations are especially rare. Still, even if these reports are widely replicated, the findings may have little immediate clinical import. For one thing, they have no diagnostic significance. In the studies reported to date, most chronic schizophrenic patients have normal-sized ventricles. Moreover, enlarged ventricles have also been observed in normal individuals. Indeed, even among psychiatric patients, ventricular enlargement is not specific to schizophrenia but has also been found in some patients with affective disorders

(Weinberger and Wyatt, in press[b]). These points are consistent with the fact that the CT findings represent nonspecific alterations in brain structure, the possible end results of numerous pathological processes and etiologies. Yet, because the findings are objective indications of a biological brain disorder in at least some schizophrenic patients, they raise important questions for further research.

Hemispheric Asymmetry

FUNCTIONAL STUDIES   Flor-Henry drew attention to the significance of hemispheric asymmetries in psychopathology, and particularly of left hemispheric dysfunction in schizophrenia. He showed that in temporal lobe epilepsy schizophrenic symptoms were frequently associated with left hemispheric or bilateral foci, while affective symptoms were frequently associated with right hemispheric foci (Flor-Henry, 1979). Subsequent studies have used EEG power spectra analysis, average evoked responses, galvanic skin responses, and direction of lateral gaze. All measures support the association of left hemispheric dysfunction with schizophrenia (Wexler, 1980). In addition, left-handedness, which in the absence of a family history of left-handedness may reflect left hemispheric insult, has been shown to be more frequent than normal in schizoaffective psychoses (Lishman and McMeekan, 1976). In monozygotic twins with at least one schizophrenic member, left-handedness is more frequent when twins are discordant for schizophrenia and presumably suffer from a less "genetic" form of illness. It is normally distributed in twins who are concordant for schizophrenia (Boklage, 1977). Furthermore, within these twinships it is the left-hander who tends to be schizophrenic (Luchins et al., 1980b).

NEUROANATOMICAL STUDIES   The human brain has a number of neuroanatomical asymmetries (Galadburda et al., 1978), some of which can be detected on CT scans (LeMay, 1976, Figure 2). These asymmetries may be relevant to left hemispheric functioning. Reversals of the normal CT asymmetry are associated with a better prognosis in global aphasias (see Naeser et al., 1981), suggesting decreased lateralization of language to the left hemisphere. Reversals have been reported, however, to be more frequent in a variety of disorders of language function: autism (Hier et al., 1978a), delayed speech acquisition (Rosenberger and Hier, 1980), and developmental dyslexia (Hier et al., 1978b). Individuals with learning disorders who also have reversed asymmetry tend to have lower verbal than performance IQ scores (Rosenberger and Hier, 1980). An increased frequency of reversals in right-handed schizophrenics, compared with nonpsychiatric controls, has been reported by two different groups (Luchins et al., 1979; Naeser et al., 1981). There is also some evidence that the presence of reversals may define a subgroup of schizophrenic patients. Schizophrenic patients with reversals (1) tend not to evidence other structural brain abnormalities on CT scans, (2) tend to have an increased frequency of HLA-A2 (Luchins et al., 1981a), and (3) tend to have lower verbal than performance IQ scores (Luchins et al., 1981b). These studies, however, await confirmation.

Findings of left hemispheric dysfunction in schizophrenic patients need to be viewed with caution on two principal grounds. First, these findings are not specific to schizophrenia. For example, left-handedness and reversed neuroanatomical asymmetries have been reported to have increased frequencies in numerous other disorders. Second, the presence of left hemispheric dysfunction does not rule out right hemispheric abnormalities. In fact, studies with CT scans (Golden et al., 1980), regional cerebral blood flow (Mathew et al., 1981), and positron emission tomography (Buchsbaum et al., 1981) all suggest bilateral abnormalities in schizophrenia. Despite such reservations, there nevertheless may be a link between disruption of normal left hemisphere function and some schizophrenic symptoms.

ENZYMATIC ALTERATIONS

Enzymatic deficiencies have been associated with many genetically determined illnesses. Since there appears to be an important genetic component to schizophrenia, the activity and structural properties of enzymes involved in neurotransmitter metabolism have been heavily studied in schizophrenic patients.

Monoamine Oxidase (MAO)

The most extensively studied enzyme, MAO, has been found to be lower in the platelets of chronic schizophrenic patients than in those of controls (reviewed by DeLisi et al., 1981b). MAO is responsible for the metabolism of several compounds of hypothesized importance to the development of schizophrenia. These include dopamine, serotonin, norepinephrine, phenylethylamine, and dimethyltryptamine. Since the initial report (Murphy and Wyatt, 1972) of decreased MAO activity in platelets of schizophrenic patients, there have been at least 44 independent studies published. They compare MAO activity in peripheral cells (platelets, lymphocytes, and skeletal muscle) of chronic schizophrenic patients with that of controls. (See Figure 3.) Thirty-one of

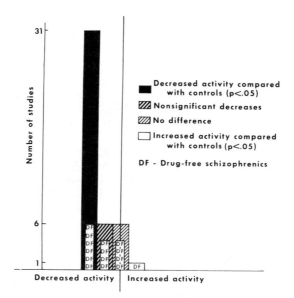

Figure 3. Bar graph composite of all published independent studies (1972 through 1980) comparing MAO activity in schizophrenic patients with controls.

these find activity is significantly lower in at least a definable subgroup of schizophrenics. Of the 13 studies in which results were not significant, six reported a trend towards a decrease (DeLisi et al., 1981b).

SUBGROUPS Among schizophrenic patients, clinical discriminators of low MAO activity have been found by some investigators to be paranoid symptomatology, the presence of auditory hallucinations, or both (Potkin et al., 1978; Adler et al., 1980; Meltzer et al., 1980).

Finally, while platelet MAO activity is probably reduced in a subgroup of chronic schizophrenic patients, perhaps paranoid and/or hallucinating patients, it does not appear to be altered in acute schizophrenics. It may, however, be elevated in schizoaffective patients (Wyatt et al., 1980).

PHYSIOCHEMICAL STUDIES The chemical mechanism for producing low MAO activity is currently under investigation. While there is some evidence for alteration in the physiochemical properties of the MAO molecule (reviewed by Wyatt et al., 1979; Abell et al., in press), there is one report, not confirmed by other studies, of a plasma inhibitor of MAO activity in schizophrenic patients (Berrettini and Vogel, 1978).

SPECIFICITY Low platelet MAO activity is not specific for schizophrenia. There have been several reports of decreased MAO activity in bipolar illness as well as alcoholism (Belmaker et al., 1980). Many other disorders have also been reported at least once to be associated with low MAO activity (DeLisi et al., 1981b).

In addition, low MAO activity, similar to that produced by MAO inhibitors, has also been found in nonpatient populations. These low MAO individuals, however, have been reported to have a greater number than normal of past psychiatric contacts and criminal convictions and higher than normal MMPI scores (Haier et al., 1980). Thus, while decreased MAO activity may not be specific to schizophrenia, it may be a factor of significance in aspects of mental illness that cross diagnostic lines.

GENETICS Considerable interest in the relevance of MAO activity to the schizophrenic process stems from the hypothesis that decreased MAO activity may represent a genetic predisposition for development of the illness (Wyatt et al., 1973). The evidence developed in support of this hypothesis is as follows. Monozygotic twins discordant for schizophrenia, as well as normal twins, have highly correlated MAO activities and dizygotic twins somewhat less, and first-degree relatives of low MAO schizophrenics are also reported to have low MAO activity (Wyatt et al., 1973; Nies et al., 1974; Berrettini et al., 1980). Böök et al. (1978) further hypothesized a dual-gene hypothesis for the inheritance of schizophrenia based on a multigenerational pedigree analysis of a multischizophrenic family. In this family, diagnosed schizophrenics had both low MAO and low dopamine-β-hydroxylase (DBH) activities compared with other family members. Recently, Baron et al. (1980) found schizophrenics with a family history of schizophrenia to have lower MAO than those with a negative family history. Several other investigators, however, have failed to confirm these findings.

Although it appears that most of the intraindividual enzyme variation in healthy individuals is genetically determined, the possibility that MAO is linked to those family members with psychiatric illness needs further exploration in careful pedigree analysis. Even if low MAO is proven to be genetically linked to schizophrenia, it is unlikely to be a sole cause. The treatment of nonpsychotic individuals with MAO inhibitors does not usually produce schizophrenia-like symptoms. Likewise, treating schizophrenic patients with MAO inhibitors has not, for the most part, made them worse. While it is far from clear that platelet MAO activity correlates with brain MAO activity or is representative of it (Murphy and Kalin, 1980), no differences in MAO activity have been found in post-mortem brains of schizophrenics compared with controls (reviewed by DeLisi et al., 1981b).

NEUROLEPTIC EFFECT Alternatively, the decreased MAO activity seen in several schizophrenic populations could be a consequence of chronic neuroleptic use, as well as other differential environmental factors. Although several earlier studies reported no effect of neuroleptics on platelet MAO activity, more recent evidence associates declines in both platelet and brain MAO activity with neuroleptic treatment (reviewed by DeLisi et al., 1981b).

A total of 15 of the 44 studied schizophrenic populations mentioned above were nonmedicated. Six of the 15 reported significantly lower mean activity in drug-free chronic schizophrenics, but all of the 15 did contain patients who had been medicated for long periods of time prior to neuroleptic withdrawal.

While reduced MAO activity is consistent with every hypothesis of schizophrenia based on biogenic amine alterations, its direct relevance to the pathogenesis of schizophrenia remains unclear. Further study of MAO activity and its relationship to other biochemical processes will help clarify the impact of these mechanisms.

Dopamine-β-Hydroxylase (DBH)

DBH, the enzyme that catalyzes the conversion of dopamine to norepinephrine, is located intracellularly in sympathetic neurons, in brain noradrenergic neurons, and in the adrenal medulla. Because of the possible role of catecholamines in psychoses, DBH activity has been studied extensively in plasma, CSF, and post-mortem brains of psychiatric patients. While Wise and Stein (1973) reported reduced DBH activity in post-mortem brains of schizophrenic patients, others have failed to confirm this finding (Wyatt, et al., 1975; Cross et al., 1978). Most studies of plasma DBH activity find no difference between schizophrenic patients and controls (DeLisi et al., 1980 and Meltzer et al., 1980), although one study finds a significant increase (Markianos et al., 1976) and one a decrease (Fujita et al., 1978). One study, while finding a correlation between CSF and plasma DBH activity, found no differences in CSF DBH activity among several psychiatric diagnostic groups (Lerner et al., 1978).

It is well known that the activity of DBH in plasma is, in part, under genetic control (Weinshilboum et al., 1975). In addition, the recent multigenerational family study by Böök et al. (1978) found that low DBH and low MAO activities were associated with schizophrenia within the family. While this finding may be an effect of neuroleptic use by the schizophrenic family members (Markianos, et al., 1976; DeLisi et al., 1981c), nevertheless DBH inhibitors, such as fusaric acid, produce significant psychopathology in normal subjects (Hartmann and Teschke, 1979), suggesting that altered DBH activity may be relevant in the pathogenesis of psychiatric disorders.

Catechol-0-methyltransferase (COMT)

While MAO is principally responsible for intraneuronal catecholamine metabolism, COMT provides the principal extraneuronal route for catecholamine inactivation. Wise et al. (1974) reported decreased brain COMT in post-mortem brains from chronic schizophrenics, but this was not confirmed in later studies (Wyatt et al., 1976; Cross et al., 1978). Several conflicting reports of alterations in erythrocyte COMT activity in psychiatric disorders have also appeared in the literature. While Matthysse et al. (1972) initially found significantly elevated mean erythrocyte COMT activity in chronic schizophrenic patients, they subsequently failed to confirm their findings in erythrocytes or fibroblasts (Groshong et al., 1978). From the data gathered in these few studies, it appears unlikely that there is a generalized deficit in COMT activity in schizophrenia.

Serum Creatinine Phosphokinase (CPK)

An elevation of serum CPK activity was first reported by Schiavone and Kaldor (1965) in schizophrenic patients and has subsequently been extensively studied, in particular by Meltzer (1979b). Studies have generally shown that newly hospitalized psychotic patients (acute and chronic schizophrenics, schizoaffectives, and affective psychotics) often have serum CPK activity that exceeds the upper limits of normal, while nonpsychotic patients less frequently show such elevations. In addition, patients with elevated serum CPK activity tend to have the more florid psychoses. Elevations range from being just above the 95-percent limit for normals to being over 200 times greater than the normal limit. The mean elevation, however, is two or three times greater than the upper limit of normals. Such elevations are usually transient, lasting only one or two days. There is also evidence of a more stable elevation of serum CPK activity in psychotic patients. When mean serum CPK activity levels throughout patients' hospitalizations have been determined, it has been found that the patients with the higher mean activities also had more frequent episodes of "true" elevations. Also, these patients' first-degree relatives frequently had elevated serum CPK activity. In conjunction with studies of serum CPK activity in monozygotic twins discordant for schizophrenia, these findings raise the possibility that serum CPK may be a genetic marker for psychosis. Family studies would help to determine whether elevated serum CPK activity actually segregates with psychosis.

MUSCLE DISORDER The elevated serum CPK activity noted in many psychotics is apparently of skeletal muscular origin. Both chromatographic and electrophoretic investigations have identified CPK as the skeletal muscle isoenzyme. Further, studies to detect elevations of brain CPK of psychotic patients have been consistently negative. Extensive histological studies in biopsies from psychotic patients have revealed abnormalities, such as an excess of atrophic fibers and Z-band streaming, findings that are consistent with the view that increases in serum CPK activity reflect muscle pathology. These histological abnormalities and the related elevations in serum CPK activity are probably secondary to an underlying neurogenic process. Studies of the branching patterns of subterminal motor nerves provide strong evidence for alpha motor neuron abnormalities in psychotics (Ross-Stanton and Meltzer, in press). There is also a correlation in psychotics between the degree of branching abnormality and the mean serum CPK activity. These findings are consistent with the view that the CNS provides some trophic input that is important in maintaining the integrity of skeletal muscle. Increased serum CPK activity has been reported in patients with several acute brain disorders including cerebrovascular disease, gliomas, anoxia, status epilepticus, brain trauma, and many others. The present evidence suggests that psychosis may have a similar effect. When seen in the context of these diverse brain disorders, however, elevated serum CPK activity and related findings do not necessarily seem relevant to the pathophysiology of a specific disorder, although they may indicate disturbed CNS function. Psychosis, it may be speculated, produces not only degeneration of peripheral neurons, as evidenced by increased branching of subterminal motor neurons, but also the degeneration of brain structures that is detected as enlarged ventricles (Ross-Stanton and Meltzer, in press).

NEUROTRANSMITTERS AND HALLUCINOGENS

Serotonin

PHYSIOLOGY Serotonin (5-hydoxytryptamine), a derivative of the amino acid tryptophan, has been associated with a number of normal and pathological processes. Serotonin is metabolized by MAO. Its product, 5-hydroxyindoleacetic acid (5-HIAA), can be measured in urine and CSF. The cell bodies of serotonergic neurons are localized in the midline raphe nuclei in lower midbrain and upper pons. Their axons are widely distributed throughout the brain.

There is believed to be a catecholamine-serotonin balance in the brain. Thus, Gerson and Baldessarini (1980) reported that increases or decreases of brain serotonin tended to decrease and increase, respectively, motor responses of animals to catecholaminergic drugs. In health, changes in catecholamine function can often be compensated for by suitable alterations in serotonergic activity.

SEROTONIN AND SCHIZOPHRENIA At least two serotonin hypotheses of schizophrenia have been proposed (Wyatt et al., 1971). One hypothesis suggests that some cases of schizophrenia might be associated with an imbalance between serotonergic systems (underactive) and dopaminergic systems (overactive) (Smythies, 1976). In contrast, the other hypothesis postulates that increased activity or abnormal metabolism of indoles may result in the production of an endogenous psychotogen (Green and Grahame-Smith, 1976). Attempts to validate these hypotheses have involved measurement of indolamines and their metabolites in schizophrenic patients, in response to pharmacologic challenges. These have often yielded conflicting or inconclusive results.

Several studies comparing CSF 5-HIAA concentrations in schizophrenic patients and controls have been performed (see Green and Grahame-Smith, 1976; Berger et al., 1980a). In a post-mortem study,

Bennett et. al. (1979) examined the now controversial view that binding levels of titrated LSD may be associated with postsynaptic serotonin receptors. They found that the levels were reduced forty percent to fifty percent in the frontal cortex of schizophrenic patients compared with controls. This change could not be attributed to the effects of the drugs that the patients had received. Other investigators, however, did not confirm these findings (Whitaker et al., 1981). Finally, increases in blood serotonin have been reported in schizophrenic patients (Freedman et al., 1981), particularly in those patients with abnormal CT scans (DeLisi et al., 1981).

Pharmacologic studies related to indoleamines have not been successful in confirming or refuting serotonergic hypotheses of schizophrenia. One of the authors (Wyatt, 1976) has reviewed the literature on the effects of neuroleptics on indoleamine functions. Although neuroleptics have some effect on serotonergic activity, the serotonergic system does not seem to be the primary site of neuroleptic action. On the basis of the serotonin-deficiency hypothesis, the clinical effects of the serotonin precursor, L-5-hydroxytryptophan (L-5-HTP), and a peripheral decarboxylase inhibitor, carbidopa, were administered to schizophrenic patients (Bigelow et al., 1979a). No significant change in the clinical status of the patients was noted with this L-5-HTP-loading strategy. Alternatively, the hypothesis of serotonergic overactivity suggests that schizophrenia might be treated with a drug such as p-chlorophenylalanine (PCPA) which inhibits tryptophan hydroxylase, the rate-limiting enzyme in the synthesis of serotonin. Since there have been few published double-blind studies with PCPA, no definitive statement can be made about the antipsychotic efficacy of this drug.

In summary, there is weak evidence suggesting a disturbance of indoleamine metabolism in schizophrenic patients. The nature and extent of such abnormalities are uncertain, but they do not appear to be of a primary etiologic significance in schizophrenia.

The Norepinephrine Hypothesis

In its simplest form the norepinephrine (NE) hypothesis of schizophrenia holds that there is a functional excess of norepinephrine in the brains of patients with schizophrenia and that this excess is related to the patient's psychopathology. This hypothesis has been tested with numerous biochemical and pharmacological approaches involving measurements of norepinephrine, its metabolites, and enzymes of synthesis and degradation, as well as its receptors in the periphery or in the brain itself. Pharmacological approaches have involved attempts to decrease psychopathology through inhibition of synthesis, monoamine depletion, and receptor blockade. Conversely, increased release and synthesis and decreased degradation have also been studied in schizophrenic patients.

BIOCHEMICAL STUDIES Direct measurements of noradrenergic function *in vivo* at present can only be done in peripheral studies. This approach assumes that functions in the periphery may shed some light on central functions. Bearing in mind the limitations of this assumption, positive findings can be categorized in three areas: increased plasma NE, enzyme abnormalities, and increased noradrenergic receptor binding. Increased plasma NE concentrations in chronic schizophrenic

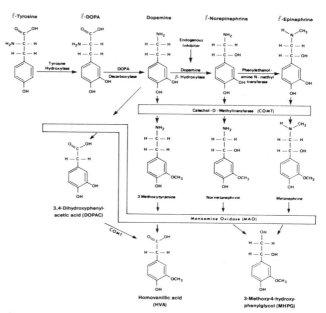

Figure 4. Metabolic pathway of norepinephrine and dopamine.

patients are thought to be an effect of neuroleptic treatment (Naber et al., in press). Three possible enzyme abnormalities (MAO, DBH, and COMT) are reviewed above. The remaining finding, increased noradrenergic receptor binding in platelets of chronic schizophrenic patients, occurs in a variety of other patients, including those with affective disorders (Kafka et al., in press). Although schizophrenic patients have been drug free at least two weeks in these studies, this period of time may not be sufficient to rid the platelet of the effect of neuroleptics. Even the association of this finding with patients with predominantly paranoid features (Jeste et al., in press) does not, in itself, rule out a neuroleptic effect. Finally, this particular binding site should be studied in post-mortem human brain, as its relevance is questionable if the finding occurs only in the platelet.

PHARMACOLOGICAL STUDIES   Another indirect approach to the study of the NE hypothesis involves pharmacological manipulations. One of the first successful pharmacological treatments of the schizophrenic syndrome involved reserpine, which depletes monoaminergic neuron terminals of dopamine, serotonin, and NE. The advent of phenothiazines and the correlation of their antipsychotic properties to their dopamine-blocking properties (Creese et al., 1976) has led to the conclusion that reserpine's antipsychotic properties are also related to its dopamine-depleting properties. Similarly, although L-dopa and amphetamine can exacerbate or mimic psychotic symptoms, for a variety of reasons their actions have been attributed to dopamine rather than to NE (reviewed by Matthysse, 1974). Reports of the therapeutic effects of propranolol in chronic schizophrenic patients has caused reexamination of the interpretations of these pharmacological findings (Yorkston et al., 1974). Attributing propranolol's efficacy to its β-adrenergic blocking properties has its problems as it appears that massive doses, far more than needed for β-blockade alone, are necessary for therapeutic benefits. Aside from the fact that the mechanism of action remains unclear, not all investigators have been able to demonstrate propranolol's benefits for schizophrenic patients (Bigelow et al., 1979b)*

CSF AND BRAIN NE   A third approach, measurement of NE in CSF, has yielded promising results. Norepinephrine concentrations in lumbar CSF of chronic paranoid schizophrenics have been observed to be elevated relative to controls (Lake et al., 1980). Whether or not lumbar CSF NE reflects brain or plasma NE or both remains to be determined. Moreover, the confounding variable of neuroleptic treatment has not been eliminated, and the finding has yet to be confirmed by other laboratories.

POST-MORTEM STUDIES   A fourth approach, post-mortem studies of noradrenergic functions, has reemerged in the last several years. An initial report of increased NE concentrations in limbic regions of paranoid schizophrenics (Farley et al., 1978) could not be confirmed by two other groups of investigators (Crow et al., 1978; Bird et al., 1979a), but a fourth group did find increased NE in the mesencephalon of paranoid schizophrenics (Carlsson et al., 1979). The two negative studies did not look at paranoid schizophrenics as a separate group, possibly obliterating differences between these subtypes. This appears to be relevant, as a larger, more recent study confirmed the initial finding and also found increased concentrations of 3-methoxy-4-hydroxyphenylglycol (MHPG), a NE metabolite in the nucleus accumbens, a limbic system nucleus, of paranoid schizophrenics (Kleinman et al., in press). Clearly, this approach has considerable promise, although questions of diagnosis, neuroleptic treatment, and the clinical relevance of these findings remain unanswered.

Although there is as yet no convincing or consistent evidence for a role of NE in the schizophrenic syndrome, there are several intriguing findings. Further consideration of this catecholamine as a pathogenic agent or marker is warranted.

The Dopamine Hypothesis

The dopamine hypothesis of schizophrenia holds that there is a functional excess of central dopaminergic activity. A secondary and supporting part of the hypothesis is that the neuroleptics act by blocking brain dopamine receptors. The role of dopamine and its relationship to schizophrenia have been well reviewed previously (Meltzer 1979b; van Kammen, 1979). The evidence supporting the dopamine hypothesis initially was derived from two findings: (1) the observation that drugs that increase brain dopamine, such as L-dopa and amphetamine, induce a "schizophrenic-like psychosis" when given in high or sustained dosages and (2) studies that show that neuroleptics block dopaminergic activity in a fashion correlated with their relative antipsychotic potency. Here we examine some of the support for the possibility that there is an excess of dopamine or that there is an increase in dopamine receptors.

*Preceptor's note: In their chapter Davis and his colleagues review the findings of 15 studies of the effect of propranolol and reaches a similar conclusion.

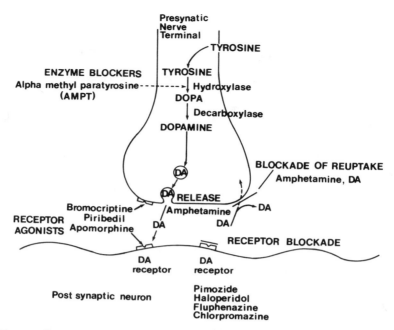

Figure 5. Schematic diagram of dopamine synapse.

CSF STUDIES A number of attempts have been made to understand central dopamine metabolism in schizophrenia. For example, Bowers (1974) measured the concentration of the dopamine metabolite, homovanillic acid (HVA), in CSF from schizophrenic patients. He pretreated his patients with probenecid, a drug that prevents HVA from leaving the CSF and thus forces HVA to accumulate. The amount of the accumulated HVA is thought to reflect dopaminergic neuronal activity or dopamine turnover. Bowers found decreased HVA concentrations in a schizophrenic group compared with a group of patients with affective disorders. If there is an overactivity of the central dopaminergic system in schizophrenic patients, one would expect that HVA would be increased, not decreased.

BRAIN DOPAMINE Bird et al. (1977; 1979a; 1979b) found increased dopamine concentrations in the nucleus accumbens and olfactory tubercle of schizophrenic brains. Several other investigators, however, could not confirm the finding in the nucleus accumbens (Kleinman et al., in press). Moreover, no consistent increase in dopamine metabolites has been found in schizophrenic brains.

DOPAMINE RECEPTORS Studies have demonstrated that psychosis can be precipitated by dosages of dopamine agonists (indirect/direct) that ordinarily would not induce a psychosis in normals (Janowsky and Davis, 1976). This implies that there are alterations in dopaminergic receptors. Also, Angrist et al. (1975) and Cotzias et al. (1976) have shown that high dosages of the dopamine agonists piribedil and apomorphine exacerbate psychosis.

Post-mortem brain studies have been used to examine the dopamine hypothesis. Several groups have found increases in dopaminergic bind-

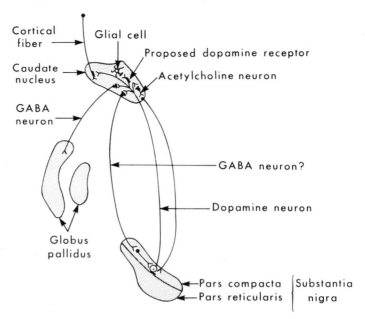

Figure 6. Schematic diagram of dopamine system projecting from substantia nigra to caudate nucleus. Similar dopamine projections go to limbic system and cortex. Heavy dark blocks at synapses indicate places where putative dopamine receptors are located. For example, the dopamine autoreceptor may be on the dendrites in the substantia nigra or on the axons in the caudate. Postsynaptic receptors are on the cortical projections to the caudate and GABA neurons projecting from the caudate.

ing sites in schizophrenic brains (Creese et al., 1975; Seeman et al., 1975; Kleinman et al., in press), while others have not (Reynolds et al., 1980; Mackay et al., 1980). Unfortunately, the data are mixed, and until further studies with larger groups of medication-free patients are conducted and more definitive results obtained, the findings can be attributed to an artifact. Further, few if any of the patients studied have had lifetimes free from neuroleptics, and administration of neuroleptics to rats has been shown to increase dopamine receptor numbers for prolonged periods after the drugs have been given. Nevertheless, if these findings are related to the etiology of schizophrenia, increased receptors are found in only some brains of schizophrenics. Crow et al. (1980) have suggested that patients with increased receptor numbers also have positive symptoms and normal-sized ventricles.

another e.g. of neuroleptic confound

AUTORECEPTORS   In recent years, it has become evident that there are dopamine receptors on dopamine neurons, although the exact location of these autoreceptors on the neuron is in dispute. Because of the dopamine autoreceptor, the presence of dopamine or dopamine-like agents will cause the neuron to slow its firing. In animals low dosages of dopamine agonists, stimulating the autoreceptor, induce hypomobility and decrease production of dopamine metabolites (Skirboll, 1979). Administration of apomorphine, a short-acting dopamine agonist, has been observed to lead to decrease of psychosis in unmedicated schizophrenics in some studies (Corsini et al., 1977a; 1977b; DiChiara et al., 1978; Smith et al., 1977) but not in all studies (Meltzer, 1979c). Recently, what might be an autoreceptor effect with the use of low dose apomorphine (0.005 mg/kg) in medicated schizophrenics has been demonstrated (Cutler et al., unpublished). Serum HVA decreased significantly following apomorphine, and there was an improvement in psychosis in three out of five of the patients. Meltzer (1980b) used a longer acting dopamine agonist, bromocriptine, in very small dosages (0.25 to 0.5 mg/d) in three schizophrenic patients and found beneficial results.

DOPAMINE DEPLETION Studies using agents such as α-methyl-paratyrosine (AMPT), a competitive inhibitor of tyrosine hydroxylase—the rate-limiting enzyme in the conversion of tyrosine to dopamine—have attempted to determine if reducing the amount of brain dopamine would decrease psychosis. Several studies showed no effect (Nasrallah et al., 1977; Gershon et al., 1967). Carlsson (1978), however, reported that AMPT did have an antipsychotic effect. It is possible that one reason for the negative results was the unresponsive nature of the illness in the patients chosen for the study (Nasrallah et al., 1980).

NEUROENDOCRINE The mesolimbic and mesocortical dopaminergic centers of the brain have been postulated to be critically involved in the schizophrenic psychosis. Development of neuroendocrine strategies for studying schizophrenia has been vigorous because of the difficulty in directly measuring central dopaminergic systems in man. As a result, the status of dopamine contained in the tuberoinfundibular neuroendocrine system of patients, as a reflection of limbic system functioning, has been examined. In addition, various neuroleptic agents have been shown to produce effects on these neurons. These effects can be readily and reliably measured by blood prolactin (PRL) and growth hormone (GH) concentrations.

Prolactin concentrations increase with neuroleptics and decrease with dopamine agonists. Initial studies attempting to confirm the dopamine hypothesis examined whether PRL concentrations in schizophrenics were different from those of controls (Meltzer et al., 1974). No significant difference was found. Clinical response and initial PRL concentrations were found to be positively correlated with neuroleptics (Meltzer and Fang, 1976). Further studies are needed to examine the relationship between PRL response to neuroleptics and clinical outcome.

From another perspective, Brown and Laughren (1981) and Laughren et al. (1979) examined PRL concentrations as a predictor of relapse in schizophrenic patients maintained on neuroleptics. They found that the lower the PRL concentrations (6.0 ng/ml), the greater the chance for relapse if the patient was withdrawn from neuroleptics. These studies may have useful clinical implications if their results can be confirmed in larger populations.

Prolactin concentrations and psychopathology in schizophrenic patients have been examined by Johnstone et al. (1977) and Kleinman et al. (submitted). Both groups found inverse relationships between the degree of psychopathology and PRL concentrations. Furthermore, when schizophrenics were separated into groups defined by normal and abnormal ventricular size, the inverse relationship was found only in the normal-sized ventricle group. This fits into the hypothesis that a group defined by normal ventricular size will have increased dopaminergic function.

The response of growth hormone (GH) to various dopamine agonists is used as a measure of possible central dopaminergic activity and responsivity. The GH response has been used as a predictor of treatment response and to determine receptor alterations.

Rotrosen et al. (1976; 1978) examined the GH response to apomorphine in acute and chronic schizophrenic patients. They found that the schizophrenics who had a blunted GH response to apomorphine were neuroleptic responders, while the schizophrenic patients with marked GH responses did not respond to neuroleptics. The patients with the exaggerated responses to 0.5 mg of apomorphine had increases in GH concentrations between 40 and 60 ng/ml. Recently, Hirschowitz and Garver (1981) examined schizophrenic patients' GH response to 0.75 mg of apomorphine administered subcutaneously. The patients they studied had a mean peak of 38.7 ng/ml of GH concentrations, were responders to lithium therapy, and were diagnosed as having a schizophreniform disorder. In addition, consistent with these results, Pandey et al. (1977) found greater apomorphine-induced GH responses in acute versus chronic schizophrenics. The implications of the findings by Rotrosen et al. (1976) and Hirschowitz and Garver (1981) may provide a useful index for predicting treatment alternatives in heterogeneous groups of schizophrenic patients.

With regard to receptor alterations, Tamminga et al. (1977) examined apomorphine and L-dopa GH and PRL response in tardive dyskinesia patients. They expected that the postulated supersensitive dopaminergic postsynaptic receptor alterations would demonstrate increased GH and PRL responses. No increases were found. This suggests that the tuberoinfundibular dopaminergic system does not show the postulated supersensitive receptor alterations in tardive dyskinesia.

The neuroendocrine strategies for studying dopaminergic mechanisms in schizophrenia appear to be less useful for PRL concentrations than initially promised. Nevertheless, the findings of Kleinman et al. (submitted) of an inverse relationship between PRL concentrations and psychopathology in schizophrenic patients with normal ventricular size are of interest and need further examination. With regard to the GH response of various dopaminergic agonists, particularly apomorphine, the findings of Hirschowitz and Garver (1981) and of Rotrosen et al. (1976), if confirmed in larger study populations, may develop into a predictor of response to neuroleptics.

In conclusion, the dopamine hypothesis of schizophrenia has stimulated important developments in the knowledge about the physiology, biochemistry, and neuroanatomy of the dopamine system in animals and man. The mixed findings that not all schizophrenic patients improve with dopamine antagonist drugs and the inconsistent results of post-mortem studies, along with recent biochemical data, encourage reformulation of the hypothesis. In the future, research should focus more on the dynamic change in receptor physiology, not merely on excess of dopamine production.*

*Preceptor's note: In their chapter Davis and his colleagues offer another discussion of the dopamine hypothesis and review the effects of neuroleptics on GH response and PRL concentrations.

Phenylethylamine (PEA)

PEA is an endogenous amine found in blood, urine, and CSF (Karoum et al., 1979). In the human brain the highest concentrations are found in the limbic system (Borison et al., 1977). PEA has been hypothesized to be of etiological importance in some schizophrenic persons because of its structural and pharmacological resemblance to amphetamine (Sandler and Reynolds, 1976; Wyatt et al., 1977). Normal persons ingesting amphetamine in sufficient doses may develop psychotic symptoms that are clinically indistinguishable from paranoid schizophrenia (Connell, 1958; Griffith et al., 1970). The overlap in symptoms makes it possible to misdiagnose amphetamine intoxication when the history of amphetamine ingestion is not known. Phenothiazines and other dopamine-blocking agents are somewhat successful in the treatment of both amphetamine intoxication and schizophrenia.

Amphetamine intoxication has been widely used as an animal model for schizophrenia. In the laboratory setting, amphetamine and PEA produce similar stereotypies in animals, although PEA is less potent and has a shorter duration of action (Borison et al., 1977; Randrup and Munkvad, 1967). The PEA- and amphetamine-induced stereotypies in animals are blocked by the neuroleptics that are clinically useful in treating schizophrenia, and the relative doses of neuroleptics required to block the stereotypies approximate the neuroleptics' relative clinical potency (Moja et al., 1978). Differences in pharmacological and behavioral effects of PEA and amphetamine in animals do exist, but the similarities are striking.

Fischer et al. (1968; 1972) were the first to measure urinary PEA excretion in psychiatric patients. They found elevated concentrations in a group of seven schizophrenic subjects and later confirmed this elevation in PEA excretion in four additional schizophrenic subjects. Suzuki and Yagi (1977) did not confirm these findings in the five schizophrenic subjects they studied. Schweitzer et al. (1975) found normal urinary PEA excretion in three acute schizophrenic subjects. Lack of sufficient assay sensitivity and specificity may have contributed to these divergent findings.

Potkin et al. (1979), using a highly specific and sensitive mass fragmentography assay, measured PEA in 24-hour urine collections from 31 chronic schizophrenic patients (16 paranoid and 15 nonparanoid) and 32 nonhospitalized normal controls. The urinary PEA excretion (ug/24 hour) was statistically significantly higher for the 16 paranoid chronic schizophrenics than for the 15 nonparanoid chronic schizophrenics and the 32 normal controls. The urinary PEA excretion of the paranoid group was more than twice that of the other two groups. The elevated PEA excretion in the paranoid group was considered not to be related to hospitalization, medication, or diet because both the paranoid and nonparanoid schizophrenics were hospitalized on identical wards for similar time periods and received comparable treatments. Further, eight patients studied on and off neuroleptics failed to demonstrate a neuroleptic effect on PEA excretion.

The paranoid-nonparanoid classification was used in a cross-cultural collaborative study conducted in Bombay, India (Jeste et al., in press). Hospitalized schizophrenic patients were subdivided into a paranoid group of 39 and a nonparanoid group of 11. Twenty-four urine samples were collected from these two groups and from a control group of psychiatrically normal persons who were hospitalized for cosmetic plastic surgery. Paranoid schizophrenics once again had the highest 24-hour PEA excretion (ug/24 hour) of the groups. While the pattern of elevations for the Indian schizophrenics and controls was similar to that for the subjects in the United States study, the absolute PEA values for all three Indian groups were lower than those for their United States counterparts. Body weight differences do not entirely explain these differences, raising the possibility of genetic, metabolic, or environmental influences. When urinary PEA excretion is expressed in ug/g creatinine, however, the paranoid groups remain the highest PEA excretors, and the differences in PEA excretion between the Indian and United States subjects disappear. The major difference in psychiatric treatment between the Indian schizophrenics and the United States schizophrenics was the longer average hospitalization for the United States patients. The Indian subjects had been hospitalized only several weeks compared with several years for the United States schizophrenics. But the fact that the United States controls had never been hospitalized argues against length of hospitalization as an important factor.

Using the same mass fragmentography assay, Karoum et al. (1979) found that a group of United States unipolar depressed patients had lower urinary PEA excretion (ug/24 hour) than the paranoid schizophrenics in the United States study, suggesting some diagnostic specificity. Nevertheless, in the original Fischer et al. study (1968), manic patients were also found to be high PEA excretors. Therefore, the question of diagnostic specificity requires further study. Even within the chronic schizophrenic population, high urinary PEA excretion is neither necessary nor sufficient for paranoid schizophrenia. The frequency of elevated PEA excretion in other paranoid and nonparanoid groups remains to be determined. Further, while a great deal is known about amphetamines' ability to produce a paranoid psychosis, the potential psychotomimetic effects of PEA in humans require elucidation.

L-γ-aminobutyric Acid (GABA)

PHYSIOLOGY GABA is formed from L-glutamic acid through the action of the enzyme L-glutamic acid decarboxylase (GAD). GABA is metabolized by GABA-glutamate transaminase (GABA-T) to succinic semialdehyde. GABA is thought to be an inhibitory neurotransmitter, with the highest concentrations found in the substantia nigra, globus pallidus, and hypothalamus. It is postulated that GABA serves to counteract central dopaminergic activity (Figure 6).

GABA AND SCHIZOPHRENIA Robert (1972) proposed that schizophrenia was associated with a deficiency of GABA, resulting in dopaminergic hyperactivity. Later, on the basis of the finding of marked reductions in GABA activity in the brains of patients with Huntington's disease, Bird (1976) and others suggested that schizophrenia, which shares some clinical features with Huntington's disease, may also be related to GABA deficits. Two ways in which investigators have tested the hypothesis of GABA'ergic hypoactivity in schizophrenia have been (1) measurement of GABA and related enzymes in the CNS of schizophrenic patients and (2) studies of the effects of putative GABA'ergic drugs on schizophrenic symptoms.

CSF   In a recent study Zimmer et al. (1980) reported that CSF concentrations of GABA were significantly higher in neuroleptic-treated schizophrenic patients compared with controls. Neuroleptic withdrawal for four weeks, however, resulted in a drop in the CSF GABA concentrations to near control values. Two post-mortem studies of the brains of schizophrenic patients and controls found no meaningful differences in the activity of GAD and in the binding associated with GABA receptors (Bennett et al., 1979; McGeer and McGeer, 1979). It should be noted that measuring the *in vivo* functional activity of enzymes associated with GABA is still not possible.

PHARMACOLOGIC CHALLENGES   Putative GABA'ergic drugs such as benzodiazepines (Haefely, 1978) have been tried in the treatment of schizophrenia. Generally, the results concerning specific antipsychotic effects have been equivocal or disappointing. Clinically, it is usually difficult to rule out the likely contribution of sedation to the apparent antipsychotic efficacy of the GABA'ergic drugs. Furthermore, Tamminga et al. (1978) reported that muscimol, a drug that excites GABA-like activity, produced a worsening of psychotic symptoms in schizophrenic patients.

To conclude, the available data do not support the hypothesis of a GABA deficit in schizophrenia. It would be premature, however, to write an obituary for that hypothesis. Further study is needed to fully understand GABA's relationship to schizophrenia.

Hallucinogens

Hallucinogens comprise a loosely related group of pharmacological compounds that, after acute administration, induce hallucinations, delusions, or both without altering sensorium. Over thirty years of extensive basic and clinical research have produced a wealth of information about the properties of many of these substances. Yet the pharmacological basis of the so-called psychedelic state remains unclear. Hallucinogens have been linked to schizophrenia in primarily three ways: (1) as a pharmacological model for the illness, (2) as exogenous etiological factors, and (3) as endogenous etiological factors.

HALLUCINOGENS AS PHARMACOLOGICAL MODELS   Overall, LSD, mescaline, and related compounds have not provided useful pharmacological models of schizophrenia. The psychedelic state is only weakly analogous to acute schizophrenia, and it cannot be concluded that it is blocked—rather than masked—in either animals or man by neuroleptic drugs. Tolerance to LSD quickly develops in most test systems. Furthermore, although LSD has effects on catecholaminergic neuronal systems, its primary actions appear to involve the median raphe system of serotonergic neurons (Freedman, 1978). This is perhaps more relevant to our understanding of dream formation than schizophrenia.

A better psychotomimetic may be phencyclidine (PCP), a drug which has hallucinogenic properties and was developed in the 1950's as a general anesthetic. In some individuals PCP induces a psychotic state phenomenologically indistinguishable from schizophrenia. Symptoms include depersonalization, paranoid delusions, fearfulness, flat affect, social withdrawal, catatonia, and violent behavior (Fauman and Fauman, 1980). The psychosis may persist for a week or longer. PCP has also been reported to exacerbate symptoms in schizophrenic patients (Luisada, 1978). From the point of view of a pharmacological model, these effects are more similar to schizophrenia than are the psychedelic states, but they do not invariably follow administration of the drug.

The pharmacological actions of PCP are protean and complicated, varying from arousal to coma and convulsions. Its psychotogenic effects probably do not reflect changes solely in the neurotransmitter systems currently related to schizophrenia, and neuroleptic drugs are not uniformly effective in blocking these effects (Freed et al., 1980). Finally, in addition to dopaminergic, noradrenergic, serotonergic, and acetylcholinergic actions (Johnson et al., 1978) PCP may involve specific brain receptor binding sites (Vincent et al., 1979; Zukin et al., 1979), but the functions of these sites are unknown.

HALLUCINOGENS AS EXOGENOUS ETIOLOGICAL FACTORS

There have been many anecdotal reports that hallucinogenic drugs precipitate psychotic episodes that persist well beyond the pharmacological half-lives of the drugs. These reports, together with extensive clinical experience, have led to the belief that chronic use of LSD, mescaline (Bowers, 1972), PCP (Smith, 1980; Fauman and Fauman, 1980), and even marijuana (Meyer, 1978) can play a primary etiological role in producing prolonged psychosis. Nevertheless, in the absence of prospective studies, we do not know the extent to which the drug effect may be a catalytic effect in a prepsychotic individual or the result of an attempt at self-medication in someone already psychotic.

HALLUCINOGENS AS ENDOGENOUS ETIOLOGICAL FACTORS

Noting the structural similarity between mescaline and norepinephrine, Osmond and Smythies (1952) proposed that abnormal methylation of neurotransmitter substances could produce endogenous hallucinogens. This led to the transmethylation hypothesis of schizophrenia (see Gillin et al., 1978). The most compelling support for this hypothesis is two fold. First, methionine, a putative methyl donor, can exacerbate schizophrenic psychosis, and second, methyl transferase enzymes capable of synthesizing hallucinogens, such as dimethyltryptamine (DMT), have been identified in human tissues. The major problem with this hypothesis is that no one has conclusively demonstrated abnormal synthesis, concentration, or metabolism of any abnormally methylated amines in schizophrenic patients. Nevertheless, a transmethylation hypothesis is still relevant to schizophrenia research, if only because there are probably other unexplored methylated compounds with potential hallucinogenic properties. It is also relevant because the psychoactive effects of a drug may vary depending upon whether it is exogenously administered or whether it exists in an endogenous form. For example, corticosteroids administered exogenously can produce mania and psychosis, while endogenous hypercortisolism, e.g., Cushing's disease, is more often associated with depression. By the same token, endogenously occurring hallucinogenic compounds may behave differently when administered in experimental tests.

DIALYSIS If a toxic factor exists in plasma of schizophrenics, then a logical treatment procedure might be the use of hemodialysis. Hemodialysis was first reported as a treatment for schizophrenia by Feer and colleagues in 1960. While subsequent uncontrolled trials have reported remarkable improvements, double-blind evaluations of this form of treatment have not proved its effectiveness (Schulz et al., 1981). Regardless of the efficacy of dialysis as a form of treatment for schizophrenia, its use has led to the finding of an abnormal polypeptide in the dialysate of these patients (Palmour et al., 1977). Other investigators, however, have been unable to confirm the presence of an abnormal polypeptide.

OTHER BIOCHEMICAL FACTORS

Endogenous Opiates

The discovery of endogenous opiate-like peptides, endorphins, in mammalian brains (Hughes, 1975) has led to hypotheses concerning their role in schizophrenia. These hypotheses have been tested using pharmacological and biochemical approaches. Pharmacological approaches have involved administration of narcotic antagonists, such as naloxone, or endorphins themselves to patients with schizophrenia. More recently, direct biochemical measurements of endorphins have been made in post-mortem studies of the brains of schizophrenic patients.

NALOXONE In initial open trials naloxone reduced psychopathology in schizophrenic patients (Gunne et al., 1977). Double-blind studies, however, have yielded mixed results.* One successful study involved an apparently unusual subtype of schizophrenic patients who had chronic unremitting auditory hallucinations. Regardless of the differing results, the therapeutic benefits are at best of modest proportions, and naloxone does not appear to constitute a major new treatment modality.

ENDORPHIN TRIALS A second approach has involved administration of endorphins to schizophrenic patients. The results of initial open trials, where β-endorphin was given to schizophrenic patients, were confusing at best (Kline et al., 1977). Subsequent double-blind controlled studies of β-endorphin given to schizophrenic patients have yielded no results to confirm significant therapeutic benefits (Berger et al., 1980b). Another endorphin, des-tyrosine-γ-endorphin, has been reported to be of benefit to schizophrenic patients (Verhoeven et al., 1979), but attempts to reproduce these findings have failed (Tamminga et al., 1981; Casey et al., 1981).

MEASUREMENTS OF ENDORPHINS Elevations of a variety of endogenous opiates have been detected in plasma and CSF of schizophrenic patients (reviewed by Berger et al., 1980b). Plasma findings have not been confirmed, and neuroleptics reportedly return elevated CSF endorphins to normal.

*Preceptor's note: For a review of studies of naloxone as a therapeutic agent, see the chapter by Davis and his colleagues.

Finally, attempts have been made to measure endorphins in post-mortem schizophrenic brains. Methionine-enkephalin concentrations in caudate nuclei were elevated in a small number of the brains of chronic undifferentiated schizophrenic patients, relative to the brains of chronic paranoid schizophrenic patients and normal controls (Kleinman et al., in press). No significant differences were found in four other brain regions (nucleus accumbens, putamen, globus pallidus, and hypothalamus). Reports that neuroleptics raise methionine-enkephalin concentrations in rat brains certainly support the idea that these elevations are drug induced. The question then arises as to why paranoid schizophrenics did not have the same elevations. Accuracy of subtype diagnosis, neuroleptic treatment, and the small number of subjects are obvious problems with this study.

Another post-mortem study has measured tritiated opiate binding in schizophrenic brain tissue (Reisine et al., 1980). Decreased opiate binding in caudate nuclei of chronic schizophrenic patients has been reported and awaits confirmation from other laboratories. The significance of this finding in light of previous neuroleptic treatment remains to be determined.

The endorphin hypothesis of schizophrenia is obviously still in its infancy. There remains considerable disagreement as to which endorphin is involved and whether it is increased or decreased. Nevertheless, the several positive findings do warrant further consideration.

Megavitamin Therapy and Orthomolecular Psychiatry

Megavitamin therapy initially was described as the use of large doses of niacin (vitamin B_3) for the treatment of schizophrenia. This treatment was based on the hypothesis that niacin acted as a methyl group acceptor, thereby preventing the formation of abnormally methylated psychotogens. Later the therapy was extended to include nicotinamide adenine dinucleotide (NAD), and ultimately it included ascorbic acid, pyridoxine (vitamin B_6), folic acid, vitamin B_{12}, and other vitamins, minerals, and dietary therapies. The name was changed to orthomolecular psychiatry to reflect the expansion in theory and treatment (Pauling, 1968). The treatment for schizophrenia is almost always added to existing pharmacological and somatic treatments, such as neuroleptics or ECT.

NIACIN (NICOTINIC ACID, VITAMIN B_3) AND NIACINAMIDE
The initial major report claiming the efficacy of nicotinic acid in the treatment of schizophrenia was published by Hoffer and colleagues (1957). The rationale was that ingestion of a strong methyl group acceptor like niacin would prevent the conversion of norepinephrine to epinephrine and the hypothesized subsequent conversion to adrenochrome and adrenolutin. In the double-blind study, patients were given 3.0 g/day of nicotinic acid and nicotinamide for thirty days, in addition to ECT as indicated. The results showed a small degree of improvement on the vitamin over placebo during the hospitalization and a decreased relapse rate in the vitamin group over the next four years. Only 13 of 74 patients, however, had remained on nicotinic acid after discharge.

A second double-blind study found improvement during hospitalization on nicotinic acid but little difference in relapse rate (Osmond and Hoffer, 1962). In a double-blind study by Denson (1962), patients received nicotinamide or placebo, in addition to ECT and neuroleptics. Those on nicotinamide had a shorter period of hospitalization. Unfortunately, methodological problems preclude strong support for these conclusions (American Psychiatric Association, 1973; Wyatt, 1974). Moreover, subsequent double-blind studies have failed to confirm the positive effects (Ashby et al., 1960; Meltzer et al., 1969; McGrath et al., 1972). Additionally, questions regarding whether *in vivo* formation of adrenochrome actually occurs and questions regarding the psychotomimetic properties of adrenochrome itself have cast doubt on the underlying rationale for the niacin treatment. Further, nicotinic acid in doses up to 3.0 g/day does not reduce the ability of stressed subjects to excrete epinephrine (methylated norepinephrine) or change the ratio of epinephrine to norepinephrine (Ellerbook and Purdy, 1970). It should be noted, however, that this latter research was performed on normal stressed subjects. Further study is required to determine the effects on schizophrenic patients.

Regardless of whether the hypothesized basis of using niacin is sound, the critical question is whether niacin treatment is useful for schizophrenic patients. Although niacin has been the cornerstone of megavitamin therapy, orthomolecular psychiatry has become highly complex, using neuroleptics, ECT, and many other vitamins and minerals. Because treatment is highly individualized, it is extremely difficult to conduct replication trials.

In an attempt to replicate the major components of orthomolecular therapy, Ban, Lehmann, and Deutsch (1977) gave twenty hospitalized chronic schizophrenic patients chlorpromazine plus megavitamins. The chlorpromazine was given in standard doses. The megavitamin treatment consisted of nicotinic acid (1.0 g to 9.0 g/day), thiamine (300 mg/day), pyridoxine (150 mg/day) hydroxycobalamine (0.5 mg/day) and ascorbic acid (1.0 g to 3.0 g/day). This 24-week, double-blind study found no statistical differences between the two groups, although there was a trend toward greater improvement in the chlorpromazine and placebo group over the chlorpromazine and megavitamin group.

The best attempts to confirm the claims for the utility of vitamin therapies were carried out by the Canadian Mental Health Association. The Canadian studies, as reviewed by the American Psychiatric Association (APA) Task Force on Vitamin Therapy (1973), found no support for the utility of nicotinic acid or nicotinamide for decreasing hospitalization, reducing the requirements for phenothiazines, or producing a more rapid response to medication. In general, the Canadian studies found no therapeutic effects in acute or chronic schizophrenia, whether the treatment was with niacin alone or was niacin combined with pyridoxine or neuroleptics. In fact, the APA Task Force, in reviewing the data, concluded that niacin and nicotinamide are not effective.

ASCORBIC ACID (VITAMIN C)   Pauling et al. (1973) found that urinary excretion of ascorbic acid was low in a group of schizophrenics. Administration of 10.0 g/day ascorbic acid for a week corrected their urinary ascorbic acid excretion to the normal range. In a double-blind study, Milner (1963) found that a predominantly schizophrenic group improved when given 1.0 g/day of ascorbic acid. Many of these patients, however, had clinical symptoms of scurvy that disappeared with ascorbic acid treatment, and most had been chronically hospitalized.

Maas, Gleser, and Gottschalk (1961) found low levels of urinary ascorbic acid in both anxious schizophrenics and neurotic patients, suggesting a relationship of low excretion of ascorbic acid to anxiety. In mice, however, pharmacological doses of ascorbic acid blocked amphetamine-induced stereotyped behavior, suggesting a possible relationship between ascorbic acid and dopamine. These findings suggest that the role of vitamin C in schizophrenia may warrant further investigation.

MINERALS Orthomolecular psychiatry also uses mineral treatment, based on the assumption that mental illness may result from an abnormal need for vitamins and minerals other than those mentioned above. Pfeiffer et al. (1973) found low blood zinc in 11 percent and high copper in twenty percent of schizophrenic outpatients but did not report using a control group. These researchers believe that as many as thirty percent of schizophrenics have elevated body and urinary pyrrole excretion. The pyrroles are hypothesized to combine with pyridoxine and zinc to produce a syndrome characterized by B_6 and zinc deficiency, symptoms of schizoaffective schizophrenia, and the physical manifestations of deficiencies. Cruz and Vogel (1978) could not consistently confirm elevated pyrrole excretion in nine schizophrenics and ten controls.

Pfeiffer and Braverman (1979) state that, in addition to the pyrrole-excreting group of schizophrenics that comprise thirty percent of the schizophrenics in their practice, two other groups exist. The histapenic group (fifty percent) has low blood histamine, high serum copper, and low folate and are treated with B_{12}, folic acid, zinc, niacin, vitamin C, and manganese. The histadelic group (twenty percent) has high blood histamine and low-normal serum copper. To assess the frequency of such biochemical groups and the degree of response to dietary treatment, double-blind studies in groups of carefully diagnosed schizophrenics are needed.

Other interest in minerals lies both in their important role as cofactors in enzymatic steps in the indole and catecholamine pathways and in their role in disorders like Menke's syndrome, Wilson's disease, and manganese poisoning, disorders which may produce psychotic symptoms. Studies of serum magnesium in schizophrenia have produced inconclusive results. Yassa and Nair (1979) found low serum magnesium in schizophrenics, compared with a group of nonpsychotic, mentally retarded patients, but they found no difference in calcium or phosphorus. Within a group of twenty schizophrenics, low serum calcium and magnesium predicted the occurrence of extrapyramidal symptoms (EPS) with low doses of neuroleptics. Further, the 16 patients that developed EPS had significantly lower drug-free serum calcium than the six patients in whom EPS did not develop.

While elevated serum copper is found in some schizophrenic patients, it is a nonspecific finding. Tyrer, Delves, and Weller (1979) report low CSF copper in schizophrenics. They interpret their findings as consistent with reduced CNS activity of the copper-dependent enzymes tyrosine hydroxylase and DBH. In a study of 76 schizophrenics and 62 normal controls, Gillin and associates (unpublished) found no differences in zinc or copper in serum, urine, CSF, hair, and gastric aspirates.

The claims of the efficacy of mineral treatments in subgroups of schizophrenics require replication in carefully designed double-blind studies.

It is clear that some psychiatric patients do have vitamin and mineral deficiencies and that these deficiencies are usually accompanied by corresponding clinical signs. Moreover, the value of vitamins, minerals, and some nutrients has been clearly established for optimal brain function. Data suggesting their utility in large doses for treating schizophrenia, however, are currently largely lacking. However, the goal of orthomolecular psychiatric therapy put forth by Pauling as "the treatment of mental disease by the provision of the optimum molecular environment for the mind, especially the optimum concentrations of substances normally present in the human body," offers much promise (Pauling, 1968, 265).

Gluten

In 1966, Dohan suggested that gluten, a component of cereal grains, may be a major pathogenic factor in the production of overt schizophrenic symptoms and that a diet limiting gluten could be of therapeutic value. Observations of improvement of symptoms coinciding with severe restrictions of gluten-containing foods (like bread and cereal grain) are consistent with Dohan's hypothesis (Dohan, 1976). Dohan provided epidemiological support with the finding of a 0.96 correlation between the rate of mental hospital admissions for female schizophrenic patients and the change in wheat consumption of Canada, Finland, Norway, and the United States during World War II. Reports of a higher than expected occurrence of celiac disease in schizophrenic patients, as well as an increase of psychotic symptoms in celiac disease patients, created further interest in the gluten hypothesis of schizophrenia.

Dohan et al. (1969) examined the effects of a cereal grain-free, milk-free diet (CMF) on relapsed schizophrenic patients. They found that the number of days of hospitalization on a locked ward decreased on the experimental CMF diet. This improvement disappeared when gluten was "secretly" added to the diet. In a subsequent investigation, Dohan et al. (1973) found that schizophrenic patients on the CMF diet were discharged twice as fast as control patients and also that response to the diet occurred early in the hospitalization. In both studies, patients were treated with standard doses of neuroleptic drugs. Singh and Kay (1976) reported that a majority of schizophrenic patients improving on a CMF diet and on neuroleptic drugs demonstrated a reversal or interruption in their therapeutic progress when wheat gluten was given in a double-blind challenge. The deleterious effects of wheat gluten were most marked in the "more seriously ill patients with a less favorable therapeutic outcome" (Singh and Kay, 1976, 402). A gluten effect on neuroleptic absorption could explain the gluten-associated deterioration, but Luchins et al. (1980a) could find no effect of dietary gluten challenge on plasma neuroleptic concentrations.

Rice et al. (1978) studied 16 chronic schizophrenic patients and found that two patients improved during a four-week period of a gluten-free, milk-free diet. One patient who had been hospitalized for

13 years improved to the point that she could be discharged to her family. Potkin et al. (in press) studied eight young chronic schizophrenics on a CMF diet, challenged with wheat gluten and placebo in a double-blind manner. Daily challenge with wheat gluten for at least five weeks produced no deterioration in clinical status in any of the patients studied.

The existence of a subgroup of gluten-intolerant schizophrenic patients remains a possibility. Ashkenazi et al. (1979) found that about half of a group of schizophrenic patients and half of a group of nonschizophrenic patients, like celiac patients, demonstrated an antigenic response to gluten in their peripheral lymphocytes, implying that they had absorbed gluten. Yet none of the psychotic patients with the antigenic response had clinical symptoms of malabsorption or the abnormal xylose tolerance seen in celiac disease. Klee et al. (1978) have demonstrated that gluten-derived polypeptides have endorphin properties. The possibility that such compounds could be absorbed through an altered gastrointestinal tract and play a role in the generation of psychotic symptoms remains an interesting speculation.

Prostaglandins

PHYSIOLOGY The prostaglandins (PG) are a group of cyclic fatty acids first discovered in 1906 by Japelli and Scafa. They possess a number of neurophysiological properties. There are three main types of PG formed from the parent compound arachidonic acid: prostaglandin A (PGA), prostaglandin E (PGE), and prostaglandin F (PGF). The relationship between prostaglandins (PGE) and neurotransmitters was demonstrated by Bergstrom and co-workers in 1964. They found that PGE_1 depressed catecholamine release. Further studies have demonstrated that catecholamines and antipsychotic agents have opposing effects on PG concentrations; catecholamines enhance and neuroleptics inhibit secretion of PG.

SCHIZOPHRENIA A connection between PG and schizophrenia has been proposed by a number of investigators. Feldberg (1976) maintained that there was a perturbation of prostaglandin metabolism in schizophrenia. Patients with the diagnosis of schizophrenia were found to have complete inhibition of production in PGE_1 in platelets as compared with nonschizophrenics (Abdulla and Harmadah, 1975). Recently, Mathé et al. (1980) found increased total PGE (PGE_1 plus PGE_2) concentrations in CSF of schizophrenic patients. Horrobin (1980) interprets the findings of Mathé et al. (1980) as being consistent with a hypothesis of a deficiency of PGE in schizophrenia. Since PGE_1 inhibits the mobilization of arachidonic acid and there may be an alternate increase in formation of PGE_2, he further suggests that Mathé et al. (1980) may have been measuring an increase in PGE_2. Alternatively, brain dysfunction could produce changes in the prostaglandins, secondary to some other aspect of the disorder.

In summary, the metabolism of the prostaglandins in the CNS, with its modulations of the various neurotransmitter systems, such as the dopaminergic, noradrenergic, and others, suggests that PG perturbation could be an etiologic factor in schizophrenia. For the most part, however, the prostaglandin-schizophrenia relationship is conjectural.

Tardive Dyskinesia

Treatment with neuroleptics is generally recognized as the single most effective therapy for schizophrenia (Davis, 1980). Yet there is a heterogeneity among schizophrenic patients in their responsiveness to neuroleptics. According to Meltzer (1979b), therapeutic response to neuroleptics may be at least partly related to biochemical subtyping of the schizophrenic syndrome. Similar considerations probably apply to the development of side effects with neuroleptics, especially the development of tardive dyskinesia.

Tardive dyskinesia may be defined as a syndrome consisting of abnormal stereotyped involuntary movements, usually of choreoathetoid type and principally affecting the mouth, face, limbs, and trunk. These effects occur relatively late in the course of drug treatment, with drug treatment being a necessary factor in their etiology (Jeste and Wyatt, in press). Tardive dyskinesia is a serious iatrogenic disorder, both because of a progressive increase in its reported prevalence, and because the dyskinesia tends to persist long after withdrawal of neuroleptics in nearly two-thirds of the afflicted patients (Jeste and Wyatt, 1981).

Only a portion of patients treated chronically with neuroleptics develop dyskinesia, suggesting that predisposing constitutional factors are also necessary for its induction. The constitutional factor that has been most convincingly shown to be related to tardive dyskinesia is age (Smith and Baldessarini, 1980). From the viewpoint of subtyping of schizophrenia, biochemical and neuropathological studies of tardive dyskinesia deserve particular attention.

BIOCHEMICAL STUDIES It is possible to speculate that those schizophrenic patients who are at risk for developing tardive dyskinesia may have somewhat different neurochemical mechanisms from those who remain nondyskinetic despite neuroleptic treatment. In other words, the dyskinetic and nondyskinetic patients may belong to different subtypes of the schizophrenic syndrome. Studies have shown that schizophrenic patients with tardive dyskinesia have significantly lower MAO activity in platelets and lymphocytes and significantly higher DBH activity in plasma, as compared with well-matched controls. In a recent study the authors compared two groups of chronic schizophrenic patients, one with and the other without tardive dyskinesia, on a number of clinical, biochemical, and neuropathological variables. (Jeste et al., in press). Discriminant function analysis showed that two of the best discriminators between the two groups of patients were platelet MAO and plasma DBH activities. This suggests that dyskinetic patients have higher catecholaminergic activity, at least in the periphery. The interpretation of these findings must await further work. It is, however, tempting to consider two possibilities. On the one hand, schizophrenic patients who demonstrate low MAO and high DBH activities before neuroleptic treatment might be at a greater risk for developing tardive dyskinesia if they do receive treatment. On the other hand, those patients who respond initially to neuroleptics with a decrease in MAO and an increase in DBH activity might be more likely to develop dyskinesia later in the course of treatment. The association between tardive dyskinesia and low platelet MAO or high DBH activity was not universal, but was seen in a majority of the schizophrenic patients with dyskinesia. Also, it is not known if biochemical changes preceded or followed the onset of tardive dyskinesia.

NEUROPATHOLOGICAL STUDIES A number of investigators believe that schizophrenic patients with brain damage may be more prone to have neuroleptic-induced tardive dyskinesia. The definitions and criteria of brain damage used by different investigators have been variable, and so are the results of studies (see Jeste and Wyatt, in press). With a possible exception of β-mitten EEG pattern, the available techniques of measuring neuropathology, including CT, have generally failed to unravel a meaningful association between tardive dyskinesia and brain damage. Refinement of the neuropathological techniques may improve the ability to detect subtle brain damage.

DISCUSSION

Findings from the recent biochemical and morphological research in schizophrenia appear to cluster together in a manner that may shed light on the disorder itself. We have identified five dimensions around which the findings seem to cluster (see Table 2). By ordering the results in this manner, we do not intend to close the door on the possibility or even the likelihood that the findings are artifacts or secondary to the schizophrenia. Clearly, the development of tardive dyskinesia is secondary to being schizophrenic and to the drugs used to treat it. Moreover, there is increasing evidence that at least part of the decrease in platelet MAO activity is due to the medications used to treat schizophrenia. It is also too early to know if some of the morphological findings observed on CT scans are also medication related, although the available data suggest that this is not the case. Even if the MAO and CT scan abnormalities turn out to be due to medications, they are still of considerable interest. Not every schizophrenic patient treated with medications has decreased platelet MAO activity, and not every patient has alterations consistent with brain atrophy on the CT scan. Also, it is a peculiar coincidence that the low MAO activity is more likely to occur in the paranoid-hallucinatory group (consistent with the amphetamine-PEA model of schizophrenia), while the abnormal CT scans are more likely to occur in the poor premorbid history patients (consistent with the theory of a slowly developing process). Thus, even if these changes are due to medications, they say something about the vulnerabilities of the patients having them.

Dimension I: No Abnormal Morphology and Dimension II: Abnormal Morphology (see Crow, 1980)

The search for morphological changes in the brains of schizophrenic patients has had a long and rich tradition (Weinberger and Wyatt, in press[a]). With the explosion of neuropharmacological knowledge, interest in morphological abnormalities smoldered from the middle 1950's to the late 1970's. Then, with the advent of CT scans, there came a burst of renewed interest, and at least five abnormalities have been found. It is not clear yet how likely it is for a patient with one kind of the atrophy-like abnormalities to have one of the others, although the patients with abnormal asymmetries seem to have little evidence of atrophy. It is also not known what histological changes correspond to the gross anatomical changes. Since all the abnormalities seen with a CT scan in schizophrenia are also seen in neurological disorders, we know none of them are specific to schizophrenia. Furthermore, even within the psychiatric diagnosis, we do not know the specificity of the abnormalities since patients with diagnoses other than the schizophrenic disorders have been little studied.

Classic neurology is based on finding a circumscribed anatomical lesion that corresponds to a specific neurological deficit. If the abnormalities seen on the CT scan are causative of schizophrenia, the upset in brain function is probably of greater complexity than those of the usual neurological disorders. Given our current knowledge of how the brain works, it is difficult to understand how abnormalities surrounding the ventricles, in the cerebral cortex, in the pons, and in the anterior cerebellar vermis, could produce the signs and symptoms of schizophrenia. But these findings, and particularly enlarged ventricles, may reflect distant or diffuse brain changes.

Dimension III: Paranoid/Hallucinatory

The classification of paranoia has been present in psychiatric literature for over one hundred years. It was Kraepelin, however, through the many editions of his textbook, who tried to determine paranoia's place in schizophrenia. Kraepelin excluded from paranoid schizophrenia patients with chronic fixed delusions if they did not evidence personality deterioration and hallucinations (paranoia) and older patients developing a paranoid disorder (paraphrenia). In his paranoid schizophrenia group he did include those patients with paranoia, thought disturbance, emotional inappropriateness, and apathy. While Bleuler and others argued that paraphrenia was really late onset schizophrenia (and they may yet turn out to be correct), as we use the term *paranoid schizophrenia*, we are primarily using Kraepelinian classifications which also correspond to DSM-III.

The paranoid/nonparanoid distinction is one that many investigators have used to subdivide types of schizophrenia. Frequently, when this distinction is made, the paranoid group of schizophrenics tends to have become ill at a slightly older age than the nonparanoid patients, but the paranoid patients are not so old as to be considered paraphrenic. Also, the paranoid patients are usually more intact and have a greater chance for partial recovery.

In several recent studies it is the presence of *hallucinations* rather than paranoia that has allowed investigators to make successful distinctions between patients. Future research will have to examine to what extent paranoia and hallucinations are independent variables. Future researchers using the paranoid/hallucinatory dimension also need to consider such parameters as age of onset, premorbid personality, relative intactness of personality, and whether the paranoia is reactive to the presence of the hallucinations.

Many authors have described how the several associations clustering in the paranoid/hallucinatory dimension might fit together in a cause-and-effect manner. While it is unclear if low MAO activity is partially a primary effect or entirely a secondary effect related to medication, reduced MAO activity might in either case significantly alter the concentration of the natural substrates for this enzyme. The endogenous substrate with the greatest affinity for the form of MAO (type B) that is decreased in the platelet of schizophrenic patients is PEA. The fact that urinary PEA was found in two studies to be elevated in

Table 2. Schizophrenia-Research Dimensions

			DIMENSIONS		
Associations	I No Abnormal Morphology	II Abnormal Morphology	III Paranoid/ Hallucinations	IV Schizoaffective	V Tardive Dyskinesia
CT Scans	No Atrophy	A = Enlarged Ventricles B = Atrophic cortex C = Atrophy Anterior cerebellar vermis D = Small pons & cerebellum	Normal or Abnormal	Abnormal lateralization; Usually no evidence of atrophy	Normal or Abnormal
Premorbid History	Good	Poor	Mixed	Good	Mixed
Positive/ Negative Symptoms	Positive predominate	Negative predominate	Positive predominate	Mixed	Either may predominate
Dementia	Usually absent	Frequent (mild)	Little	None	Variable
I.Q. Scores	Usually Normal	Low	Usually Normal	Lower verbal than performance scores	Mixed
Course	Acute to unremitting	Unremitting	Relapsing to unremitting	Acute and relapsing	Usually unremitting
Neurological Signs	Usually absent	Frequently present	Stereotypy	Usually absent	Always present
Smooth-Pursuit Eye tracking	Usually good	Poor	Usually good	?	?

DIMENSIONS

Associations	I No Abnormal Morphology	II Abnormal Morphology	III Paranoid/ Hallucinations	IV Schizoaffective	V Tardive Dyskinesia
Neuroleptic response	Good	Poor	Variable	Good	Usually good (tardive dyskinesia)
Lithium response	Poor	Poor	Poor	Good with neuroleptics	Poor (tardive dyskinesia)
Response to Dopamine Agonists	Worse	Little change	?	?	Worse at large dosages; Variable at small dosages
Serum CPK	Normal	Normal	Normal	High	Normal
Platelet MAO Activity	Variable	Variable	Low	High	Low
Plasma DBH	Normal	Normal	Normal	?	High
CSF and Brain NE	Normal	Normal	High	?	?
Urine PEA	Variable	Variable	Low	?	?
HLA-type	Nonspecific	Nonspecific	?	Frequently HLA-A2	?

paranoid schizophrenic patients is of considerable interest, because PEA and amphetamine are structurally similar and produce many of the same behavioral effects.

↑ PEA
↓
↓ MAO
↓
↑ norep
↓
↑ schiz.

PEA recently has been shown to increase norepinephrine in the CSF of monkeys and in the brains of rats (Wyatt et al., in press). Furthermore, one of the areas of the brain where PEA has been found to increase norepinephrine, the nucleus accumbens, is the same brain area where norepinephrine has been found to be increased in paranoid schizophrenic patients. Finally, there is a suggestion that some neuroleptics work by blocking norepinephrine receptors and that propranolol, a β-adrenergic blocking agent, might be useful in treating some schizophrenic patients. This chain of events—from decreased MAO activity to increased brain norepinephrine—must be further explored.

Dimension IV: Schizoaffective

The term *schizoaffective* has meant many things since it was first used by Kasanin (1933). The title "The Acute Schizoaffective Psychoses" and content of Kasanin's paper indicate that he meant the term to mean a short-lasting illness which was an amalgam of symptoms from both the schizophrenic and affective disorders and which might have multiple recurrences. Since Kasanin's paper, schizoaffective has been thought variously to be a subtype of schizophrenia, a subtype of the affective disorders, a bridge between the two, or an entirely separate entity. A number of recent studies indicate that the proper placement of the schizoaffective disorder belongs more with the affective disorders than with schizophrenia (Abrams and Taylor, 1976; Pope et al., 1980). To a large degree, the research upon which these studies was based used very narrow criteria for diagnosing schizophrenia and gave the affective disorders more breadth. These studies, therefore, may be biased by their underinclusive criteria for schizophrenia and their overinclusive criteria for the affective disorders. The correctness of their conclusions awaits further study.

There are two groups of patients who are given the diagnosis of schizoaffective. One group of patients generally has a good short-term treatment response and a good long-term outcome. Another often has a poor prognosis and generally does not respond either to neuroleptics alone or to lithium alone, although they may respond to neuroleptics and lithium in combination (Bigelow et al., 1981).

What these two groups of patients have in common is the presence of both affective and schizophrenic symptoms. While the more chronic group probably never has full recovery between serious episodes, the groups also share some cyclicity of behavior. Determining where the schizoaffective dimension belongs as a subtype of the major psychoses and distinguishing more precisely between its acute and chronic forms is beyond the scope of this discussion but will be important to do when more data become available.

Dimension V: Tardive Dyskinesia

This dimension obviously runs orthogonally to the other dimensions, in that it is a reaction to treatment with neuroleptic medications. A patient has to be schizophrenic or have some other disorder that needs treatment with neuroleptics prior to developing tardive dyskinesia. The value of keeping tardive dyskinesia as a separate dimension, at least for the time being, is that the dimension encourages gathering important information about the physiology of the brains of the patients who develop tardive dyskinesia. Further, since there are overlapping hypotheses about the causes of schizophrenia and the causes of tardive dyskinesia, keeping tardive dyskinesia as a separate dimension may have a heuristic value.

CONCLUSION

The dimensions just described do not provide the clinician with material support, but are designed to provide a framework for ordering the diverse research being amassed in schizophrenia. Biochemical and morphological research on schizophrenia cannot yet give clinicians sound advice on how to prevent, lessen, or cure schizophrenia. Indeed, the substantial advances made in psychopharmacological treatment have developed in spite of our primitive state of knowledge of how the brain works and our especially limited knowledge of the cognitive and affective processes that are disrupted in schizophrenia.

Although studies of schizophrenia have increased our understanding of human biologic function, there is much left to be learned. Despite psychopharmacological treatment advances, our techniques for reducing or curing schizophrenia, at present, are limited. We are still unable to remove the excessive financial and emotional burdens of the schizophrenic patient, the patient's family, the clinician, and society. With our paucity of knowledge and working tools, necessity dictates that we continue to treat the full spectrum of patients similarly. In time, however, research efforts will provide the profound insight needed to lessen this burden and will give the clinician tools that are based on a fuller understanding of the disorder.

Introduction to the Treatment of the Schizophrenic Disorders
by Robert Cancro, M.D., Med.D.Sc.

The material presented in the earlier chapters, describing certain of the issues concerning how the schizophrenic disorders are conceptualized, diagnosed, and understood etiologically, forces the reader to several conclusions. The many different illnesses included under the rubric of the schizophrenic disorders differ strikingly. The people who are diagnosed as having a schizophrenic disorder vary in their premorbid personality, family history, age of onset, rapidity of onset, severity and kind of presenting symptoms, response to treatment, course of illness, and outcome. Because the diagnostic category represents a syndrome, the etiology varies as well. Every parameter which can vary does. This leads to the fundamental risk that the people so diagnosed become vulnerable to the fads and fantasies of the moment. The history of the treatment of these patients reveals that they have indeed been subjected to every conceivable assault and insult (Cancro, 1979). A knowledge of the ways in which schizophrenic patients have been injured in the guise of treatment will lead the clinician to a more humble and cautious therapeutic approach.

There can be no single treatment for these multiple disorders, which share their signs and symptoms selectively and intermittently. There must be many treatments. Yet, the recognition of the multiplicity of approaches does not mean that just any treatment approach is worth trying. Before all else the clinician must prevent harm, particularly since these patients do tend to recover in the long run. But not only must treatment be carefully chosen, it is also necessary to administer different treatments at the same time. It is highly improbable that a patient with a schizophrenic psychosis will respond rapidly to a single pure modality of intervention. Psychiatrists should be familiar with a number of different modalities and how best to integrate them into a comprehensive and consistent treatment plan.

This section reviews but three broad categories of treatment. These three are, nevertheless, of vital importance and are those in which psychiatrists and other mental health professionals have consistently shown the greatest interest. Drs. Douglas Heinrichs and William Carpenter review individual psychotherapy, and Dr. Samuel Keith and Ms. Susan Matthews discuss group and family therapy. In their review of pharmacotherapy, Dr. John Davis and his colleagues have prepared the longest chapter. The length of this chapter does not reflect an inherent verbosity on the part of biologic psychiatrists but rather illustrates the fact that there is more scientific knowledge available about the biology of living systems than about their psychosocial functioning. Together, the three chapters provide a very useful and comprehensive survey of the three treatment modalities.

Chapter 13

The Psychotherapy of the Schizophrenic Disorders
by Douglas W. Heinrichs, M.D. and William T. Carpenter, Jr., M.D.

INTRODUCTION

The authors conceive of psychotherapy as a treatment in which the relationship between the patient and the therapist is key. The relationship provides a context and a vehicle for the patient to develop some degree of self-understanding, with the belief that this understanding will facilitate therapeutic change. Therapy usually entails an articulation of psychodynamic patterns and pathogenic factors rooted in early experience. The critical ingredient, however, is the use of a relationship to encourage the patient to make a cognitive and affective reappraisal of the self and of his or her situation.

Workers committed to intensive psychotherapy of schizophrenia now work in isolation from those espousing other therapeutic strategies, paralleling the reduced interest and status for psychotherapy in general psychiatry and the growing defensiveness in the writings of psychotherapy advocates. Among the possible contributing factors are the growing interest in biologic models of etiology, the success of antipsychotic drugs, the increased emphasis on rigorous empirical research, and a public policy that spreads fixed mental health resources across the largest possible number of patients.

THE RISE OF BIOLOGIC AND GENETIC THEORIES OF THE ETIOLOGY OF SCHIZOPHRENIA

Biologic and genetic factors are important parts of the puzzle of schizophrenic etiology. In the ongoing nurture-nature debate, evidence for this has frequently been linked with the assumption that etiology should define treatment (Soskis, 1972). The argument that conditions with somatic etiology require somatic treatment and those with psychologic etiology require psychologic treatment is inaccurate. Nevertheless, linkage of etiology and treatment remains an important influence, not only in the thinking of many proponents of somatic treatments but among many advocates of psychotherapy as well. Hilde Bruch, for instance, in discussing historical considerations at a recent conference on the psychotherapy of schizophrenia, stated, "The treatment a mentally ill person receives depends to a large extent on the therapist's theoretical conceptions about the nature of the illness. In schizophrenia, there has been a continuous controversy around the question of whether its origin was of a psychological or an organic nature" (Bruch, 1980b, 3). She went on to state, "If you hold the assumption that schizophrenia is an unchangeable, organic illness, then psychotherapy will not be useful and will be very ineffective" (Bruch, 1980a, 71).

As long as proponents of psychotherapy accept the etiology-treatment link, their discomfort and defensiveness in response to the growing evidence for biologic and genetic factors in the origins of schizophrenia are understandable. However, there has been a growing realization that etiology itself is complex and must be conceptualized in terms of the interaction of multiple factors, some which are genetic and biologic and others which are psychologic and environmental in nature (Strauss and Carpenter, 1981). Furthermore, there is growing appreciation of the fact that even conditions involving organic factors can be significantly altered by psychologic and environmental means. Proponents of psychotherapy may acknowledge a role for organic factors in etiology while remaining vague about the nature of biologic factors.

It is here that the problem arises. While evidence continues to accumulate that permits progressively more specific hypotheses about the biologic deficit, the same has not occurred with respect to psychologic factors. Since most psychologic theories locate the problem in early parent-child interaction, one would expect to be able to demonstrate clear abnormalities in the organization and interaction of the families of schizophrenics. A number of such abnormalities have, in fact, been proposed based either on theoretical premises or clinical experience. However, as several recent reviews have noted, the vast majority of empirical attempts to differentiate the families of schizophrenics from other families have been either unsuccessful or inconsistent. The primary exception, communication deviance, is an intriguing variable that lends itself to several interpretations including a genetic one (Goldstein and Rodnick, 1975; Liem, 1980).

While current evidence makes it difficult to justify a psychotherapeutic approach to schizophrenia on any specific pathogenic pattern of parent-child interaction early in life, there are two alternate rationales. One is to justify it on the basis of an empirical demonstration of its efficacy. Another is to relate the psychotherapeutic mechanism to current functional abnormality and to conceptualize the illness in relation to current functioning. Fortunately, considerably more can be said here than with respect to etiology. Schizophrenics may find stressful life events disorganizing. They generally have difficulty forming and sustaining relationships with others. They frequently experience a deadening of their affective life and suffer from anhedonia. Sense of purpose and motivation are disturbed. Information processing is impaired, and accurate perception and interpretation of the environment are impeded. Based on these and other aspects of schizophrenic dysfunction, psychotherapeutic methods and goals may seem reasonable from a variety of perspectives. For example, engaging the patient in a stable, predictable, and unthreatening therapeutic relationship can be valuable in light of the social withdrawal and avoidance that tend to characterize the illness. The importance of the therapist's perspective in helping the patient to interpret reality with minimal distortion follows logically from the patient's difficulties in the realistic assessment of his or her environment. The patient's vulnerability to stress argues for psychotherapy to help the patient internalize a broader repertoire of coping strategies.

THE IMPLICATIONS OF ANTIPSYCHOTIC DRUGS

While the question of etiology has played an important role in theoretical discussions of schizophrenia, the single factor having the most profound impact on practice has been the development of antipsychotic drugs. Clinical trials suggested and clinical experience has proven that it is possible to treat many schizophrenic psychoses more effectively and less extensively with drugs than without. Not every schizophrenic patient responds to or requires antipsychotic drugs, but the majority does benefit from them. Initially, advocates of psychotherapeutic treatments were inclined to dismiss the drugs as forms of behavioral control that interfered with the psychotherapeutic process. This early polarization between psychotherapists and pharmacotherapists contributed to the view that these two treatments were in competition. Consequently, the demonstration of the efficacy of one is frequently experienced as a threat to the other. Although even the most enthusiastic pharmacotherapist does not regard medication as a comprehensive treatment in schizophrenia, the widespread use of antipsychotic drugs, combined with advances in social psychiatry, has, in fact, challenged the relevancy of the traditional psychotherapeutic approach. The setting for treatment has changed profoundly. Periods of severe psychosis have been shortened. Brief hospitalizations have replaced long-term hospital-based care. The patient returns to the community, and, if treatment is continued, it most often is in a public clinic in which therapeutic resources are limited.

This contrasts sharply with the traditional notion of psychotherapeutic work with the schizophrenic patient. Such work usually has implied intensive involvement between patient and therapist over many years. The patient was expected to have, especially early in the treatment, extended phases of regression, as well as hostile and negativistic reactions to the therapist. The gradual working through and resolution of such phases was seen as an important element in successful therapy. Extended periods of regression would require considerable management, often in a hospital setting. Similarly, the hospital setting could guarantee that the therapist had continued access to the patient, even when the patient was hostile and rejecting. Such a model is not appropriate in today's usual treatment setting and, incidentally, was never really available to the majority of patients. Quite apart from the question of validity of traditional models of psychotherapy, the manner in which they have usually been practiced is no longer directly applicable to the typical schizophrenic patient. Thus, it has become necessary to demonstrate that psychotherapeutic strategies can be effectively modified to deal with the current treatment setting.

In addition, the development of antipsychotic drugs has shown the importance of defining therapeutic efficacy in more specific terms, namely, by indicating which dimensions of symptomatology are benefited by a given treatment, which are unaffected, and which, if any, are made worse (Carpenter, 1980). Antipsychotic drugs have proven to be powerful in reducing and preventing psychotic symptoms, but they have not been clearly efficacious in dealing with the interpersonal and occupational limitations of patients or with deficit symptoms. Psychotherapy, on the other hand, has failed to define specific treatment domains and is contrasted with medication in the domains most relevant to drug effects, not those that might be most relevant to psychotherapy. Psychotherapy does compare poorly with antipsychotic drugs in rapid reduction of psychotic symptoms, but the relative effects of each treatment on social functioning and deficit symptoms are relatively unexplored (Carpenter et al., 1980).

Finally, the advent of antipsychotic drugs greatly weakens the final rationale for psychotherapy: when all else fails, try psychotherapy. This rationale may remain valid for the subset of patients who are not responsive to current medication, but the vast majority of patients are helped by drugs. The question then becomes how much additional benefit can be obtained from psychotherapy in resolving residual symptoms of the illness. Although such symptoms may often significantly impair the schizophrenic's functioning, attempting psychotherapy is no longer the obvious solution, given its cost and the uncertainty of its results.

The emergence of antipsychotic drugs requires a new framework for thinking about psychotherapy. Psychotherapeutic strategies now have a role in a more comprehensive treatment strategy, and they focus on those objectives to which psychotherapy can make unique contributions. Treatment is now done in a context that permits a rapid return to some level of independent functioning and must have a reasonable likelihood of success at an acceptable cost. Finally, it must be sufficiently acceptable to the patient that continuity of care is facilitated.

THE QUESTION OF THE EFFICACY OF PSYCHOTHERAPY

The new emphasis on collecting psychiatric research data in accordance with standards that generally apply to research in the biomedical sciences contrasts sharply with the traditional method of accruing new knowledge in psychotherapy. The traditional method relies heavily on the detailed case study followed by theoretical elaboration and is strong when the goal is to illustrate an approach or to generate hypotheses, but weak when the researcher seeks persuasive evidence.

Psychotherapy advocates frequently argue that the standard biomedical and social science research paradigms are not applicable and that a number of factors make rigorous research more difficult in this area. Traditional psychotherapies with schizophrenics require an extensive duration of treatment before benefits are likely to be objectively evident. Efficacy testing is therefore onerous and the use of untreated controls untenable for such long periods. Furthermore, the double-blind controlled experiment is not possible, since both patient and therapist are aware of the amount of time spent together and what occurs during their interaction. Moreover, in psychotherapy research, the experimental treatment itself is assumed to operate by psychological mechanisms so that the distinction between the experimental treatment and the placebo is not clear. The mode of action of psychotherapy is not known with certainty and, therefore, cannot be excluded with certainty in the placebo condition. Although these and other factors make controlled research in psychotherapy considerably more difficult and complex than clinical trials with pharmacologic agents, they are not in principle insurmountable.

Beyond such inherent limitations, a number of additional factors have apparently discouraged psychotherapy advocates from subjecting their model of treatment to controlled empirical assessment. The long tradition of appeals to authority in psychiatry has resulted in psychotherapists' tendency to construe clinical observations and derived theory as unquestionable truths for which there is no need for further verification. Psychotherapists may also reject experimental research because they feel it destroys the uniqueness, richness, and complexity of the clinical experience, a feeling which may be valid when study results are viewed as exhausting all the useful information to be derived from the clinical setting. However, the experimental task does require extracting from and simplifying the complexity of a natural experience to permit examination of the relationship between a small, finite number of the many variables involved. Finally, psychotherapists are reluctant to embrace experimental research which seems to test their personal worth. If a pharmacotherapist finds that a particular drug is not efficacious, neither his person nor his career is challenged. He simply searches for an alternative pharmacologic intervention. With the psychotherapist, however, who has frequently been trained exclusively in one modality, the prospect of finding that the sort of treatment that he or she provides is of little or no value has major personal and professional ramifications.

As a result of these and other factors, very little empirical research on the psychotherapy of schizophrenia has been systematically conducted by knowledgeable psychotherapists, and the limited work that has been accomplished has not used designs optimal for testing the hypothesized effects of psychotherapy. Generally, the psychotherapist has taken the limited role of criticizing existing studies and explaining why the studies did not demonstrate beneficial effects for psychotherapy (Carpenter and Heinrichs, 1980).

The authors have conducted a comprehensive review of the existing research (Heinrichs and Carpenter, 1981).* Six of the more influential studies have results which are far from encouraging (May and Tuma, 1965; May, 1968; May et al., 1976; Karon and Vanderbos, 1972; Grinspoon et al., 1972; Rogers et al., 1967; Bookhammer et al., 1966; and

*Preceptor's note: The studies are also reviewed in the chapter by Davis and his colleagues.

Marks et al, 1968). Only two of the six studies purport to demonstrate any value for psychotherapy. But since most have significant methodological flaws, the verdict remains unsettled. The chronic nature and small size of study samples, a lack of standardization of treatments, insufficient randomization, and even a questionable quality of treatment undermine the utility of one or more of the studies. The psychotherapy advocate can therefore argue that the case against psychotherapy has not been firmly established.

With the difficulty in justifying psychotherapy on the basis of etiology, and given the fact that the development of other treatments, especially drugs, greatly weakens the argument that anything is worth a try irrespective of costs or uncertainty of outcome, the empirical demonstration of efficacy continues to be an important challenge. Investigators familiar with the complexities of psychotherapeutic work should conduct the studies, and studies should be designed to maximize the likelihood of defining beneficial effects should they exist. The following are some principles the authors believe should be employed in designing such studies:

(1) *Selection of subjects appropriate to treatment.* The schizophrenic disorders are extremely heterogeneous, and it is highly unlikely that any one treatment will benefit patients in all the classifications. Subjects and their controls should be good candidates for the treatment(s) in question. Fortunately, there is some consensus on which schizophrenic patients will be good candidates for psychotherapy. A panel of experts compiled the following for the seminars sponsored by the National Institute of Mental Health:

> Schizophrenic patients who tend to profit the most from individual psychotherapy are young and intelligent (I.Q. above low-normal), "reactive," and present during their first break in an acute manner. They have a past history of achievement at work and in other creative activity, as well as some success in interpersonal, especially heterosexual relationships. They are motivated and tend to experience pain or the sense of struggle and definitely see themselves in need of help. They often appear to be striving actively for higher levels of functioning, and exhibit some degree of the following capacities: Self observation, problem solving, integrating experience, self control and delay (Gunderson and Mosher, 1975, xxi).

(2) *Selection of subjects in appropriate phase of illness.* Since schizophrenic illness varies over time, the selection of patients in the appropriate phase of illness is crucial to testing the efficacy of any treatment. For instance, the studies referred to focus on treating psychotic, hospitalized patients. Given the established value of antipsychotic drugs in this phase of illness, as well as the intuitive sense that psychotherapy is likely to be especially valuable in helping the patient with social dysfunction and deficit symptoms, outpatient treatment may be the more appropriate setting for testing psychotherapeutic efficacy. Yet the literature contains no reports of adequate studies of traditional psychotherapy in the outpatient setting.

(3) *Establishment of sufficient outcome measures.* It is important to consider various domains of outcome independently when assessing treatment effects. Only by assessing a spectrum of outcome areas can an investigator ensure that an important benefit is not being missed and determine in which areas the treatment has no effect or may, in fact, be harmful. Outcome assessment in schizophrenia research has tended to emphasize psychotic symptoms and to neglect

deficit symptoms and the interpersonal and intrapsychic consequences of illness.

(4) *Provision of sufficient levels and duration of treatment.* It is essential that clinical trials of any treatment be of adequate dose and duration to maximize the likelihood of benefit occurring. With pharmacologic trials, the duration can often be quite brief, sometimes hours to days. In psychotherapeutic trials, considerably longer periods are undoubtedly necessary (see Hogarty et al., 1973; 1974a; 1974b).

(5) *Conceptualization of treatment strategies.* It is extremely important to overcome the assumption of competition between therapeutic modalities and to design studies so that optimal combinations of therapeutic strategies can be assessed. The work of Hogarty and his co-workers (1973; 1974a; 1974b) and Goldstein et al. (1978) is instructive. Here a positive interaction between drugs and major role therapy was demonstrated. If investigators limit their designs to simple drugs-versus-psychotherapy trials, interactions between treatments will not be discovered and understood.

ISSUES OF PUBLIC POLICY

Few societies have granted public support for psychotherapy, and the U.S. government and various supporters of health care are presently scrutinizing support for psychotherapy in general. Limited resources in the public sector seem incompatible with highly personalized mental health care. Psychotherapy with schizophrenic patients is expensive and labor intensive. Yet, many medical treatments that go unquestioned are considerably more costly and of undetermined value. As with psychotherapy with schizophrenic patients, the majority of medical treatments have not been validated by controlled clinical trials (Herrington, 1980). Immobilizing a fracture, for instance, can be seen as obviously beneficial in the absence of a controlled trial. There are other treatment strategies that are so well grounded on indisputable facts of anatomy, physiology, or biochemistry that they are intuitively acceptable to persons educated in the field.

Psychotherapy is problematic in this regard. Its mechanism of action is frequently seen as improbable, if not mystical. In the absence of a well-established basic science of behavioral or mental events, therapeutic strategies are frequently justified by appeals to highly abstract and contestable models of mental functioning. Many aspects of psychotherapy could alternatively be justified on the basis of relatively atheoretical concepts (Carpenter and Heinrichs, 1980). It seems reasonable, for instance, that a schizophrenic person who has difficulty in interpreting his or her environment without distortion could benefit from ongoing exchanges with an individual trained to help the patient clarify the ambiguities of the environment.

Formulations such as these not only make psychotherapy more understandable, but can also serve as a basis for developing hypotheses about psychotherapy that can subsequently be tested empirically. They also bear on the question of whether psychotherapy should be supported until definitive empirical assessment of its efficacy is available. The authors believe it is a misapplication of methodologic rigor to maintain that no treatment be employed unless its value has been established in controlled clinical trials. It seems a more reasonable policy to continue to use the as yet "unproven" therapeutic strategies if they fit with common sense, if they have an intuitive relationship to acceptable treatment goals, and if they appear unlikely to incur untoward risk or expense.

A second difficulty facing psychotherapy in establishing its legitimacy is that it lacks many of the external trappings that usually distinguish medical treatment from other human activities. It involves neither giving a pill nor using specialized equipment. It does not even require a physician. In many cases, it is difficult to distinguish psychotherapy from the background experience of benign human interactions. This is made more difficult because so much of the potency of psychotherapy is thought to reside in personal characteristics of the therapist rather than in specific aspects of the therapeutic technique. These intrinsic problems are worsened by the holistic and nonspecific models of psychotherapy. Finally, there is little precision in the definition of what ingredients of the psychotherapeutic process are beneficial and what techniques are proper in the conduct of psychotherapy.

Although there will inevitably always be difficulties in this area, it behooves advocates of psychotherapy, whenever possible, to define with precision the active ingredients of psychotherapy, the conditions for their optimal administration, the minimum required training for the psychotherapist, the specific target symptoms for which therapy is indicated, and the groups of patients for whom psychotherapy is contraindicated. Recent progress in this area is reflected in the study of affective disorders (Rush and Beck, 1978; Weissman, 1974; 1979; Klerman et al., 1974).

CLINICAL GUIDELINES

In the absence of adequate empirical descriptions of the long-term psychotherapy of the schizophrenic disorders, the best guidance on the subject may still be the careful descriptions of the psychotherapeutic process (Will, 1968; Fromm-Reichman, 1950; Searles, 1965) and the observations of the long-term course of schizophrenic disorders (Bleuler, 1978; Ciompi, 1980). While these works do not deal with the issue of proof of therapeutic efficacy, they do clarify the need, the nature of the aims, and the likely generalized and nonspecific effects of treatment. For a variety of reasons, it has been difficult to apply traditional psychotherapy to a broad range of schizophrenic patients. As discussed above and elsewhere (Carpenter and Heinrichs, 1980), the declining influence of psychodynamic psychiatry and the failure of leading spokespersons for psychotherapy in schizophrenia to integrate their treatment techniques with other modalities have prevented articulating a workable model for a comprehensive therapy which appeals to the good sense of the typical clinician.

A Developmental-Interactive Model

The authors propose using a *developmental-interactive* model of schizophrenia for integrating the wide range of data relevant to understanding etiology, pathogenesis, clinical manifestation, and therapeutic approaches (Strauss and Carpenter, 1981). This medical model incorporates the broad range of data and the general systems theory as articulated by Engel (1977; 1980). Although the etiology of schizophrenia remains enigmatic, the model posits that the interaction of social, psychological, and biological factors over time shapes an individual's vulnerability to illness. In the vulnerable individual, precipitating or triggering factors may then be defined. In the person with manifest illness, an additional range of factors relevant to course of illness will be appreciated. The interactive model requires the simultaneous consideration of various treatments and negates espousing one therapy to the exclusion of others. Consequently, the clinician must integrate psychotherapy with other psychosocial approaches and view the psychosocial aspect of treatment as one of several domains of therapy. The broad-based training of the psychiatrist is especially useful here and argues against relinquishing psychotherapeutic work to clinicians whose training is more narrowly based.

The developmental-interactive model of schizophrenia revolves around the core feature of an ongoing and informative clinical relationship between the doctor and the schizophrenic patient. The therapeutic approaches to be integrated vary among patients and for each patient over time. Diagnosis and evaluation for treatment necessarily involve a comprehensive appreciation of both psychopathology and strengths of the personality. Since many schizophrenic patients have remarkable difficulty in communicating the essence of their experience, this may be a time-consuming process.

Establishing the Relationship

Establishing the relationship not only provides a basis for an ongoing accumulation of relevant data, but the process itself may be therapeutic. The patient has an opportunity to relate highly personal and perplexing experiences to a known individual and to appreciate the nature and purpose of various interventions within the context of the relationship. These factors may decrease the sense of isolation and estrangement that is so much a part of the schizophrenic process. It is self-evident that the clinician must be skilled in interviewing and establishing a dyadic relationship and appreciative of the phenomenological processes whereby one individual gains intimate familiarity with the experiences of another (Jaspers, 1968). A highly specific theoretical approach is disadvantageous, at least in the initial stages, since the clinician must suspend judgment and minimize presuppositions in order to appreciate the unique effect of psychopathologic processes on the individual patient.

Any model for psychotherapy with the schizophrenic patient must recognize that the patient is likely to have limited financial resources, may have had a number of hospitalizations for acute psychotic episodes or acute exacerbations of psychotic symptoms, and may, after a relatively brief hospitalization of days or weeks, have been discharged to outpatient care in a state of at least partial remission.

In establishing a therapeutic alliance with such a patient, whether it is during a brief hospitalization or shortly after discharge, the first task is to develop a shared view of the illness. This can help the patient move quickly to being a willing participant in the therapeutic endeavor and can avert early termination. The development of such a shared view is usually facilitated by exploring together the range of the illness experiences and what they mean to the patient.

At times, the patient and therapist will be able to agree readily on what aspects of the patient's experience are pathologic. At other times, the patient will have great difficulty in recognizing or acknowledging the manifestations of the illness. Even here, the patient and the therapist can develop a shared view of the consequences of certain aspects of the patient's behavior. For instance, a patient who insists on the veracity of his or her delusional beliefs might nonetheless be able to understand that acting on those beliefs in certain ways inevitably results in undesirable consequences. At times, this is an adequate shared beginning.

Based on this perspective, the therapist and patient can proceed to develop a series of common goals. It is helpful to make these goals relatively specific and to go beyond holistic statements such as "getting well." Discussion should then focus on the rationale for the range of treatment that the therapist is considering and should relate the treatment possibilities to the specific goals that the therapist and patient have together agreed to pursue. The patient will thus understand the role of the therapy itself, medication, rehabilitative group experiences, and other special programs.

Very often some of the initial phase of treatment must focus on concrete problems and stressors in the patient's life. Frequently, therapy begins at a time when the patient is returning from a brief hospitalization and is facing disruption in relationships to family and friends, a precarious financial future, and the need for a place to live. Therapy cannot proceed productively until these concrete issues are adequately resolved. Although the therapist may delegate certain parts of this resolution to others, the therapist should keep intimately involved in the planning and monitor the progress closely.

For those patients returning to live with their family, a comfortable and consistent relationship between the therapist and the patient's family should be established quickly. The patient and therapist may have to negotiate about the role the family is to play. The family should feel that they are allies with the therapist and patient, because accepting the patient back into the home often places a considerable burden on the family. In the authors' experience, traditional approaches to family therapy can make the family feel blamed and criticized for the patient's illness, and a psychoeducational approach seems a useful alternative (Anderson et al., 1980). Frequently, families of schizophrenic patients have been excluded from previous treatment experiences and have been largely uninformed about the nature of the patient's illness, the rationale of various treatments, and the likely prognosis. They may previously have received little practical advice on how to deal with manifestations of the patient's illness in the home. Providing such information generates a marvelous context for the therapist to establish a nonthreatening collaborative relationship with the family.

Long-term Concerns

Once the therapeutic relationship is solidly established and work begins on the individualized goals, treatment must also focus on a number of enduring tasks. First is the avoidance of psychotic relapse whenever possible. Here the use of antipsychotic drugs, either continuously or intermittently, generally plays an important part. In addition, it is useful for patient and therapist to study past episodes carefully in order to identify external events or internal conflicts that operate as stressors to the patient. Therapy should try to reduce the impact of these factors, and both patient and therapist should maintain an ongoing vigilance for their reappearance or intensification. Patient and therapist should also develop a careful understanding of the earliest signs and symptoms that may suggest impending decompensation. Although such prodromal features vary immensely between patients, a given patient usually manifests considerable similarity from episode to episode.

A second task of enduring importance in therapy with schizophrenic patients is to combat ongoing deficit symptoms and impaired functioning. Existing somatic treatments have been particularly unsatisfying with these problems, and psychosocial intervention would intuitively seem to be extremely valuable. Although there is, in fact, little empirical evidence to argue for its efficacy or to indicate precisely what therapeutic strategies are most helpful, several approaches emerge from an understanding of typical impairments. The therapeutic process is a unique opportunity for the schizophrenic patient to experience an ongoing and intense human relationship that is consistent but not rigid, intimate but not intrusive, and supportive but not thwarting of the patient's stirring toward autonomy. As such, the relationship provides a laboratory in which the patient can experiment with and then reflect upon relating to others and upon the relationship issues that have become so awesome and intimidating in his or her everyday life.

Beyond this, the therapeutic relationship is a context in which the therapist and the patient can identify specific deficiencies in interpersonal skills and coping strategies. Once these are identified, approaches can be developed to increase the patient's adaptive capacities. Sometimes these approaches may be highly structured behavioral training programs in either individual or group settings. At other times the patient may have strong inhibitions and anxieties limiting his or her level of functioning, and these may relate to long-standing internal conflicts, coupled with distortions of the interpersonal environment. These issues should be addressed in the context of the psychotherapy.

In still other instances, concrete realities may serve as formidable obstacles to the patient's efforts to increase functioning. The therapist must be cognizant of such obstacles and be willing to manipulate the environment where possible and appropriate. The belief that a patient must take responsibility for his or her own life and the fear that the therapist may be gratifying the patient's excessive longing for passivity and dependency makes the therapist reluctant to assist directly in bringing about reasonable environmental changes. Yet these very changes could sometimes maximize the patient's chances to achieve a higher level of functioning. Throughout the entire process, the therapist must help the patient to titrate realistically his or her performance expectations and to avoid the extremes of resigned acceptance of dysfunction on the one hand, and unrealistic and frustrating plans on the other.

While all else is being done, the therapist must never forget the importance of sustaining the relationship. All other goals depend upon this. The therapist must be particularly sensitive to the emergence of negative transference issues that, if unchecked, can drive the patient from treatment. Attention to positive transference is usually not as urgent, but the therapist should note any unrealistic idealized transferences. When the patient sees the therapist as having exaggerated power, bitter disillusionment can follow as the therapist seems to fall short of the excessive expectations. One expectation of the patient should, within reason, be fulfilled; namely, that the therapist will be available to the patient at times of crisis or stress. The schizophrenic patient's limitations in binding affect and the tendency to disorganize under stress means that, at times, a therapist's intervention cannot be delayed until the next scheduled appointment or sometimes even until the next morning without serious consequence.

The availability principle also applies to the termination of therapy. Most schizophrenics need an enduring relationship, although it may vary in intensity over time. Some patients will internalize the accomplishments of therapy so well that they can function for long periods of time without direct contact with the therapist. Nevertheless, given the enduring nature of the schizophrenic illness, at least as a vulnerability, the patient should feel free to recontact the therapist at times of need, even after the regular psychotherapy has ended.

Summary

How do the above model and clinical notions relate to the traditional psychodynamic models of psychotherapy with schizophrenics? While they represent a modification and a broadening of the approach, they incorporate an understanding of the patient in psychodynamic terms, and they use that understanding to guide the choice and timing of the various therapeutic strategies. Furthermore, psychodynamically based exploratory therapy can assume an important role with many patients at various points in their treatment. Such exploration must, however, always be firmly rooted in reality, must emphasize correcting patients' distortions about themselves and others, and must avoid unnecessary regression. As an added caution in the case of psychodynamic explorations, clinicians should recall that the articulation and exploration of inner conflicts are stressful, and, like all stressors, increase the patient's risk for symptomatic exacerbation.

From these observations two final implications follow. First, when the treatment incorporates psychodynamically based exploration, both the patient and the therapist must be especially alert to early signs of impending decompensation. Antipsychotic drugs or other concurrent interventions may be useful for decreasing the patient's vulnerability to psychosis. Second, any decision to explore a conflict-laden area with the patient must be justified by the anticipation of a clear benefit in light of the particular patient and the nature of the conflict. Conflict areas in some cases may already be highly active and near consciousness, working as powerful stressors to overwhelm and disorganize the patient. In such cases, careful exploration of such issues is not likely to make matters significantly more disruptive and promises to reduce the patient's ongoing stress once matters are adequately resolved. In other cases, ongoing conflicts are powerful inhibitors to the patient's general functioning and encourage social withdrawal and avoidance of others. At such times, exploratory work around the conflicts may free the patient to achieve increased levels of functioning. A psychodynamic approach to psychotherapy can finally be very helpful with the psychological and social sequelae of the schizophrenic illness. It can help the schizophrenic patient deal with the massive loss in self-esteem, the isolation and ostracism from society, and the chronic demoralization and despair such patients experience.

The model presented here is intended to address the needs of the modal schizophrenic patient in the setting that is currently the most typical. This does not imply that the more traditional model for psychotherapy with schizophrenic patients has no place. That model, which stresses long-term, intensive work with patients, often in the context of lengthy hospitalizations and reduced emphasis on pharmacologic

treatments, remains the best hope for certain patients. Those unfortunate patients with severe, chronic forms of the schizophrenic
illness, who fail to respond appreciably to any other treatments, may
benefit from that mode. Finally, traditional psychotherapy has also
been and remains a uniquely powerful source of information about the
subjective experience of the schizophrenic patient and the complex
workings of his inner world. As such, it is a valuable research tool,
yielding information important to all professionals working with
schizophrenic patients.

CONCLUSIONS

The various recent challenges to psychotherapeutic work with schizophrenic patients do not constitute an indictment of psychotherapy in
principle, but do raise serious questions about the applicability of
traditional models of intensive therapy to the typical schizophrenic
patient. While recognizing the great value that has accrued from that
tradition, as well as the continuing role of such intensive work in select
circumstances, the authors have suggested a modified clinical model,
more suited to the typical schizophrenic patient in need of treatment
today. The model allows psychotherapeutic strategies to be integrated
into a comprehensive treatment approach that is based on a thorough
phenomenologic understanding of the individual patient.

Chapter 14

Group, Family, and Milieu Therapies and Psychosocial Rehabilitation in the Treatment of the Schizophrenic Disorders
by Samuel J. Keith, M.D. and Susan M. Matthews

INTRODUCTION

The term *schizophrenia* has many different meanings and seems to
have no unifying concept. While for many disorders the diagnosis
provides a unifying concept by bringing together conceptual understanding, etiologic discrimination, and treatment implications, the
diagnosis of schizophrenia unfortunately falls short in this regard. Much
of the difficulty comes from our having no means of validating the
diagnosis for this major health problem. The absence of independent
validation has led to an extensive effort to establish the reliability of the
diagnosis by selecting those symptoms which can be rated consistently.
Yet even the very best reliability will fail to bring validity to the
diagnosis. No single variable and no cluster of biologic, psychophysiologic, psychologic, or social variables can be found in all schizophrenics or only in schizophrenics. The basic heterogeneity of the
disorder appears inescapable.

DIAGNOSIS

From the time of Kraepelin and Bleuler, diagnosis has assumed an
ascendant position in research on schizophrenia. This follows from the
basic assumption that because certain symptoms occur in com-

binations with a recognizable frequency, researchers may be able to discover common etiologies, treatments, or even prevention strategies. The categorization of symptoms is often important in establishing a diagnosis in general medicine, as in the case of an infectious disease such as measles or a neurological disease such as amyotrophic lateral sclerosis. For symptoms to be useful in diagnosis, however, they must be capable of being reliably rated, regardless of their conceptual relationship to the disease. Indeed, until rating variability is reduced, we can never be sure that phenomenologically similar populations are being addressed. Consequently the findings of different investigators cannot be compared.

There are, however, certain limitations to making improved symptom reliability the sole means for creating a classification. An example from general medicine can illustrate this point. Applying the principles of reliable classification to coughing, one could reliably classify it on the basis of frequency (number of coughs per minute), depth of inspiratory effort preceding it, force of expiratory effort associated with it, association with fever, and so forth. But would any of this lead to a better understanding of the pathophysiology of coughing? The etiology of coughing can range from centralized brain tumor, to ear infections, to postnasal drip, to bronchogenic carcinoma. The reliability or frequency of association of the symptoms which occur in conjunction with coughing does little to improve our understanding of etiology or pathophysiology.

The schizophrenic disorders can be similarly examined. DSM-III lists six specific forms of hallucinations or delusions, several areas of deterioration to be compared to previous levels of functioning, a minimum duration, and prodromal and residual phases, and, within the prodromal and residual phases, cites eight specific kinds of symptoms (American Psychiatric Association, 1980). What does this level of detail add to our understanding of schizophrenia and our clinical treatment of it? Whether it will increase understanding is in doubt, and because DSM-III offers so little treatment guidance to practicing clinicians, its contribution to clinical treatment is also in doubt. An alternate way of organizing our current knowledge about the nosology of schizophrenia fits better with our current treatment repertoire and promises to add more to our understanding of the phenomenon.

Drawing from the work of Hughlings Jackson on the evolution/dissolution theory, Strauss, Carpenter, and Bartko (1974) have presented a rather compelling argument for there being three groupings of problems associated with schizophrenic symptoms. Based on precursors and prognosis, problems are grouped as positive symptoms, negative symptoms, and disorders of personal relationships. *Positive symptoms* refer to symptoms of schizophrenia which characterize it by their presence, i.e., hallucinations and delusions. *Negative symptoms* refer to those symptoms which characterize it by their absence, i.e., lack of goal directed behavior, blunting of affect, and so forth. *Disordered personal relationships* refer to patterns of asociality, withdrawal, and lack of close personal ties. Positive symptoms can develop over a short period of time, may represent reactions to biologic or socioenvironmental causes, and have nonspecific response and minimal prognostic importance. Negative symptoms, on the other hand, develop over an extended period of time, are conceptualized as either the source of chronicity or the result of it, and are prognostically important. Disordered personal relationships also develop over the long term, but are conceptualized as interactive processes of uncertain etiology; they are prognostically important for functioning and for both negative and positive symptomatology. This conceptual framework aids in the following examination of the relative contributions of various approaches to treating schizophrenia.

TREATMENT

Although advances in psychopharmacology and psychosocial treatments combined to produce a major revolution in the treatment of schizophrenia in the 1950's, the ensuing two decades have seen a parallel, but distinctly separate, development of knowledge about these two elements of treatment. The well-designed, rigorous clinical trials of neuroleptics have produced an imposing body of data pointing to their efficacy in the control of the positive symptoms of schizophrenia. Almost no one would question that positive symptomatology is profoundly affected by pharmacologic treatment. Further, controlled studies of maintenance chemotherapy demonstrate a decided advantage to those assigned to receive drugs as compared with those assigned to placebo. In a review of 29 studies of relapse prevention with antipsychotic medication, Davis et al. (1980) found a striking difference in relapse rates between patients maintained on drugs (19 percent) and those on placebo (55 percent). Another way of stating these findings is that twenty percent will relapse, even with drugs, and that 45 percent will not relapse, even without drugs. Moreover, it should be noted that relapse is primarily accounted for and generally measured by the recurrence of the positive symptoms of schizophrenia, not very often by negative symptoms or disordered personal relationships.

Psychosocial treatments, with their high consumption of time and dollars, have proved more difficult to assess and are clearly not viewed with the enthusiasm that they once were. The reasons for this are myriad. At least three, however, deserve noting. The first is our need for a magical cure. Schizophrenia is a disorder of terrifying magnitude. The disability that schizophrenia causes and the fear that irrational behavior engenders in all of us have prompted many people to search for a "silver bullet" for schizophrenia. Of the many positive things one can say about psychosocial treatments, their resemblance to anyone's concept of "silver bullets" is remote.

Second are the administrative, political, and fiscal decisions that have made short-term hospital treatment a reality of our times. Many psychosocial treatments by their very nature do not lend themselves to brief application at a time when florid positive symptomatology is present.

Third, although positive symptomatology is the least enduring and least prognostic aspect of schizophrenia, it is the most dramatic and characteristic aspect. A treatment which is successful with these symptoms therefore becomes a treatment standard against which other treatments are measured. Most psychosocial treatments are aimed either at ameliorating negative symptoms or at improving social competence, not at alleviating positive symptoms. Therefore, if the severity of positive symptoms is examined alone, the comparison of drug effects with the effects of psychosocial treatments is simply not valid. Rather, it is like comparing the effects of surgery with the effects of physical rehabilitation in the case of a broken hip or the effects of insulin versus diet on diabetes. The debate over whether drugs are better or worse than psychosocial treatments in schizophrenia is similarly meaningless.

Long-Term Pharmacologic Treatment

Pharmacologic treatments are undoubtedly effective in treating the positive symptoms of schizophrenia. Such treatments are, however, only a part of the outcome in what we know as schizophrenia. In terms of the long-term disability, they may in fact be a very small part.

If neuroleptics were one hundred percent safe and had no serious short- or long-term side effects, then any contribution they could make to effective treatment would be sufficient justification for their general use. But we know after almost three decades of experience with neuroleptic treatment that this is not the case. In the acute short-term treatment of the positive symptoms of the schizophrenic disorders, the many extrapyramidal side effects of neuroleptics are either controllable with other medication, tolerable to the patient, or reversible after treatment is discontinued. The long-term effects, such as corneal deposits, retinopathy, and tardive dyskinesia, are considerably more serious and resistant to treatment. Unfortunately, for at least one of the long-term side effects, tardive dyskinesia, there is presently no effective treatment other than prevention, and neuroleptic treatment may mask its appearance until treatment is discontinued.

The assignment to long-term pharmacotherapy should always be considered in light of these risks and may also be aided by our knowledge that response to neuroleptic treatment falls along a continuum. We know or can infer from extensive reviews of the literature (Davis, 1976; Gardos and Cole, 1976) that a patient may fall into one of four hypothetical response groups. A patient either responds to drugs and takes them; or responds to drugs but doesn't take them; or doesn't respond to drugs but takes them; or doesn't respond to drugs and doesn't take them.

(1) *Responds to drugs and takes them.* A patient with this response presumably represents the majority (sixty percent) who are considered to be at high risk of relapse if withdrawn from neuroleptics. These patients do need to be maintained on medication, but they must be monitored carefully for the development of tardive dyskinesia.

(2) *Responds to drugs but doesn't take them.* For many years, most treatment failures in schizophrenia were attributed to the fact that patients who needed them had not taken their medications. However, a recent study by Schooler et al. (1980) casts considerable doubt on the assumption that noncompliance is the major contributor to relapse. Guaranteeing compliance through the use of injectable fluphenazine decanoate, Schooler et al. found no significant difference in relapse rates between patients receiving injectable and those receiving oral forms of medication. Although there may yet be patients who need drugs but refuse to take them, they are probably fewer than was formerly believed.

(3) *Doesn't respond to drugs but takes them.* It is critically important to identify patients in this category. Not only is drug treatment not helpful for them, but because of the risk of developing tardive dyskinesia, it is actually deleterious. Such patients may constitute a significant percentage of the chronically mentally ill, who are by definition either nonresponsive or minimally responsive to neuroleptics. Some support for this notion can be found in a study by Paul et

al. (1972). They reported that discontinuing drug treatment in a group of chronically hospitalized and medicated patients produced no detrimental results. Indeed, drug withdrawal enabled the patients to participate better in their social rehabilitation programs. When dealing with patients who are doing well on medication, clinicians worry with good reason about the risk of relapse without medication. In the case of chronic patients who are not doing well on drugs, however, a trial without medication, especially in the presence of an active psychosocial treatment, would seem to be quite desirable and relatively risk free.

(4) *Doesn't respond to drugs and doesn't take them.* A patient in this group has either recovered from the disorder without drugs and does not take them, or has simply not responded to drugs and therefore discontinued taking them. Psychosocial or other alternative treatments either have been or will be crucially important for patients such as this.

While these groupings could eventually be useful for reducing some of the long-term risks of pharmacotherapy and for identifying patients for whom alternate means of treatment may be most important, two caveats are in order. First, we cannot yet make these treatment group assignments precisely in individual cases. And second, as noted earlier, the pharmacologic agents currently available to us are effective only for positive symptoms. Since we are unlikely to find any new drugs which will impact on negative symptoms and disordered interpersonal relationships, we must continue to rely on psychosocial interventions to bring about improvements in these areas. Even when pharmacotherapy is indicated for the long-term prevention of the positive symptomatology that so often characterizes a relapse, other treatments are indicated for negative symptoms and relationship problems.

The following examination of psychosocial treatments of schizophrenia relies on studies identified in a previous review (Mosher and Keith, 1980) and the relatively few articles which have appeared since then. As evidenced by a recent review of the outcome research (Carpenter et al., 1981), overall outcome reporting is too nonspecific and too heavily weighted toward positive symptomatic relief to provide a useful means of evaluating treatments not directed toward the overt manifestations of psychosis. Examining the research from the standpoint of negative symptomatology and disordered relationships, as well as positive symptomatology, may give us new optimism about psychosocial treatments and permits us to identify where our treatment approaches need to be made more effective.

GROUP THERAPY

Among the psychosocial treatment modalities, group therapy has been the focus of the greatest amount of research. Some compelling reasons exist for group therapy as a choice of treatment. The ratio of the patients seen to the professional staff time involved is high. The range of types of approaches is broad. And techniques used in individual psychotherapy, the flagship of psychosocial treatments, can be adapted to it. But the reasons for the popularity of group therapy are also its major handicaps.

The idea that group therapy is a less expensive treatment risks its being seen as less desirable and prestigious and consequently being delegated to the lower status and less highly trained professionals. Yet we know that the effectiveness of group therapy or any other psychosocial therapy depends in large part on the positive expectations and regard in which it is held. A treatment assignment to group therapy for the sole reason of cost-effectiveness cannot be expected to produce much positive gain.

The broad range of types of group therapies presents a problem of a different sort. What people mean by *group therapy* differs widely. The research literature contributes to this confusion. Rarely do the studies provide thorough descriptions of the type of treatment utilized.

Finally, the application or transplantation of the techniques of individual psychotherapy may or may not be effective. Therapy must be modified for people depending on their problems with regard to positive and negative symptoms and social competence. While such fine tuning is possible in individual psychotherapy, it may not be as easy in group therapy. We should not, therefore, confuse the ease of extrapolation from one technique to another with its effectiveness.

Group therapy is ubiquitous in both inpatient and outpatient treatment programs for schizophrenia. It is hard to conceive of an inpatient unit that does not have group therapy or at least a group meeting that is supposed to be therapeutic, but research results offer little support to the group modality. Inpatient treatment of any kind generally occurs at a time when positive symptomatology or social disorganization is at its highest point. As we have learned from milieu studies, a stimulus-decreasing environment is most useful in the early stages of acute symptomatology. Since group therapy is in fact the opposite of stimulus reducing, it may be counterproductive early in treatment. To be effective in an inpatient population, group therapy should begin after the resolution of the most flagrant psychotic symptoms, be focused on current problems in a structured fashion, and follow the patient into the community as an available and ongoing treatment. From a practical standpoint in today's short-term hospitalizations, it may be difficult if not impossible to begin group therapy with an inpatient. Moreover, there is some evidence that inpatient group therapy is not beneficial for schizophrenics (Prince et al., 1973). Thus, it may be best to introduce an inpatient into an outpatient therapy group after the florid symptoms have remitted but prior to discharge from the hospital.

When group therapy begins after discharge, groups which are moderately supportive and directed at problems of daily living are apparently more successful than individual therapy, whether the goal is to improve socialization (Donlan et al., 1973; O'Brien et al., 1972) or vocational adjustment (Purvis and Miskimims, 1970). Finally, other studies have shown that only those groups which employ drugs are able to achieve a reduction in positive symptoms (Borowski and Talwinski, 1969; Claghorn, 1974; O'Brien et al., 1972).

For a modality that is in such wide use and has been the subject of such intense research for the past twenty years, these minimal conclusions can only be described as disappointing. The general enthusiasm for group therapy as a solitary means of treatment finds little if any support. Even as an ancillary treatment, with goals restricted to socialization and direct problem solving, its contribution to reducing negative symptoms and improving social competence is more theoretical than actual. Whether or not these limited conclusions stem from a lack of specificity and differentiation in type of group, type of patient, type of therapist, and type of outcome to be expected, the next generation of research studies on group therapy would do well to attend to these problems and to draw from the lessons learned about them in the research on family and milieu therapy.

FAMILY THERAPY

Approaches to family therapy in the treatment of schizophrenia have developed from two general philosophical stances. One viewpoint is that the family, through a number of possible mechanisms, plays a causal role in schizophrenia. Another is that the family acts as a system to maintain schizophrenia in one of its members.

Those who purport that the family is itself an etiologic factor include Fromm-Reichmann, with her concept of the cold, aloof "schizophrenogenic mother" (Fromm-Reichmann, 1948); Lidz with his idea of patterns of marital schisms and skew (Lidz et al., 1957); and Singer and Wynne with their observations on disordered intrafamilial communication patterns (Singer and Wynne, 1966). Each of these understandings of the family's role in the causation of schizophrenia has its supporters, but they are the subject of continuing controversy (Hirsch and Leff, 1971; 1975).

Those who see the family acting as a system to maintain schizophrenia in a member include Jackson and Riskin, and more recently the British group of Birley, Brown, Vaughn, Hirsch, and Leff. This particular approach to families has recently been strengthened by reports of increased schizophrenic relapse in families characterized by an emotional attitude referred to as expressed emotion (EE). EE is a hostile, critical, and overinvolved attitude evidenced by the relatives of schizophrenics. It has been shown that patients in families with high EE relapse at significantly higher rates than those in families with low EE and that medications, while reducing the rate of relapse, can by no means offset it (Vaughn and Leff, 1976).

Based on these two theoretical approaches, there are three areas where family therapy could have an impact on schizophrenia. It could serve as a primary prevention strategy, a treatment and evaluation strategy at onset of the symptomatic period, or a maintenance therapy to prevent relapse. The primary prevention idea is clearly the most appealing but is unfortunately also the least well developed. The combination of our current inability to predict who will develop schizophrenia, the difficulty of doing research on family dynamics, and the pejorative implications of family etiologic theories have all contributed to a lack of progress in this area.

The second strategy, intervention at the onset of the psychotic process, can be considered secondary prevention and is also appealing. Although some interventions have produced positive results, the number of studies has been small. Furthermore, the drug effect is either impossible to evaluate because pharmacotherapy is not discussed, or the drug effect predominates because outcome measures focus on drug-sensitive positive symptomatology or relapse. In some interventions, the treatment may have been too short in duration to produce long-term progress in negative symptoms or social competence (Goldstein et al., 1978; Langsley et al., 1968).

The third strategy, prevention of relapse, has evolved from the view of the family as a system for maintaining the schizophrenic illness. Here, carefully designed approaches to schizophrenia and the family have drawn upon previous research and have specified therapeutic goals appropriate to psychosocial treatment. Two particularly promising approaches are discussed. Anderson, Hogarty, and Reiss developed the first such approach at the University of Pittsburgh. They title their approach a "psycho-educational family treatment" (Anderson et al., 1980) and postulate that the "core deficit" in schizophrenia is in the manner in which schizophrenics process stimuli. This deficit, they believe, is constantly present, not only during the actively psychotic state. Combining their impressions from both the family dynamics literature and the attention-processing literature, they conclude, "An individual who has difficulties controlling the intensity and processing of stimuli would be likely to exhibit a diminished tolerance for interpersonal stress in general and for these complex, ambiguous, or intense family communications in particular" (Anderson et al., 1980, 492).

Drawing from the work of the British investigators on EE and from their own work which showed that "contention in the patient's household" was correlated to relapse (Hogarty et al., 1979), these investigators have created a family intervention program with four components. (1) An *educational component* provides the family with practical information to permit more rational decision making about the patient and reduces intrafamilial anxiety by clarifying misconceptions about schizophrenia and providing realistic goals and expectations. (2) A *stress reduction component* instructs families on means to increase structure and decrease familial disorganization. (3) A focus on *familial social networks* aims to defuse internal (frequently critical) attention on the patient by increasing family involvement in interpersonal, avocational, and vocational contacts. (4) An *individualized component* permits addressing issues that are specifically relevant to a given family. The patient is included in the therapy after the remission of acute positive symptoms.

Julian Leff of the British group (Leff, 1979) has developed a second approach to family therapy from a systems perspective. This approach draws heavily on his own work with EE. Hypothesizing that it is the family as a system which leads to relapse in the patient, Leff treats the family to the exclusion of the patient. The rationale for this is to interrupt the cycle of control that the patient exercises in dominating family problem discussions and to eliminate the stress the patient experiences when confronted by the high EE relatives. His approach uses a multiple family treatment strategy, combining families with high EE with families with low EE. On the effectiveness of his approach, Leff concludes:

> It is too early to comment on the effectiveness of our form of family therapy, but we have already seen our expectations being fulfilled in the group setting. The high EE relatives are intolerant of the patient's behavior at home, which leads to angry confrontations. By contrast the low EE relatives show a tolerant, even collusive, attitude toward the patient's symptoms and retain a remarkable ability to make light of the most fraught situations. There is no hint of blaming or criticizing the patient. We have already seen modifications of the attitudes of high EE relatives during their participation in the group, which makes us guardedly optimistic about the outcome of this study (Leff, 1979, 230).

There is some question as to whether these two treatment approaches are addressing positive symptoms, on the one hand, or negative symptoms and social competence on the other. On the one hand, both of these treatments are designed to prevent relapse, a phenomenon associated with positive symptoms. Moreover, the British approach goes so far as to exclude the identified patient from the treatment itself, a condition that makes it hard to conceive of the treatment as a means of improving negative symptoms and social competence. On the other hand, some feel, as the authors do, that EE is an interactive phenomenon. It is a response certain families have to their frustration with the patient's apathy and withdrawal. In other words, EE may be a measure of a family's level of intolerance of a schizophrenic member's negative symptoms and lack of social competence. The differences in the two approaches to family therapy revolve around the issue of whether to address the negative symptoms while using the same treatment mechanism to increase tolerance to them, or whether to do so through two separate mechanisms, one directed at the patient and the other at the family context.

The enthusiasm with which the authors view this area does not, thus far, stem from the results achieved, since results are not yet available. Further, the general applicability of family therapies will be restricted by the fact that not all schizophrenic patients have families who are available and willing to participate in therapy. The authors' enthusiasm stems rather from their appreciation of the thoughtful consideration of research findings which underlies the design of these treatments. In this regard, the family treatment research is providing the field with a model that it would do well to emulate in other modalities.*

MILIEU TREATMENT

Like family therapy, milieu treatment has experienced a growth in new knowledge since the late 1960's. When May reported the results of his elegant study in 1968, the impact of milieu therapy for unmedicated schizophrenic patients was seriously questioned. It now appears that successful milieu treatment requires the specification of milieu typologies for specific aspects of schizophrenia. No longer can it be maintained that any milieu, well meaning though it may be, is useful for treating all facets of schizophrenia. For instance, it is known from a number of sources that some forms of milieu, while acceptable for addressing negative symptoms, may be quite deleterious for positive symptoms.

When patients present the acute, positive symptoms of schizophrenia, four milieu characteristics can be related to successful treatment. (1) Three separate investigators have identified *high patient/staff interaction* as significant for the acutely disorganized patient (Kellam et al., 1967; Linn, 1970; Ellsworth, in press). The high degree of flexibility, one-to-one contact, and attention to individual patient characteristics that this characteristic permits is shown not only in positive symptom reduction, but also in improved interpersonal functioning after discharge. For this to occur the milieu must be small, have a sufficient number of staff, offer flexibility in length of stay, and have an accepting, supportive staff that views their role as contributing to treatment outcome.

(2) The *democracy of the unit* has also been associated with successful treatment of positive symptoms. A nonhierarchical, responsive, and responsible decision-making process has also been related to community tenure and adjustment. The sharing of responsibilities and

*Preceptor's note: For a further discussion of family factors and EE, see the chapter by Liberman.

the involvement of middle-level staff in decisions add to the affiliative, morale-enhancing effectiveness of milieu treatment (Ellsworth et al., 1971; Smith and King, 1975). A striking example of a milieu in which great attempts have been made to eliminate hierarchical structure is the Soteria project where psychotropic medication is rarely used (Mosher et al., 1973; 1975; Mosher and Menn, 1978; Mosher, 1972). This milieu has been able to achieve reductions in positive symptoms equal to those achieved by a unit using medication and has also demonstrated superior results in reducing negative symptoms as measured by vocational levels and independent living adjustment after discharge.

(3) *Stimulus-decreasing strategies* can apparently contribute to the reduction of positive symptoms. It has become increasingly clear that positive schizophrenic symptoms are adversely affected by over-stimulating and dynamic milieus. The studies of Van Putten and May (1976) on inpatient units, of Linn et al. (1979; 1980) in foster care homes and day treatment centers, and of Goldberg et al. (1977) in outpatient settings have all identified the deleterious effects of milieu intensity on positive symptoms. Clinically, it would appear that multi-source stimuli (e.g., community ward meetings), stimuli with multiple or confused meaning (e.g., family meetings), and dynamic inter-personal environments (e.g., rapidly changing staff assignments) need to be carefully controlled.

(4) A *problem-oriented approach* appears to be a final beneficial milieu characteristic when symptomatology is positive (Moos et al., 1973). This practical day-to-day approach is concrete and less likely to be interpersonally overstimulating.

As compared with the foregoing reports on milieu effects on positive symptoms, there has been much less work reported concerning effects on negative symptoms. But the research that has been done is impor-tant and of high quality. From one of the most carefully designed studies ever undertaken, Paul and Lentz (1977) have reported that the milieu characteristics most useful with chronic patients are those which make the greatest use of structure, organization, high expec-tations, and a specific behavioral change orientation. By extending their program to their patients in the community, they achieved relapse rates of less than five percent over a two-year period, and patients improved on a number of negative symptoms. The somewhat sobering fact that only ten percent of the patients could live completely independently does not diminish the achievement. That these patients made the gains they did in providing for basic needs and in socialization and recreation is truly remarkable, considering that they had a current hospitalization mean of 14.4 years. The interaction of drugs with the psychosocial treatment is also noteworthy. Paul et al. (1972) found that among the chronically hospitalized patients, the discontinuation of neuroleptics increased the patients' adaptation and ability to participate in the treatment regimen. Since any patient who establishes chronic resi-dency in a hospital in this time of emphasis on short-term hos-pitalization can almost be called a drug nonresponder by definition, this illustrates how discontinuation of drugs may prove beneficial.

The different effects of differing milieu typologies on various aspects of schizophrenia are complex, but results to date do offer clues toward increasing the specificity of our treatment approaches. The interaction with drugs in this particular modality remains an open issue, and future studies should attempt to demonstrate the power of a milieu to enable a reduction or elimination in the amount of medication, particularly where patients have obviously not responded to pharmacotherapy.

PSYCHOSOCIAL REHABILITATION

Psychosocial rehabilitation services owe their inception to a group of patients who organized in the late 1940's to meet what they considered their important but neglected need for rehabilitation. These services respond directly to negative symptoms and deficits in interpersonal competence in the schizophrenic population. In general, these services have been initiated when positive symptoms have resolved, but as in physical rehabilitation, it is now apparent that such efforts should begin early in the treatment process.

The overall goal is to reintegrate the psychiatrically disabled patient into the community by maintaining and augmenting whatever level of functional independence he or she has been able to achieve. Rehabilitation has generally focused on social support, independent living, and vocational skills. Results of research on the chronic patient population underline the population's need for rehabilitation programs. An extensive review of the findings by Anthony and his associates (1978) showed baseline readmission figures of thirty percent to forty percent after six months, 35 percent to fifty percent after one year, and sixty percent to 75 percent after three to five years. As for employment, most studies indicate only a ten percent to thirty percent rate of independent employment at follow-up, regardless of the time period studied.

To date, little controlled comparative research has been carried out on the impact that comprehensive psychosocial rehabilitation services have on the high rates of recidivism and unemployment. Beard and his associates (1978) recently reported on a five-year follow-up study. Clients of Fountain House, who received an active outreach program for the initial two years, had significantly lower rehospitalization rates at one, two, and five years than control subjects. Those Fountain House clients who were hospitalized spent forty percent fewer days in the hospital than did the rehospitalized control subjects. The data also indicate that the more contact the patients had with the program, the less likely they were to be rehospitalized. As in many studies of psychosocial treatment programs, though, any differences in pharmacotherapy between experimental and control groups were not described, and specific areas of expected rehabilitation impact were not addressed.

Other research on psychosocial rehabilitation programs has focused on services provided by aftercare clinics. These clinics, which usually offer some form of therapeutic or casework contact in addition to medication, have been shown to reduce readmission rates (Anthony et al., 1972). These positive results reflect a combination of factors: the effects of both the drugs and the additional services and of the type of patients who attend. Hogarty and his associates (1976) reported that patients who received major role therapy (i.e., casework with an experienced social worker) plus drugs had significantly better social adjustment than those who received drugs alone. The contribution of major role therapy was not immediately apparent: a beneficial effect first became evident at 18 months and was somewhat stronger at 24 months.

From this study and another by Wing's group (1970), we can also extend the knowledge about the effects of overstimulation. Hogarty et al. (1976) reported that the major role therapy had negative effects in the first eight months, and Wing reported that positive symptoms increased when patients were involved in a highly stimulating rehabilitation program. From this we can infer that it may be advisable to introduce a rehabilitation program in stages, carefully graduating the intensity of the program and monitoring the patient for early signs of decompensation. In a comparative study of ten day hospitals, Linn et al. (1979) found that success in treating chronic schizophrenic patients correlated with programs that had an emphasis on occupational therapy in a sustained environment, but not with programs which had a high patient turnover.

Chronicity, as defined by the number of previous hospitalizations, length of last hospitalization, psychotic vs. nonpsychotic diagnoses, and previous employment status, has been shown to predict outcome in aftercare clinic populations (Kirk, 1976). Kirk reported that the recidivism rate of patients who had a high level of chronicity decreased as the number of visits increased to above six. In contrast, the recidivism rate of patients who had a low level of chronicity was not affected by an increasing number of visits. Based on the results of this study, the Fountain House results, and another recent study (McCranie and Mizell, 1978), it is tempting to conclude that aftercare treatment is most effective with those chronic patients who maintain a continuing relationship with the program.

Transitional facilities, halfway houses, and day centers are other major components of psychosocial rehabilitation that have been shown to be effective in reducing recidivism as long as the patient remains in contact with the facility (Anthony, 1972). In an examination of the results achieved in transitional facilities, Rog and Raush (1975) found data to suggest a lower recidivism rate for residents of halfway houses, although they noted an almost complete absence of controlled studies. Other successful programs, rather than using a transitional facility to reduce readmissions, have assigned a community worker to give discharged patients practical help in adjusting to life outside the hospital (Katkin et al., 1971; 1975; Weinmann, 1975).

That psychosocial rehabilitation will expand and have an increasing impact on treatment programs is clear. But the humanitarian goals and the logic of the treatment approach are becoming less and less compelling as reasons for that expansion. In our increasingly fiscally accountable society, research and evaluation are more compelling than goals and logic. The field needs baseline data on employment and levels of adjustment, as well as more complex information on skill gains, quality of life, satisfaction with services, patient-program fit, and patient-society benefits.

CONCLUSIONS

In a previous review one of the authors and a colleague (Mosher and Keith, 1979) concluded that in general we know more about the utility of psychosocial treatments than has been acknowledged. This conclusion is still valid. Indeed, an examination of the impact of psychosocial treatments on the areas they would be expected to affect, negative symptoms and interpersonal skills, produces considerable evidence to support the conclusion. What is also apparent from this examination is that the technologies for assessing treatment impact in this area are underdeveloped. Measuring the presence or absence of a positive symptom or the rate of readmission to a hospital is far easier and more reliable than assessing negative symptoms and interpersonal competence. We should not, however, emulate the example of the apocryphal drunk who looks for his lost watch near the lamppost because the light is better there than where he lost it.

Schizophrenia is not solved by positive symptom reduction and freedom from hospitalization. The nonproductive lives that so frequently persist beyond these desirable outcomes are far more important. Intervening effectively with schizophrenic patients requires that we abandon our bimodal approach to the treatment of schizophrenia—drugs vs. psychosocial treatment. Acknowledging that both are useful—perhaps for different aspects, perhaps at different times, perhaps in ways we have not yet considered—will be a major step toward a better life for our patients.

Chapter 15

Recent Advances in the Pharmacologic Treatment of the Schizophrenic Disorders
by John M. Davis, M.D., Philip Janicak, M.D., Sidney Chang, M.D., Karen Klerman

ANTIPSYCHOTICS

When chlorpromazine (CPZ) or comparable doses of other antipsychotics were given in therapeutic dosages, they were found to be more effective than placebo in the treatment of schizophrenic patients. Figure 1 presents the results of the collaborative double-blind study No. 1 of the National Institute of Mental Health (NIMH) (Davis, 1976; Cole, Goldberg, and Davis, 1966).

This discovery led to a dramatic change in the treatment of psychotic patients and coincided with a significant shift of large populations out of mental institutions (Figure 2).

There is no evidence that one class of neuroleptics is more effective than any other. Insofar as is known, all subtypes of schizophrenia respond equally to all antipsychotic drugs (Goldberg et al. 1967; 1972). The suggestions made by some researchers that a given subtype may respond differentially to a given drug have not stood the test of cross-validation. The assertions have never been proven that hyperexcitable patients respond best to CPZ because it is a sedating phenothiazine, and that withdrawn patients respond best to an alerting phenothiazine, such as fluphenazine or trifluoperazine. Although evidence from the NIMH collaborative studies (Goldberg et al., 1967; 1972) indicated that a second-order factor labeled "apathetic and retarded" predicts a differentially good response to CPZ, this finding did not withstand the test of cross-validation. Mechanistically, because all antipsychotic drugs block dopamine receptors and are theo-

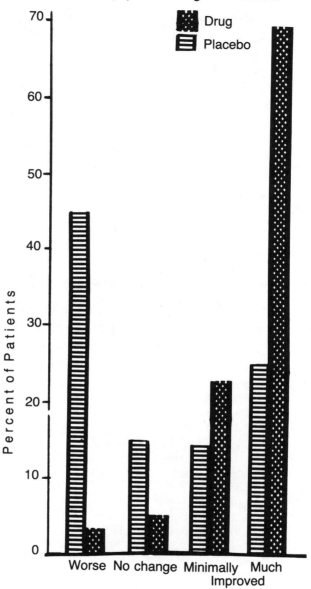

Figure 1. Results of treatment of schizophrenics with antipsychotic drugs or placebo presented as the percent of patients who are much improved, who are minimally improved, who do not change, or who become worse, as determined by a reanalysis (Davis, 1976) of data in NIMH Collaborative Study No. 1 (Cole, Goldberg, and Davis, 1966).

retically acting through the same mechanism, it is reasonable to expect that when given in comparable doses, they would be equally effective for all subtypes of schizophrenia.

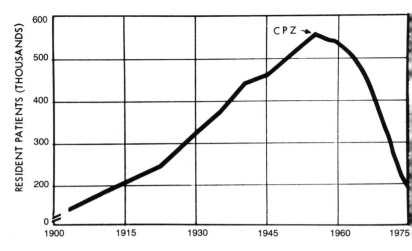

Figure 2.   Number of hospitalized patients from 1900 to 1975.

New Antipsychotics

DIHYDROINDOLONES   Molindone (Moban) belongs to the indole category of antipsychotics (dihydroindolones). In a carefully controlled study, Clark and his co-workers (1970a) found that molindone was clearly superior to placebo on evaluations done by both the physicians and the nurses. Gallant and Bishop (1968) found molindone slightly less effective than trifluoperazine on the Global Rating Scale as scored by nurses, although the difference was not statistically significant. Freeman and Frederick (1969) found the standard drug's efficacy exactly equal to molindone, whereas Simpson et al. (1971) found molindone slightly superior to trifluoperazine, but the finding was not statistically significant. In total, six controlled studies, including two hundred patients, found molindone approximately equal to the standard drug (see Table 1 for the results of five studies).

Molindone was reported slightly superior in one study, equal in three studies, and slightly inferior in two studies; but none of these differences was statistically significant. Since molindone does not inhibit the norepinephrine uptake pump, unlike CPZ, it would not interfere with the hypotensive action of guanethidine. Molindone does not cause weight gain.

DIBENZOXAZEPINE   Loxapine (Loxitane) is in the dibenzoxazepine chemical category of antipsychotics (Filho et al., 1975). Clark et al. (1972a; 1975; 1977) first compared loxapine, CPZ, and placebo in chronic schizophrenics and then compared loxapine, trifluoperazine, and placebo in newly admitted schizophrenics. They found loxapine superior to placebo. Van Der Velde and Kiltie (1975) and Selman and his co-workers (1976) also found loxapine to be statistically superior to placebo. Charalampous et al. (1974), however, failed to find loxapine superior to placebo.

The authors have previously used the Box Score Method of summarizing the number of positive or negative studies, but more recently, believing this to be insensitive, have devised a better way to summarize the results of different studies. Most double-blind, controlled projects

Table 1. Molindone Studies And Their Results

Author	Subjects and Treatment Duration	Dose Ratio STD/New	Patient Improvement			Overall Results
Clark et al., 1970a	Chr. Schiz. 12 weeks	10:1	Mol: +3, −12	CPZ: +8, −6	Pla: 0, −14	Mol>Pla Mol=CPZ CPZ>Pla
Gallant and Bishop, 1968	Chr. Schiz. 9 weeks	1:1	Mol: +3, −9	Tri: +6, −6		Mol=Tri
Ramsey et al., 1970	Chr. Schiz. 12 weeks	1:2				Mol=Tri
Freeman and Frederick, 1969	Chr. Schiz. 8 weeks	1:2	Mol: +8, −12	Tri: +10, −8		Mol=Tri
Simpson et al., 1971	Acute Schiz. 4 weeks	1:2	Mol: +11, −16	Tri: +9, −16		Mol=Tri

report the number of patients who do well on a given drug and the number of patients who have a poor response. They also generally report these parameters for the standard drug or placebo. These data can be manipulated through statistical techniques designed by Fleiss and Mantel especially for combining data from different studies (Fleiss, 1981). When the loxapine and placebo data from all studies are combined, the probability is significant to $p = .00002$ that loxapine is superior to placebo.

Shopsin et al. (1972a) found loxapine slightly inferior to standard neuroleptics, whereas Steinbook et al. (1973) found loxapine superior to standard neuroleptics in some measures but not in all. Charalampous et al. (1974) found loxapine less effective than thiothixene. It is important to consider Charalampous's results, but even when they are included, loxapine appears almost precisely equal to the standard drug in its antipsychotic action. A new drug should be slightly better than a standard drug in some studies and slightly worse in some studies, due simply to the random nature of measurement error. If one omits the occasional negative study, a new drug can falsely be made to look better than it is. In 22 of the 24 studies, with 857 patients investigated under controlled conditions (see Table 2), 63 percent of patients did well on loxapine and 63 percent on standard drugs. Thus, using the authors' statistical technique, loxapine is essentially equal to standard neuroleptics.

DIBENZODIAZEPINE   The dibenzodiazepine, clozapine, deserves special mention for two reasons. First, it is no longer available for research use in this country because of serious problems with a-granulocytosis. Second, while it was in use, it demonstrated no evidence of extrapyramidal symptoms (EPS) or tardive dyskinesia (Shopsin et al., 1979). An agent with more specific effect on the mesolimbic system, thus sparing the dopaminergic neurons of the corpus striatum, would certainly be a significant advance in our ability to treat with antipsychotics.

DIPHENYLBUTYRYLPIPERIDINES   Although the agents penfluridol and pimozide, both representatives of the diphenylbutyrylpiperidine category, are not yet available in this country, they have been marketed in Europe for some time. Penfluridol is an orally administered antipsychotic with a duration of action of one week. In essence, it is equal to either oral or depot fluphenazine for maintenance (Quitkin et al., 1978). Pimozide is one of the purest dopamine antagonistic drugs available, and there is a large body of literature which supports this agent's antipsychotic efficacy in the treatment of both acute and chronic schizophrenia. Since it has been particularly well studied for maintenance, there is no doubt that it is an effective drug for prophylaxis.

Special Issues in the Use of Antipsychotics

PLASMA LEVELS   Most experienced clinicians know that the therapeutic dose for a given individual can vary tremendously, and this has led to a consideration of blood levels of antipsychotics as one explanation for the variance. The basic assumption underlying the plasma level studies is that the rate of metabolism, as well as other factors, may affect the quantity of the drug that actually reaches the receptor site. When an antipsychotic agent is given at a constant dose to different individuals, therefore, different amounts of the drug reach the receptor because of interindividual differences in metabolism. From this it follows that a plasma level-clinical response curve, on the one hand, and a plasma level-toxicity curve, on the other hand, are both dose-response curves (Figure 3). Combining them additively results in an inverted U-shaped curve, which is a visual representation of the *therapeutic window.* Below the window, the amount of drug that reaches the receptor site is insufficient to produce the desired clinical response. Above the window, either toxicity occurs or a paradoxical pharmacological response or both.

A good way of examining the dose-therapeutic-efficacy relationship is to consider it as essentially a dose-response curve, but clinical pharmacologic parameters determine how much drug reaches the receptor site. Unfortunately, methods for measuring blood levels of antipsychotics are technically complex, and it will take many years of refinement before such levels are used routinely in clinical practice. Evidence from several laboratories suggests that patients with low plasma levels fail to have an adequate clinical response, and some evidence (albeit more limited), suggests that a few patients fail to respond with high plasma levels (Curry et al., 1970a; 1970b; Davis et al., 1978; Garver et al., 1976; 1977; Smith et al., 1977a; 1979a; 1979b; Wode-Helgodt et al., 1977; 1978). Although these studies support a correlation between plasma levels and clinical response, most are methodologically unsound, and there is not enough evidence to support clinical use of plasma level at this time.

HIGH-DOSAGE PHENOTHIAZINE TREATMENT Hot debate surrounds the use of high-dosage antipsychotics which are thought to act more quickly or benefit the refractory patient. When patients do not improve as a result of normal doses of antipsychotic drug medication, psychiatrists often wonder whether a higher than normal dose would cause a remission in their disease. Now that it is clear that massive doses or megadoses of such agents as trifluoperazine, haloperidol, perphenazine, and fluphenazine can be safely given, e.g., 700 or 1,000 mg, various studies have been conducted to determine if loading doses will produce a more rapid result in schizophrenic patients.

In collaboration with Ericksen et al. (1978), the authors investigated two questions. (1) Compared to a normal dose, does a high loading or digitalizing dose produce a more rapid improvement in the first five days of treatment? (2) Is the final result after three weeks better than the result that would have been achieved had a normal dose been used? The study found that a five-day loading dose of 60 mg of intramuscular haloperidol was no more effective than 15 mg given orally every day. The study compared the two treatments over five days and at three weeks. After the first five days, the high-dose group was tapered to a normal dose of 15 mg of haloperidol. This group was compared to a normal-dose group, which received 15 mg of haloperidol throughout the three weeks of the study. The therapeutic outcomes at both five days and three weeks were identical (see Figures 4, 5).

In both groups thought disorder improved equally, the only difference being that there were more side effects, particularly dystonia, in the loading-dose group.

Table 2. Loxapine Studies and Their Results

Author	Subjects and Treatment Duration	Dose Ratio STD/New	Patient Improvement			Overall Results
Clark et al., 1975	New. Schiz.* 4 weeks	1:2	Lox +2 -11	Tri +2 -10	Pla 0 -12	Lox>Pla Lox=Tri Tri>Pla
Charalampous et al., 1974	Subacute Schiz. 4 weeks	10:25	Lox +10 -9	Thio +14 -3	Pla +10 -8	Lox=Pla Lox<Thio Thio=Pla
Clark et al., 1972	Chr. Schiz. 12 weeks	10:1	Lox +7 -10	CPZ +2 -15	Pla 0 -16	Lox>Pla Lox=CPZ CPZ>Pla
Moyano, 1975	Chr. Schiz. 12 weeks	1:2	Lox +14 -11		Tri +9 -14	Lox=Tri
Van Der Velde and Kiltie, 1975	New Schiz.* 6 weeks	10:25	Lox +17 -7	Thio +17 -10	Pla +6 -19	Lox>Pla Lox=Thio Thio=Pla
Bishop and Gallant, 1970	Chr. Schiz. 10 weeks	1:2	8 weeks Lox +3 -9		Tri +3 -9	
Steinbook et al., 1973	New. Schiz.* 6 weeks	1:2	Lox>CPZ on some measures but CPZ slightly but not significant>Lox on CGI			

Study	Diagnosis	Ratio	Loxapine	Comparator	Result
Shopsin et al, 1972a	New. Schiz.* 3 weeks	10:1	Lox + 2 / -13	CPZ + 8 / - 7	CPZ>Lox
Schiele, 1975	Chr. Schiz. 12 weeks	10:1	Lox + 9 / -16	CPZ +10 / -14	Lox = CPZ
Moore, 1975	New. Schiz.* 12 weeks	10:1	Lox +21 / - 7	CPZ +14 / -15	Lox>CPZ
Smith, Jackson, Personal Communication	New. Schiz.* 4 weeks	1:2	Lox + 6 / - 6	Tri + 6 / - 6	Lox = Tri
Denber, 1970	New. Schiz.* 6 weeks	1:1	Lox +11 / - 9	Tri +11 / - 9	Lox = Tri
Simpson and Cuculic, 1976	New. Schiz.* 4 weeks	1:2	Lox + 7 / -17	Tri + 4 / -15	Lox = Tri
Paprochi and Versiani, 1977	Acute Schiz. 5 weeks	1:10	Lox +10 / - 7	Hal +15 / - 3	Lox = Hal
Dube, 1976	New. Schiz.* 12 weeks	9:3	Lox +24 / - 2	CPZ +25 / - 1	Lox = CPZ
Seth et al, 1979	Chr. Schiz. 12 weeks	1:2	Lox N = 33	Tri N = 31	Lox = Tri

Table 2. Continued

Author	Subjects and Treatment Duration	Dose Ratio STD/New	Patient Improvement		Overall Results
Vyas and Kalla, 1980	Chr. Schiz. 24 weeks	10:1	Lox +13 − 2	CPZ +15 0	Lox = CPZ
Malih and Kumar, 1980	New. Schiz.* 4 weeks	2.5:10	Lox +23 − 3	Tri +24 − 2	Lox = Tri
Fruens-gaard et al., 1978	Acute Schiz. 3-11 weeks	34:54	Lox + 8 − 1	Per + 7 − 1	Lox = Per
Fruens-gaard et al., 1978	Chr. Schiz. 12 weeks	90:81	Lox + 3 − 6	Per + 5 − 6	Lox = Per
Fruens-gaard et al., 1977	Acute Schiz. 3 days	1:10	Lox +14 − 1	Hal +15 0	Lox = Hal
Kiloh et al., 1976	Acute Schiz. 12 weeks	3:5	Lox +24 − 1	Tri +20 −11	Lox = Tri
Arib, 1974	Chr. Schiz. 13 weeks	1:2	Lox +16 − 9	Tri +19 − 6	Lox = Tri
Selman et al., 1976	New Schiz.* 12 weeks	2:25	Lox +26 − 2	Hal +22 − 4	Pla +17 − 8	Lox = Hal>Pla

*Newly Admitted Schizophrenic

THEORETICAL CONCEPT OF THERAPEUTIC WINDOW

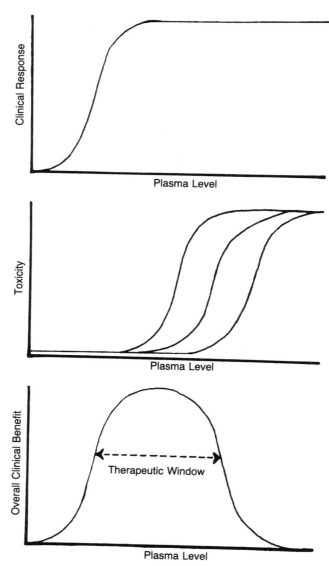

Figure 3. Schematic hypothetical relationship between plasma level and clinical response; between plasma level and toxicity; and between plasma level and overall clinical benefit (Davis, Ericksen, and De-kirmenjian, 1978).

Donlon et al. (1978) conducted a similar study testing the effects of rapid treatment of psychosis with fluphenazine. For up to seven days they studied 32 patients who were receiving either a standard dose of 20 mg or 80 mg per day. Neborsky, Janowsky, and their co-workers (1981) did a similar high dose vs. moderate dose study and found that the different doses produced an identical rate of improvement.

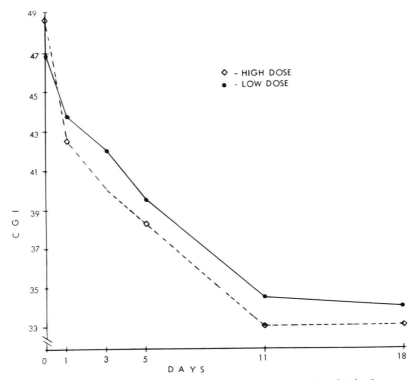

Figure 4. Rate of improvement of patients receiving high dose or standard dose of haloperidol on the Clinical Global Index (CGI) (Ericksen, Hurt, Holzman, and Davis, unpublished data).

Goldberg and his collaborators (1972), in a study comparing the efficacy of 60 mg and 600 mg of trifluoperazine, found the two treatments to be equally effective. Similarly, Quitkin et al. (1975) showed that a dose of 1 200 mg fluphenazine a day is no better than 30 mg a day. Studies of chronic patients have yielded similar results (Itil et al., 1970a; 1971; Brotman et al., 1969).

Gardos and his co-workers (1974) compared 10 mg vs. 40 mg of thiothixene (440 mg of CPZ equivalence vs. 1,760 mg of CPZ equivalence) and found the two doses essentially equal in effectiveness. Prien, Levine, and Cole (1969) found 15 mg of trifluoperazine (equivalent to 535 mg of CPZ) to be just as effective as 80 mg of trifluoperazine (2,800 mg CPZ equivalence). That finding probably indicates that 535 mg (CPZ equivalent) are close to the maximal effective doses of trifluoperazine, so that an extra-high dose did not produce additional improvement in the chronically ill population they studied. However, Clark et al. (1970b; 1972b) showed that doses of 300 mg or less of CPZ are probably below the effective therapeutic dose for chronically ill patients (600 mg are better than 300 mg, which are better than 150 mg). Prien and Cole (1968) found that a high dose was superior to a low dose when comparing 2,000 mg of CPZ with 300 mg of CPZ in chronic schizophrenic patients. This study suggests that when a low dose is less effective than a high dose, the low dose must be below the optimal point on the dose-response curve.

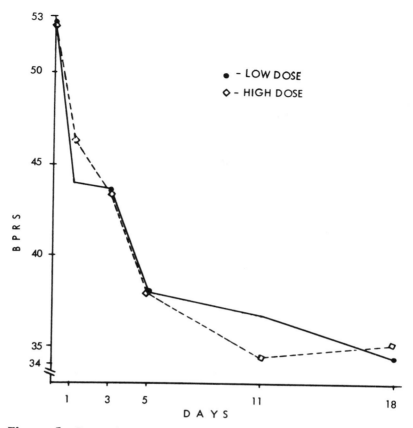

Figure 5. Rate of improvement of patients receiving high dose or standard dose of haloperidol on the Brief Psychiatric Rating Scale (BPRS) (Ericksen, Hurt, Holzman, and Davis, unpublished data).

Simpson and co-workers (1968) also did dose-response studies of butaperazine, investigating 24 chronically regressed schizophrenic patients, randomly assigned to four groups investigated under nonblind conditions. One group was started at 5.0 mg of butaperazine a day (55.5 mg CPZ equivalence), and the other groups started at doses of 40, 80, and 120 mg (444, 888, and 1,333 mg CPZ equivalence). During this early part of the trial, the patients who received 5.0 mg of butaperazine tended not to do as well as patients who received a higher initial dose.

It is important to differentiate between the use of moderately high doses, such as double the normal dose used by Prien and Cole (1968), and the megadose strategy used by Quitkin et al. (1975), who used 100 times the normal dose. A modest increase in dose, such as double or quadruple the normal recommended amount, may be beneficial to some acute or subacute schizophrenics, and greater increases may help a few more patients. In the authors' judgment, dose information should be conceptualized using the model of a dose-response curve. In general, doses below approximately 500 mg of CPZ seem to be on the linear portion of the dose-response curve. Doses above 600 mg of CPZ seem to be above the linear portion of the dose-response curve. Since there are not enough studies to define the dose-response curve of antipsychotics precisely, the curve can only be approximated within limits of plus or minus 100 mg of CPZ equivalent. The authors estimate that the dose-response curve starts to flatten out around 500 mg of CPZ.

A mean dose-response curve from a group study averages the individual curves of many patients. The mean curve is made up of many different individual responses to different doses. Plasma level differences undoubtedly account for part of the individual variations, as do patients' clinical conditions. Some individuals may have dose-response curves skewed to the left and others to the right. Furthermore, an individual's dose-response curve could shift from one time to another, depending on the intensity of his or her clinical state. Some patients may be fast metabolizers and have very low plasma levels and, hence, very low brain levels, their curves are skewed to the right of the mean. High-dose strategy may be useful in treating these treatment-resistant patients. Some patients may have slow metabolisms, high plasma levels, and dose-response curves that are skewed to the left, and such patients should be treated with low doses. The foregoing discussion of mean dose-response curves is intended to give the reader a feel for the *average* dose-response curve of antipsychotics, taking into account the limitations of our present information and recognizing individual differences.

MAINTENANCE TREATMENT   More than 35 double-blind studies show that maintenance antipsychotic drugs prevent relapse. Most of these studies lasted from four to six months. Thirty-three of these studies report findings on the number of patients who relapsed or failed to relapse on placebo or on maintenance medication (Table 3). Of the total of 3,606 patients in the studies, twenty percent relapsed on drug, whereas 53 percent relapsed on placebo. Intuitively, with such a large sample of patients, and with a drug-placebo difference of 33 percent, one would anticipate that the combined results are statistically significant. The Mantel method for combining data from studies proved that the results were, in fact, highly statistically significant ($p < 10^{-100}$).

In a descriptive sense, patients clearly do gradually relapse over time. To determine whether the relapse rate is constant over time, the authors have analyzed the data from three well-controlled studies (Caffey et al., 1964; Hogarty and Goldberg, 1973; 1974; Prien and Cole, 1968). The relapse rates, here defined as the percentages of patients who relapsed each month, appear in the bottom panels of Figures 6, 7, 8. Note that the relapse rate does seem to be constant over time. If a relapse rate of ten percent per month were constant over time and if the patient population numbered one hundred, then in the first month, ten would relapse and ninety unrelapsed patients would remain. In the next month, ten percent of ninety or nine would relapse, leaving 81. In the next month, ten percent of 81 or eight would relapse, and 73 unrelapsed patients would remain.

This is much the same as compound interest: as interest compounds, interest earns interest. In mathematics, this is referred to as an exponential function. The authors' laboratory was the first to propose that the rate of relapse demonstrated by patients might be expressed as an exponential function (Davis, 1975; 1976), and, accordingly, to correct for the fact that each month a smaller absolute number remains in the study. In the top panels of Figures 6, 7, and 8, the number of patients not relapsed is plotted vs. time (a semi-log plot), using data from the same

Table 3. Antipsychotic Prevention of Relapse

	No. of patients	Relapse on placebo	Relapse on drug	Difference in relapse rate (placebo-drug)
Caffey	250	45%	5%	40%
Prien	762	42%	16%	26%
Prien	325	56%	20%	36%
Schiele	80	60%	3%	57%
Adelson	281	90%	49%	41%
Morton	40	70%	25%	45%
Baro	26	100%	0%	100%
Hershon	62	28%	7%	21%
Rassidakis	84	58%	34%	24%
Melynk	40	50%	0%	50%
Schauver	80	18%	5%	13%
Freeman	94	28%	13%	15%
Whitaker	39	65%	8%	57%
Garfield	27	31%	11%	20%
Diamond	40	70%	25%	45%
Blackburn	53	54%	24%	30%
Gross	109	58%	14%	44%
Englehardt	294	30%	15%	15%
Leff	30	83%	33%	50%
Hogarty	361	67%	31%	36%
Troshinsky	43	63%	4%	59%
Hirsch	74	66%	8%	58%
Chien	31	87%	12%	75%
Gross	61	65%	34%	31%
Rifkin	62	68%	7%	61%
Clark	35	78%	27%	51%
Clark	19	70%	43%	27%
Kinross-Wright	40	70%	5%	65%
Andrews	31	35%	7%	28%
Wistedt	38	63%	38%	25%
Cheung	28	62%	13%	49%
Levine, P.O.	33	59%	33%	26%
Levine, I.M.	34	30%	18%	12%

Summary statistics: $p < 10^{-100}$ (Chi-square = 470.3; df = 1)

Sources: Davis, 1975; Levine et al., 1978; Wistedt, 1981.

three double-blind, controlled studies. The data produce an excellent fit to an exponential function and suggest that a constant percentage of patients relapse each month. Expressed this way, the data of Hogarty

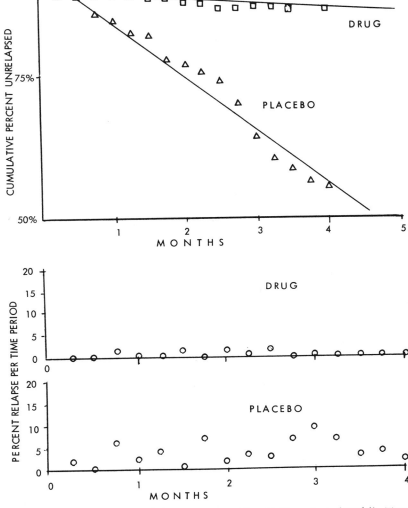

Figure 6. Reanalysis of data presented by Caffey et al. (1964). Top panel presents cumulative percent of schizophrenics unrelapsed on drug or on placebo vs. time. Bottom panel presents the percent of patients who relapsed in each time period (number of patients relapsing vs. number of patients unrelapsed at beginning of that period).

and Goldberg (1973; 1974) indicate that antipsychotic drugs reduce relapses by a factor of 2.5. This is a substantial degree of prophylaxis, especially since the sample had a history of chronic relapsing schizophrenia. About half of those who had relapsed had stopped taking their medication. If one were to assume that all these patients relapsed as a result of not having taken their medication, then the drug-induced reduction of relapse would take on a factor of 5.0. But since some of the patients actually have relapsed while on medication and then later stopped taking their medication because of the psychosis, the factor of 5.0 must be viewed with qualification.

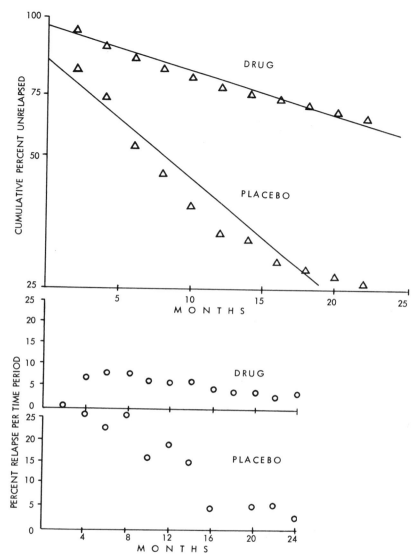

Figure 7. Reanalysis of data of Hogarty and Goldberg (1973; 1974). Top panel presents cumulative percent of patients unrelapsed on drug and placebo. Bottom panel presents percentage of patients relapsing per time period (number of patients relapsed divided by number of patients as yet unrelapsed at beginning of that particular time period).

Despite the apparent efficacy of the drugs, in a long-term, chronic situation it would be desirable to manage patients without medication in order to prevent tardive dyskinesia. In an effort not to medicate any chronic schizophrenic patient unnecessarily, Morgan and Cheadle (1974) picked 74 of 475 such patients as possibly suitable for a drug-free trial. Only five of these patients remained off drugs. The relapse of the other 69 patients occurred at an average of about four-and-a-half months off drugs, indicating that most chronic schizophrenics are at risk for relapse without medication.

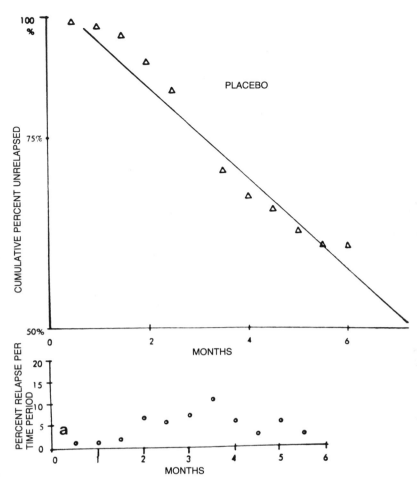

Figure 8. Reanalysis of data of Prien and Cole (1968). Top panel presents cumulative percent of patients unrelapsed vs. time. Bottom panel presents the percent of patients relapsing per time period (number of patients relapsing in a given time period divided by number of patients as yet unrelapsed at the beginning of that time period).

Since fifty percent of patients relapse with drugs and fifty percent do not, some have claimed, fifty percent of patients do not need medication. This is not an accurate way to think about relapses. With the relapse rate of ten percent per month, a study lasting four or five months will, indeed, find that about fifty percent of the patients relapse. But if the study lasted one year, 75 percent of the patients would relapse. If it lasted two years, 87 percent of the patients would relapse. The fact that fifty percent of the patients do not relapse by four months does not mean that they will never relapse and, hence, do not need medication. A more accurate approach to maintenance data is to consider whether the relapse rate is constant over time. If it is constant over time, then it is better to conceptualize the relapse phenomenon in terms of the relapse rate rather than in terms of the absolute number of patients who relapse. As noted, the data from various studies do fit an exponential function better than a linear function, but in a long trial there may be a ceiling effect. That is, as well as patients who are at risk for relapse and who do relapse, there may be patients who will never relapse, and the curve should flatten out. In the Hogarty and Goldberg study (1973; 1974), the relapse occurred at a constant rate until about 18 months when the curve began to flatten out (see Figure 7). By 18 months, however, so few patients were in the study that the empirically observed relapse rate may not be accurate. Because of this, Hogarty et al. (1976) examined the relapse rate of the same group of patients who had been studied for two years or more. Although there were not enough patients in the placebo group, there were an appreciable number of patients in the drug-treated group who were available for investigation. When those patients had their antipsychotic drugs discontinued, they relapsed in an exponential manner, with a rate quite similar to that they had observed initially.

MAINTENANCE TREATMENT—*Choice of Depot Fluphenazine Preparations.* Between the two forms of fluphenazine for depot administration, fluphenazine enanthate and fluphenazine decanoate, one could conceivably be superior to the other.

Findings from six studies provide evidence that fluphenazine decanoate appears to be slightly more potent but essentially equal to the enanthate formulation (Hogarty et al., 1979; Kane et al., 1978; Schooler and Levine, 1978; Schooler et al., 1979; Levine et al., 1980; del Guidice et al., 1975; Van Praag and Dois, 1973). EPS are seen slightly less often among patients receiving decanoate, as indicated by Donlon et al. (1978). Differences between these two preparations of depot fluphenazine are very marginal, but insofar as these slight differences may be real, fluphenazine decanoate appears to have some marginal advantages.

Low-Dose Maintenance Treatment. During the chronic maintenance therapy of schizophrenia, clinicians must balance the risk of patients relapsing without adequate medication against the risk of their developing tardive dyskinesia, assuming the latter is dose dependent. Using the fluphenazine decanoate, Kane et al. (1979a; 1979b) randomly assigned partially remitted outpatient schizophrenics to a low-dose group (1.25 to 5.0 mg biweekly) or to a standard-dose group (12.5-50 mg biweekly). The cumulative relapse rate was significantly higher in the low-dose group. Many of these relapses on low doses are, it should be noted, easily treated by increasing the dose, and they rarely lead to hospitalization.

New Maintenance Medications. A team of French investigators (Simon et al., 1978) compared the effects of standard neuroleptics fluphenazine decanoate, and pipotiazine palmitate (also a depot neuroleptic) among patients assigned at random to one of the three treatments. They found that the two depot formulations were as effective as the oral medication.

The antipsychotic penfluridol, administered orally once each week, has been compared with fluphenazine decanoate and found equally efficacious (Quitkin et al., 1978).

Haloperidol decanoate injectable has become available in Europe and can be given once every month. Roose (1981) has reported that monthly injections of haloperidol decanoate in 34 psychotic patients who had previously received biweekly injections of fluphenazine decanoate were of similar or superior efficacy. Based on two open trials, Meco et al. (1981) and Darondel and Fengler (1981), reported that haloperidol decanoate monthly injections were at least as effective as oral haloperidol. In these two studies, dosages of the monthly haloperidol decanoate were calculated by oral dose of haloperidol multiplied by a factor of 20. The dosage of haloperidol decanoate used in the three studies was 75 to 200 mg every four weeks.

Mechanisms of Action

BIOLOGICAL All clinically effective antipsychotics block the neurotransmitter, dopamine, at postsynaptic membrane receptor sites in the CNS (Carlsson, 1978; Horn and Snyder, 1971). Dopamine blockade in the mesolimbic system is thought to be responsible for the antipsychotic effect of these agents. In the corpus striatum, this same process is thought to cause the neuroleptic side effects (or EPS) associated with the antipsychotics. Since Parkinsonian side effects are caused by antipsychotic drugs, and since Parkinson's disease involves a dopamine deficiency, it is reasonable to assume that these side effects are produced by the drugs' blockade of dopamine. When central dopamine receptors are blocked by the antipsychotic agents, dopamine synthesis is increased until tolerance develops over a course of a few weeks. These findings have led to the dopamine hypothesis of schizophrenia.

The potency of antipsychotic agents to block dopamine receptors as measured by dopamine binding *in vitro* strongly parallels the potency of these drugs in man. There is a quantitative correspondence between the dose necessary for treating schizophrenia in man and the dose *in vitro* that blocks dopamine binding (Seeman et al., 1975; 1976; Snyder et al., 1975; Creese et al., 1976). Clinical potency and dopamine binding both correlate with pharmacological and behavioral evidence of dopamine receptor-blocking properties. Furthermore, the isomer of flupenthixol that blocks dopamine receptors is a potent antipsychotic in humans, but the isomer that does not block dopamine receptors is ineffective in schizophrenia (Johnstone et al., 1978).

If the antipsychotic drugs do benefit schizophrenia by blocking dopamine at the receptor site, reducing the amount of dopamine in the brain with an inhibitor of dopamine synthesis could conceivably potentiate the action of the antipsychotic drugs. Indeed, if dopamine synthesis is blocked with α-methyl-paratyrosine, the amount of antipsychotic agents necessary for a beneficial effect in schizophrenia is reduced (Carlsson, 1978). This is consistent with the evidence that these particular agents produce their antipsychotic action by means of an interaction with dopamine. Although reserpine and tetrabenazine have antipsychotic properties, compared to phenothiazine derivatives these agents are not as effective. They interfere with the storage of many biogenic amines, such as serotonin, norepinephrine, or dopamine, by compromising the integrity of the storage vesicles. In the laboratory the authors found apomorphine to have an antipsychotic action, presumably produced by its property of stimulating presynaptic receptors to reduce dopamine synthesis and release (Smith et al., 1977b; Tamminga et al., 1978). Corsini et al. (1977) found a similar effect.

If decreasing the dopaminergic activity benefits schizophrenic patients, it would seem that increasing dopaminergic activity could aggravate their condition. Dopamine receptor stimulants, such as bromocriptine, lisuride, and legatrile, can produce psychotic symptoms. Psychomotor stimulants, such as amphetamine, methylphenidate, and cocaine, are potent releasers of dopamine, and they also block its reuptake. It is well known that large doses of an amphetamine-type drug or cocaine can cause a paranoid schizophrenic-like episode in normal volunteers or addicts. Janowsky et al. (1973) reported that small intravenous doses of methylphenidate (0.5 mg/kg) can produce a marked worsening of preexisting psychosis in patients with active schizophrenic illness. The phenomenon of substantially worsening a preexisting psychosis may be a different one from that of producing a typical paranoid psychosis in the nonschizophrenic subject. A patient's psychosis worsens both qualitatively and quantitatively in the direction of his or her preexisting psychosis. Thus, catatonic and hebephrenic schizophrenics become more catatonic and hebephrenic, without showing paranoid symptoms. In the order of potency, methylphenidate is more potent than D-amphetamine, which itself is more potent than L-amphetamine. Methylphenidate releases central intraneuronal stores of norepinephrine and dopamine from the reserpine-sensitive pool.

As we have summarized above, there is some evidence which suggests the role for dopamine as a hypothetical transmitter which may be involved in schizophrenia. Certainly, there is excellent evidence that the antipsychotic drugs produce their therapeutic benefit in schizophrenia through their property of dopamine blockade. Nonetheless, although the dopamine hypothesis of schizophrenia is an interesting speculation, in the absence of direct evidence that an abnormality of dopamine is involved, we must clearly recognize that the biochemical basis of schizophrenia is unknown at this time.*

PSYCHOLOGICAL A common mistake is to think of the antipsychotic drugs as a special type of sedative. The label antischizophrenic also may be misleading, since the drugs are also effective in psychotic depression, mania, and organic psychosis. Antipsychotic drugs do not produce a state of tranquility in either a normal or a psychotic person. If antipsychotics acted through sedation, the more sedative drugs would be shown to be more effective, but antipsychotics that are maximally stimulating are just as effective as antipsychotics that are maximally sedating. Antipsychotics, in fact, have a normalizing effect. For example, they slow down excited patients and speed up retarded states. They also lessen typical schizophrenic symptoms, such as hallucinations and delusions (see Table 4).

The approach of a biological psychiatrist to the quantitation of schizophrenic symptoms is essentially Kraepelinian. Existing rating scales quantitate the symptoms of schizophrenia, and the antipsychotic drugs ameliorate these symptoms across the board. In this sense, then, the descriptive term *antipsychotic* conveys the results of the lessening of the symptomatology as observed in quantitative studies. Both Kraepelin and Bleuler discussed the thought disorder frequently found in schizophrenic patients, but Bleuler particularly emphasized the

*Preceptor's note: See also the chapter by Wyatt and his colleagues for a further discussion of the dopamine hypothesis.

Table 4. Effect of Phenothiazines on Symptoms in Schizophrenia

	V.A. Study No. 1	V.A. Study No. 3	Kurland and Richardson, 1966	NIMH-PSC No. 1	Gorham and Pokorny, 1964 (vs. Group Psychotherapy)
Fundamental symptoms					
Thought disorder	++	++	++	++	++
Blunted affect-indifference	++	++		++	+
Withdrawal-retardation	++	++	0	++	++
Autistic behavior-mannerisms	++	++	0	++	+
Accessory symptoms					
Hallucinations	++	++	+	+	0
Paranoid ideation	0	++	0	+	+
Grandiosity	0	0	0	0	+
Hostility-belligerence	++	++	H.R.	+	+
Resistiveness-uncooperativeness	++	++	H.R.	++	++
Nonschizophrenic symptoms					
Anxiety-tension agitation	0	0	H.R.	+	0
Guilt depression	++	0	0	0	0
Disorientation				0	
Somatization					0

+ + symptom areas showing marked drug-control group differences

+ areas showing significant but less striking differences

0 areas not showing differential drug superiority

H.R. heterogeneity of regression found on analysis of covariance of the measures indicated. This invalidates this particular statistical procedure but does not mean that there was no drug effect (Cole et al, 1966).

Source: Cole et al, 1966.

thought disorder as being fundamental to the schizophrenic process. Thought disorder does not necessarily occur in all schizophrenics, nor are one or more of the various thought disorders necessary for the diagnosis of a Schizophrenic Disorder. A recently developed quantitative instrument enables the researcher to assess thought disorder and to evaluate its intensity in a blind fashion (Johnston and Holzman, 1979). To determine whether or not antipsychotic drugs benefit the thought disorder of schizophrenic patients as well as they do the symptoms of schizophrenia, Holzman, Hurt, and Davis measured the drug-induced improvement in schizophrenic symptoms and difference in thought disorders, before and after the drug treatment. The results indicated that antipsychotic drugs produced a marked reduction in the various symptoms of schizophrenia, as well as in the thought disorder. The disordered thinking improved within the same time course and to the same degree as the schizophrenic symptoms (Figure 9).

Spohn and his co-workers (1977) studied the effect of antipsychotic drugs on chronic schizophrenic patients. After a six-week placebo washout period, patients were randomly placed either on placebo or on CPZ. CPZ reduced their overestimation and fixation time on a perceptual task and increased their accuracy of perceptual judgment. Since

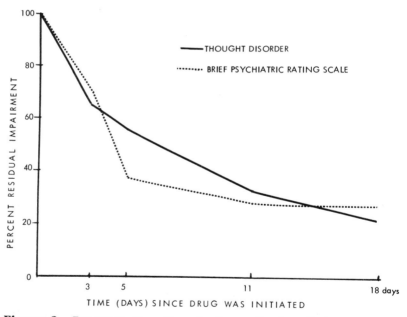

Figure 9. Response to antipsychotic medication (haloperidol) in schizophrenic patients as measured by the Holzman Thought Disorder Index and the Brief Psychiatric Rating Scale (BPRS). On each measure, psychopathology is assigned a value of 100% prior to drug treatment and then the improvement is expressed as the percent of 100% on these two indices at each assessment time. The rate of improvement of BPRS and of thought disorder parallel each other, and at the end of the three-week study, the extent of improvement is approximately equal, the residual psychopathology present at that time being reduced from 100% to 25% (Hurt, Holzman, and Davis, unpublished data).

the common denominator of those tests may be the ability to attend appropriately to the task at hand, CPZ seemed to enhance the patients' concentration and attention. The attentional dysfunction, information-processing impairment, and autonomic dysfunction were normalized by the antipsychotic drug, but they were not normalized by placebo. Hence, the normalization process about which psychologists have speculated may be associated with the psychological abnormalities that underlie schizophrenia. Empirically, antipsychotic drugs seem not only to reduce typical symptoms of schizophrenia, like hallucinations, but also to lessen the characteristic thought disorder and to have a normalizing effect on various common perceptual, cognitive, or autonomic dysfunctions.

Neuroendocrine Effects

In the past few years, we have made striking advances in our understanding of how antipsychotics affect the endocrine system (Agnoli et al., 1979; Alfredsson et al., 1979; Brown et al., 1976b). Evidence suggesting that the locus of antipsychotic effects on prolactin is at the pituitary, findings concerning the effects of antipsychotics on prolactin, and the effects of antipsychotics on the other hormones (Casacchia et al., 1979) are especially germane.

PROLACTIN—*Locus of Prolactin Changes:* Dopaminergic systems external to the blood brain barrier (BBB) are likely loci for the regulation of plasma prolactin. The finding that domperidone (a drug which does not pass the BBB) elevates prolactin levels in man provides evidence for this hypothesis (Brown et al., in press; Brown, 1977; Pourmond et al., 1980). In addition, since dopamine does not cross the BBB, it is of interest that infusions of dopamine decrease plasma levels (Besses, 1975; Leblanc et al., 1976). Furthermore, administration of carbidopa, a peripheral decarboxylase inhibitor which lowers peripheral dopamine levels, elevates prolactin (Brown et al., 1976a).

Antipsychotic Drugs' Effects on Prolactin: Many investigators have noted the very rapid prolactin response to neuroleptics (Busch, 1979; Kolakowska et al., 1979; Langer et al., 1977b; Rubin and Forster, 1980; Rubin and Hays, 1978). Depot intramuscular neuroleptics also elevate prolactin (Huws and Groom, 1977). Drugs that block dopamine receptors in various test systems are clinically potent neuroleptics in man. The marked relationship between dose of drug in man and the ability of various antipsychotic drugs to bind to dopamine receptors is a clue as to how neuroleptics help schizophrenics. Plasma prolactin is one measure of dopamine blockade in man at a pituitary level. Antipsychotics stimulate prolactin secretion in rats, whereas apparently similar structures of drugs without antipsychotic actions do not increase prolactin (Clemens, 1974).

Langer (1979) and Langer et al. (1977a; 1977b; 1978) and Gruen et al. (1978a; 1978b) compared the potency of neuroleptics for stimulating prolactin to the drugs' clinical potency in schizophrenia. The authors plotted both Langer's and Gruen's data and found that the dose necessary to benefit schizophrenia is higher than the dose necessary to increase prolactin in man. Crowley and MacDonald (1981) administered thioridazine or thiothixene in a ratio of 25:1 and found that the two neuroleptics produced comparable increases in prolactin. Cotes et al. (1978) found that α-flupenthixol produced improvement in schizophrenia and increased prolactin, whereas β-flupenthixol produced neither improvement in schizophrenia nor an increase in prolactin. The α-isomer is active in blocking dopamine in animal preparations. Sedvall (1979) noted that melperone elevated prolactin much less than thiothixene. If prolactin elevation and antipsychotic dose were highly correlated, then at an equal antipsychotic dose both melperone and thiothixene would be expected to elevate prolactin to the same degree. CPZ was found to elevate prolactin less than equivalent thiothixene.

Clozapine (600 mg/day) either failed to elevate prolactin or produced only a small effect (Sedvall, 1979; Sachar et al., 1976; Meltzer et al., 1979; and Lal and Nair, 1979). Sulpiride is more potent in elevating prolactin levels than in ameliorating psychotic symptoms (Crosignani et al., 1977; Mielke et al., 1977; Mancini et al., 1976; Muller et al., 1979), although in therapeutic doses it clearly has some antipsychotic properties (Cassano et al., 1975; Rama-Rao et al., 1981; Toru et al., 1972; Mielke et al., 1977). Thus, both clozapine and sulpiride depart somewhat from the parallelism.

In general, there is a partial parallel between the antipsychotic drugs' ability to block dopamine receptors as measured in a variety of systems, including the pituitary, and their clinical potency in man. Certain discrepancies may be explained by a drug's poorer penetration into the brain than into the pituitary, but this may not be of great theoretical interest. A high affinity to specific receptors in the mesolimbic system and relatively low affinities in other systems may be important clues to the mechanism of action of different antipsychotics. Overall, the wide variety of assays of dopamine receptor blockade (direct measure of receptor binding, pituitary effects, animal behavior, and EPS) show an excellent correlation with clinical dose, consistent with the theory that antipsychotic drugs produce their behavioral effects in schizophrenia by blocking dopamine receptors.

Since patients can develop tolerance to the effects of many drugs, investigators have asked if patients develop specific tolerance to the ability of neuroleptics to elevate plasma prolactin. If this were so, prolactin levels would return to normal despite continued doses of neuroleptics. Several authors fail to find a decrease in prolactin levels after neuroleptic treatment of approximately one month (Gruen et al., 1978a; 1978b; Meltzer et al., 1977). Generally, since these studies increased the neuroleptic doses over time, any decrease due to tolerance could have been canceled out. Over eighty days of treatment, Mielke, Gallant, and Kessler (1977) found no development of tolerance to the prolactin-elevating properties of sulpiride. During the same period, they did observe a hint of development of tolerance for conventional neuroleptics. The patients on conventional neuroleptics showed a fifty percent reduction of prolactin at this time, but this finding was not statistically significant.

While almost one hundred percent of patients treated acutely with a small dose of neuroleptic have a substantial (two hundred or three hundred percent) elevation in prolactin levels, only about fifty percent of patients treated with long-term neuroleptics have elevated prolactin levels. Table 5 presents prolactin values found by various researchers in patients treated with long-term antipsychotics. The authors have some preliminary evidence that the types of patients who become very chronic (ten to twenty years in the hospital) have lower plasma levels than do newly admitted patients on comparable doses of neuroleptics

Table 5. Prolactin Value (PRL) in Patients Treated with Long-Term
Antipsychotics

	Number of Patients with Elevated PRL	Number of Patients with Normal PRL
Arato et al. (1979)	15	12
Martin Du Pan (1979)	10	10
De Rivera et al. (1976)		
Young Male	8	4
Young Female	11	1
Old Male	7	5
Old Female (48 yr +)	8	6
Wilson et al. (1973)	35	13
Beumont et al. (1974a; 1974b)		
Female with Lactation	13	3
Male	0	5
Postmenopausal Female	3	1
Naber (1979; 1980c)		
Male	0	23
Female	6	29
Naber (1980a; 1980b)		
Male	0	12
Female	1	9
Cohen et al. (1979)	1	3
Kolakowska et al. (1981)*		
Male	10	3
Female	2	0
Kolakowska et al. (1979)		
Male	2	2
Female	4	3
Wiles et al. (1980)		
Male	6	3
Female	2	0
	144	147

*Patients on long-term (1 yr. +) continuous medication

(Smith et al., 1977a; 1979a). One reason that patients develop chronicity may be that they are fast metabolizers of neuroleptic drugs, never build up a therapeutic plasma level, and hence never receive adequate treatment. Whether or not this is true, tolerance cannot be definitively dealt with until patients are studied both under conditions of acute treatment and following long-term drug treatment. In addition to basal prolactin levels, Naber and his co-workers (1980a; 1980b; 1980c) studied thyrotropin-stimulated prolactin levels. In both studies the levels were increased approximately 53 ng/ml in men and approximately 80 ng/ml in women, providing evidence that the pituitary had sufficient reserve to increase prolactin levels. Parenthetically, there is no evidence that increase in prolactin levels leads to breast cancer (Schyve et al., 1978). Women have much higher antipsychotic prolactin levels than men (Judd et al., 1978b; Goode et al., 1980; Buckman and Peake, 1973).

Use of Prolactin Level as Plasma Level: Some have suggested using steady-state prolactin levels as measures instead of antipsychotic plasma levels, because the antipsychotics produce a fairly quantitative rise in prolactin. A number of studies have correlated prolactin levels to antipsychotic plasma levels, and the correlations vary from essentially zero to very high. Considering all correlations from the various studies, the mean correlation between prolactin level and plasma level is approximately 0.50 (Ohman and Axelsson, 1978; Ohman et al., 1980; Linnoila et al., 1980; Nikitopoulou et al., 1976; Rama-Rao et al., 1980; Brown and Laughren, 1981; Rubin, 1980; Rubin et al., 1976; Rubin and Hays, 1978; 1979; Rubin and Forster, 1980; Hays and Rubin, 1981).

Gruen and his co-workers (1978a; 1978b) suggest that there might be a ceiling effect in the prolactin dose-response curve. Ohman and Axelsson (1978) and Ohman et al. (1980) investigated this possibility, studying a group of patients who received both low-dose and moderate-dose thioridazine. In doing a dose-response curve, since patients' plasma levels differ widely, it is important to have steady-state values of the same patient at two different doses. Performing a separate, independent statistical analysis, the authors examined their data on patients who had dose increases of 200 mg from approximately 200 mg to approximately 400 mg, and then from approximately 600 mg to 800 mg. On the average, prolactin levels at the lower doses went from 46 ng/ml to 73 ng/ml, a difference of 27 ng. At the higher dose, plasma levels were essentially identical: the level of increment from approximately 600 to approximately 800 mg averaged 0.65 ng/ml. This finding clearly indicates a ceiling effect. Kolakowska et al. (1981) also find evidence for a ceiling effect. Since the ceiling effect may begin to occur above approximate CPZ equivalent doses of 600 mg, prolactin levels could conceivably be of some value for defining the lower end of the therapeutic window.

TARDIVE DYSKINESIA AND ENDOCRINE EFFECTS Tardive dyskinesia is hypothesized to be caused by a supersensitivity of striatal dopamine receptors. Since it is presumably caused by an increased number of receptor sites secondary to an assumed chronic denervation caused by dopamine blockade of neuroleptics (Lemberger and Crabtree, 1979), one would expect an increase in the number of dopamine receptor sites in the pituitary after chronic neuroleptic treatment. It would follow that patients with tardive dyskinesia would have lower basal prolactin levels and a greater magnitude of decrease in serum prolactin following apomorphine or dopamine administration.

Friend et al. (1978) found that binding of haloperidol to rat pituitary was decreased following chronic haloperidol treatment. The authors' group (Tamminga et al., 1976; 1977) used apomorphine and dopa as a provocative agent to stimulate growth hormone (GH) or to reduce prolactin. They found that chronic schizophrenics with or without tardive dyskinesia had slightly lower prolactin levels in response to these stimulants than did controls. Similarly, chronic schizophrenics with and without tardive dyskinesia had a sluggish response to dopa- or apomorphine-stimulated GH test. These data are not consistent with expected changes. Ettig et al. (1976) had similar findings.

Asnis et al. (1979) found that prolactin levels in tardive dyskinesia patients were similar to those of controls after neuroleptic withdrawal or patients later given a neuroleptic challenge. Jeste et al. (1981) investigated 12 patients with tardive dyskinesia and 12 matched controls. Of the controls, eight were chronic schizophrenics and four had organic brain syndromes. All patients were on a stable dose of neuroleptic or had been drug free for one month. The levels of plasma prolactin and GH did not differ significantly from those of controls. Parenthetically, it has been suggested that tardive dyskinesia has clinical and biochemical features of depression (Rosenbaum, 1979).

EFFECTS ON GH Antipsychotic drugs would be expected to lower GH levels (either basal GH levels or stimulated GH levels). Since GH levels are already low, it may be hard to demonstrate that any agent would lower them further, and results are, not surprisingly, somewhat inconsistent. Many authors have found that antipsychotic drugs produce a slight lowering in GH levels (Collu et al., 1975; Masala et al., 1977; Sherman et al., 1971; Saldanha et al., 1972; Beumont et al., 1974a; 1974b; Tyson and Friesen, 1973; Benjamin et al., 1969; Kleinberg and Frantz, 1971; Mielke et al., 1977; Rubin and Hays, 1978; Beg et al., 1979). But the lowering effect is modest, and the results are somewhat inconsistent. In general, the antipsychotic drugs have little effect on basal level, but insofar as they do have an effect, it tends to be a very slight decrease.

Studies have also evaluated antipsychotics' effects on GH response to provocative tests. Both Sherman et al. (1971) and Chalmer and Bennie (1978) found that antipsychotics lower insulin-stimulated GH, but Saldanha et al. (1972) had inconsistent results. However, Beumont (1974a; 1974b) did not find such blunting. Schwimm et al. (1976) found that pimoxide blunted the GH response to arginine and exercise. Several groups found a slight decrease in the GH response to dopa, but this was not always statistically significant (Collu et al., 1975; Masala et al., 1977; Mims et al., 1975). Rotrosen and his co-workers (1979) found that haloperidol blocked the GH response to apomorphine. Clarenback and his co-workers (1978) found a slight but not statistically different decrease in the sleep-induced GH peak. In general, in most but not all studies, antipsychotics do blunt the GH response to provocative tests.

PROPHYLACTIC ANTIPARKINSONIAN DRUGS

In general, the authors do not advocate using prophylactic anti-parkinsonian drugs unless previous experience with a given patient specifically indicates that they will be needed. Generally, antiparkinsonian drugs should be used to treat Parkinsonian symptoms when they develop. Several studies do indicate that they have some prophylactic value. Hanlon et al. (1966) conducted one of the few studies which was approximately designed to investigate the efficacy of antiparkinsonian drug treatment. In this controlled study patients were assigned to one of two groups, a group which received antiparkinsonian agents plus perphenazine, and a group which received a placebo plus perphenazine. Only ten percent of subjects in the first group displayed EPS, as compared with 27 percent of the subjects in the second group, a marked contrast. Chien et al. (1974) divided chronic schizophrenics into three groups. The first group received fluphenazine enanthate, plus daily antiparkinsonian drugs; the second group received antiparkinsonian drugs for five days following each fluphenazine injection; and the third group was not given any antiparkinsonian medication. Side effects occurred in eight percent to twenty percent of patients in the first two treatment groups and were treated accordingly. In the third group 54 percent of patients displayed parkinsonian symptomatology. Additional support for this finding is furnished by the longitudinal work of Lapolla and Nash (1965). Most patients apparently do not develop EPS, but in the minority who do, antiparkinsonian drugs may prevent the occurrence of some fifty percent to 75 percent of these side effects.

There is some clinical evidence that a tolerance to EPS develops over the course of several months of treatment. A number of studies have investigated chronic schizophrenics, who are almost invariably on a combination of antiparkinsonian and antipsychotic medication. When the antiparkinsonian medication is discontinued, only a relatively small minority of the patients (ten percent to forty percent) develop EPS (Klett and Caffey, 1972; Lapolla and Nash, 1965; Orlov et al., 1971; Peckhold et al., 1971). Many of these patients may have been unnecessarily placed on prophylactic antiparkinsonian drugs. As well as having had no EPS when these drugs were discontinued, they might never have developed EPS in the first place.

To the degree that patients develop tolerance to the ability of antipsychotics to produce EPS, it may be postulated, the antiparkinsonian drugs which may have been indicated in the first few months should routinely be gradually discontinued after three or four months. It is important to discontinue antiparkinsonian drugs gradually to avoid rebound. One can begin the drug again if the patient develops EPS. In general, the authors treat patients with antipsychotic drugs alone, add antiparkinsonian drugs as indicated, and later discontinue the antiparkinsonian drugs. The prophylactic antiparkinsonian drugs are useful in special cases, such as when a patient would be expected to have EPS based on past response to a given drug. This practice obviously differs from the blanket use of prophylactic antiparkinsonian drugs.

OTHER PHARMACOLOGIC AGENTS AND THE ROLE OF ECT

Propranolol

This agent has had many uses in general medicine and more recently in psychiatry. Atsmon et al. (1970; 1976; 1978) in Jerusalem first found it potentially useful in the treatment of schizophrenia. Since then, a number of open and controlled studies have hinted at the possible clinical usefulness of propranolol and other β-adrenergic blockers in the treatment of psychotic states (see Table 6).

Most recently, Yorkston et al. (1981) reported the results of a double-blind, randomly assigned study comparing propranolol (670 mg) to CPZ (300 mg peak). The patients on propranolol did about as well as those on CPZ. The fact that such low doses of CPZ were used casts some doubt on the results. The dose of propranolol was also low, less than that used in many of the open studies. Although far from conclusive, the data do indicate a possible role for the β-adrenergic blockers in the treatment of schizophrenic disorders, and confirmation studies are needed.

Table 6. β-Adrenergic Blockers in the Treatment of Schizophrenic Spectrum Disorders

Source	No. Pts.	Drug & Dosage	Diagnosis	Results		
					PROP	CPZ
Atsmon et al. (1970; 1971; 1972; 1978) *open*	44	propranolol (high doses)	mixed psychoses	18 marked imp. 12 some imp. 14 no imp.		
Yorkston et al. (1974; 1976a; 1976b; 1978b) *open*	55	propranolol (max) (160–3000)	mixed psychoses	17 remission on propranolol		
Yorkston et al. (1978a; 1981) *double-blind, random assignment*	46	propranolol (peak dose 670) CPZ (peak dose 300)	newly admitted schizophrenics	Remitted Marked Moderate Minimal Unchanged Worse	2 6 4 7 3 2	4 6 3 2 6 1
Belmaker et al. (1979) *open*	10	propranolol	schizophrenia	3 mild imp. 5 no change 2 worse		
Volk et al. (1972) *open*	8	oxprenolol (max) (770-3600)	mixed psychoses	1 paranoid schizo-phrenic not responsive 1 agitated depressive not responsive 3/3 manics responded 2/3 schizoaffective responded		
Gardos et al. (1973) *open*	8	propranolol (max) (770–2880) adequate dose	chronic schizophrenia	No imp. on propranolol		
	6					
Shopsin et al. (1975) *open*	4	propranolol	acute schizophrenics	No imp. in any of 4 pts.		

Study	N	Treatment/Dose	Diagnosis	Results
von Zerssen (1976) *open*	17	propranolol (max) (160–3780)(900–1400) oxprenolol (max) (1480–4720)	mixed psychoses	6/8 improved or in remission 4/6 sl. improved 3 no effect
Yorkston et al. (1977; 1978a) *double-blind, controlled*	14	propranolol (7) (max) 450 placebo (7) combined with antipsychotics	schizophrenia	propranolol with antipsychotic superior to antipsychotic alone
Rackensperger et al. (1976) *open*	6	propranolol 280–2320	manic	4 pts. responded
Rackensperger et al. (1974) *placebo-controlled*	5	oxprenolol or propranolol	acute schizophrenia	0/5 responded
Hanssen et al. (1978) *open*	6	2 wks. drug-free; 2-4 wks. propranolol alone; after 2-4 wks. 5 pts. received propranolol alone; 1 pt. received propranolol and phenothiazine	schizophrenia (refractory to previous treatment)	with propanolol alone 1 good 2 sl. imp. 1 no change 1 worse
Lindstrom and Persson (1980) *double-blind, random sequence* placebo vs. propranolol 50% received drug first, 50% vice versa	12	11 flupenthixol decanoate + propranolol 1 propranolol alone dose: 1280–1928	antipsychotic-refractory schizophrenia	imp. on propranolol relative to placebo: 1 mod. imp. 2 sl. imp. 3 very sl. imp. 3 no change 3 worsened
Hirsch et al. (1981) *open*	9	D-propranolol mean dose: 1329	schizophrenics	7/9 imp.
Elizur et al. (1979a; 1979b) *open*	10	propranolol mean dose: 1600	nonresponding schizophrenics	4/10 imp.

The fact that propranolol does not increase serum prolactin levels or induce EPS suggests a biochemical action different from dopamine blockade. This opens the way for new and perhaps quite disparate theories regarding the neurobiology of schizophrenia (Gruzelier et al., 1981; Stam, 1971; Steiner et al., 1973; Cuche and Deniker, 1980). Data are insufficient to justify a nonresearch use of propranolol, but they do warrant further controlled studies. One interpretation of the results of combined trials of propranolol and antipsychotics is that propranolol may increase antipsychotic plasma levels. A rise in plasma levels of CPZ has been reported (Peet et al., 1980). Parenthetically, CPZ can inhibit propranolol metabolism.

Lithium Carbonate

A number of open and controlled studies have indicated a potential use for lithium either alone or in combination with neuroleptics for the treatment of Atypical Psychoses, Schizophreniform Disorders, and Schizoaffective Disorders (see Table 7).

An empirical trial is warranted in patients refractory to neuroleptic treatment alone or who are unable to tolerate neuroleptics because of side effects or other medical contraindications. Initial evidence also supports the hypothesis that some psychotic patients with "good" prognoses (e.g. Atypical Psychosis and Schizophreniform Disorder) may be manifesting variants of a manic disorder: they often show high lithium ratios, a putative marker for Affective Disorder and do respond well to treatment with lithium (David Garver, personal communication). Extremely disturbed patients, such as classic manics, atypical manics, or schizoaffectives may require temporary antipsychotic medication in an emergency. Some clinicians use the antipsychotic medications initially and switch to lithium. Others begin treatment with lithium plus antipsychotics and discontinue the antipsychotics after a few days.

At this time, the authors prefer lithium for the definitive treatment of typical and atypical manic patients because of an apparently better qualitative result. If a patient responds to lithium and evidence suggests that the diagnosis may be mania, lithium is also the maintenance treatment. Even when an extremely disturbed patient requires antipsychotics for emergency treatment, the switch to lithium alone occurs in the acute phase. At that point, the response to lithium can have both diagnostic and prognostic implications and can also achieve a better qualitative result.

An important question is which medication to use for the basis of prophylaxis. The naturalistic study of Angst et al. (1970) indicates the prophylactic properties of lithium in schizoaffectives. Some of the patients who present with typical schizophrenic symptoms have been thought for years to be in the schizophrenic spectrum. Sometimes these patients are diagnosed Schizophreniform Disorder or Brief Reactive Psychosis. Notably, the patients sometimes called "schizophrenics with good prognosis" or "reactive schizophrenics" do not have the progressive downhill course of the typical process schizophrenic with childhood asociality. Such schizophrenics with good prognosis often have affective features in their family histories. More work is needed to clarify the diagnosis and drug treatment of patients in the schizoaffective, brief psychotic reaction, or schizophreniform spectrum. Whether some have a variant of mania, a variant of schizophrenia, a unique disorder, or all of these, there may be a role for lithium treatment.

Lithium alone is clearly ineffective in most patients with core schizophrenia. For the few core schizophrenics who are misdiagnosed manic-depressives or in some unique category, this may not hold true, but results with the typical core schizophrenic are disappointing. Two studies (Small et al., 1975 and Growe et al., 1979) do hint that adding lithium to conventional antipsychotics may be of some modest benefit to some core schizophrenics.

Antidepressants and Antipsychotics

Unfortunately, adding tricyclic antidepressants to antipsychotics does not produce an appreciable effect in extremely retarded or chronic, burnt-out schizophrenics. Adding antidepressants to neuroleptics is indicated in schizoaffective patients with an admixture of affective (depressive) and schizophrenic symptoms (Casey et al., 1961; Prusoff et al., 1978; 1979; Michaux et al., 1966; Brockington et al., 1978; Hanlon et al., 1964; Hanson et al., 1979).

Naloxone

Several well-controlled studies report improvement of hallucinations in hallucinatory schizophrenic patients following intravenous high-dose naloxone administration (see Table 8). This evidence, coupled with the fact that those studies which have shown negative results tended either to be less well controlled or used lower doses of naloxone, lend credence to this agent's positive effect on hallucinating schizophrenic patients. Many questions do remain unanswered, and continued investigation in this area seems quite reasonable from the perspectives of both treatment and theory.

The Role of ECT

Two excellent recent reviews come to essentially similar conclusions about ECT (American Psychiatric Association, 1978; Salzman, 1980). First, most of the research on the effectiveness of ECT in schizophrenia is so methodologically flawed that few valid conclusions can be drawn. Second, although ECT does appear to be effective in treating certain types of schizophrenic patients, it has been relegated to a secondary role behind antipsychotic drug treatment. Third, further well-controlled research is indicated to clarify the role of ECT in the treatment of schizophrenic disorders. May (1975) found ECT almost as effective as antipsychotics in treating first-admission schizophrenic patients. ECT has also been found useful in combination with antipsychotics (Smith et al., 1967). In two reports Murillo and Exner found that ECT produced significant improvement in process schizophrenics who were refractory to drugs (Murillo and Exner, 1973; Exner and Murillo, 1977). For the present, the clinician should consider ECT as a possible treatment in schizophrenia under three conditions—when there are immediate life-threatening circumstances, such as "lethal" catatonia or suicidal preoccupation; when it may help reduce dosages of medications for those patients who need megadoses of antipsychotics to control their symptoms; and when schizophrenic disorders are refractory to other more standard regimens.

Table 7. Lithium in the Treatment of Schizophrenic Spectrum Disorders

Source	No. Pts.	Treatment	Diagnosis	Results
Alexander et al. (1979) *longitudinal study*	13	lithium: drug free-lithium 3 wks; drug free 1 wk.	schizophrenic disorder	7/13 imp receiving lithium 4/7 relapsed after lithium withdrawal
Prien et al. (1972) *controlled, random assignment*	83	lithium or CPZ	excited schizoaffective disorder	CPZ significantly better in 41 highly active schizoaffective pts.; CPZ = lithium in 40 mildly excited schizoaffective pts.
Angst et al. (1970) *longitudinal naturalistic*	72	lithium: course on lithium compared to course before lithium	schizoaffective	Frequency of admission on lithium vs. before lithium: 36 imp. 28 no change 8 worse

Study	N	Treatment	Diagnosis	Results
Small, et al. (1975) *placebo-controlled crossover*	22	lithium + neuroleptics	chronic schizophrenia	Pts. benefited significantly while on lithium vs. placebo
Forssman and Walinder, (1969) *anecdotal*	27	lithium	atypical psychoses	18/27 imp.
Shopsin, et al. (1972b) *double-blind controlled*	21	lithium or CPZ	schizophrenia	Pts. did much worse on lithium than CPZ
Growe et al. (1979) *double-blind, placebo-controlled, crossover*	8	lithium or placebo + neuroleptic	6-schizophrenia 2-schizoaffective	No significant change in 7 of 8 scales of the psychotic Inpatient Profile; sl. decr. on Psychotic Excitement Scale
Hirschowitz et al. (1980) *open*	31	lithium	schizophrenia	8/10 do well 1/21 do poorly

Table 8. Naloxone in the Treatment of Schizophrenic Disorders

Source	No. Pts.	Treatment & Dose	Diagnosis	Results
*Gunne et al. (1977) *single-blind, placebo-controlled*	4	naloxone (0.4 mg)	chronic schizophrenia	Temporary decrease or abolish auditory hallucinations
Freeman and Fairburn (1981) *double-blind, crossover, placebo-controlled*	13	naloxone (1.6 mg) or placebo	schizophrenia	No difference
*Berger et al. (1981) *placebo-controlled, double-blind, crossover*	14	naloxone (10 mg)**	chronic, male schizophrenics	Significant decrease in hallucination with naloxone
Davis et al. (1977) *randomized, double-blind, placebo*	14	naloxone (0.4–10 mg)	schizophrenia	No overall improvement with naloxone
Lipinski et al. (1979) *double-blind, placebo-controlled, crossover design*	9	naloxone (1.6 mg)	schizophrenia	No clear significant difference
*Lehman et al. (1979) *single-blind double-blind*	6	naloxone (10 mg)**	chronic, male schizophrenics	Significant decrease in tension item in BPRS
	5	naloxone (10 mg)**		Total BPRS score improved with naloxone
*Watson et al. (1978) *double-blind, crossover*	11	naloxone (10 mg)** 5/11 on concurrent neuroleptics	schizophrenia	Significant decrease in hallucinations
Kurland et al. (1977) *randomized, placebo, double-blind*	12	naloxone (0.4–1.2 mg) + concurrent neuroleptics	schizophrenia (hallucinating)	No change in hallucinatory experience

Study	N	Drug (dose)	Diagnosis	Result
Janowsky et al. (1977) *double-blind, crossover design, placebo control*	8	naloxone (1.2 mg) + concurrent neuroleptics	male schizophrenics	No significant difference in BPRS scores
Volavka et al. (1977) *double-blind, placebo-controlled semi-random*	7	naloxone (0.4 mg)	schizophrenia	No significant difference in BPRS scores
*Emrich et al. (1977) *controlled double-blind*	20	naloxone (4.0 mg)**	schizophrenia (hallucinating and/or delusional)	Significant decrease in schizophrenic symptoms in 12/20 pts.
Verhoeven et al. (1981) *double-blind, placebo-controlled*	10	naloxone (20 mg)	5 schizophrenic 5 manic	No therapeutic effect
Emrich et al. (1979) *double-blind, placebo-controlled*	20	naloxone (24.8 mg)	schizophrenia (hallucinating)	No effect
Mielke and Gallant (1977) *open*	6	naltrexone (250 mg) 9 days	schizophrenia	No therapeutic effect
Simpson et al. (1977) *single-blind*	6	naltrexone (100–800 mg) 8 wks.	schizophrenia	No therapeutic effect
Gitlin and Rosenblatt (1978) *single-blind*	3	naltrexone (50–100 mg) 14 days	schizophrenia	No therapeutic effect
Hertz et al. (1978) *double-blind, crossover*	20	naloxone (4 mg i.v.)	schizophrenia	No therapeutic effect

Table 8. Continued

Source	No. Pts.	Treatment & Dose	Diagnosis	Results
Janowsky et al. (1978) *double-blind, crossover*	12	naloxone (20 mg i.v. infusion 30–90 min. duration)	manic	Attenuated manic symptom
Orr and Oppenheimer (1978) *single-blind*	1	naloxone (0.4 mg)	schizophrenic (hallucinating)	Decrease in hallucinations
Dysken and Davis (1978) *single-blind*	1	naloxone (20 mg single dose)	catatonic schizophrenic	No effect
Abrams et al. (1978) *open*	1	naloxone (1.2 i.v. single dose)	catatonic schizophrenic	No effect
Schenk et al. (1978) *open*	14	naloxone (0.4 to 30 min. or 1.6–9 mg/day 1–21 days)	catatonic schizophrenics	11/14 responded acutely 7/14 responded chronically
Ragheb et al. (1980) *open*	5	naltrexone (100–300 mg) 3 wks; (1-wk. placebo washout)	schizophrenia (hallucinating)	2/5 responded
Gunne et al. (1979) *double-blind, placebo crossover*	10	naloxone (0.8 mg i.v. 100 mg/day) 4-wk. study 2 wks. on drug 2 wks. on placebo	schizophrenia (hallucinating) on neuroleptic	1/10 responded to naloxone No change overall (1 pt. did moderately better on naltrexone, 4 sl. worse, 5 no change)

*better controlled
**higher dosage

THE ROLE OF PSYCHOTHERAPIES IN THE TREATMENT OF SCHIZOPHRENIA

A Dual Mechanism Theory

American psychiatrists are divided in their opinions on the efficacy of psychotherapy in schizophrenia. These differences are due, in part, to the existence of several theories concerning the cause of schizophrenia. If we place these theories on a spectrum, at one end is the position that schizophrenia is an exclusively biochemical disorder and that psychotherapy is at best irrelevant and at worst harmful.

Diametrically opposed is the theory that schizophrenia is a purely psychological disorder and that organic treatments are simply palliative and may actually interfere with the process of working through psychological conflicts. Adherents of this perspective recommend long-term hospital treatment with intensive psychotherapy and without drugs. This theory implies that psychotherapy administered without drugs acts directly on the classic schizophrenic symptoms of hallucinations, catatonic posture, delusions, ideas of reference and so forth, and also helps with intrapsychic and social adjustment.

The authors suggest a dual mechanism theory. They hypothesize that psychotropic drugs would benefit a CNS circuit involved in the disease process, normalizing the classic symptoms. If these symptoms improved, a secondary improvement in some social skills might be expected to occur, but this would be less definitive and less well related to the disease process. Drugs cannot be expected to induce social skills or warmer, more empathetic human relationships. But insofar as the symptoms of schizophrenia interfere with social functioning, the drugs can be expected to reduce such interference and allow the patient to regain preexisting social skills. Psychotherapy, on the other hand, can reduce intrapsychic conflict. Patients with schizophrenia, like all of us, have the normal range of psychological problems. Indeed, since schizophrenics may come from disordered families, and since the disease itself may interfere with interpersonal functioning, one would expect that schizophrenics would have ample opportunities to develop such problems.

This mode of thinking about drugs and psychotherapy suggests a role for both. Psychotherapy may help interpersonal problems directly and may secondarily benefit biological processes. Drugs that help the symptoms of schizophrenia may have a secondary effect on interpersonal functioning. Toward further exploration of this dual theory, the interpersonal dimension should be considered separately from the symptom dimension, since this will facilitate our analyzing differential effects of treatment.

If the psychologically focused theories were exclusively true, one would expect that, although the drugs might have some temporary sedative function, the psychotherapy would in the long run be much more effective both in relation to narrowly defined variables reflecting schizophrenic symptoms and in relation to intrapsychic and interpersonal variables. If schizophrenia were a truly biologic disorder, the drug treatment would benefit the symptomatic variables, and psychological treatments would have no effect on anything. According to the dual mechanism theory, the drugs should produce a good effect on symptoms, and the psychological treatment should affect the social and intrapsychic functioning of the patient.

A Review of the Literature

Only studies that meet certain methodologic requirements are reviewed here. The most important methodologic rule is randomization. In any controlled study, randomization is extremely important. Randomization must not be manipulated to get good prognosis patients into a particular treatment group. Such manipulation has occurred throughout the history of medicine. The preferred patient would be assigned to the new treatment group, while to the old treatment group would be assigned treatment-resistant, poor prognosis patients. Studies of this type are not included, since the results are clearly invalid.

Parenthetically, none of the studies reviewed controls for the demand characteristics of the situation. Ideally, properly done psychotherapy studies should compare psychotherapy against a psychological placebo of similar demand characteristics, short of sham psychotherapy. A methodology which includes blind evaluation needs to be developed.

MENDOTA STATE STUDY. Rogers and his co-workers (1967) conducted a study at Mendota State Hospital involving eight hospitalized, chronic patients and eight acute patients who had been hospitalized less than eight months. These 16 patients were matched to 16 additional patients (eight chronic and eight acute) and to 16 normal controls on the basis of sex, age, and socioeconomic status. One-half of the patients were randomly assigned to the psychotherapy group. Both groups may have received drugs, but the type, dosage, and any other details are not mentioned.

This study found that psychotherapy had no effect on the schizophrenic symptoms. In addition, overall change score for the TAT showed no statistically significant difference between the psychotherapy and nonpsychotherapy groups. (Some subscales of the TAT did show a difference.) The schizophrenics receiving psychotherapy did demonstrate a decreasing need to deny their own experience and a greater appropriateness in emotional expression. There was a slight tendency for the psychotherapy group to spend less time outside the hospital during the follow-up. In discussions of the study, May (1974) and May and Tuma (1970) have noted that if initial differences among subjects are controlled by covarying for initial differences in ego strength, the probability that this follow-up difference may occur by chance would be less than 0.25.

LINDBERG STUDY. Lindberg (1981) conducted an eight-year study of 14 schizophrenics who received both intensive psychotherapy and neuroleptic medication and a control group of 13 schizophrenics who received only drug treatment. The patients were not randomly assigned to either group; rather, the control group was matched to the experimental group. Without random assignment, some systematic effect could have altered the prognosis of patients in either group. Although the psychotherapy-plus-drug group did remain out of the hospital a greater number of days, the difference was not statistically significant. What is striking is that the patients in both groups spent a substantial amount of time in the hospital each year, approximately the same amount of time per group over the eight-year period of time.

KANAS STUDY. Comparing insight-oriented group psychotherapy with an activities-oriented task group or a controlled condition for acute psychotic patients, Kanas et al. (1980) found that no group showed any particular advantage in the initial phase of the hospitalization. Within the group psychotherapy condition, however, the more psychotic patients scored worse.

LAING STUDY. R.D. Laing, an antimedical theorist, conducted a study on family-oriented therapy with hospitalized schizophrenics. In a report of the results, he and his colleagues note that 25 percent of the patients received no "tranquilizers" at all (Esterson, Cooper, and Laing, 1965). This implies that 75 percent of the patients did receive tranquilizers. One might even hypothesize that Laing and his co-workers used a somewhat looser definition of schizophrenia than is common in Great Britain and may have treated a population consisting of 25 percent borderline personality disorders and 75 percent narrowly diagnosed schizophrenics. It is even possible that all of the core schizophrenics received tranquilizers.

KARON STUDY. Karon et al. compared the results of psychotherapy with and without drugs, versus no psychotherapy (Karon and O'Grady, 1969; Karon and Vandenbos, 1970; 1972). Many of the patients in the control group were transferred very quickly to what appeared to be a chronic facility. Thus, any difference in results might be due to the quality of care in the chronic state hospital rather than to the psychotherapy. Another problem was that three of the 11 patients studied in the psychotherapy-without-drug group received some drugs. May and Tuma have reviewed the many serious methodologic problems of this study (May and Tuma, 1970; Tuma and May, 1975).

ROSEN STUDY. Rosen (1947; 1953) stated that the direct analytic technique produced improvement in 37 cases of deteriorated schizophrenia. He defined improvement first as the ability to live comfortably outside an institution. Second, improvement entailed achieving such psychological integrity, emotional stability, and character structure that the patient could withstand as much environmental assault as is expected of a person who has never experienced a psychotic episode.

Five years later in a follow-up study, Horwitz et al. (1958) were able to identify 19 of the 37 patients treated by Rosen. They found that 37 percent of these patients were not diagnosed as schizophrenic, but rather had been initially diagnosed as primarily psychoneurotic, or in one case as manic-depressive. Another patient was cured after her thyroid was removed. The remainder were considered schizophrenic, and during the ten years that followed Rosen's treatment, 75 percent of these patients had two to five admissions to a mental hospital.

Rosen continued his work, treating another 14 patients (Bookhammer et al., 1966). In this study, certain patients were designated as controls, according to a scheme where every third patient was sent to Rosen and the other two were designated controls. Since this does not involve a sufficient element of randomization, a further group of controls was selected from a similar population. But this, too, is far different from random assignment. The five-year follow-up, however, indicated that while 57 percent of Rosen's patients were rated as improved, 62 percent of the controls were also rated as improved (Bookhammer et al., 1966).

GRINSPOON STUDY.   At the Massachusetts Mental Health Center, a small group of chronically ill schizophrenic patients were treated by senior psychoanalysts and psychoanalytically oriented psychotherapists (Grinspoon et al., 1968; 1972; Messier et al., 1969). Grinspoon and his colleagues assigned patients at random to initial drug or placebo in a crossover design. Patients receiving psychotherapy plus thioridazine showed greater improvement than when they received psychotherapy alone. In fact, patients' behavior deteriorated when a placebo was substituted for thioridazine. Many therapists have objected to phenothiazine treatment because they fear it will block emotional involvement. This study, however, demonstrated just the opposite effect. Patients seemed more involved with their psychotherapists when receiving phenothiazines than they did when receiving no drug. In addition, they seemed more involved with the outside world and more aware of recent events, such as President Kennedy's death or the absence of the psychotherapist or the ward physician.

GREENBLATT STUDY.   Greenblatt and his co-workers (1965) at the Massachusetts Mental Health Center found that psychological interventions are necessary to effect any treatment plan, precipitate discharge, or facilitate successful reintegration into the community. They compared four variations of drug and social therapies. Patients were divided into drug and nondrug groups, and each of these two groups was in turn subdivided into two groups—intensive (high) social therapy and minimal (low) social therapy. Patients at the Center received the high social therapies, which consisted of a variety of psychotherapies, social work, occupational therapies, psychodrama, and total-push therapies. The low social therapies were administered to chronic patients in a state hospital. The results are presented in Table 9.

A clear-cut drug effect was demonstrated. In terms of symptomatic improvement, the patients who received drugs in both milieus showed greater improvement. There was a slight nonsignificant trend toward greater symptomatic improvement in the drug-plus-high-social therapy group (33 percent) than in the drug-plus-low-social-therapy group (23 percent). Patients who continuously received both social and drug therapy were more likely to leave the hospital. After 36 months, 13 patients from the high-social-therapy group were living in the community, as compared with five from the low-social-therapy group. Of these 13 patients, all but one had received drug as well as social therapy during the initial six-month treatment period. After the initial six nonproductive months without drug treatments, the group receiving high social therapy and no drugs was treated with high social therapy plus drugs for six months. In spite of having high social therapy for a full year and drugs for six months, this group never did catch up with the original drug-plus-high-social-therapy group. Being without drugs for the initial six-month period may have had a harmful carry-over effect in these patients.

O'BRIEN STUDY.   O'Brien et al. (1972) compared patients randomly assigned to group or individual therapy upon discharge from a state mental hospital. Evaluating outcome at 12 and 24 months of treatment,

Table 9. Results of Four Treatments
in Chronic Schizophrenia (Greenblatt et al., 1965)

	High Social Therapy[a]	Low Social Therapy[b]
Percentage Showing High Improvement at 6 Months Evaluation		
Drug therapy	33	23
No drug therapy	0	10
Percentage Discharged after 6 to 9 Months		
Drug therapy	27	9
No drug therapy for 6 months	7	5
Percentage Showing High Improvement after 36 Months		
Drug therapy	35	19
No drug therapy for 6 months	26	6

[a]Patients transferred to the Massachusetts Mental Health Center.
[b]Patients remained in state hospitals.

they found that the group-therapy group did significantly better on both social factors and symptomatic ratings. The readmission rate, however, did not differ between the two groups.

CLAGHORN STUDY. Claghorn and his co-workers (1974) assigned outpatient schizophrenics on maintenance medication to group therapy or no group therapy. Group therapy did not alter these patients' symptomatology, but projective testing showed they made greater gains on such variables as insight.

GOLDSTEIN STUDY. Goldstein and his co-workers (1978), in a home treatment program after brief hospitalization, demonstrated that family therapy had a statistically significant effect on continuing the initial therapeutic gains. In this study, 104 young, acute schizophrenics were randomly assigned to one of four groups: low dose (6.25 mg every two weeks) or moderate dose (25 mg every two weeks) of fluphenazine decanoate and family therapy or no family therapy for an eight-week trial. Patients were initially hospitalized for two weeks (mean 14 plus or minus six days) and then spent the following six weeks in outpatient family therapy. Since it was only a two-week hospitalization, the patient's acute illness may not have been completely remitted by the time of discharge, and the psychological support and family therapy care could have been acting on the process of recovering from the acute episode. The results indicated a clear dose-response relationship. Relapse was prevented significantly by moderate doses of fluphenazine, and family therapy had a modest positive influence. Since it takes six weeks or more for acute treatment to become effective, the meaning of the term *relapse* here is different from its meaning in long-term maintenance studies. Relapse here refers to a partially remitted patient, discharged after two weeks, who then deteriorates rather than continuing to improve (see Table 10).

HOGARTY STUDY. Hogarty et al. (1973; 1974a; 1974b) studied the effect of psychotherapy in combination with drug or placebo on both

Table 10. Rate of Relapse
According to Treatment Group (Goldstein et al., 1978)

| | At Six Weeks | | | |
| | Relapses | | No Relapses | |
	Mod. Dose	Low Dose	Mod. Dose	Low Dose
Family Therapy	0	2	23	21
No Family Therapy	3	5	26	16
	Six Weeks to Six Months			
	Relapses		No Relapses	
	Mod. Dose	Low Dose	Mod. Dose	Low Dose
Family Therapy	0	3	23	20
No Family Therapy	1	3	28	18

the level of posthospital adjustment and the number of relapses. Although they found a large drug-placebo difference, intervening psychotherapy had little effect on the number of relapses. After a year, 73 percent of the placebo-without-psychotherapy group and 63 percent of the placebo-with-psychotherapy group had relapsed, but only 33 percent of the drug-maintenance group and 26 percent of the drug-maintenance-with-psychotherapy group had relapsed. With those patients who received drugs and failed to relapse, psychotherapy resulted in improved social functioning in such areas as "relationships in and out of the home." The psychotherapy-without-drug group did poorly. This indicates that psychotherapy improves social functioning when given in the follow-up period concurrently with drug treatment.

MAY STUDIES. May (1968) and May et al. (1976a; 1976b; 1981) performed a particularly interesting and important study comparing the outcome of five treatment programs on a group of hospitalized first-admission schizophrenics. The ECT treatment group is discussed above, and the remaining four are discussed here. They were treated either with phenothiazine alone, psychotherapy alone, psychotherapy plus phenothiazines, or neither psychotherapy nor phenothiazines. In general, the maximal improvement was produced by phenothiazines alone or phenothiazines plus psychotherapy. The drug treatments, whether given alone or in combination with psychotherapy, increased the release rate, shortened the length of the hospital stay, decreased the necessity for use of sedatives or hydrotherapy, and produced more beneficial changes in clinical status, including a change toward a more healthy rating on the Menninger Health-Sickness Scale. Table 11 presents several of the more important results.

While some have suggested that psychotherapy may have a dramatic beneficial effect on some patients and make others substantially worse, May and his co-workers found that the presence or absence of psychotherapy did not significantly alter the variance of outcomes. (In this study, the therapists were either residents or had been out of residency a short period of time. The average length of therapists' experience at the midpoint of each patient's psychotherapeutic treatment was 3.8 years, with a range of two months to 12 years.)

Table 11. Assessment of Outcome in Schizophrenic Patients Treated with and without Antipsychotic Drugs and Psychotherapy (May, 1978)

	NO DRUGS		DRUG	
	No Psychotherapy	Psychotherapy	No Psychotherapy	Psychotherapy
Percent released	59	64	95	96
Nurses' rating MACC total	38	38	48	48
Nurses' Menninger Health-Sickness rating	26	23	29	30
Nurses' rating of idiosyncractic symptoms (125-X)*	37	29	66	74
Therapists' symptom rating (50-X)*	22	21	27	27
Psychoanalysts' rating of insight	3.4	3.3	3.7	4.1

*A higher number reflects greater improvement. In order to have the two scales fit with this convention, scores were subtracted from an arbitrary constant.

The most important aspect of these findings is not the initial therapeutic effect but rather the follow-ups at three, four, and five years. During the follow-up periods, treatment was given on a clinical basis. Patients could receive any therapy their physicians wished to give. In spite of the fact that all patients did receive treatment during the follow-up periods, their outcomes differed markedly. Using the number of days spent in the hospital after release from the hospital as the index of remission, the researchers found a very large drug effect (see Figure 10).

Both of the two drug groups did much better than the two no-drug groups. A particularly important finding is that the patients who were not treated with drugs spent approximately twice as many days in the hospital after discharge than those who were treated with drugs. Since all the patients could have any treatment after the controlled portion of the study was over, differences in their subsequent course were based

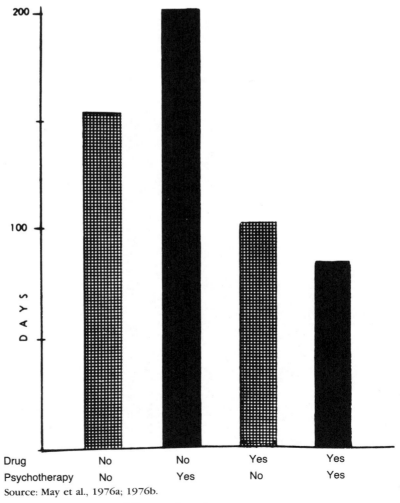

| Drug | No | No | Yes | Yes |
| Psychotherapy | No | Yes | No | Yes |

Source: May et al., 1976a; 1976b.

Figure 10. Three-years follow-up after release.

on whether they did or did not receive drugs during their initial hospitalization. Thus, denying drugs during serious acute episodes may do harm which can persist over a three-to five-year period.

These findings must, however, be viewed in the context of the limited course of psychotherapy received by patients in the study. Patients in the drug-plus-psychotherapy group, for example, received psychotherapy from relatively inexperienced therapists and had only 24 hours more psychotherapy than the drug-alone group. Hence, the results may not reflect a fair test of the effects of psychotherapy. The authors, however, did find that the therapists' experience and general clinical ability were not related to outcome (May et al., 1968).

Figure 11 and Figure 12 present the results for the one-year and the three-year follow-up period (May et al., 1981). Patients who initially received drugs did substantially better at both follow-up periods than did the patients who did not receive drugs. Statistical analysis did not show a significant effect of psychotherapy but did show a significant drug effect.

Another meaningful index of functioning a few years after relapse is the proportion of time a patient works for pay. A rating of two was used to indicate half-time work and a rating of three to indicate more than half-time work. The results can be expressed in a fourfold table, giving the mean rating for working for pay under drug or no-drug conditions and under psychotherapy or no-psychotherapy conditions (Table 12). As the table shows, psychotherapy had a negative effect on patient's

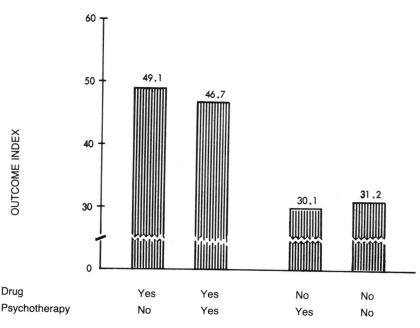

| Drug | Yes | Yes | No | No |
| Psychotherapy | No | Yes | Yes | No |

Values for outcome index (higher number = better outcome) are the average for each group.

Source: May et al., 1981.

Figure 11. Treatment group vs. outcome index (one-year follow-up).

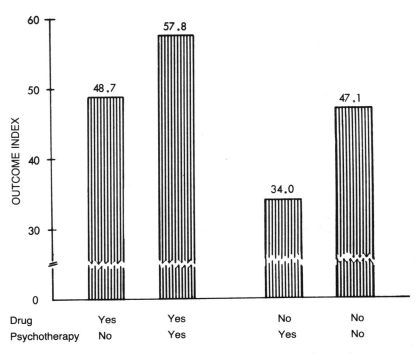

Values for outcome index (higher number = better outcome) are the average for each group.

Source: May et al., 1981.

Figure 12. Treatment group vs. outcome index (three-year follow-up).

time spent working for pay. More significant statistically was the positive effect that drugs had on this measure of functioning.

If psychotherapy does produce a dramatic effect, and if it is most likely to affect interpersonal and intrapsychic variables, one would expect to see maximum effects in patients rated initially as undergoing successful treatment and later assessed on the basis of variables related to interpersonal relations and adjustment. In this subgroup of patients, patients receiving psychotherapy plus drugs had poorer interpersonal

Table 12. Mean Rating on Working for Pay at Two Years

	Psychotherapy	No Psychotherapy	Psychotherapy Effect (p = .07)
Drug	1.8	2.3	− .5
No Drug	1.2	1.6	− .4
Drug Effect (p = .009)	.6	.7	

Source: May et al., 1981.

relationships with others outside of the family setting and had significantly poorer social adjustment than patients who received drugs alone (May et al., 1981). Similarly, in the no-drug group, those who received psychotherapy did significantly worse than those in the no-psychotherapy group. Furthermore, during the follow-up period, those patients who were successful in psychotherapy alone were substantially less successful on most outcome variables than those patients who were rated as successful in all other forms of therapy.

LENGTH OF STAY AND TYPE OF SETTING: A REVIEW OF STUDIES

An issue related to the effects of psychotherapy in schizophrenia is the length of stay and the setting for inpatient treatment. At the end of World War II, the community psychiatry movement led to an increased interest in the length of hospitalization and alternatives to hospital care (Sommer and Weinberg, 1944). Only recently have there been studies assigning patients who would normally be hospitalized to alternative treatment, such as a day hospital, foster care, family home treatment, or brief hospitalization. Control groups receive regular length hospitalization. Generally speaking, populations are mixed, but since many include a large percentage of schizophrenics, they are appropriate for review here. In one of the classic studies, Pasamanick (1967) found that drug treatment is clearly an important part of the nonhospital or minimal hospital treatment of severely ill schizophrenic patients. In another of the classic studies in this area, Langsley et al. (1968; 1971) randomly assigned patients to family crisis therapy or to a control group of regular hospital treatment. In general, the patients in family therapy did about as well as the hospital controls, and on some variables they did better. Wilder and his co-workers (1966) used a similar design to compare day-hospital patients to conventional hospital patients. Again, the day-hospital patients did as well or slightly better than the regular hospital patients. Some of the newer studies are reviewed below.

LANGLEY PORTER STUDY. Glick and his co-workers (1974; 1975; 1976; 1979) performed a random-assignment study of the effect of short- and long-term hospitalization. The short-term group received three to four weeks of treatment, and the long-term group received 13 to 17 weeks of treatment. After four weeks of treatment, the short-term group did better compared to the long-term treatment group. However, the long-term group did improve between the fourth week and the time of discharge several months later. Overall better results may have been obtained in the long-term group because the short-term group was not measured after a comparable time. At the two-year follow-up, both groups did about the same on many measures, but at one year the long-term group showed an edge on some measures. Long-term patients, it should be noted, received maintenance antipsychotic drugs more frequently and at substantially higher dosages and also received a greater number of psychotherapy visits after discharge from the hospital.

On the chance that more patients who would be predicted to have unfavorable prognoses had been assigned to the short-term treatment group, Glick and Hargreaves (1979) performed an analysis of covariance to adjust for prognostic variables, as well as posthospital treatment. Although the results on many outcome variables are similar between the short-term and the long-term group, the long-term treatment group still does slightly better on certain variables at one year. At two years, however, there is little difference between the two treatments. Table 13 presents the results on certain variables after appropriate covariant analysis.

CAFFEY STUDY. In a collaborative Veterans Administration (VA) hospital study, Caffey et al. (1968; 1971) compared three groups: a standard group, a short-term hospital group, and a second standard group who were followed after release in a manner similar to the short-term group. The short-term group did better at three weeks than the long-term groups.

WASHBURN STUDY. Washburn and his co-workers (1977a; Vannicelli et al., 1978) did a particularly important study in which they assigned patients randomly to a day-hospital setting or to an inpatient setting. Both settings were located at McLean Hospital. The subjects were patients who would normally be assigned to an inpatient setting, but who were not sufficiently homicidal, suicidal, or incapable of forming a treatment alliance to make inpatient care an absolute necessity. Evaluations of psychopathology every six months for 18 months to two years showed equal improvement in the two groups. The only psychopathologic measure where there was a clear-cut difference was subjective distress. Here, the day patients showed significantly more improvement than the inpatients. On several measures of social adjustment at the various follow-up periods, the authors found no significant difference between the two treatment modalities. On most measures of social judgment, though, the day-hospital group showed a significantly better community adjustment. Furthermore, patients in this group seemed to place less of a burden on the family and were more satisfied with their care.

HERZ STUDY. Herz et al. (1971; 1975; 1976; 1977; 1980) and Reibel and Herz (1976) studied the effects of length of hospitalization on outcome in a community mental health center. They randomly assigned patients to three treatment groups: one standard-hospital group

Table 13.　Langley Porter Study
Outcome at Two Years After Covariate Adjustment
for Prehospital Prognosis and Posthospital Treatment

	Short	Long	
Health-Sickness Rating Scale*	38.0	40.7	NS
Psychiatric Evaluation Form** (Severity of Illness)	3.6	3.4	NS
Katz Adjustment Scale** (Relative Rating of Social Performance)	31.0	30.9	NS
Historical Information Form** (Global Scale)	.2	.2	NS

*　　Higher number = good outcome
**　Lower number = good outcome

Source: Glick and Hargreaves, 1979.

with a full-length hospitalization of several months, and two brief-hospitalization groups, one with and one without transitional day care. The brief-treatment groups did slightly better initially, returning more quickly to their normal social roles. Overall, the few differences between the groups generally favored the brief-treatment group over the standard-treatment group. There was no significant difference in readmission rate.

OTHER STUDIES.   Knight et al. (1980) and Platt et al. (1981) report on a randomized controlled trial of brief hospital admission. They found that clinical outcome was slightly, but not significantly, better in the brief-admission group. Kennedy and Hird (1980) randomly allocated patients to a brief-admission ward and a usual length hospitalization ward. The total therapeutic gain in the two groups was approximately equal.

In a VA cooperative study to evaluate the effectiveness of foster care as an alternative to continued hospitalization (Linn et al., 1977), 572 males (75 percent schizophrenic) were randomly assigned to either foster care preparation or to continued hospitalization. Patients' social functioning, mood, activity, and overall adjustment were studied before assignment, at placement, and four months later. Within four months after being placed in foster care, foster care subjects showed significant improvement as compared with the hospital controls, particularly in the areas of functioning and overall adjustment. Stein and Test (1980) performed an extensive evaluation of community treatment vs. hospital treatment, using a random assignment of patients, approximately fifty percent of whom were schizophrenic. On several variables, the community group did better. Fenton and Struening (1978) assigned patients to a home treatment group and a regular hospital group. On measures of psychopathology the two groups were almost exactly equal.

OVERVIEW

Although many studies have introduced psychotherapy, there is no evidence that psychotherapy without drugs produces an etiologic cure in any subgroup of schizophrenics. In some studies, schizophrenics do better on psychosocial ratings after both drug and psychological treatments. A close inspection of these results suggests that the social therapies help to make psychosocial gains possible because the drugs have normalized the schizophrenic process. Indeed, applying the psychological treatments without drugs may be analogous to using physical therapy on someone with a broken leg before applying a cast! Physical therapy before casting would probably worsen the patient's condition, while it would be appropriate and helpful after the cast had enabled initial healing.

For the viewpoint that drugs are harmful and that psychotherapy without drugs will get better results than psychotherapy with drugs, there is no supportive evidence. Patients receiving psychotherapy without drugs do no better than patients receiving psychotherapy with drugs. In fact, patients receiving psychotherapy alone do much worse than appropriate controls receiving drugs.

It is important to point out that in dealing with any statistical study, one is dealing with the results for a sample of patients. Moreover, although a generalization may hold true for the average patient, the individual patient may be an exception. The evidence does not rule out the possibility that a subgroup of patients who present with apparent schizophrenic symptomatology may, indeed, respond well to psychotherapy alone. But the possibility that such a group could exist does not prove that it does exist. Similarly, a statistically brief hospital treatment or alternate placement appears to be equal to or perhaps even slightly better than longer hospital treatment, but there may be certain patients for whom a hospital stay of several months would be indicated.

The best way to maximize the psychotherapy effect may be to focus it on the posthospital outpatient treatment. Both psychological treatment and drugs should begin in the hospital, and the patient should be discharged with adequate maintenance drug treatment. Over the course of years, outpatient psychotherapy should affect patients' intrapsychic and interpersonal functioning and improve how they deal with the real world. Thus, the greatest psychotherapy effect may appear as the cumulative effect of years of outpatient treatment.

Bibliographies to Part II

Bibliography for the Introduction

Bleuler, E.P. "Dementia Praecox oder die Gruppe der Schizophrenien." In *Handbuch der Psychiatrie*, 4th ed., edited by G. Aschaffenburg. Leipzig: Franz Deuticke, 1911.

Cancro, R., and Pruyser, P.W. "A Historical Review of the Development of the Concept of Schizophrenia." *Bulletin of the Menninger Clinic* 34 (1970): 61–70.

Kraepelin, E. *Psychiatrie. Ein Lehrbuch für Studierende und Ärzte*, 6th ed. Leipzig: Barth, 1899.

Morel, B.A. Études Cliniques: Traité Théorique et Pratique des Maladies Mentales. Paris: Masson, 1852–1853.

Bibliography for Chapter 9

Barton, R. *Institutional Neurosis.* Bristol: Wright, 1959.

Bleuler, M. "The Long-Term Course of the Schizophrenic Psychoses." *Psychological Medicine* 4 (1974): 244–254.

Brown, G.W., Monck, E.M., Carstairs, G.M., and Wing, J.K. "Influence of Family Life on the Course of Schizophrenic Illness." *British Journal of Preventive and Social Medicine* 16 (1962): 55–68.

Carpenter, W.T., Jr., and Strauss, J.S. "Diagnostic Issues in Schizophrenia." In *Disorders of the Schizophrenic Syndrome*, edited by L. Bellak. New York: Basic Books, 1979.

Chodoff, P., and Carpenter, W.T., Jr. "Psychogenic Theories of Schizophrenia." In *Schizophrenia: Biological and Psychological Perspectives*, edited by G. Usdin. New York: Brunner/Mazel, 1975.

Ciompi, L. "Catamnestic Long-Term Study on the Course of Life and Aging of Schizophrenics." *Schizophrenia Bulletin* 6 (1980): 606–618.

Cooper, J.E., Kendell, R.E., Gurland, B.J., Sharpe, C., Copeland, J.R.M., and Simon, R. *Psychiatric Diagnosis in New York and London.* Maudsley Monograph Series #20. London: Oxford University Press, 1972.

Docherty, J.P., vanKammen, D.P., Siris, S.G., and Marder, S.R. "Stages of Onset of Schizophrenic Psychosis." *American Journal of Psychiatry* 135 (1978): 420–426.

Gunderson, J. "A Re-evaluation of Milieu Therapy for Nonchronic Schizophrenic Patients." *Schizophrenia Bulletin* 6 (1980): 64–69.

Harding, C.M., and Brooks, G.W. "Longitudinal Assessment for a Cohort of Chronic Schizophrenics Discharged 20 Years Ago." *Psychiatric Journal of the University of Ottawa* 5 (1980): 274–278.

Harrow, M., Grinker, R.R., Silverstein, M.L., and Holzman, P. "Is Modern-Day Schizophrenic Outcome Still Negative?" *American Journal of Psychiatry* 135 (1978): 1156–1162.

Herz, M.A., and Melville, C. "Relapse in Schizophrenia." *American Journal of Psychiatry* 137 (1980): 801–805.

Heston, L.L. "The Genetics of Schizophrenia and Schizoid Disease." *Science* 167 (1970): 249–256.

Hogarty, G.E., Goldberg, S.C., Schooler, N.R., and Ulrich, R.F. "Drug and Sociotherapy in the Aftercare of Schizophrenic Patients. II. Two-Year Relapse Rates." *Archives of General Psychiatry* 31 (1974): 603–608.

Huber, G., Gross, G., and Schuttler, R. "A Long-Term Follow-up of Schizophrenia: Psychiatric Course of Illness and Prognosis." *Acta Psychiatrica Scandinavica* 52 (1975): 49–57.

Karasu, T.B., and Skodol, A.E. "VIth Axis for DSM III: Psychodynamic Evaluation." *American Journal of Psychiatry* 137 (1980): 607–610.

Kendler, K., Gruenberg, A., and Strauss, J. "An Independent Analysis of the Copenhagen Sample of the Danish Adoption Study of Schizophrenia: IV. Childhood Social Withdrawal and Adult Schizophrenia." *Archives of General Psychiatry*, submitted.

Kuriansky, J.B., Gurland, B.J., Spitzer, R.L., and Endicott, J. "Trends in the Frequency of Schizophrenia by Different Diagnostic Criteria." *American Journal of Psychiatry* 134 (1977): 631–636.

Langfeldt, G. "Schizophrenia: Diagnosis and Prognosis." *Behavioral Science* 14 (1969): 173–182.

Leff, J.P. "Schizophrenia and Sensitivity to the Family Environment." *Schizophrenia Bulletin* 2 (1976): 556–574.

McGlashan, T.H., and Carpenter, W.T., Jr. "An Investigation of the Postpsychotic Depressive Syndrome." *American Journal of Psychiatry* 133 (1976): 14–19.

Rodnick, E.H., and Goldstein, M.J. "Premorbid Adjustment and the Recovery of Mothering Functioning in Acute Schizophrenic Women." *Journal of Abnormal Psychology* 83 (1974): 623–628.

Rosenthal, D., Wender, P.H., Kety, S.S., Welner, J., and Schulsinger, F. "The Adopted-Away Offspring of Schizophrenics." *American Journal of Psychiatry* 128 (1971): 87–91.

Schneider, K. *Clinical Psychopathology*, translated by M. Hamilton. New York: Grune & Stratton, 1959.

Sneznevsky, A.V. "The Symptomatology, Clinical Forms and Nosology of Schizophrenia." In *Modern Perspectives in World Psychiatry*, edited by J.G. Howells. London: Oliver & Boyd, 1968.

Stierlin, H. "Bleuler's Concept of Schizophrenia: A Confusing Heritage." *American Journal of Psychiatry* 123 (1967): 996–1001.

Strauss, J.S. "A Comprehensive Approach to Psychiatric Diagnosis." *American Journal of Psychiatry* 132 (1975): 1193–1197.

Strauss, J.S., and Carpenter, W.T., Jr. "The Prognosis of Schizophrenia: Rationale for a Multidimensional Concept." *Schizophrenia Bulletin* 4 (1978): 56–67.

Strauss, J.S., and Carpenter, W.T., Jr. *Schizophrenia.* New York: Plenum, 1981.

Strauss, J.S., Loevsky, L., Glazer, W., and Leaf, P. "Organizing the Complexities of Schizophrenia."

Journal of Nervous and Mental Disease 169 (1981): 120–126.

Watt, N.F. "Patterns of Childhood Social Development in Adult Schizophrenics." *Archives of General Psychiatry* 35 (1978): 160–165.

Wing, J.K., and Brown, G.W. *Institutionalism and Schizophrenia.* Cambridge: Cambridge University Press, 1970.

Bibliography for Chapter 10

Cancro, R. "Overview of Schizophrenia." In *The Comprehensive Textbook of Psychiatry 3d ed.,* edited by H.I. Kaplan, A.M. Freedman, and B.J. Sadock. Baltimore: Williams & Wilkins, 1980.

Fischer, M. "Genetic and Environmental Factors in Schizophrenia." *Acta Psychiatrica Scandinavica,* Supplement 238, 1973.

Gottesman, I.I., and Shields, J. "Schizophrenia in Twins: 16 Years' Consecutive Admissions to a Psychiatric Clinic." *British Journal of Psychiatry* 112 (1966): 809–818.

Gottesman, I.I., and Shields, J. "A Critical Review of Recent Adoption, Twin, and Family Studies of Schizophrenia: Behavioral Genetics Perspectives." *Schizophrenia Bulletin* 2 (1976): 360–401.

Heston, L.L. "Psychiatric Disorders in Foster Home Reared Children of Schizophrenic Mothers." *British Journal of Psychiatry* 112 (1966): 819–825.

Kallmann, F.J. *The Genetics of Schizophrenia.* New York: Augustin, 1938.

Kallmann, F.J. "The Genetic Theory of Schizophrenia: An Analysis of 691 Schizophrenic Twin Index Families." *American Journal of Psychiatry* 103 (1946): 309–322.

Kety, S.S., Rosenthal, D., Wender, P.H., and Schulsinger, F. "The Types and Prevalence of Mental Illness in the Biological and Adoptive Families of Adopted Schizophrenics." In *The Transmission of Schizophrenia,* edited by D. Rosenthal and S.S. Kety. Oxford: Pergamon Press, 1968.

Kety, S.S., Rosenthal, D., Wender, P.H., Schulsinger, F., and Jacobsen, B. "Mental Illness in the Biological and Adoptive Families of Adopted Individuals Who Have Become Schizophrenic: A Preliminary Report Based on Psychiatric Interviews." In *Genetic Research in Psychiatry,* edited by R.R. Fieve, D. Rosenthal, and H. Brill. Baltimore: Johns Hopkins University Press, 1975.

Kringlen, E. *Heredity and Environment in the Functional Psychoses.* London: Heinemann, 1967.

Lindelius, R. "A Study of Schizophrenia: A Clinical, Prognostic, and Family Investigation." *Acta Psychiatrica Scandinavica,* Supplement 216, (1970).

Pollin, W., Allen, M.G., Hoffer, A., Stabenau, J.R., and Hrubec, Z. "Psychopathology in 15,909 Pairs of Veteran Twins." *American Journal of Psychiatry* 126 (1969): 597–609.

Rosenthal, D., Wender, P.H., Kety, S.S., Schulsinger, F., Welner, J., and Ostergaard, L. "Schizophrenics' Offspring Reared in Adoptive Homes." In *The Transmission of Schizophrenia,* edited by D. Rosenthal and S.S. Kety. Oxford: Pergamon Press, 1968.

Rüdin, E. *Zur Vererbung und Neuentstehung der Dementia Praecox.* Berlin: Springer Verlag, 1916.

Schultz, B. "Zur Erbpathologie der Schizophrenie." *Zeitschrift für die gesamte Neurologie und Psychiatrie* 143 (1932): 175–293.

Slater, E. "A Review of Earlier Evidence on Genetic Factors in Schizophrenia." In *The Transmission of Schizophrenia,* edited by D. Rosenthal and S.S. Kety. Oxford: Pergamon Press, 1968.

Slater, E., and Shields, J. "Psychotic and Neurotic Illness in Twins." *Medical Research Council Special Report Series,* No. 278. London: Her Majesty's Stationery Office, 1953.

Stephens, D.A., Atkinson, M.W., Kay, D.W.K., Roth, M., and Garside, R.F. "Psychiatric Morbidity in Parents and Sibs of Schizophrenics and Nonschizophrenics." *British Journal of Psychiatry* 127 (1975): 97–108.

Tienari, P. "Psychiatric Illnesses in Identical Twins." *Acta Psychiatrica Scandinavica,* Supplement 171, 1963.

Tienari, P. "Schizophrenia in Monozygotic Male Twins." In *The Transmission of Schizophrenia,* edited by D. Rosenthal and S.S. Kety. Oxford: Pergamon Press, 1968.

Tsuang, M.T., Fowler, R.C., Cadoret, R.J., and Monnelly, E. "Schizophrenia Among First-Degree Relatives of Paranoid and Nonparanoid Schizophrenics." *Comprehensive Psychiatry* 15 (1974): 295–302.

Wender, P.H., Rosenthal, D., Kety, S.S., Schulsinger, F., and Welner, J. "Cross-Fostering: A Research Strategy for Clarifying the Role of Genetic and Experiential Factors in the Etiology of Schizophrenia." *Archives of General Psychiatry* 30 (1974): 121–128.

Bibliography for Chapter 11

Adebimpe, V.R. "Overview: White Norms and Psychiatric Diagnosis of Black Patients." *American Journal of Psychiatry* 138 (1981): 279–285.

Anthony, W.W., Cohen, M.R., and Vitalo, R. "The Measurement of Rehabilitation Outcome." *Schizophrenia Bulletin* 4 (1978): 365–383.

Birley, J.L.T., and Brown, G.W. "Crises and Life Changes Preceding the Onset or Relapse of Acute Schizophrenia." *British Journal of Psychiatry* 116 (1970): 327–333.

Bland, R.C., and Orn, H. "Schizophrenia: Sociocultural Factors." *Canadian Journal of Psychiatry* 26 (1981): 186–188.

Brenner, M.H. *Mental Illness and the Economy.* Cambridge: Harvard University Press, (1973).

Brown, G.W., and Birley, J.L.T. "Crises and Life Changes and the Onset of Schizophrenia." *Journal of Health and Social Behavior* 9 (1968): 203–214.

Brown, G.W., Bones, M., Dalison, B., and Wing, J.U. *Schizophrenia and Social Care.* London: Oxford Univ. Press, (1966).

Carpenter, L., and Brockington, I.F. "A Study of Mental Illness in Asians, West Indians and Africans Living in Manchester." *British Journal of Psychiatry* 137 (1980): 201–205.

Cheetham, R.W.S., and Griffiths, J.A. "Errors in the Diagnosis of Schizophrenia in Black and Indian Patients." *South African Medical Journal* 59 (1981): 71–75.

Eaton, W.W. "A Formal Theory of Selection for Schizophrenia." *American Journal of Sociology* 86 (1980): 149–158.

Eaton, W.W., and Larry, J.C. "Mental Health and Occupational Mobility in a Group of Immigrants." *Social Science and Medicine* 12 (1978): 53–58.

Falloon, I.R.H. "Communication and Problem-Solving Skills Training With Relapsing Schizophrenics and Their Families." In *Family Therapy and Major Psychopathology,* edited by M.R. Lansky. New York: Grune & Stratton, 1981.

Falloon, I.R.H., Watt, D.C., and Shepherd, M. "The Social Outcome of Patients in a Trial of Long-Term Continuation Therapy in Schizophrenia: Pimozide vs. Fluphenazine." *Psychological Medicine* 8 (1978): 265–274.

Falloon, I.R.H., Liberman, R.P., Lillie, R., and Vaughn, C.E. "Family Therapy of Schizophrenics at High Risk for Relapse." *Family Process* 20 (1981): 211–221.

Garmezy, N. "Children at Risk: The Search for the Antecedents of Schizophrenia." *Schizophrenia Bulletin* 8 (1974): 14–90.

Gittleman-Klein, R., and Klein, D.F. "Premorbid Social Adjustment and Prognosis in Schizophrenia." *Journal of Psychiatric Research* 7 (1969): 35–53.

Goldstein, A.A. *Structured Learning Therapy.* New York: Academic Press, 1973.

Greco, M.A., and Stein, L.I. "An Alternative to Hospitalization Program: The Contributions of a Rehabilitation Approach." *Rehabilitation Counseling Bulletin* 24 (1980): 85–93.

Hersen, M., and Bellack, A.S. "A Multiple Baseline Analysis of Social Skills Training in Chronic Schizophrenics." *Journal of Applied Behavior Analysis* 9 (1976a): 239–245.

Hersen, M., and Bellack, A.S. "Social Skills Training for Chronic Psychiatric Patients: Rationale, Research Findings, and Future Directions." *Comprehensive Psychiatry* 17 (1976b): 559–580.

Huffine, C.L., and Clausen, J.A. "Madness and Work: Short- and Long-Term Effects of Mental Illness on Occupational Careers." *Social Forces* 57 (1979): 1049–1062.

Jacobs, S., and Myers, J. "Recent Life Events and Acute Schizophrenic Psychosis: A Controlled Study." *Journal of Nervous and Mental Disease* 162 (1976): 75–87.

Kasanin, J. and Rosen, Z.A. "Clinical Variables in Schizoid Personalities." *Archives of Neurology and Psychiatry* 30 (1933): 538–566.

Karno, M., and Edgerton, R.B. "The Perception of Mental Illness in a Mexican-American Community." *Archives of General Psychiatry* 20 (1969): 233–238.

Kohn, M.L. "The Interaction of Social Class and Other Factors in the Etiology of Schizophrenia." *American Journal of Psychiatry* 133 (1976): 177–180.

Kohn M.L., and Clausen, J.A. "Social Isolation and Schizophrenia." *American Sociological Review* 20 (1955): 265–273.

Kokes, R.F., Strauss, J.S., and Klorman, R. "Premorbid Adjustment in Schizophrenia: Concepts, Measures, and Implications Part II. Measuring Premorbid Adjustment: The Instruments and Their Development." *Schizophrenia Bulletin* 3 (1977): 186–213.

Leff, J.P., and Wing, J.U. "Trial of Maintenance Therapy in Schizophrenia." *British Medical Journal* 3 (1971): 599–604.

Leff, J.P., and Vaughn, C.E. "The Interaction of Life Events and Relatives' Expressed Emotion in Schizophrenia and Depressive Neurosis." *British Journal of Psychiatry* 136 (1980): 146–153.

Leff, J.P., Hirsch, S.R., Gaird, R., Rolides, P.D., and Stevens, B.S. "Life Events and Maintenance Therapy in Schizophrenic Relapse." *British Journal of Psychiatry* 123 (1973): 659–660.

Lehman, S. "The Social Ecology of Natural Supports." In *Community Mental Health: A Behavior Ecological Perspective,* edited by A. Jeger and R.W. Slotnick. New York: Plenum Publishing Corp., 1980.

Levine, J., and Zigler, E. "The Essential-Reactive Distinction in Alcoholism." *Journal of Abnormal Psychology* 81 (1973): 242–249.

Liberman, R.P., Falloon, I.R.H., and Aitchison, R.A. "Multiple Family Group Therapy for Schizophrenics at Risk for Relapse." *Schizophrenia Bulletin,* submitted.

Liberman, R.P., King, L.W., DeRisi, W.J., and McCann, M. *Personal Effectiveness: Guiding People to Assert Themselves and Improve Their Social Skills.* Champaign: Research Press, 1975.

Liberman, R.P., Lillie, F., Falloon, I.R.H., Harpin, E., and Hutchison, W. "Multiple Baseline Analysis of Social Skills Training With Schizophrenics." *Archives of General Psychiatry,* submitted.

Liberman, R.P., McCann, M., and Wallace, C.J. "Generalization of Behavior Therapy With Psychotics." *British Journal of Psychiatry,* 129 (1976): 490–496.

Liberman, R.P., Wallace, C.J., Vaughn, C.E., Snyder, K.S., and Rust, C. "Social and Family Factors in the Course of Schizophrenia." In *Psychotherapy of Schizophrenia: Current State and New Directions,* edited by J. Strauss and M. Bowers. New York: Plenum Publishing Corp. 1980.

Liberman, R.P., Wallace C.J., Falloon, I.R.H., and Vaughn, C.E. "Interpersonal Problem-Solving Therapy for Schizophrenics and Their Families." *Comprehensive Psychiatry,* in press.

Lipton, F.R., Cohen, C.I., Fischer, E., and Katz, S.E. "Schizophrenia: A Network Crisis." *Schizophrenia Bulletin* 7 (1981): 144–181.

Littlewood, R., and Lipsedge, M. "Some Social and Phenomenological Characteristics of Psychotic Immigrants." *Psychological Medicine* 11 (1981): 289–302.

Ludwig, A. "The Disabled Society." *American Journal of Psychotherapy* 35 (1981): 5–15.

Marsella, A.J., and Snyder, K.K. "Stress, Social Supports, and Schizophrenic Disorders: Toward an Interactional Model." *Schizophrenia Bulletin* 7 (1981): 152–163.

Mednick, S.A., and Schulsinger, F. "Factors Related to Breakdown in Children at High Risk for Schizophrenia." In *Life History Research in Psychopathology,* edited by M. Roff and D.F. Ricks. Minneapolis: University of Minnesota Press, 1970.

Mosher, L., and Keith. S.J. "Research on the Psychosocial Treatment for Schizophrenia: A Summary

Report." *American Journal of Psychiatry* 136 (1979): 623–631.

Paul, G.L., and Lentz, R. *Psychosocial Treatment for Chronic Mental Patients.* Cambridge: Harvard University Press, 1977.

Platt, J.J., and Siegel, J. "MMPI Characteristics of Good and Poor Social Problem-Solvers Among Psychiatric Patients." *Journal of Psychology* 94 (1976): 245–251.

Platt, J.J., Siegel, J.J., Siegel, J.M., and Spivack, G. "Do Psychiatric Patients and Normals See the Same Solutions as Effective in Solving Interpersonal Problems?" *Journal of Consulting and Clinical Psychology* 43 (1975): 307.

Quitkin, F., Rifkin, A., and McKay, L. "Scapegoating in Hospitalized Adolescents: A Behavioral Phenomenon Associated With Schizophrenia With Premorbid Asociality." *Archives of General Psychiatry* 28 (1973): 680–682.

Robin, A., Copas, J.B., and Freeman-Browne, D.L. "Problem Areas and Mental and Behavioral Status in Schizophrenia, Neurosis and Depression." *Journal of Nervous and Mental Disease* 168 (1980): 412–418.

Rushing, W.A., and Ortega, S.T. "Socioeconomic Status and Mental Disorder: New Evidence and a Sociomedical Formulation." *American Journal of Sociology* 84 (1979): 1175–1200.

Sartorius, N., Jablensky, A., and Shapiro, R. "Two Year Follow-Up of the Patients Included in the WHO International Pilot Study of Schizophrenia." *Psychological Medicine* 7 (1977): 529–541.

Schulsinger, H. "A Ten-Year Follow-Up of Children of Schizophrenic Mothers: Clinical Assessment." *Acta Psychiatrica Scandinavica* 53 (1976): 371–386.

Shepherd, M. *A Study of the Major Psychoses in an English County.* London: Chapman & Hall, 1957.

Simmons, O.G. *Work and Mental Illness.* New York: Wiley, 1965.

Spivack, G., Platt, J.J., and Shure, M.B. *The Problem-Solving Approach to Adjustment.* San Francisco: Jossey-Bass, 1976.

Spring, B. "Stress and Schizophrenia: Some Definitional Issues." *Schizophrenia Bulletin* 7 (1981): 23–33.

Stein, L.I., and Test, M.A. (Eds.) *Alternatives to Mental Hospital Treatment.* New York: Plenum Publishing Corp., 1978.

Strauss, J.S., and Carpenter, W.T. "The Prediction of Outcome in Schizophrenia II. Relationship Between Predictor and Outcome Variables." *Archives of General Psychiatry* 31 (1974): 37–42.

Streiner, D.L., Norman, G.R., McFarland, A.H., and Roy, R.G. "Quality of Life Events and Their Relationship to Strain." *Schizophrenia Bulletin* 7 (1981): 34–42.

Torrey, E.F. "Epidemiology." In *Disorders of the Schizophrenic Syndrome,* edited by L. Bellak. New York: Basic Books, 1979.

Trower, P., Bryant, B., and Argyle, M. *Social Skills and Mental Health.* Pittsburgh: University of Pittsburgh Press, 1978.

Tsuang, M.I. "Social Effects of Schizophrenia and Affective Disorders." In *The Social Consequences of Psychiatric Illness,* edited by L.N. Robins, P.J. Clayton, and J.K. Wing. New York: Brunner-Mazel, 1980.

Vaughn, C.E., and Leff, J.P. "The Influence of Family and Social Factors on the Course of Psychiatric Illness." *British Journal of Psychiatry* 129 (1976): 125–137.

Vaughn, C.E., Snyder, K.S., Liberman, R.P., and Falloon, I.R.H. "Family Factors in Schizophrenic Relapse." *Schizophrenia Bulletin* in press.

Wallace, C.J., Nelson, C.J., Liberman, R.P., Aitcheson, R.A., Lukoff, D., and Ferris, C. "A Review and Critique of Social Skills Training With Schizophrenic Patients." *Schizophrenia Bulletin* 6 (1980): 42–63.

Watt, D.C., and Szulecka, T.K. "The Effect of Sex, Marriage, and Age at First Admission on the Hospitalization of Schizophrenics During Two Years Following Discharge." *Psychological Medicine* 9 (1979): 529–539.

Waxler, N.E. "Is Outcome for Schizophrenia Better in Non-Industrial Societies?" *Journal of Nervous and Mental Disease* 167 (1979): 144–158.

Weaver, J.L. "Mexican-American Health Care Behavior." *Social Science Quarterly* 54 (1973): 85–102.

Wing, J.K. "The Social Context of Schizophrenia." *American Journal of Psychiatry* 135 (1978): 1333–1339.

Wing, J.K., Cooper, J.E., and Sartorius, N. *The Measurement and Classification of Psychiatric Symptoms.* London: Cambridge University Press, 1974.

Zigler, E., and Phillips, L. "Social Competence and Outcome in Psychiatric Disorder." *Journal of Abnormal and Social Psychology* 63 (1961): 264–271.

Zubin, J., and Spring, B. "Vulnerability: A New View of Schizophrenia." *Journal of Abnormal Psychology* 86 (1977): 103–126.

Bibliography for Chapter 12

Abdulla, Y.H., and Hamadah, K. "Effect of ADP on PGE_1 Formation in Blood Platelets From Patients With Depression, Mania and Schizophrenia." *British Journal of Psychiatry* 127 (1975): 591–595.

Abell, C.W., Fritz, R.R., Landowski, J., Bessman, J.D. Castellane, S., Boeringa, J.A., and Rose, R.M. "Studies of MAO Concentration and Activity in Schizophrenic Patients." In *Proteins of the Nervous System: Structure and Function.* New York: Alan R. Liss Inc., in press.

Abrams, R., and Taylor, M.A. "Mania and Schizo-Affective Disorder, Manic Type: A Comparison." *American Journal of Psychiatry* 133 (1976): 1445–1447.

Adler, S.A., Gottesman, I.I., Orsulak, P.J., Kizuka, P.P., and Schildkraut, J.J. "Platelet MAO Activity: Relationships to Clinical and Psychometric Variables." *Schizophrenia Bulletin* 6 (1980): 226–231.

Albrecht, P., Torrey, E.F., Boone, E., Hicks, J., and Daniel, N. "Raised Cytomegalovirus-Antibody Levels in Cerebrospinal Fluid of Schizophrenic Patients." *Lancet* ii (1980): 769–772.

American Psychiatric Associaton. *A Report of the APA Task Force on Vitamin Therapy in Psychiatry: Megavitamin and Orthomolecular Therapy in Psychiatry.* Washington, D.C.: American Psychiatric Association, 1973.

Amkraut, A., Solomon, G.F., Allansmith, M., Mc-Clellan, B., and Rappaport, M. "Immunoglobulins and Improvement in Acute Schizophrenic Reactions." *Archives of General Psychiatry* 28 (1973): 673–677.

Ananth, J.V., and Minn, K. "Chlorpromazine-Induced Systematic Lupus Erythematosus." *Canadian Medical Association Journal* 108 (1973): 680.

Angrist, B.M., Thompson, H., Shopsin, B., and Gerson, S. "Clinical Studies with Dopamine Receptor Stimulants." *Psychopharmacologia* 44 (1975): 273–280.

Ashby, W.R., Collins, G.H., and Bassett, M. "The Effects of Nicotinamide and Placebo on the Chronic Schizophrenic." *Journal of Mental Science* 106 (1960): 1555–1559.

Ashkenazi, A., Krasilowsky, D., Levin, S., Idar, D., Kalian, M., Or, A., Ginat, Y., and Halperin, B. "Immunologic Reaction of Psychotic Patients to Fractions of Gluten." *American Journal of Psychiatry* 136 (1979): 1306–1309.

Averback, P. "Lesions of the Nucleus Ansae Peduncularis in Neuropsychiatric Disease." *Archives of Neurology* 38 (1981): 230–235.

Baldwin, J.A. "Schizophrenia and Physical Disease." *Psychological Medicine* 9 (1979): 611–618.

Ban, T.A., Lehman, H.E., and Deutsch, M. "Negative Findings with Megavitamins in Schizophrenic Patients: Preliminary Report." *Communications in Psychopharmacology* 1 (1977): 119–122.

Baron, M., and Levitt, M. "Platelet Monoamine Oxidase Activity: Relation to Genetic Load of Schizophrenia." *Psychiatry Research* 3 (1980): 69–74.

Belmaker, R.H., Bracha, H.S., and Ebstein, R.P. "Platelet Monoamine Oxidase in Affective Illness and Alcoholism." *Schizophrenia Bulletin* 6 (1980): 320–323.

Bennett, J.P., Enna, S.J., Bylund, D.B., Gillin, J.C., Wyatt, R.J., and Snyder, S.H. "Neurotransmitter Receptors in Frontal Cortex of Schizophrenics." *Archives of General Psychiatry* 36 (1979): 927–934.

Bergen, J.R., Grinspoon, L., Pyle, H.M., Martinez, J.L., and Pennell, R.B. "Immunologic Studies in Schizophrenic and Control Subjects." *Biological Psychiatry* 15 (1980): 369–379.

Bergen, J.R., Mittag, T.W., Frohman, C.E., Arthur, R.E., and Freeman, H. "Plasma Factors in Schizophrenia: Cooperative Study." *Archives of General Psychiatry* 18 (1968): 471–476.

Berger, P.A., Faull, K.F., Kilkowski, J., Anderson, P.J., Kraemer, H., Davis, K.L., and Barchas, J.D. "CSF Monoamine Metabolites in Depression and Schizophrenia." *American Journal of Psychiatry* 137 (1980a) 174–180.

Berger, P.A., Watson, S.J., Akil, H., Elliott, G.R., Rubin, R.T., Pfefferbaum, A., Davis, K.L., Barchas, J.D. and Li, C.H. "B-Endorphin and Schizophrenia." *Archives of General Psychiatry* 37 (1980b): 635–640.

Berrettini, W.H., Benfield, T.C., Schmidt, A.D., Ladman, R.K., and Vogel, W.H. "Platelet Monoamine Oxidase in Families of Chronic Schizophrenics." *Schizophrenia Bulletin* 6 (1980): 235–237.

Berrettini, W.H., and Vogel, W.H. "Evidence for an Endogenous Inhibitor of Platelet MAO in Chronic Schizophrenia." *American Journal of Psychiatry* 135 (1978): 605–607.

Bigelow, L.B., Walls, P., Gillin, J.C., and Wyatt, R.J. "Clinical Effects of 5-Hydroxytryptophan Administration in Chronic Schizophrenic Patients." *Biological Psychiatry* 14 (1979a): 53–67.

Bigelow, L.B., Weinberger, D.R., and Wyatt, R.J. "Synergism of Combined Lithium-Neuroleptic Therapy: A Double-Blind Placebo Controlled Case Study." *American Journal of Psychiatry* 138 (1981): 81–83.

Bigelow, L.B., Zalcman, S., Kleinman, J.E., Weinberger, D.R., Luchins, D., Tallman, J., Karoum, F., and Wyatt, R.J. "Propranolol Treatment of Chronic Schizophrenia: Clinical Response, Catecholamine Metabolism and Lymphocyte B-Receptor." In *Catecholamine Basic and Clinical Frontiers,* edited by E. Usdin, I. Kopin, and J. Barchas. New York: Pergamon Press, 1979b.

Bird, E.D. "The Clinical Significance of Disturbances in the Central GABA System." In *Neurotransmission and Disturbed Behavior,* edited by H.M. Van Praag, and J. Bruinvels. New York: S.P. Medical and Scientific Books, 1976.

Bird, E.D., Spokes, E.G., Barnes, J., Mackay, A., Iversen, L., and Shepherd, M. "Increased Brain Dopamine and Reduced Glutamic Acid Decarboxylase and Choline Acteyltransferase Activity in Schizophrenia and Related Psychoses." *Lancet* ii (1977): 1157–1159.

Bird, E.D., Spokes, E.G., and Iversen, L.L. "Brain Norepinephrine and Dopamine in Schizophrenia." *Science* 204 (1979a): 93–94.

Bird, E.D., Spokes, E.G., and Iversen, L.L. "Increased Dopamine Concentration in Limbic Areas of Brain From Patients Dying with Schizophrenia." *Brain* 102 (1979b): 347–360.

Bleuler, E. *Dementia Praecox or The Group of Schizophrenias.* New York: International Universities Press, 1950.

Boklage, C. "Schizophrenia, Brain Asymmetry Development and Twinning: Cellular Relationship with Etiological and Possibly Prognostic Implications." *Biological Psychiatry* 12 (1977): 19–35.

Böök, J.A., Wetterberg, L., and Modryewska, K. "Schizophrenia in a North Swedish Geographical Isolate 1900–1977: Epidemiology, Genetics and Biochemistry." *Clinical Genetics* 14 (1978): 373–394.

Borison, R.L., Lemus, F., Reyes, M., Havdala, H., and Diamond, B. "Regional Localization of 2-Phenylethylamine in Human Brain." *Research Communications in Psychology, Psychiatry, and Behavior* 2 (1977): 193–201.

Bowers, M. "Acute Psychosis Induced by Psychotomimetic Drug Abuse." *Archives of General Psychiatry* 27 (1972): 439–440.

Bowers, M. "Central Dopamine Turnover in Schizophrenia Syndrome." *Archives of General Psychiatry* 31 (1974): 50–54.

Brown, W., and Laughren, T. "Low Serum Prolactin and Early Relapse Following Neuroleptic Withdrawal." *American Journal of Psychiatry* 138 (1981): 237–239.

Buchsbaum, M., Kessler, R., Bunney, W.E., Cappelletti, J., Coppola, R., Flynn, R., Goble, J.C., Manning, R.G., van Kammen, D.P., Rigal, F., Waters, R., Sokoloff, L, and Ingvar, D. "Positron Emission Tomography and EEG in Schizophrenia." *American Psy-*

chiatric Association, 134th Annual Convention, New Orleans, May, 1981.

Carlsson, A. "Antipsychotic Drugs, Neurotransmitters and Schizophrenia." *American Journal of Psychiatry* 135 (1978): 164–173.

Carlsson, A. *Catecholamines: Basic and Clinical Frontiers.* New York: Pergamon Press, 1979.

Carp, R. "The Search for an Infectious Agent: Approaches Explored for Multiple Sclerosis." *Birth Deficits: Original Article Series* 14 (1978): 89–109.

Casey, D.E., Korsgaard, S., Gerlach, J., Jorgensen, A., and Simmelsgaard, H. "Effect of Des-Tyrosine-Gamma-Endorphin in Tardive Dyskinesia." *Archives of General Psychiatry* 38 (1981): 158–160.

Connell, P.H. *Amphetamine Psychosis, Maudsley Monographs No. 5.* London: Oxford University Press, 1958.

Corsini, G., Del Zompom, M., Manconi, S., Cianchetti, C., Mangoni, A., and Gessa, G.L. "Sedative, Hypnotic and Antipsychotic Effects of Low Doses of Apomorphine in Man." *Advances in Biochemistry and Psychopharmacology* 16 (1977a): 645–648.

Corsini, G., Del Zampo, M., Manconi, S., Piccardi, M.P., Onali, P.L., and Mangoni, A. "Evidence for Dopamine Receptors in the Human Brain Mediating Sedation and Sleep." *Life Sciences* 20 (1977b): 1613–1618.

Cotzias, G.C., Papavasilow, P.S., Totosa, E., Mendez, J.S., and Bello Midina, M. "Treatment of Parkinson's Disease with Apomorphine: Possible Role of Growth Hormone." *New England Journal of Medicine* 294 (1976): 567–572.

Creese, I. Burt, D.R., and Snyder, S.H. "Dopamine Receptor Binding. Differentiation of Agonist and Antagonist States with (^{3}H)-Dopamine and (^{3}H) Haloperidol." *Life Sciences* 17 (1975): 1715–1720.

Creese, I., Burt, D.R., and Snyder, S.H. "Dopamine Receptor Binding Predicts Clinical and Pharmacological Potencies of Antischizophrenic Drugs." *Science* 192 (1976): 481–483.

Cross, A.J., Crow, T.J., Killpack, W.S., Longdon, A., Owen, F., and Riley, G.J. "The Activities of Brain Dopamine-B-Hydroxylase and Catechol-O-Methyltransferase in Schizophrenics and Controls." *Psychopharmacology* 59 (1978): 117–121.

Crow, T.J. "Molecular Pathology of Schizophrenia: More Than One Disease Process?" *British Medical Journal* 280 (1980): 66–68.

Crow, T.J., Ferrier, I.N., Johnston, E.C., Macmillan, J.F., Owens, D.G., Parry, R.P., and Tyrrell, D.A.J. "Characteristics of Patients with Schizophrenia or Neurological Disorder and Virus-Like Agent in Cerebrospinal Fluid." *Lancet* I (1979): 842–844.

Crow, T.J., Owen, F., Cross, A.J., Lofthourse, R., and Longden, A. "Brain Biochemistry in Schizophrenia." *Lancet* I (1978): 36–37.

Cruz, R., and Vogel, W. "Pyroluria: A Poor Marker in Schizophrenia." *American Journal of Psychiatry* 135 (1978): 1239–1241.

Davis, G.C., Buchsbaum, M.S., and Bunney, W.E., Jr. "Research in Endorphins and Schizophrenia." *Schizophrenia Bulletin* 5 (1979): 244–250.

Davis, J.M. "Antipsychotic Drugs." In *Comprehensive Textbook of Psychiatry, 3d ed.,* edited by H.I. Kaplan, A.M. Freedman, B.J. Sadock. Baltimore: Williams & Wilkins, 1980.

Davison, R., and Bagley, C. "Schizophrenia-Like Psychoses Associated With Organic Disorders of the Central Nervous System: A Review of the Literature." In *Current Problems in Neuropsychiatry,* edited by R.N. Herington. Ashford, England: Headley Brothers, 1969.

DeLisi, L.E., Neckers, L.M., Weinberger, D.R., and Wyatt, R.J. "Whole Blood Serotonin Concentrations in Schizophrenic Patients." *Archives of General Psychiatry* 38 (1981b): 647–654.

DeLisi, L.E., Wise, C.D., Bridge, T.P., Potkin, S., Phelps, B., and Wyatt, R.J. "Monoamine Oxidase and Schizophrenia." In *Biological Markers for Mental Illness.* New York: Pergammon Press, 1981a.

DeLisi, L.E., Weinberger, D.R., Potkin, S.G., Neckers, L., and Wyatt, R.J. "Quantitative Determination of Immunoglobulins in CSF and Plasma of Chronic Schizophrenic Patients." *British Journal of Psychiatry,* in press.

DeLisi, L.E., Wise, C.D., Bridge, T.P., Rosenblatt, J.R., Wagner, R.L., Morihisa, J., Karson, C., Potkin, S.G., and Wyatt, R.J. "The Effect of Neuroleptic Medication on Platelet Monoamine Oxidase Activity *In Vivo* and *In Vitro.*" *Psychiatry Research* 4 (1981c): 95–107.

DeLisi, L.E., Wise, C.D., Potkin, S.G., Zalcman, S., Phelps, B., Lovenberg, W., and Wyatt, R.J. "Dopamine-B-Hydroxylase, Monoamine Oxidase and Schizophrenia." *Biological Psychiatry* 15 (1980): 899–907.

Denson, R. "Nicotinamide in the Treatment of Schizophrenia." *Diseases of the Nervous System* 23 (1962): 167–172.

DiChiara, G., Corsini, G.U., Mereu, G.P., Tissari, A., and Gessa, G.L. "Self-Inhibitory Dopamine Receptors: Their Role in the Biochemical and Behavioral Effects of Low Doses of Apomorphine." *Advances in Biochemical Psychopharmacology* 19 (1978): 275–292.

Dohan, F.C. "The Possible Pathogenic Effect of Cereal Grains in Schizophenia-Celiac Disease as a Model." *Acta Neurologica* 31 (1976): 195–205.

Dohan, F.C., and Grasberger, J.C. "Relapsed Schizophrenics: Earlier Discharge from Hospital After Cereal-Free, Milk-Free Diet." *American Journal of Psychiatry* 130 (1973): 686–688.

Dohan, F.C., Grasberger, J.C., Lowell, F.M., Johnston, H.T., and Aregast, A. "Relapsed Schizophrenics: More Rapid Improvement on a Milk and Cereal-Free Diet." *British Journal of Psychiatry* 115 (1969): 595–596.

Domino, E.F., Krause, R.R., Thiessen, M.M., and Batsakes, J.G. "Blood Protein Fraction Comparisons of Normal and Schizophrenic Patients." *Archives of General Psychiatry* 32 (1975): 717–721.

Doust, J.W.L. "Psychiatric Aspects of Somatic Immunity: Differential Incidence in the Histories of Psychiatric Patients." *British Journal of Social Medicine* 6 (1952): 49–67.

Ellerbook, R.C., and Purdy, M.D. "Capacity of Stressed Humans Under Megadoses of Nicotinic Acid to Synthesize Methylated Compounds." *Diseases of the Nervous System* 31 (1970): 196–197.

Fauman, M.A., and Fauman, B.J. "Chronic Phencyclidine Abuse: A Psychiatric Perspective." *Psychopharmacology Bulletin* 16 (1980): 70–75.

Farley, I.J., Price, K.S., McCullough, E., Deck, J.H.N., Hordynski, W., and Hornykiewicz, O. "Norepinephrine in Chronic Paranoid Schizophrenia: Above-Normal Levels in Limbic Forebrain." *Science* 200 (1978): 456–458.

Feer H., Thoelin, H., and Massini, M.A. "Hemodialysis in Schizophrenia." *Comprehensive Psychiatry* 1 (1960): 338–344.

Feldberg, W. "Possible Association of Schizophrenia With a Disturbance in Prostaglandin Metabolism: A Physiological Hypothesis." *Psychological Medicine* 6 (1976): 359–369.

Ferguson, R.M., Schnudtke, J.R., and Simmons, R.L. "Effects of Psychoactive Drugs on *In Vitro* Lymphocyte Activation." In *Neurochemical and Immunologic Components in Schizophrenia,* edited by J. Mudge. New York: A.R. Liss, 1978.

Fessel, W.J., Hirata-Hibi, M. "Abnormal Leukocytes in Schizophrenics." *Archives of General Psychiatry* 9 (1963): 601–613.

Fessel, W.J., and Solomon, G.F. "Psychosis and Systemic Lupus Erythematosus: A Review of the Literature and Case Reports." *California Medicine* 92 (1960): 266–270.

Fieve, R.R., Blumenthal, B., and Little, B. "The Relationship of Atypical Lymphocytes, Phenothiazines, and Schizophrenia." *Archives of General Psychiatry* 15 (1966): 529–534.

Fischer, E., Heller, B., and Miro, A. "B-Phenylethylamine in Human Urine." *Arzneimittel-Forschung* 18 (1968): 1486–1489.

Fischer, E., Spatz, H., Saavedra, J.M., Reggiani, H., Mira, A., and Heller, B. "Urinary Elimination of Phenylethylamine." *Biological Psychiatry* 5 (1972): 139–147.

Fisman, M. "The Brain Stem in Psychosis." *British Journal of Psychiatry* 126 (1975): 414–422.

Flor-Henry, P. "On Certain Aspects of the Localization of the Cerebral Systems Regulating and Determining Emotion." *Biological Psychiatry* 14 (1979): 677–698.

Freed, W.J., Weinberger, D.R., Bing, L. and Wyatt, R.J. "Neuropharmacological Studies of Phencyclidine (PCP)-Induced Behavioral Stimulation in Mice." *Psychopharmacology* 71 (1980): 291–297.

Freedman, D.X., Belenduik, K., Belenduik, G.W., and Crayton, J.W. "Blood Tryptophan Metabolism in Chronic Schizophrenics." *Archives of General Psychiatry* 38 (1981): 655–662.

Freedman, D.X., and Halaris, A.E. "Monoamines and the Biochemical Mode of Action of LSD at Synapses." In *Psychopharmacology: A Generation of Progress,* edited by M.A. Lipton, A. DiMascio, and K.F. Killam. New York: Raven Press, 1978.

Friedman, S.B., Cohen, J. and Iker, H. "Antibody Response to Cholera Vaccine. Differences Between Depressed Schizophrenic and Normal Subjects." *Archives of General Psychiatry* 16 (1967): 312–315.

Frohman, C.E., Arthur, R.E., and Gottlieb, J.S. "Distribution and Mechanism of Action of the Anti-S Protein in Human Brain." *Biological Psychiatry* 7 (1973): 53–61.

Frohman, C.E., Harmison, C.R., Arthur, R.E., and Gottlieb, J.S. "Confirmation of a Unique Plasma Protein in Schizophrenia." *Biological Psychiatry* 3 (1971): 113–121.

Frohman, C.E., Latham, K.L., Beckett, P.G.S., and Gottlieb, J.S. "Evidence of a Plasma Factor in Schizophrenia." *Archives of General Psychiatry* 2 (1960): 255–262.

Funkenstein, D.H. "Psychophysiologic Relationship of Asthma and Urticaria to Mental Illness." *Journal of Nervous and Mental Disease* 12 (1950): 377–385.

Fuyita, D., Ito, T., Maruta, K., Teradaira, R., Beppu, H., Nakagama, Y., Kato, Y., Nagatsu, T., and Kato, T. "Serum Dopamine-B-Hydroxylase in Schizophrenic Patients." *Journal of Neurochemistry* 30 (1978): 1569–1572.

Galadburda, A., LeMay, M., Kemper, T., and Geschwind, N. "Right-Left Asymmetries in the Brain." *Science* 199 (1978): 852–856.

Gershon, S., Hekimian, L.J., Floyd, A. Jr., and Hollister, L.E. "Alpha-Methyl-P-Tyrosine (AMPT) in Schizophrenia." *Psychopharmacologia* 11 (1967): 189–194.

Gerson, S.C., and Baldessarini, R.J. "Motor Effects of Serotonin in the Central Nervous System." *Life Sciences* 27 (1980): 1435–1451.

Gillin, J.C., Stoff, D.M., and Wyatt, R.J. "Transmethylation Hypothesis: A Review of Progress." In *Psychopharmacology: A Generation of Progress,* edited by M.A. Lipton, A. DiMascio, and K.F. Killam. New York: Raven Press, 1978.

Golden, C., Graber, B., Coffman, J., Berg, R., Bloch, S., and Brogam, D. "Brain Density Deficits in Chronic Schizophrenia." *Psychiatry Research* 3 (1980): 179–184.

Gove, P.B. *Webster's Third New International Dictionary of the English Language Unabridged.* Springfield, Mass.: G. & C. Merriam Company, 1978.

Gowdy, J.M. "Immunoglobulin Levels in Psychotic Patients." *Psychosomatics* 21 (1980): 751–756.

Gregg, D. "The Paucity of Arthritis Among Psychotic Cases." *American Journal of Psychiatry* 95 (1939): 853–858.

Green, R.A., and Grahame-Smith, D.G. "Effects of Drugs on the Processes Regulating the Functional Activity of Brain 5-Hydroxytryptamine." *Nature* 260 (1976): 487–491.

Griffith, J.D., Cavanaugh, J.H., and Oates, J.A. "Psychosis Induced by the Administration of d-Amphetamine to Human Volunteers." In *Psychotomimetic Drugs,* edited by D.H. Efron. New York: Raven Press, 1970.

Groshong, R., Baldessarini, R.J., Gibson, A., Lipinski, J.F., Axelrod, D., and Pope, A. "Activities of Types A and B MAO and Catechol-O-Methyltransferase in Blood Cells and Skin Fibroblasts of Normal and Chronic Schizophrenic Subjects." *Archives of General Psychiatry* 35 (1978): 1198–1205.

Gunne, L.M., Lindstrom, L., And Terenius, L. "Naloxone-Induced Reversal of Schizophrenic Hallucinations." *Journal of Neural Transmission* 40 (1977): 13–19.

Haase, A.T., Ventura, P., Gibbs, C.J., Jr., and Tortellotte, W.W. "Measles Virus Nucleotide Sequences: Defection by Hybridization *In Situ.*" *Science* 212 (1981): 672–675.

Haefely, W.E. "Central Actions of Benzodiazepines: General Introduction." *British Journal of Psychiatry* 133 (1978): 231–238.

Haier, R.J., Buchsbaum, M.S., Murphy, D.L., Gottesman, I.I., and Coursey, R.D. "Psychiatric Vulnerability, Monoamine Oxidase, and the Average Evoked Potential." *Archives of General Psychiatry* 37 (1980): 340–345.

Halonen, P., Rimon, R., Arohonka, K., and Jantti, V. "Antibody Levels to Herpes Simplex Type I, Measles and Rubella Viruses in Psychiatric Patients." *British Journal of Psychiatry* 125 (1974): 461–465.

Hartmann, E. and Keller-Teschke, M. "The Psychological Effects of Dopamine-Beta-Hydroxylase Inhibition in Normal Subjects." *Biological Psychiatry* 14 (1979): 455–462.

Heath, R.G., Guschwan, A.F., and Coffey, J.W. "Relation of Taraxein to Schizophrenia." *Diseases of the Nervous System* 31 (1970): 391–395.

Heath, R.G., and Krupp, I.M. "Schizophrenia as an Immunologic Disorder: Demonstration of Antibrain Globulins by Fluorescent Antibody Techniques." *Archives of General Psychiatry* 16 (1967b): 1–9.

Heath, R.G., and Krupp, I.M. "The Biologic Basis of Schizophrenia: An Autoimmune Concept." In *The Molecular Basis of Some Aspects of Mental Activity.* New York: Academic Press, 1967a.

Heath, R.G., Martens, S., Leach, B.E., Cohen, M., and Angel, C. "Effect on Behavior in Humans with the Administration of Taraxein." *American Journal of Psychiatry* 114 (1957): 14–24.

Hier, D., LeMay, M., and Rosenberger, P. "Autism Associated with Reversed Cerebral Asymmetry." *Neurology* 28 (1978a): 348–349.

Hier, D., LeMay, M., Rosenberger, P., and Perlo, V. "Developmental Dyslexia: Evidence for a Subgroup with a Reversal of Cerebral Asymmetry." *Archives of Neurology* 35 (1978b): 90–92.

Hirschowitz, J., and Garver, D.L. "Postsynaptic Sensitivity, Lithium and the Schizophrenias." *Proceedings of the 134th American Psychiatric Association Meeting.* New Orleans, May 1981.

Hoffer, O., Osmond, H., and Callbeck, M.J. "Treatment of Schizophrenia with Nicotinic Acid and Nicotinamide." *Journal of Clinical and Experimental Psychopathology* 18 (1957): 131–158.

Horrobin, D. "Prostaglandins and Schizophrenia." *Lancet* I (1980): 706–707.

Hughes, J. "Isolation of an Endogenous Compound from the Brain with Pharmacological Properties Similar to Morphine." *Brain Research* 88 (1975): 295–308.

Jankovic, B.D., Jakulic, S., and Horvat, J. "Cell-Mediated Immunity and Psychiatric Diseases." *Periodic Biology* 81 (1979): 219–220.

Janowsky, D., and Davies, J. "Methylphenidate, Dextroamphetamine and Levamphetamine Effects on Schizophrenic Symptoms." *Archives of General Psychiatry* 33 (1976): 304–308.

Japelli, G., and Scafa, G.M. "Sur Les Effects Des Injections Intra-veineuses D'Estrait Prostatique De Chiem." *Arch It Al Biology* 45 (1906): 165–172.

Jeste, D.V., Doongaji, D.R., Sheth, A.S., Apte, J.S., Potkin, S.G., Karoum, F., Panjwani, D., Datta, M., Thatte, R., and Wyatt, R.J. "Paranoid Schizophrenia: Cross-Cultural Test of a Biochemical Hypothesis." *British Journal of Psychiatry,* in press.

Jeste, D.V., Kleinman, J.E., Potkin, S.G., Luchins, D., and Weinberger, D.R. *"Ex Uno Multi:* Subtyping the Schizophrenic Syndrome." *Biological Psychiatry,* in press.

Jeste, D.V., and Wyatt, R.J. "Changing Epidemiology of Tardive Dyskinesia: An Overview." *American Journal of Psychiatry* 138 (1981): 297–309.

Jeste, D.V., and Wyatt, R.J. *Understanding and Treating Tardive Dyskinesia.* New York: Guilford Press, in press.

Johnson, K.M. "Neurochemical Pharmacology of Phencyclidine." In *Phencyclidine Abuse: An Appraisal.* National Institute of Drug Abuse Research Monograph 21, DHEW Publication No. (78–728). Washington, D.C.: U.S. Government Printing Office, 1978.

Johnstone, E.C., and Whaley, K. "Antinuclear Antibodies in Psychiatric Illness: Their Relationship to Diagnosis and Drug Treatment." *British Medical Journal* 2 (1975): 724–725.

Johnstone, E.C., Crow, T.J., Frith, C.D., Stevens, M., Keel, L., and Husband, J. "The Dementia of Dementia Praecox." *Acta Psychiatrica Scandinavica* 57 (1978): 305–324.

Johnstone, E.C., Crow, T.J., and Mashiter, K. "Anterior Pituitary Hormone Secretion in Chronic Schizophrenia—An Approach to Neurohumoral Mechanisms." *Psychological Medicine* 7 (1977): 223–228.

Kafka, M.S., van Kammen, D.B., Kleinman, J.E., Nirenberger, J.I., Siever, L.J., Uhde, T.W., and Polinsky, R.J. "Alpha Adrenergic Receptor Function in Schizophrenia, Affective Disorders and Some Neurological Disease." *Communications in Psychopharmacology* in press.

Kamp, Van H. "Nuclear Changes in the White Blood Cells of Patients with Schizophrenic Reactions." *Journal of Neuropsychiatry* 4 (1962): 1–3.

Karoum, F., Nasrallah, H., Potkin, S.G., Chuang, L.W., Moyer-Schwing, J., Phillips, I., and Wyatt, R.J. "Mass Fragmentography of Phenylethylamine, m- and p-Tyramine and Related Amines in Plasma, Cerebrospinal Fluid, Urine, and Brain." *Journal of Neurochemistry* 33 (1979): 201–212.

Kasanin, J. "The Acute Schizoaffective Psychoses." *American Journal of Psychiatry* 123 (1933): 90–97.

Kerbikov, O.V. "Immunologic Reactivity in Schizophrenia as Influenced by Some Modern Drugs." *Annals of the New York Academy of Sciences* 92 (1961): 1098.

Kinney, D., and Jacobsen, B. "Environmental Factors in Schizophrenia: New Adoption Study Evidence." In *The Nature of Schizophrenia,* edited by L.C. Wynne, R.L. Cromwell, and S. Matthysse. New York: John Wiley and Sons, 1978.

Klee, W.A., Ziovdrov, C., and Streaty, R.A. "Exorphins: Peptides With Opioid Activity Isolated from Wheat Gluten and Their Possible Role in the Etiology of Schizophrenia." In *Endorphins in Mental Health Research,* edited by E. Usdin, W.E. Bunney, and N.S. Kline. New York: Oxford U. Press, 1979.

Kleinman, J.E., Karoum, F., Rosenblatt, J.E., Gillin, J.C., Hong, J., Bridge, T.P., Zalcman, S., Storch, F., del Carmen, R., and Wyatt, R.J. "Postmortem Neurochemical Studies in Chronic Schizophrenia." In *Biological Markers in Psychiatry and Neurology,* edited by I. Hanin, and E. Usdin. Oxford: Pergamon Press, in press.

Kleinman, J.E., Weinberger, D.R., Rogol, A.O., Bigelow, L.B., Klein, S.T., Gillin, J.C., and Wyatt, R.J. "Relationships Between Plasma Prolactin Concentrations and Psychopathology in Chronic

Schizophrenia." *Archives of General Psychiatry*, submitted.

Kline, N.S., Li, C.H., Lehmann, H.E., Lajtha, A., Laski, E., and Cooper, T. "B-Endorphin-Induced Changes in Schizophrenic and Depressed Patients." *Archives of General Psychiatry* 34 (1977): 1111–1113.

Koliaskina, G., Kushner, S., and Gaskin, L. "Certain Immunological Changes in Schizophrenic Patients." In *Biological Research in Schizophrenia*, edited by D. Lozovskii. Russia: 1967.

Koliaskina, G., Tsutsulkovskaya, M., Domashneva, I., Mazina, T., Kielholz, P., Gastpar, M., Bunney, W., Rafaelsen, O., Heltberg, J., Coppen, A., Hippus, H., Koecherl, B., and Vartanian, F. "Antithymic Immune Factor in Schizophrenia. A World Health Organization Study." *Neuropsychobiology* 6 (1980): 349–355.

Kraepelin, E. *Dementia Praecox and Paraphrenia*. New York: Robert E. Krieger Publishing Company, Inc., 1971.

Lake, R.C., Sternberg, D.E., van Kammen, D.P., Ballenger, J.C., Ziegler, M.G., Post, R.M., Kopin, I.J., and Bunney, W.E., "Schizophrenia: Elevated Cerebrospinal Fluid Norepinephrine." *Science* 207 (1980): 331–333.

Laughren, T.P., Brown, W.A., and Williams, B.W. "Serum Prolactin and Clinical State During Neuroleptic Treatment and Withdrawal." *American Journal of Psychiatry* 136 (1979): 108–110.

LeMay, M. "Morphological Cerebral Asymmetries of Modern Man, Fossil Man, and Nonhuman Primates." *Annals of the New York Academy of Science* 280 (1976): 349–366.

Lerner, P., Goodwin, F.K., van Kammen, D.P., Post,R.M., Major, L.F., Ballenger, J.C., and Lovenberg, W.C. "Dopamine-Beta-Hydroxylase in Cerebrospinal Fluid of Psychiatric Patients." *Biological Psychiatry* 13 (1978): 685–694.

Libíková, H., Pogády, J., Kutinova, L., Breir, S., and Matis, J. "Early and Delayed Skin Reactivity to Soluble Antigens of Herpes Virus Hominus I in Psychiatric Patients and Guinea Pigs." *Acta Virology* 24 (1980): 279–290.

Liedeman, R.R., and Prilipko, L.L. "The Behavior of T Lymphocytes in Schizophrenia." *Birth Defects* 14 (1978): 365–377.

Lishman, W.A., and McMeekan, E.R.L. "Hand Preference Patterns in Psychiatric Patients." *British Journal of Psychiatry* 129 (1976): 158–166.

Lovett, L.C., Virich, T.J., Simms, B.G., and Goldstein, A.L. "Effects of Chlorpromazine on Antibody Production *In Vitro.*" In *Neurochemical and Immunologic Components in Schizophrenia*, edited by D. Bergsma and A. Goldstein. New York: A.R. Liss, Inc., 1978.

Luchins, D.J., Freed, W.J., Potkin, S.G., Rosenblatt, J.E., Gillin, J.C., and Wyatt, R.J. "Wheat Gluten and Haloperidol." *Biological Psychiatry* 15 (1980a): 819–820.

Luchins, D.J., Pollin, W., and Wyatt, R.J. "Laterality in Monozygotic Schizophrenic Twins: An Alternative Hypothesis." *Biological Psychiatry* 15 (1980b): 87–93.

Luchins, D.J., Weinberger, D.R., Torrey, E.F., Johnson, A., Rogentine, N., and Wyatt, R.J. "HLA-A2 Antigen in Schizophrenic Patients With Reversed Cerebral Asymmetry." *British Journal of Psychiatry* 138 (1981a): 240–243.

Luchins, D.J., Weinberger, D.R., and Wyatt, R.J. "Reversed Cerebral Asymmetry in Schizophrenia." *American Psychiatric Association, 134th Annual Convention*, New Orleans, May 1981b.

Luchins, D.J., Weinberger, D.R., and Wyatt, R.J. "Schizophrenia: Evidence of a Subgroup With Reversed Cerebral Asymmetry." *Archives of General Psychiatry* 36 (1979): 1309–1311.

Luisada, P.V. "The Phencyclidine Psychosis: Phenomenology and Treatment." National Institute of Drug Abuse Research Monograph 21. DHEW Publication No. (78–728). Washington, D.C.: U.S. Government Printing Office, 1978.

Maas, J.W., Glesser, G.C., and Gottschalk, L.A. "Schizophrenia, Anxiety and Biochemical Factors." *Archives of General Psychiatry* 4 (1961): 109–118.

Mackay, A.V., Bird, E., Spokes, E.G., Rossor, M., Iversen, L., Creese, I., and Snyder, S.H., "Dopamine Receptors and Schizophrenia: Drug Effect or Illness?" *Lancet* ii (1980): 915–916.

Markianos, E.S., Nystrom, I., Reichel, H., and Matusek, N. "Serum Dopamine-Beta-Hydroxylase in Psychiatric Patients and Normals. Effects of D-Amphetamine and Haloperidol." *Psychopharmacology* 50 (1976): 259–267.

Mathé, A.A., Sedvall, G., Weisel, F.A., and Nyback, H. "Increased Content of Immunoreactive Prostaglandin E in Cerebrospinal Fluid of Patients with Schizophrenia." *Lancet* 1 (1980): 16–18.

Mathew, R., Meyer, J., Francis, D., Schoolar, J., Weinman, M. and Mortel, K. "Regional Cerebral Blood Flow in Schizophrenia: A Preliminary Report." *American Journal of Psychiatry* 138 (1981): 112–113.

Matthysse, S. "Dopamine and the Pharmacology of Schizophrenia: The State of the Evidence." *Journal of Psychiatric Research* 11 (1974): 107–113.

Matthysse, S., Baldessarini, R.J. "S-Adenosylmethionine and Catechol-O-Methyltransferase in Schizophrenia." *American Journal of Psychiatry* 128 (1972): 1310–1312.

McGrath, S.D., O'Brien, P.F., Power, P.J., and Shea, J.R. "Nicotinamide Treatment of Schizophrenia." *Schizophrenia Bulletin* 5 (1972): 74–76.

McGreer, E.G., and McGreer, P.L. "GABA-Containing Neurons in Schizophrenia, Huntington's Chorea and Normal Aging." In *GABA-Neurotransmitters*, edited by P. Korsgarrd-Larsen, J. Scheel-Krüger, H. Kofod. New York: Academic Press, 1979.

McGuffin, P. "What Have Transplant Antigens Got to do with Psychosis?" *British Journal of Psychiatry* 136 (1980): 510–512.

Meltzer, H.Y. "Biochemical Studies in Schizophrenia." In *Disorders of the Schizophrenia Syndrome*, edited by L. Bellak. New York: Basic Books, 1979b.

Meltzer, H.Y. "Biology of Schizophrenic Subtypes: A Review and Proposal for Method of Study." *Schizophrenia Bulletin* 5 (1979a): 460–479.

Meltzer, H.Y. "Clinical Evidence for Multiple Dopamine Receptors in Man." *Communications in Psychopharmacology* 3 (1979c): 457–470.

Meltzer, H.Y., and Fang, V.S. "The Effect of Neuroleptics on Serum Prolactin in ·Schizophrenic Patients." *Archives of General Psychiatry* 33 (1976): 279–286.

Meltzer, H.Y., Nask, S.J., and Tong, C. "Serum Dopamine-B-Hydroxylase Activity in Schizophrenia." *Biological Psychiatry* 15 (1980): 781–788.

Meltzer, H.Y. "Relevance of Dopamine Autoreceptors for Psychiatry: Preclinical and Clinical Studies. *Schizophrenia Bulletin* 6 (1980): 456–475.

Meltzer, H.Y., Sachar, E., and Frantz, A.G. "Serum Prolactin Levels in Unmedicated Schizophrenic Patients." *Archives of General Psychiatry* 31 (1974): 564–569.

Meltzer, H.Y., Shader, R., and Grinspoon, L. "The Behavioral Effects of Nicotinamide Adenine Dinucleotide in Chronic Schizophrenia." *Psychopharmacologia* (Berl) 15 (1969): 144–152.

Meyer, R.E. "Behavioral Pharmacology of Marihuana." In *Psychopharmacology: A Generation of Progress,* edited by M.A. Lipton, A. DiMascio, and K.F. Killam. New York: Raven Press, 1978.

Milner, G. "Ascorbic Acid in Chronic Psychiatric Patients: A Controlled Trial." *British Journal of Psychiatry* 109 (1963): 294–299.

Moja, E.A., Stoff, D.M., Gillin, J.C., and Wyatt, R.J. "Neuroleptics Attenuate Stereotyped Behavior Induced by Beta-Phenylethylamine in Rats." *Biological Psychiatry* 13 (1978): 291–295.

Molholm, H.B. "Hyposensitivity to Foreign Protein in Schizophrenic Patients." *Psychiatric Quarterly* 16 (1942): 565–571.

Murphy, D.L., and Kalin, N.H. "Biological and Behavioral Consequences of Alterations in Monoamine Oxidase Activity." *Schizophrenia Bulletin* 6 (1980): 355–367.

Murphy, D.L., and Wyatt, R.J. "Reduced Platelet Monoamine Oxidase Activity in Chronic Schizophrenia." *Nature* 238 (1972): 225–226.

Murphy, H.B.M., and Raman, A.C. "The Chronicity of Schizophrenia in Indigenous Tropical Peoples." *British Journal of Psychiatry* 118 (1971): 489–497.

Naber, D., Finkbeiner, C., Fischer, H., Zander, K.J., and Ackenheil, M. "Effect of Long-Term Neuroleptic Treatment of Prolactin and Norepinephrine Levels in Serum of Chronic Schizophrenics: Relations to Psychopathology and Extrapyramidal Symptoms." *Psychoneurobiology,* in press.

Naeser, M., Levine, H., Benson, F., Stuss, D., and Weir, W. "Frontal Leukotomy Size and Hemispheric Asymmetries on Computerized Tomographic Scans of Schizophrenics with Variable Recovery." *Archives of Neurology* 38 (1981): 30–37.

Nasrallah, H., Donnelly, E.F., Bigelow, L.B., Rivera-Calimlim, L., Rogol, A., Potkin, S.G., Rauscher, F.P., Wyatt, R.J. and Gillin, J.C. "Inhibition of Dopamine Synthesis in Chronic Schizophrenia." *Archives of General Psychiatry* 34 (1977): 649–655.

Nasrallah, H., Kleinman, J.E., Weinberger, D.R., Gillin, J.C. and Wyatt, R.J. "Cerebral Ventricular Enlargement and Dopamine Synthesis Inhibition in Chronic Schizophrenia." *Archives of General Psychiatry* 37 (1980): 1427.

Nies, A., Robinson, D.S., Harris, L.S., and Lamborn, K.R. "Comparison of Monoamine Oxidase Substrate Preference in Twins, Schizophrenics, Depressives, and Controls." *Advances in Biochemical Psychopharmacology* 12 (1974): 159–170.

Nyland, H., Naess, A., and Lunde, H. "Lymphocyte Subpopulations in Peripheral Blood from Schizophrenic Patients." *Acta Psychiatrica Scandinavica* 61 (1980): 313–318.

Osmond, H., and Hoffer, A. "Massive Niacin Treatment in Schizophrenia: Review of a Nine-Year Study." *Lancet* 1 (1962): 316–319.

Osmond, H., and Smythies, J. "Schizophrenia: A New Approach." *Journal of Mental Sciences* 98 (1952): 309–315.

Palmour, R.M., Ervin, F.R., Wagemaker, H., and Cade, R. "Characterization of a Peptide Derived from the Serum of Psychiatric Patients." *Annual Meeting Soc. Neurocir.* (Abst.), 1977.

Pandey, G.N., Garver, D.L., Tamminga, C., Ericksen, S., Ali, S., and Davis, J.M. "Postsynaptic Supersensitivity in Schizophrenia." *American Journal of Psychiatry* 134 (1977): 518–521.

Pauling, L. "Orthomolecular Psychiatry." *Science* 160 (1968): 216–271.

Pauling, L., Robinson, A.B., and Oxley, S.S. "Results of a Loading Test of Ascorbic Acid, Niacinamide and Pyridoxine in Schizophrenic Subjects and Controls." In *Orthomolecular Psychiatry: Treatment of Schizophrenia,* edited by D. Hawkins, and L. Pauling. San Francisco: W.H. Freeman and Company, 1973.

Pfeiffer, C.C., and Braverman, E. "Folic Acid and Vitamin B_{12} Therapy of Low Histamine High Copper Biotype of Schizophrenia." In *Folic Acid in Neurology, Psychiatry, and Internal Medicine,* edited by M.I. Botez, and E.H. Reynolds. New York: Raven Press, 1979.

Pfeiffer, C.C., Iliev, V., and Goldstein, L. "Blood Histamine, Basophil Counts, and Trace Elements in the Schizophrenias." In *Orthomolecular Psychiatry: Treatment of Schizophrenia,* edited by D. Hawkins, and L. Pauling. San Francisco: W.H. Freeman and Company, 1973.

Pope, H.G., Lapinski, J.F., Cohen, B.M., and Axelrod, D.T. "Schizoaffective Disorder: An Invalid Diagnosis? A Comparison of Schizoaffective Disorder, Schizophrenia, and Affective Disorder." *American Journal of Psychiatry* 137 (1980) 921–927.

Potkin, S.G., Cannon, E.H., Murphy, D.L. and Wyatt, R.J. "Are Paranoid Schizophrenics Biologically Different from Other Schizophrenics?" *New England Journal of Medicine* 29 (1978): 61–66.

Potkin, S., Karoum, F., Chuang, L.W., Cannon-Spoor E., Philips, I., and Wyatt, R.J. "Phenylethylamine in Paranoid Chronic Schizophrenia." *Science* 200 (1979):470–471.

Potkin, S., Weinberger, D.R., Nasrallah, H.A., Luchins, D.J., Kleinman, J.E., Bigelow, L.B., Linnoila, M., Bjornsson, T.D., Carman, J.S., Gillin, J.C., and Wyatt R.J. "Wheat Gluten Challenge in Schizophrenic Patients." *American Journal of Psychiatry* in press.

Pulkkinen, E. "Immunoglobulins, Psychopathology and Prognosis in Schizophrenia." *Acta Psychiatrica Scandinavica* 56 (1977): 173–182.

Randrup, A., and Munkvad, I. "Stereotyped Activities Produced by Amphetamine in Several Animal Species and Man." *Psychopharmacologia* 1 (1967): 300–310.

Raskin, D., and Frank, S. "Herpes Encephalitis with Catatonic Stupor." *Archives of General Psychiatry* 31 (1974): 544–546.

Reisine, T.D., Rossor, M.M., Spokes, E., Iversen, L.L. and Yamamura, H.I. "Opiate and Neuroleptic Receptor Alterations in Human Schizophrenic Brain Tissue." In *Receptors for Neurotransmitters and Peptides Hormones*, edited by G. Pepen, M.J. Kuha, and S.J. Enna. New York: Raven Press, 1980.

Reynolds, G.P., Reynolds, L.M., Reideren, P., Jellinga, K., and Gabrill, E. "Dopamine Receptors and Schizophrenia: Drug Effect or Illness?" *Lancet* ii (1980): 1281.

Rice, J.R., Ham, C.H., and Gore, W.E. "Another Look at Gluten in Schizophrenia." *American Journal of Psychiatry* 135 (1978): 1417–1418.

Rimon, R., Halonen, P., Puhakka, P., Laitinen, L., Marttila, R., and Salmela, L. "Immunoglobulin G Antibodies to Herpes Simplex Type I Virus Detected by Radioimmunoassay in Serum and Cerebrospinal Fluid of Patients with Schizophrenia." *Journal of Clinical Psychiatry* 40 (1979): 241–243.

Robert, E. "An Hypothesis Suggesting That There is a Defect in the GABA System in Schizophrenia." *Neurosciences Research Program Bulletin* 10 (1972): 468–481.

Rosenberger, P., and Hier, D. "Cerebral Asymmetry and Verbal Intellectual Deficits." *Annals of Neurology* 8 (1980): 300–304.

Ross-Stanton, J., and Meltzer, H.Y. "Motor Neuron Branching Patterns in Psychotic Patients." *Archives of General Psychiatry*, in press.

Rotrosen, J., Angrist, B.M., Gershon, S., Sachar, E.J., and Halpen, F. "Dopamine Receptor Alteration in Schizophrenia: Neuroendocrine Evidence." *Psychopharmacology* 51 (1976): 1–17.

Rotrosen, J., Angrist, B.M., and Paquin, J. "Neuroendocrine Studies with Dopamine Agonist in Schizophrenia." *Psychopharmacology Bulletin* 14 (1978): 14–17.

Sandler, M., and Reynolds, G.P. "Does Phenylethylamine Cause Schizophrenia?" *Lancet* 1 (1976): 70–71.

Saunders, J.C., and Muchmore, E. "Phenothiazine Effect on Human Antibody Synthesis." *British Journal of Psychiatry* 110 (1964): 84.

Schiavone, D.J., and Kaldor, J. "Phosphokinase Levels and Cerebral Disease." *Medical Journal of Australia* 2 (1965): 790–792.

Schulz, C.S., van Kammen, D.P., Balow, J.E., Flye, M.W., and Bunney, W.E., Jr. "Dialysis in Schizophrenia: A Double-Blind Evaluation." *Science* 211 (1981): 1066–1068.

Schweitzer, J.W., Friedhoff, A.J., and Schwartz, R. "Phenylethylamine in Normal Urine: Failure to Verify High Values." *Biological Psychiatry* 10 (1975): 277–285.

Seeman, P.P., Chau-Wang, M., Tederco, J., and Wong, K. "Brain Receptors for Antipsychotic Drugs and Dopamine: Direct Binding Assays." *Proceedings of the National Academy of Science*, 1975, 4376–4380.

Singh, M.M., and Kay, S.R. "Wheat Gluten as a Pathogenic Factor in Schizophrenia." *Science* 191 (1976): 401–402.

Skirboll, L.R., Grace, A.A., and Bunney, B.S. "Dopamine Auto and Postsynaptic Receptors: Electrophysiological Evidence for Differential Sensitivity to Dopamine Agonists." *Science* 206 (1979): 80–82.

Smith, D.E. "A Clinical Approach to the Treatment of Phencyclidine (PCP) Abuse." *Psychopharmacology Bulletin* 16 (1980): 67–70.

Smith, J.M., and Baldessarini, R.J. "Changes in Prevalence, Severity, and Recovery in Tardive Dyskinesia With Age." *Archives of General Psychiatry* 37 (1980): 1368–1373.

Smith, R.C., Tamminga, C.A., and David J.M. "Effect of Apomorphine on Schizophrenic Symptoms." *Journal of Neural Transmission* 40 (1977): 171–176.

Smythies, J.R. "Recent Progress in Schizophrenia Research." *Lancet* 2 (1976): 136–139.

Solomon, G.F., Allansmith, M., McClellar, B., and Amkraut, A. "Immunoglobulins in Psychiatric Patients." *Archives of General Psychiatry* 20 (1969): 272–277.

Solomon, G.F., Rubbo, S.D., and Batchelder, E. "Secondary Immune Response to Tetanus Toxoid in Psychiatric Patients." *Journal of Psychiatric Research* 7 (1970): 201.

Stevens, J. "Neuropathic Findings in Schizophrenia." *Society of Biological Psychiatry*, New Orleans, 1981.

Strahilevitz, M., Fleishman, J., Fischer, G., Harris, R., and Narasimhachari, N. "Immunoglobulin Levels in Psychiatric Patients." *American Journal of Psychiatry* 133 (1976): 772–777.

Suzuki, S., and Yagi, K. "Fluorometric Assay for B-Phenylethylamine in Human Urine." *Clinica Chimica Acta* 78 (1977): 401–410.

Tamminga, C.A., Crayton, J.W., and Chase, T.N. "Muscimol: GABA Agonist Therapy in Schizophrenia." *American Journal of Psychiatry* 135 (1978): 746–747.

Tamminga, C.A., Smith, R.C.,, Randey, G., Froham, L.A., and Davis, J.M. "A Neuroendocrine Study of Supersensitivity in Tardive Dyskinesia." *Archives of General Psychiatry* 34 (1977): 1199–1203.

Tamminga, C.A., Tighe, P.J., Chase, T.N., DeFraites, G.E., and Schaffer, M.H. "Des-tyrosine-gamma-endorphine Administration in Chronic Schizophrenics." *Archives of General Psychiatry* 38 (1981): 167–168.

Torrey, E.F. *Civilization and Schizophrenia*. New York: Jason Aronson, 1980.

Torrey, E.F., and Peterson, M. "The Viral Hypothesis of Schizophrenia." *Schizophrenia Bulletin* 2 (1976): 136–146.

Torrey, E.F., Peterson, M.R., Brannon, W.L., Carpenter, W.T., Post, R.M., and van Kammen, D.P. "Immunoglobulins and Viral Antibodies in Psychiatric Patients." *British Journal of Psychiatry* 132 (1978): 342–348.

Torrey, E.F., Torrey, B., and Peterson, M. "Seasonality of Schizophrenic Births in the United States." *Archives of General Psychiatry* 34 (1977): 1065–1070.

Tyrer, S.P., Delves, H. T., and Malcolm, P.I. "CSF Copper in Schizophrenia." *American Journal of Psychiatry* 136 (1979): 937–939.

Tyrrell, D.A.J., Parry, R.P., Crow, T.J., Johnstone, E., and Ferrier, I.N. "Possible Virus in Schizophrenia and Some Neurological Disorders." *Lancet* 1 (1979): 839–841.

van Kammen, D.P. "The Dopamine Hypothesis of Schizophrenia Revised." *Psychoneuroendocrinology* 4 (1979): 37–46.

Vartanian, M.E., Koliaskina, G.I., Lozovsky,D.V., Burbaeva, G.S., and Ignator, S.A. "Aspects of Humoral and Cellular Immunity in Schizophrenia." *Birth Defect* 14 (1978): 339–364.

Vaughn, W.T., Sullivan, J.C., and Elmadjan, F. "Immunity of Schizophrenia: Survey of the Ability of Schizophrenic Patients to Develop Active Immunity Following Injection of Pertussis Vaccine." *Psychosomatic Medicine* 11 (1949): 328–332.

Verhoeven, W.M.A., van Praag, H.M., van Ree, J.M., and de Vied, D. "Improvement of Schizophrenic Patients Treated with (des-Tyrl)- gamma-endorphin (DT-gamma-E)." *Archives of General Psychiatry* 36 (1979): 294–298.

Vincent, J.P., Kartalovski, B., Geneste, P., Kamenka, J.M., and Lazduski, M. "Interaction of Phencyclidine ('Angel Dust') With a Specific Receptor in Rat Brain Membranes." *Proceedings of the National Academy of Science* 76 (1979): 4678–4682.

Weinberger, D.R., Bigelow, L.B., Kleinman, J.E., Klein, S.T., Rosenblatt, J.E., and Wyatt, R.J. "Cerebral Ventricular Enlargement in Chronic Schizophrenia: An Association With Poor Response to Treatment." *Archives of General Psychiatry* 37 (1980a): 11–13.

Weinberger, D.R., Cannon-Spoor, E., Potkin, S.G., and Wyatt, R.J. "Poor Premorbid Adjustment and CT Scan Abnormalities in Chronic Schizophrenia." *American Journal of Psychiatry* 137 (1980b): 1410–1413.

Weinberger, D.R., and Wyatt, R.J. "Cerebral Morphology in Schizophrenia: *In Vivo* Studies." In *Schizophrenia As A Brain Disease*, edited by F. Henn, and H. Nasrallah. New York: Oxford University Press, in press[a].

Weinberger, D.R., and Wyatt, R.J. "Cerebral Ventricular Size: A Biological Marker for Subtyping Chronic Schizophrenia." In *Biological Markers in Psychiatry and Neurology*, edited by P.I. Hanin and E. Usdin. New York: Pergamon Press, in press[b].

Weinshilboum, R.M., Schrott, H.G., Raymond, F.A., Weidman, W.H., and Elveback, C.R. "Inheritance of Very Low Serum Dopamine-Beta-Hydroxylase Activity." *American Journal of Human Genetics* 27 (1975): 573–585.

Wertheimer, N.M. "Rheumatic Schizophrenia." *Archives of General Psychiatry* 4 (1961): 579–596.

Wexler, B. "Cerebral Laterality and Psychiatry: A Review of the Literature." *American Journal of Psychiatry* 137 (1980): 279–291.

Whitaker, P.M., Crow, T.J., and Ferrier, I.N. "Tritiated LSD Binding in Frontal Cortex in Schizophrenia." *Archives of General Psychiatry* 38 (1981): 278–280.

Wise, C.D., Baden, M.M., and Strin, L. "Post Mortem Measurement of Enzymes in Human Brain: Evidence of a Central Noradrenergic Deficit in Schizophrenia." *Journal of Psychiatric Research* 11 (1974): 185–198.

Wise, C.D., Stein, L. "Dopamine-B-hydroxylase Deficits in the Brains of Schizophrenic Patients." *Science* 181 (1973): 344–347.

Wyatt, R.J. "Biochemistry and Schizophrenia: (Part IV) The Neuroleptics—Their Mechanism of Action: A Review of the Biochemical Literature." *Psychopharmacology Bulletin* 12 (1976): 5–50.

Wyatt, R.J. "A Comment to Linus Pauling's Megavitamin and Orthomolecular Therapy in Psychiatry." *American Journal of Psychiatry* 131 (1974): 1258–1262.

Wyatt, R.J., Gillin, J.C., Stoff, D.M., Moja, E.A., and Tinklenberg, J.H. "B-Phenylethylamine (PEA) and the Neuropsychiatric Disturbances." In *Neuroregulators and Psychiatric Disorders*, edited by E. Usdin, J. Barchas, and D. Hamburg. New York: Oxford University Press, 1977.

Wyatt, R.J., Karoum, F., Stoff, D.M., Weinberger, D.R., Luchins, D.J., and Jeste, D.V. "Monoamine Oxidase, Phenylethylamine, Norepinephrine, and Schizophrenia." *Clinical Genetics,* in press.

Wyatt, R.J., Murphy, D.L., Belmaker, R., Cohen, S., Donnelly, C.H., and Pollin, W. "Reduced Monoamine Oxidase Activity in Platelets: A Possible Genetic Marker for Vulnerability to Schizophrenia." *Science* 179 (1973): 916–918.

Wyatt, R.J., Potkin, S.G., Bridge, T.P., Phelps, B.H., and Wise, C.D. "Monoamine Oxidase in Schizophrenia: An Overview." *Schizophrenia Bulletin* 6 (1980): 199–207.

Wyatt, R.J., Potkin, S.G., and Murphy, D.L. "Platelet Monoamine Oxidase Activity in Schizophrenia: A Review of the Data." *American Journal of Psychiatry* 136 (1979): 377–385.

Wyatt, R.J., Schwartz, M.D., Erdelyi, E., and Barchas, J.D. "Dopamine-B-Hydroxylase Activity in Brains of Chronic Schizophrenic Patients." *Science* 187 (1975): 368–369.

Wyatt, R.J., Termini, B.A., and Davis, J. "Biochemical and Sleep Studies of Schizophrenia: A Review of the Literature." *Schizophrenia Bulletin* 4 (1971): 10–66.

Yassa, R., and Nair, N.P.V. "Plasma Magnesium in Chronic Schizophrenia." *International Psychopharmacopsychiatry* 14 (1979): 57–64.

Yorkston, N.J., Zaki, S.A., Malik, M.K.U., Morrison, R.C., and Havard, C.W.H. "Propranolol in the Control of Schizophrenia Symptoms." *British Medical Journal* 14 (1974): 633–635.

Zarrabi, M.H., Zucker, S., Miller, F., Derman, R.M., Romano, G.S., Hartnett, J.A., and Varma, A.O. "Immunologic and Coagulation Disorders in Chlorpromazine Treated Patients." *Annals of Internal Medicine* 91 (1979): 194–199.

Zimmer, R., Teelken, A.W., Meier, K.D., Ackenheil, M., and Zander, K.J. "Preliminary Studies of CSF Gamma-Aminobutyric Acid Levels in Psychiatric Patients Before and During Treatment with Different Psychotropic Drugs." *Progress in Neuropsychopharmacology* 4 (1980): 613–620.

Zukin, S.R., and Zukin, S.R. "Specific ^{3}H-Phenycylidine Binding in Rat Central Nervous System." *Proceedings of the National Academy of Science* 76 (1979): 5372–5376.

Bibliography for the Introduction to the Treatment of the Schizophrenic Disorders

Cancro, R. "The Schizophrenic Syndrome: Its Dubious Past and Its Certain Future." *The Hillside Journal of Clinical Psychiatry* 1 (1979): 39–56.

Bibliography for Chapter 13

Anderson, C.M., Hogarty, G.E., and Reiss, D.J. "Family Treatment of Adult Schizophrenic Patients: A Psycho-Educational Approach." *Schizophrenia Bulletin* 6 (1980): 490–505.

Bleuler, M. *The Schizophrenic Disorders: Long-Term Patient and Family Studies,* translated by S.M. Clemens. New Haven: Yale University Press, 1978.

Bookhammer, R.S. "A Five-Year Clinical Follow-Up of Schizophrenics Treated by Rosen's Direct Analysis." *American Journal of Psychiatry* 123 (1966): 602–604.

Bruch, H. "General Discussion." In *The Psychotherapy of Schizophrenia,* edited by J.S. Strauss, M. Bowers, T.W. Downey, S. Fleck, S. Jackson, and I. Levine. New York: Plenum Publishing Corp., 1980a.

Bruch, H. "Psychotherapy in Schizophrenia: Historical Considerations." In *The Psychotherapy of Schizophrenia,* edited by J.S. Strauss, M. Bowers, T.W. Downey, S. Fleck, S. Jackson, and I. Levine. New York: Plenum Publishing Corp., 1980b.

Carpenter, W.T. "Clinical Research Methods Applicable to the Study of Treatment Effects in Chronic Schizophrenic Patients." In *Perspectives in Schizophrenic Research: Presentations and Sessions of the VA Advisory Conference on Chronic Schizophrenia, Harpers Ferry, W.VA., 1979,* edited by C.F. Baxter, and T. Melnechuk. New York: Raven Press, 1980.

Carpenter, W.T., and Heinrichs, D.W. "The Role of Psychodynamic Psychiatry in the Treatment of Schizophrenic Patients." In *The Psychotherapy of Schizophrenia,* edited by J.S. Strauss, M. Bowers, T.W. Downey, S. Fleck, S. Jackson, and I. Levine. New York: Plenum Publishing Corp., 1980.

Carpenter, W.T., Heinrichs, D.W., and Hanlon, T.E. "Methodologic Standards for Treatment Outcome Research in Schizophrenia." *American Journal of Psychiatry* 138 (1981): 465–471.

Chodoff, P., and Carpenter, W.T. "Psychogenic Theories of Schizophrenia." In *Schizophrenia: Biological and Psychological Perspectives,* edited by G. Usdin. New York: Brunner/Mazel, Inc., 1975.

Ciompi, L. "The Natural History of Schizophrenia in the Long Term." *British Journal of Psychiatry* 136 (1980): 413–420.

Engel, G.L. "The Need for a New Medical Model: A Challenge for Biomedicine." *Science* 196 (1977): 129–136.

Engel, G.L. "The Clinical Application of the Biopsychosocial Model." *American Journal of Psychiatry* 137 (1980): 535–544.

Fromm-Reichmann, F. *Principles of Intensive Psychotherapy.* Chicago: University of Chicago Press, 1950.

Goldstein, M.J., and Rodnick, E.H. "The Family's Contribution to the Etiology of Schizophrenia: Current Status," *Schizophrenia Bulletin* 14 (1975): 48–63.

Goldstein, M.J., Rodnick, E.H., Evans, J.R., May, P.R.A., and Stinzberg, M.R. "Drug and Family Therapy in the Aftercare of Acute Schizophrenics." *Archives of General Psychiatry* 35 (1978): 1169–1177.

Grinspoon, L., Ewalt, J.R., and Shader, R.I. *Schizophrenia: Pharmacotherapy and Psychotherapy.* Baltimore: Williams & Wilkins Co., 1972.

Gunderson, J.G., and Mosher, L.R. "Introduction." In *Psychotherapy of Schizophrenia.* New York: Jason Aronson, 1975.

Heinrichs, D.W., and Carpenter, W.T. "The Efficacy of Individual Psychotherapy: A Perspective and Review of Controlled Outcome Studies." In *The American Handbook of Psychiatry, Vol. 7,* edited by S. Arieti. New York: Basic Books, 1981.

Herrington, B.S. "Klerman Weighs Role in Therapy Efficacy Study." *Psychiatric News* 15 (1980): 10.

Hogarty G.E., and Goldberg, S.C. "Drug and Sociotherapy in the Aftercare of Schizophrenic Patients." *Archives of General Psychiatry* 28 (1973): 45–64.

Hogarty, G.E., Goldberg, S.C., Schooler, N.R., Ulrich, R.F. "Drug and Sociotherapy in the Aftercare of Schizophrenic Patients. II. Two-Year Relapse Rates." *Archives of General Psychiatry* 31 (1974a): 603–608.

Hogarty, G.E., Goldberg, S.C., Schoder, N.R., the Collaborative Study Group. "Drug and Sociotherapy in the Aftercare of Schizophrenic Patients. III. Adjustment of Nonrelapsed Patients." *Archives of General Psychiatry* 31 (1974b): 609–618.

Jaspers, K. *General Psychopathology,* translated by J. Hoenig, and M.W. Hamilton. Chicago: University of Chicago Press, 1968.

Karon, B.P., and Vanderbos, G.R. "Experience, Medication and the Effectiveness of Psychotherapy with Schizophrenics: A Note on Drs. May and Tuma's Conclusion." *British Journal of Psychiatry* 116 (1970): 427–428.

Karon, B.P., and Vanderbos, G.R. "The Consequences of Psychotherapy for Schizophrenic Patients." *Psychotherapy: Theory, Research, and Practice* 9 (1972): 111–119.

Klerman, G.L., DiMascio, A., Weissman, M., Prusoff, B., and Paykel, E.S. "Treatment of Depression by Drugs and Psychotherapy." *American Journal of Psychiatry* 131 (1974): 186–191.

Liem, J.H. "Family Studies of Schizophrenia: An Update and Commentary." In *Special Report: Schizophrenia 1980,* National Institute of Mental Health. 82–108.

Marks, J. Sonoda, B., Schalock, R. "Reinforcement Versus Relationship Therapy for Schizophrenics." *Journal of Abnormal Psychology* 73 (1968): 397–402.

May, P.R.A. *Treatment of Schizophrenia.* New York: Science House, 1968.

May, P.R.A., and Tuma, A.H. "Treatment of Schizophrenia: An Experimental Study of Five Treatment Methods." *British Journal of Psychiatry* 111 (1965): 503–510.

May, P.R.A., and Tuma, A.H. "Methodological Problems in Psychotherapy Research: Observations on the Karon-Vandenbos Study of Psychotherapy and Drugs in Schizophrenia." *British Journal of Psychiatry* 117 (1970): 569–570.

May, P.R.A., Tuma, A.H., and Dixon, W. "Schizophrenia—A Follow-Up Study of Results of Treatment." *Archives of General Psychiatry* 33 (1976): 474–478.

May, P.R.A., Tuma, A.H., Yale, C., Potzpan, P., and Dixon, W. "Schizophrenia—A Follow-Up Study of Results of Treatment: II. Hospital Stay Over Two to Five Years." *Archives of General Psychiatry* 33 (1976): 481–486.

Rogers, C.R., Gendlin, E.T., Kiesler, D.J., and Truax, C.R. *The Therapeutic Relationship and Its Impact.* Madison: University of Wisconsin Press, 1967.

Rush, A.J., and Beck, A. "Adults With Affective Disorder." In *Behavior Therapy in the Psychiatric Setting,* edited by M. Hersen. Baltimore: Williams & Wilkins, 1978.

Searles, H.F. *Collected Papers on Schizophrenia and Related Subjects.* New York: International Universities Press, 1965.

Soskis, D.A. "A Survey of Psychiatric Opinion on Schizophrenia." *Comprehensive Psychiatry* 13 (1972): 573–580.

Strauss, J.S., and Carpenter, W.T. *Schizophrenia,* edited by S.M. Woods. New York: Plenum Publishing Corp., 1981.

Weissman, M. "The Psychological Treatment of Depression. Evidence for the Efficacy of Psychotherapy Alone, in Comparison With, and in Combination With Pharmacotherapy." *Archives of General Psychiatry* 36 (1979): 1261–1269.

Weissman, M., Klerman, G.L., Paykel, E.S., Prusoff, B., and Hanson, B. "Treatment Effects on the Social Adjustment of Depressed Patients." *Archives of General Psychiatry* 30 (1974): 771–778.

Weissman, M., Prusoff, B.A., DiMascio, A., Neu, C., Goklaney, M., and Klerman, G.L. "The Efficacy of Drugs and Psychotherapy in the Treatment of Acute Depressive Episodes." *American Journal of Psychiatry* 136 (1979): 555–558.

Will, O.A., Jr. "Schizophrenia and Psychotherapy." In *Modern Psychoanalysis,* edited by J. Marmor. New York: Basic Books, 1968.

Bibliography for Chapter 14

American Psychiatric Association. *Diagnostic and Statistical Manual of Mental Disorders, 3d ed.* Washington, D.C.: American Psychiatric Association 1980.

Anderson, C.M., Hogarty, G.E., and Reiss, D.J. "Family Treatment of Adult Schizophrenic Patients: A Psycho-Educational Approach." *Schizophrenia Bulletin* 6 (1980): 490–505.

Anthony, W.A., Buell, G.J., Sharratt, S., and Althoff, M.E. "The Efficacy of Psychiatric Rehabilitation." *Psychological Bulletin* 78 (1972): 447–456.

Anthony, W.A., Cohen, M.R., and Vitalo, R. "The Measurement of Rehabilitation Outcome." *Schizophrenia Bulletin* 3 (1978): 365–383.

Beard, J.H., Malamud, T.J., and Rossman, E. "Psychiatric Rehabilitation and Long-Term Rehospitalization Rates: The Findings of Two Research Studies." *Schizophrenia Bulletin* 4 (1978): 622–635.

Borowski, T., and Tolwinski, T. "Treatment of Paranoid Schizophrenics With Chlorpromazine and Group Therapy." *Diseases of the Nervous System* 30 (1969): 201–202.

Carpenter, W.T., Jr., Heinrichs, D.W., and Hanlon, T.E. "Methodologic Standards for Treatment Outcome Research in Schizophrenia." *American Journal of Psychiatry* 138 (1981): 465–471.

Claghorn, J.L., Johnstone, E.E., Cook, T.H. and Itschner, L. "Group Therapy and Maintenance Treatment of Schizophrenics." *Archives of General Psychiatry* 31 (1974): 361–365.

Davis, J.M. "Overview: Maintenance Therapy in Psychiatry: I. Schizophrenia." *American Journal of Psychiatry* 132 (1975): 1237–1245.

Davis, J.M., Schaffer, C.B. K., Grant, A., Kinard, C., and Chan, C. "Important Issues in the Drug Treatment of Schizophrenia." *Schizophrenia Bulletin* 6 (1980): 70–87.

Donlon, P.T., Rada, R.T., and Knight, S.W. "A Therapeutic Aftercare Setting for 'Refractory' Chronic Schizophrenic Patients." *American Journal of Psychiatry* 130 (1973): 682–684.

Ellsworth, R.B. "Characteristics of Effective Treatment Settings." In *Psychiatric Milieu and the Therapeutic Environment,* edited by O. Will, J. Gunderson, and L. Mosher. New York: Jason Aronson, Inc., in press.

Ellsworth, R., Maroney, R., Klett, W., Gordon, H., and Gunn, R. "Milieu Characteristics of Successful Psychiatric Treatment Programs." *American Journal of Orthopsychiatry* 41 (1971): 427–441.

Fromm-Reichmann, F. "Notes on the Development of Treatment of Schizophrenia by Psychoanalytic Psychotherapy." *Psychiatry* 11 (1948): 263–273.

Gardos, G., and Cole, J.O. "Maintenance Antipsychotic Therapy: Is the Cure Worse Than the Disease?" *American Journal of Psychiatry* 133 (1976): 32–36.

Goldberg, S.G., Schooler, N.R., Hogarty, G.E., and Roper, M. "Prediction of Relapse in Schizophrenic Outpatients Treated by Drug and Sociotherapy." *Archives of General Psychiatry* 34 (1977): 171–184.

Goldstein, M.J., Rodnick, E.H., Evans, J.R., May, P.R.A., and Steinberg, M.R. "Drug and Family Therapy in the Aftercare of Acute Schizophrenics." *Archives of General Psychiatry* 35 (1978): 1169–1177.

Hirsch, S.R., and Leff, J.P. *Abnormalities in the Parents of Schizophrenics.* Maudsley Monograph No. 22. London: Oxford University Press, 1975.

Hirsch, S.R., and Leff, J.P. "Parental Abnormalities of Verbal Communication in the Transmission of Schizophrenia." *Psychological Medicine* 1 (1971): 118–127.

Hogarty, G.E., Goldberg, S.C., and the Collaborative Study Group. "Drugs and Sociotherapy in the Aftercare of Schizophrenic Patients. One Year Relapse Rates." *Archives of General Psychiatry* 28 (1973): 54–64.

Hogarty, G.E., Goldberg, S.C., and Schooler, N.R. "Drug and Sociotherapy in the Aftercare of Schizophrenic Patients. III. Adjustment of Nonrelapsed Patients." *Archives of General Psychiatry* 31 (1974b): 609–618.

Hogarty, G.E., Goldberg, S.C., Schooler, N.R., Ulrich, R.F. and the Collaborative Study Group. "Drug and Sociotherapy in the Aftercare of Schizophrenic Patients: II. Two Year Relapse Rates." *Archives of General Psychiatry* 31 (1974a): 603–608.

Hogarty, G.E., Schooler, N.R., Ulrich, R.F., Mussare, F., Ferro, P., and Herron, E. "Fluphenazine and Social Therapy in the Aftercare of Schizophrenic Patients—Relapse Analyses of a Two-Year Controlled Study of Fluphenazine Decanoate and Fluphenazine Hydrochloride." *Archives of General Psychiatry* 36 (1979): 1238–1294.

Hogarty, G.E., Ulrich, R.F., Goldberg, S.G., and Schooler, N.R. "Sociotherapy and the Prevention of

Relapse Among Schizophrenic Patients: An Artifact of Drug?" In *Evaluation of Psychological Therapies: Psychotherapies, Behavior Therapies, and their Interactions,* edited by R. Spitzer and D. Klein. Baltimore: Johns Hopkins University Press, 1976.

Katkin, S., Ginsburg, M., Rifkin, M.H., and Scott, J.T. "Effectiveness of Female Volunteers in the Treatment of Outpatients." *Journal of Counseling Psychology* 18 (1971): 97–100.

Katkin, S., Zimmerman, V., Rosenthal, J., and Ginsburg, M. "Using Volunteer Therapists to Reduce Hospital Readmissions." *Hospital and Community Psychiatry* 26 (1975): 151–153.

Kellam, S.G., Goldberg, S.C., Schooler, N.R., Berman, A., and Schmelzer, J.L. "Ward Atmosphere and Outcome of Treatment of Acute Schizophrenia." *Journal of Psychiatric Research* 5 (1967): 145–163.

Kirk, S.A. "Effectiveness of Community Services for Discharged Mental Hospital Patients." *American Journal of Orthopsychiatry* 46 (1976): 646–659.

Langsley, D.G., Pitman, F.S., Machotka, P., and Flomenhaft, K. "Family Crisis Therapy—Results and Implications." *Family Process* 7 (1968): 145–158.

Leff, J.P. "Developments in Family Treatment of Schizophrenia." *Psychiatric Quarterly* 51 (1979): 216–232.

Levine, D.S., Levine, D.R. *The Cost of Mental Illness—1971.* U.S. Department of Health, Education and Welfare, Alcohol, Drug Abuse and Mental Health Administration, National Institute of Mental Health, Rockville, Maryland. Series B, No. 7, 1975.

Lidz, T., Cornelison, A.R., Fleck, S., and Terry, D. "The Intrafamilial Environment of the Schizophrenic Patient. I. The Father." *Psychiatry* 20 (1957): 329–342.

Linn, L. "State Hospital Environment and Rates of Patient Discharge." *Archives of General Psychiatry* 23 (1970): 346–351.

Linn, M.W., Caffey, E.M., Jr., Klett, C.J., Hogarty, G., and Lamb, R. "Day Treatment and Psychotropic Drugs in the Aftercare of Schizophrenic Patients. *Archives of General Psychiatry* 36 (1979): 1055–1066.

Linn, M.W., Klett, C.J., and Caffey, E.M., Jr. "Foster Home Characteristics and Psychiatric Patient Outcome." *Archives of General Psychiatry* 37 (1980): 129–132.

May, P.R.A. *Treatment of Schizophrenia* New York: Science House, 1968.

McCranie, E.W., and Mizell, T.A. "Aftercare for Psychiatric Patients: Does it Prevent Rehospitalization?" *Hospital and Community Psychiatry* 29 (1978): 587–684.

Moos, R.H., Shelton, R., and Petty, C. "Perceived Ward Climate and Treatment Outcome." *Journal of Abnormal Psychology* 82 (1973): 291–298.

Mosher, L.R. "A Research Design for Evaluating a Psychosocial Treatment of Schizophrenia." *Hospital and Community Psychiatry* 23 (1972): 229–234.

Mosher, L.R., and Keith, S.J. "Psychosocial Treatment: Individual, Group, Family, and Community Support Approaches." *Schizophrenia Bulletin* 6 1980): 10–41.

Mosher, L.R. and Keith, S.J. "Research on the Psychosocial Treatment of Schizophrenia: A Summary Report." *American Journal of Psychiatry* 136 (1979): 623–631.

Mosher, L.R., and Menn, A. "Community Residential Treatment for Schizophrenia: Two Year Follow-Up Data." *Hospital and Community Psychiatry* 29 (1978): 715–723.

Mosher, L.R., Menn, A., and Matthews, S. "Soteria: Evaluation of a Home-Based Treatment for Schizophrenia." *American Journal of Orthopsychiatry* 45 (1975): 455–467.

Mosher, L.R., Reifman, A., and Menn, A. "Characteristics of Non-Professionals Serving as Primary Therapists for Acute Schizophrenics." *Hospital and Community Psychiatry* 24 (1973): 391–396.

O'Brian, C., Hamm, K., Ray, B., Pierce, J., Luborsky, L., and Mintz, J. "Group vs. Individual Psychotherapy with Schizophrenics." *Archives of General Psychiatry* 27 (1972): 474–478.

Paul, G.L., and Lentz, R.J. *Psychosocial Treatment of Chronic Mental Patients: Milieu vs. Social Learning Programs.* Cambridge, Harvard University Press, 1977.

Paul, G.L, Tobias, L.L., and Holly, B.L. "Maintenance Psychotropic Drugs in the Presence of Active Treatment Programs: A 'Triple-Blind' Withdrawal Study with Long-Term Mental Patients." *Archives of General Psychiatry* 27 (1972): 106–115.

Prince, R.M., Jr., Ackerman, R.E., and Barksdale, B.S. "Collaborative Provisions of Aftercare Services." *American Journal of Psychiatry* 130 (1973): 930–932.

Purvis, S.A., and Miskimins, R.W. "Effects of Community Follow-Up on Post-Hospital Adjustment of Psychiatric Patients." *Community Mental Health Journal* 6 (1970): 374–382.

Rog, D.J., and Raush, H.L. "The Psychiatric Halfway House. How is it Measuring Up?" *Community Mental Health Journal* 11 (1975): 162–166.

Schooler, N.R., Levine, J., Severe, J.B., Brauzer, B. DiMascio, A., Klerman, G., and Tuason, V. "Prevention of Relapse in Schizophrenia: An Evaluation of Fluphenazine Decanoate." *Archives of General Psychiatry* 37 (1980): 16–24.

Singer, M.T., and Wynne, L.C. "Communication Styles in Parents of Normals, Neurotics, and Schizophrenics." *Psychiatric Research Reports* 20 (1966): 25–38.

Smith, C.G., and King, J.A. *Mental Hospitals: A Study in Organizational Effectiveness.* Lexington, Mass.: Lexington Press, 1975.

Strauss, J.C., Carpenter, W.T., Jr., and Bartko, J.J. "Part III. Speculations on the Processes that Underlie Schizophrenic Symptoms and Signs." *Schizophrenia Bulletin* II (1974): 61–69.

Van Putten, T., and May, P.R.A. "Milieu Therapy of the Schizophrenias." In *Treatment of Schizophrenia, Progress and Prospects,* edited by L.J. West, and D.E. Flinn. New York: Grune & Stratton, 1976.

Vaughn, C.E., and Leff, J.P. "The Influence of Family and Social Factors on the Course of Psychiatric Illness." *British Journal of Psychiatry* 129 (1976): 125–137.

Weinman, B. "Chronics Make it in the Community." *Innovations* 2 (1975): 23–33.

Wing, J.K., and Brown, G.W. *Institutionalism and Schizophrenia* New York: Cambridge University Press, 1970.

Yolles, S.F., and Kramer, M. "Vital Statistics." In *The Schizophrenia Syndrome*, edited by L. Bellak and L. Loeb. New York: Grune & Stratton, 1969.

Bibliography for Chapter 15

Abrams, A., Braff, D., Janowsky, D., Hall, S., and Segal, D. "Unresponsiveness of Catatonic Symptoms to Naloxone Pharmacopsychiatry." *Pharmacopsychiatry* 11 (1978): 177–179.

Agnoli, A., Ruggieri, S., Baldassarre, M., Forchetti, C., Cerone, G., Falaschi, P., Frajese, G., Rocco, A., and D'Urso, R. *Neuroendocrinology: Biological and Clinical*, edited by A. Polleri, and R.M. McLeod. London: Academic Press, 1979.

Akil, H., Watson, S.J., Berger, P.A., and Bachas, J.D. "Endorphins, B-LPH, and ACTH: Biochemical and Anatomical Studies." In *Advances in Biochemical Psychopharmacology*, edited by E. Costa, and E. Trabucchi. New York: Raven Press, 1978.

Alexander, P.E., van Kammen, D.P., Bunney, W.E. "Antipsychotic Effects of Lithium in Schizophrenia." *American Journal of Psychiatry* 136 (1979): 283–287.

Alfredsson, G., Wresel, F.A., and Skett, P. "Levels of Chlorpromazine and Its Active Metabolites in Rat Brain and the Relationship to Central Monoamine Metabolism and Prolactin Secretion." *Psychopharmacology* 53 (1979): 1378.

American Psychiatric Association. *Task Force Report 14-Electroconvulsive Therapy.* Washington, D.C.: American Psychiatric Association, 1978.

Angst J., Weis, P., Grof, P., Baastrup, P.C., and Schou, M. "Lithium Prophylaxis in Recurrent Affective Disorders." *British Journal of Psychiatry* 116 (1970): 604–614.

Arato, M., Erdos, M., Polgar, M. "Endocrinological Changes in Patients With Sexual Dysfunction Under Long-Term Neuroleptic Treatment." *Pharmakopsychiatrie* 12 (1979): 426–431.

Arib, M. "Long-Term Treatment of the Chronic Schizophrenic Patient." A Scientific Exhibit.

Asnis, G.M., Sachar, E.J., Langer, G., Halpern, F.S., and Fink, M. "Normal Prolactin Responses in Tardive Dyskinesia." *Psychopharmacology* 66 (1979): 247–250.

Atsmon, A. "Early Observations of the Effect of Propranolol on Psychotic Patients." *Advances in Clinical Pharmacology* 12 (1976): 86–90.

Atsmon, A., and Blum, I. "Treatment of Acute Porphyria Variegata With Propranolol." *Lancet* 24 (1970): 196–197.

Atsmon, A., Blum, I. "The Discovery." In *Propranolol and Schizophrenia*, edited by E. Roberts, and P. Amacher. New York: Alan Liss, Inc., 1978.

Atsmon, A., Blum, I., Steiner, M., Latz, A., and Wijsenbeek, H. "Further Studies With Propranolol in Psychotic Patients." *Psychopharmacologia* 27 (1972): 249–254.

Atsmon, A., Blum, I., Wijsenbeek, H., Maoz, P., Steiner, M., and Zielgelman, G. "The Short-Term Effects of Adrenergic-Blocking Agents in a Small Group of Psychotic Patients." *Psychiatria Neurologia Neurochirurgia* 74 (1971): 251–258.

Baro, F., Brugmans, J., Dom, R., and Van Lommel, R. "Maintenance Therapy of Chronic Psychotic Patients With a Weekly Oral Dose of R 16341." *Journal of Clinical Pharmacology* 10 (1970): 330.

Beg, A.A., Varma, K.V., and Dash, R.J. "Effect of Chlorpromazine on Human Growth Hormone." *American Journal of Psychiatry* 136 (1979): 914–916.

Belmaker, R.H., Ebstein, R.P., Dasberg, H., Levy, A., Sadvall, G., and Van Praag, H.M. "The Effects of Propranolol Treatment in Schizophrenia on CSF Amine Metabolites and Prolactin." *Psychopharmacology* 63 (1979): 293–296.

Benjamin, F., Casper, D.J., and Kolodny, H.H. "Interactive Human Growth Hormone in Condition Associated With Galactorrhea." *Obstetrics and Gynecology* 34 (1969): 34–39.

Berger, P., Watson, S., Akil, H., and Barchas, J. "The Effects of Naloxone in Chronic Schizophrenia." *American Journal of Psychiatry* 138 (1981) 913–915.

Besses, G.S., Burrow, G.N., Spaldling, S.M., and Donabedian, R.K. "Dopamine Infusion Acutely Inhibits the TSH and Prolactin Reponse to TRH." *Journal of Clinical Endocrinology and Metabolism* 14 (1975): 985–988.

Beumont, P.J.V., Corker, C.S., Friesen, H.G., Kolakowska, T., Mandelbrote, B.M., Marshall, J., Murray, M.A.F., and Wiles, D.H. "The Effect of Phenothiazines on Endocrine Function: II. Effects in Men and Post-Menopausal Women." *British Journal of Psychiatry.* 124 (1974a): 420–430.

Beumont, P.J.V., Gelder, M.G., Friesen, H.G., Harris, G.W., MacKinnon, P.C.B., Mandelbrote, B.M., and Wiles, D.H. "The Effects of Phenothiazines on Endocrine Function: I. Patients With Inappropriate Lactation and Amenorrhea." *British Journal of Psychiatry* 124 (1974b): 413–419.

Beumont, P., Bruwer, J., Pimstone, B., Vinik, A., and Utian, W. "Bromocriptine in the Treatment of Phenothiazine-Induced Galactorrhea." *British Journal of Psychiatry* 126 (1975): 285–288.

Bishop, M.P., and Gallant, D.M. "Loxapine: A Controlled Evaluation in Chronic Schizophrenic Patients." *Current Therapeutic Research.* 12 (1970): 594.

Bookhammer, R.S., Meyers, R.W., Schober, C.C., and Piotrowski, Z.A. "A Five-Year Follow-Up Study of Schizophrenic Patients." *Current Therapeutic Research* 12 (1966): 594.

Brambilla, F.A., Guerrini, A., Guastalla, A., Rovere C., and Riggi, F. "Neuroendocrine Effects of Haloperidol Therapy in Chronic Schizophrenia." *Psychopharmacologia* 44 (1975): 17–22.

Brambilla, F., Guerrini, A., Riggi, F., and Ricardi, F. "Psychoendocrine Investigation in Schizophrenia: Relationship Between Pituitary-Gonadal Function and Behavior." *Diseases of the Nervous System* 34 (1974): 362–368.

Brockington, L., Kendell, R., Kellett, J., Curry, S., and Wainwright, S. "Trials of Lithium, Chlorpromazine and Amitriptyline in Schizoaffective Patients." *British Journal of Psychiatry* 133 (1978) 162–168.

Brokshank, B.W.L., MacSweeney, D.A., Johnson A.L., Cunningham, A.E., Wilson, D.A., and Copper, A "Androgen Excretion and Physique in Schizophrenia." *British Journal of Psychiatry* 117 (1970) 413–420.

Brotman, R.K., Muzekari, L.H., and Shanken, P.M. "Butaperazine in Chronic Schizophrenic Patients: A Double-Blind Study." *Current Therapeutic Research* 11 (1969): 5.

Brown, G.M., Garfinkel, P.E., Warsh, J.J., and Stancer, H.C. "Effect of Carbidopa on Prolactin, Growth Hormone and Cortisol Secretion in Man." *Journal of Clinical Endocrinology and Metabolism* 43 (1976a): 236–239.

Brown, G.M., Seeman, P., and Lee, T. "Dopamine/Neuroleptic Receptors in Basal Hypothalamus and Pituitary." *Endocrinology* 99 (1976b): 1407–1410.

Brown, G.M., Verhaegen, H., and van Wimersna Greidanus, T.B. "Endocrine Effects of Domperidone: A Peripheral Dopamine Blocking Agent." *Journal of Clinical Endocrinology,* in press.

Brown, W.A. "Psychological and Neuroendocrine Response to Methylphenidate." *Archives of General Psychiatry,* 34 (1977): 1103–1108.

Brown, W.A., and Laughren, T.P. "Low Serum Prolactin and Early Relapse Following Neuroleptic Withdrawal." *American Journal of Psychiatry* 138 (1981): 237–239.

Buckman, M.T., and Peake, G.T. "Estrogen Potentiation of Phenothiazine-Induced Prolactin Secretion in Man." *Journal of Clinical Endocrinology and Metabolism* 37 (1973): 977–979.

Busch, D.A., Fang, V.S., and Meltzer, H.Y. "Serum Prolactin Levels Following Intramuscular Chlorpromazine: Toward Three-Hour Response as Predictors of Six-Hour Response." *Journal of Psychiatric Research* 1 (1979): 153–159.

Caffey, E.M., Diamond, L.S., Frank, T.V., Grasberger, J.C., Herman, L., Klett, C.J., and Rothstein, D. "Discontinuation of Reduction of Chemotherapy in Chronic Schizophrenics." *Journal of Chronic Diseases* 17 (1964): 347.

Caffey, E.M., Galbrecht, C.R., and Klett, C.J. "Brief Hospitalization and Aftercare in the Treatment of Schizophrenia." *Archives of General Psychiatry* 24 (1971): 81–86.

Caffey, E.M., Jones, R.B., Diamond, L.S., Burton, E., and Bowen, W.T. "Brief Hospital Treatment of Schizophrenia: Early Results of a Multiple Hospital Study." *Hospital and Community Psychiatry* 19 (1968): 282–287.

Camanni, E., Genazzini, A.R., Massara, F., LaRosa, R., Cocchi, D., and Müller, E.E. "Prolactin-Releasing Effect of Domperidone in Normoprolactinemic and Hyperprolactinemic Subjects." *Neuroendocrinology* 30 (1980): 2–6.

Carlsson, A. "Antipsychotic Drugs, Neurotransmitters and Schizophrenia." *American Journal of Psychiatry* 135 (1978): 164.

Carscallen, H.B., Rochman, H., and Lovegrove, T.D. "High-Dosage Trifluoperazine in Schizophrenia." *Canadian Psychiatric Association Journal* 13 (1968): 459.

Casacchia, M., Meco, G., Carchedi, F., and DiCeglie, M. "Neurochemical Side Effects of Antipsychotic Drugs." In *Neuroendocrine Correlates in Neurology and Psychiatry,* edited by E.E. Müller, and A. Agnoli. Amsterdam: Elsevier Press, 1979.

Casey, J.F., Hollister, L.E., Klett, C.J., Lasky, J.J., and Caffey, E.M. "Combined Drug Therapy of Chronic Schizophrenics. Controlled Evaluation of Placebo,

Dextro-Amphetamine, Imipramine, Isocarboxazid and Trifluoperazine Added to Maintenance Doses of Chlorpromazine." *American Journal of Psychiatry* 117 (1961): 998.

Cassano, G.B., Castrogiovanni, P., Conti, L., and Bonollo, L. "Sulpiride vs. Haloperidol in Schizophrenia: A Double-Blind Comparative Trial." *Current Therapeutic Research* 17 (1975): 189–201.

Chalmers, R.J., and Bennie, E.H. "The Effect of Fluphenazine on Basal Prolactin Concentrations." *Psychological Medicine* 8 (1978): 483–486.

Charalampous, K.D., Freemesser, G.F., Malev, J., and Ford, K. "Loxapine Succinate: A Controlled Double-Blind Study in Schizophrenia." *Current Therapeutic Research* 16 (1974): 829–837.

Cheung, H.K. "Schizophrenics Fully Remitted on Neuroleptics for 3–5 Years." *British Journal of Psychiatry* 138 (1981): 490–494.

Chien, C.P., and Cole, J.O. "Supervised Cooperative Apartments." *American Journal of Psychiatry* 130 (1973): 156–159.

Chien, C.P., DiMascio, A., and Cole, J.O. "Antiparkinsonian Agent and Depot Phenothiazine." *American Journal of Psychiatry* 131 (1974): 86.

Claghorn, J., Johnston, E., Cook, T., and Itschner, L. "Group Therapy and Maintenance Treatment of Schizophrenia." *Archives of General Psychiatry.* 31 (1974): 361–385.

Clarenback, P., Prunkl, R., Riegler, M., and Cramer, A. "Effects of Haloperidol on Afternoon Sleep and the Secretion of Growth Hormone in Man." *Neuroscience* 3 (1978) 345–348.

Clark, M.L., Huber, W.K., Sakata, K., Fowles, D.C., and Serafetinides, E.A. "Molindone in Chronic Schizophrenia." *Clinical Pharmacology and Therapeutics* 11 (1970a): 680.

Clark, M.L., Huber, W.K., Sullivan, J., Wood, F., and Costiloe, J.P. "Evaluation of Loxapine Succinate in Chronic Schizophrenia." *Diseases of the Nervous System* 33 (1972a): 783.

Clark, M.L., Paredes, A., Costiloe, J.P., Fulkerson, F.G., and Wood, F. "Evaluation of Two Dose Levels of Loxapine Succinate in Chronic Schizophrenia." *Diseases of the Nervous System* 38 (1977): 10.

Clark, M.L., Paredes, A., Costiloe, J.P., Wood, F., and Barrett, A. "Loxapine in Newly Admitted Chronic Schizophrenic Patients." *Journal of Clinical Pharmacology* 15 (1975): 286.

Clark, M.L. Ramsey, H.R., Ragland, R.E., Rahhal, D., Serafetinides, E.A., and Costiloe, P. "Chlorpromazine in Chronic Schizophrenia: Behavioral Dose Response Relationship." *Psychopharmacologia* 18 (1970b): 260.

Clark, M.L., Ramsey, H.R., Rahhal, D.K., Serafetinides, E.A., Wood, F.D., and Costiloe, J.P. "Chlorpromazine in Chronic Schizophrenia." *Archives of General Psychiatry* 27 (1972b): 479.

Clemens, J.A., Smalstig, E.G., and Sawyer, B.D. "Antipsychotic Drugs Stimulate Prolactin Release." *Psychopharmacology* 40 (1974): 123–127.

Cohen, K.L., Cooper, R.A., and Altshul, S. "Prolactin Levels in Tardive Dyskinesia." *New England Journal of Medicine* 300 (1979): 46.

Cole, J.O., and Davis, J.M. "Antipsychotic Drugs." In *The Schizophrenic Syndrome,* edited by L. Bellak and L. Leob. New York: Grune & Stratton, 1969.

Cole, J.O., Goldberg, S.C., and Davis, J.M. "Drugs in the Treatment of Psychosis: Controlled Studies." In *Psychiatric Drugs,* edited by P. Solomon. New York: Grune & Stratton, 1966.

Cole, J.O., Goldberg, S.C., and Klerman, G.L. "Phenothiazine Treatment in Acute Schizophrenia." *Archives of General Psychiatry* 10 (1964): 246.

Collu, R., Chourmard, G., Jones, B.D., and Annable, L. "Dopaminergic Control of Prolactin Release in Humans: Absence of Neuroleptic-Induced Hypersensitivity." *Clinical Research* 26 (1978): 840.

Collu, R., Jequier, J.C., Leboeuf, J., Ducharme, J.R. "Endocrine Effects of Pimozide. A Specific Dopaminergic Blocker." *Journal of Clinical Endocrinology and Metabolism* 41 (1975): 981–984.

Corsini, G.U., DelZompo, M., Maconi, S., Chianchetti, C., Mangoni, A. "Sedative, Hypnotic and Antipsychotic Effect of Low Doses of Apomorphine in Man." In *Symposium on Non-Striatal Dopaminergic Neurons,* edited by E. Costa, and G.L. Gessa. New York: Raven Press, 1977.

Cotes, P.J., Crow, T.J., Johnstone, E.C., Bartlett, W., and Bourne, R.C. "Neuroendocrine Changes in Acute Schizophrenia as a Function of Clinical State and Neuroleptic Medication." *Psychological Medicine* 8 (1978): 657–665.

Creese, I., Burt, D.R., Snyder, S.H. "Dopamine Receptors and Average Clinical Doses." *Science* 194 (1976): 546.

Crosignani, P.G., Reschini, E., Peracch, M., Lombroso, G.C., Mattei, A., and Caccamo, A. "Failure of Dopamine Infusion to Suppress the Plasma Prolactin Response to Sulpiride in Normal and Hyperprolactinemic Subjects." *Journal of Clinical Endocrinology and Metabolism* 45 (1977): 841–844.

Crowley, T.J., and Hydinger-MacDonald, M. "Mobility, Parkinsonism, and Prolactin With Thiothixene and Thioridazine." *Archives of General Psychiatry* 38 (1981): 668–675.

Cuche, H., and Deniker, P. "Psychiatric Uses of Beta Blockers." *Pharmakopsychiatrie* 13 (1980): 267–272.

Curry, S.H., Janowsky, D.S., Davis, J.M., and Marshall, J.H.L. "Factors Affecting Chlorpromazine Plasma Levels in Psychiatric Patients." *Archives of General Psychiatry* 22 (1970a): 209.

Curry, S.H., Marshall, J.H.L., Davis, J.M., and Janowsky, D.S. "Chlorpromazine Plasma Levels and Effects." *Archives of General Psychiatry* 22 (1970b): 289–296.

Czernik, A., and Kleesiek, K. "Effects of Depot Neuroleptics on Pituitary Hormones." *Nervenarzt* 50 (1979): 527–553.

Darondel, A., and Fengler, B. "Open Study of Haldol Decanoate in Psychotic Syndromes." *Proc. III World Congress of Biological Psychiatry.* June, 1981.

Davis, G.C., Bunney, W.E., Jr., DeFraites, E.G., Kleinman, J.E., Van Kammen, D.D., Poot, R.M., and Wyatt, R.J. "Intravenous Naloxone Administration in Schizophrenia and Affective Illness." *Science* 197 (1977): 74–76.

Davis, J.M. "Dose Equivalence of the Antipsychotic Drugs." *Journal of Psychiatric Research* 11 (1974): 65–69.

Davis, J.M. "Overview: Maintenance Therapy in Psychiatry: Schizophrenia." *American Journal of Psychiatry* 132 (1975): 1237.

Davis, J.M. "Comparative Doses and Costs of Antipsychotic Medication." *Archives of General Psychiatry* 33 (1976): 858.

Davis, J.M. "Recent Developments in the Drug Treatment of Schizophrenia." *American Journal of Psychiatry* 133 (1976): 208–214.

Davis, J.M. "Dopamine Theory of Schizophrenia: A Two-Factor Theory." In *The Nature of Schizophrenia,* edited by L.C. Wynne. New York: John Wiley and Sons, 1978.

Davis, J.M., and Chang, S. "Does Psychotherapy Alter the Course in Schizophrenia?" In *Controversies in Psychiatry,* edited by J.P. Brady and H.K.H. Brodie. New York: Saunders, 1978.

Davis, J.M., Ericksen, S.E., and Dekirmenjian, H. "Plasma Levels of Antipsychotic Drugs and Clinical Response." In *Psychopharmacology: A Generation of Progress,* edited by M.A. Lipton, A. DiMascio, and K.R. Killiam. New York: Raven Press, 1978.

del Guidice, J., Clark, W., and Gocka, E. "Prevention of Recidivism of Schizophenics Treated with Fluphenazine Enanthate." *Psychosomatics* 16 (1975): 32–36.

Denber, H. "Oxilapine vs. Trifluoperazine." *Psychopharmacology Bulletin* 6 (1970): 93–94.

DeRivera, J.L., Lal, S., Ettig, P., Hontela, S., Muller, H.F., and Friesen, H.G. "Effect of Acute and Chronic Neuroleptic Therapy on Serum Prolactin Levels in Men and Women of Different Age Groups." *Clinical Endocrinology* 5 (1976): 273–282.

Donlon, P., Meadow, A., Tupin, J., and Wahby, M. "High vs. Standard Dosage Fluphenazine HCI in Acute Schizophrenia." *Journal of Clinical Psychiatry* 39 (1978): 800.

Dotti, A., Lostia, O., Rubino, I.A., Bersani, G., Carilli, L., and Zorretta, D. "The Prolactin Response in Patients Receiving Neuroleptic Therapy. The Effect of Fluphenazine Decanoate." *Progress in Neuro-Psychopharmacology* 5 (1981): 69–77.

Dube, K.C., and Kumar, N. "Loxapine Succinate: A Comparative Study With Chlorpromazine." *Current Therapeutic Research* 19 (1976): 653.

Dysken, M.W., and Davis, J.M. "Naloxone in A-mylobarbitone Responsive Catatonia." *British Journal of Psychiatry* 133 (1978): 476–480.

Elizur, A., Segal, S., Yenet, A., and Ben-David, M. "Prolactin Response and Extrapyramidal Side Effects During Propranolol and Neuroleptic Drug Treatment in Chronic Schizophrenic Patients." *Israel Annals of Psychiatry* 17 (1979a): 318–327.

Elizur, A., Segal, Z., Yeret, A., Davidson S., and Atsmon, A. "Antipsychotic Effect of Propranolol on Chronic Schizophrenics." *Psychopharmacologia* 60 (1979b): 189–194.

Emrich, H.M. "Über eine mögliche Rolle von Endorphinen bei psychischen Krankheiten." *Arzneimittel-Forschung/Drug Research* 28 (1978): 1270–1273.

Emrich H.M., Cording, C., Piree, S., Kolling, A., Zerssen, D.V., and Hertz, A. "Indication of an Antipsychotic Action of the Opiate Antagonist Naloxone." *Pharmakopsychiatrie Neuro-Psychopharmakologie* 10 (1977): 265–270.

Emrich, H.M., Holt, V., Laspe, H., Fischler, M., Heinemann, H., Kissling, W., Zerssen, D.V., and Herz, A.

"Studies on a Possible Pathological Significance of Endorphins in Psychiatric Disorders." In *Neuro-Psychopharmacology*, edited by B. Saletu, P. Berner, and L. Hollister. New York: Permagon Press, 1979.

Ericksen, S., Hurt, S.W., Chang, S., and Davis, J. "Haloperidol Dose, Plasma Levels and Clinical Response: A Double Blind Study." *Psychopharmacology Bulletin* 14 (1978): 15.

Esterson, A., Cooper, D.G., and Laing, R.D. "Results of Family-Oriented Therapy With Hospitalized Schizophrenics." *British Medical Journal* 2 (1965): 1462–1465.

Ettig, P., Nair, N.P.V., Lal, S., Cervantes, P., and Guyda, H. "Effect of Apomorphine on Growth Hormone and Prolactin Secretion." *Journal of Neurology, Neurosurgery and Psychiatry* 39 (1976): 870–876.

Exner, J., and Murillo, L. "A Long-Term Follow-Up of Schizophrenics Treated with Regressive ECT." *Diseases of the Nervous System* 38 (1977): 162.

Fenton, F.R., and Struening, E.L. "A Comparative Trial of Home and Hospital Psychiatric Care." *Archives of General Psychiatry* 36 (1978): 1074–1079.

Filho, V.V., Caldeira, M.V.N., and Bueno, J.R. "The Efficacy and Safety of Loxapine Succinate in the Treatment of Schizophrenia: A Comparative Study." *Current Therapeutic Research* 18 (1975): 476–490.

Fleiss, J.F. *Statistical Methods for Rates and Proportions*. New York: Wiley and Sons, 1981.

Forssman, H., and Walinder, J. "Lithium Treatment on Atypical Indication." *Acta Psychiatrica Scandinavica* Suppl. 207 (1969): 34–39.

Freeman, C.P.L., and Fairburn, C.G. "Lack of Effect of Naloxone and Schizophrenic Auditory Hallucinations." *Psychological Medicine* 11 (1981): 405–407.

Freeman, H. and Frederick A.N. "Comparison of Trifluoperazine and Molindone in Chronic Schizophrenic Patients." *Current Therapeutic Research* 11 (1969): 670–676.

Friend, W.C., Brown, G.M., Jawahier, G., Lee, T., and Seemen, P. "Effect of Haloperidol and Apomorphine on Dopamine Receptors in Pituitary and Striatum." *American Journal of Psychiatry* 135 (1978): 839–841.

Fruensgaard, K., Korsgaard, S., Jorgensen, H., and Jensen, K. "Loxapine vs. Haloperidol Parenterally in Acute Psychosis With Agitation: A Double-Blind Study." *Acta Psychiatrica Scandinavica* 56 (1977): 256.

Fruensgaard, K., Wollenberg, J., Hansen, K., Fenbor, C., and Sihm, F. "Current Medicine and Research Opinions." [sic] 5 (1978): 601–607.

Gallant, D.M., and Bishop, M.P. "Molindone: Controlled Evaluation in Chronic Schizophrenic Patients." *Current Therapeutic Research* 10 (1968): 441–447.

Gardos, G. "Are Antipsychotic Drugs Interchangeable?" *Journal of Nervous and Mental Disease* 159 (1978): 343.

Gardos, G., Cole, J.O., Volicer, L., Orzack, M.H., and Oliff, A.C. "A Dose-Response Study of Propranolol in Chronic Schizophrenics." *Current Therapeutic Research* 15 (1973): 314–323.

Gardos, G., Orzack, M., Finn, G., and Cole, J.O. "High and Low Dose Thiothixene Treatment in Chronic Schizophrenia." *Diseases of the Nervous System* 35 (1974): 53.

Garver, D.L., Davis, J.M., Dekirmenjian, H., Jones, F.D., Casper, R., and Haraszti, J. "Pharmacokinetics of Red Blood Cell Phenothiazine and Clinical Effects." *Archives of General Psychiatry* 33 (1976): 862.

Garver, D.L., Dekirmenjian, H., Davis, J.M., Casper, R., and Ericksen, S. "Neuroleptic Drug Levels and Therapeutic Response: Preliminary Observations With Red Blood Cell-Bound Butaperazine." *American Journal of Psychiatry* 134 (1977): 304.

Gitlin, M., and Rosenblatt, M. "Possible Withdrawal From Endogenous Opiates in Schizophrenics." *American Journal of Psychiatry* 135 (1978): 377–378.

Glick, I.D., Hargreaves, W.A., Drues, J., and Showstack, J.A. "Short vs. Long Hospitalization: A Controlled Study. IV. One Year Follow-Up Results for Schizophrenic Patients." *American Journal of Psychiatry* 133 (1976): 509–514.

Glick, I.D., Hargreaves, W.A., and Goldfield, M.D. "Short vs. Long Hospitalization: A Prospective Controlled Study. I. The Preliminary Results of a One-Year Follow-Up of Schizophrenics." *Archives of General Psychiatry* 30 (1974): 363–369.

Glick, I.D., Hargreaves, W.A., Raskin, M., and Kutner, J. "Short vs. Long Hospitalization: A Prospective Controlled Study. II. Results for Schizophrenic Inpatients." *American Journal of Psychiatry* 132 (1975): 385–390.

Glick, J.D., and Hargreaves, W.A. *Psychiatric Hospital Treatment for the 1980's*. Lexington: Lexington Books, 1979.

Goldberg, S.C., Frosch, W.A., Drossman, A.K., Schooler, N.R., and Johnson, G.F.S. "Prediction of Response to Phenothiazines in Schizophrenia: A Cross-Validation Study." *Archives of General Psychiatry* 26 (1972): 367.

Goldberg, S.C., Mattsson, N., Cole, J.O., and Klerman, G.L. "Prediction of Improvement in Schizophrenia Under Four Phenothiazines." *Archives of General Psychiatry* 16 (1967): 107.

Goldberg, S.C., Schooler, N., Hogarty, G., and Roper, M. "Prediction of Relapse in Schizophrenic Outpatients Treated by Drug and Sociotherapy." *Archives of General Psychiatry* 34 (1977): 171.

Goldstein, M., Rodnick, E., Evans, J., May, P., and Steinberg, M. "Drug and Family Therapy in the Aftercare of Acute Schizophrenics." *Archives of General Psychiatry* 35 (1978): 1169.

Goode, D.J., Meltzer, H.Y., and Fang, S. "Short Communication: Increased Serum Prolactin Levels During Phenothiazine Treatment of Six Postpartum Women." *Psychoneuroendocrinology* 5 (1980): 345–351.

Gorham, D.R., and Pokorny, A.D. "Effects of Phenothiazine and/or Group Psychotherapy With Schizophrenics." *Diseases of the Nervous System* 25 (1964): 77.

Greenblatt, M., Solomon, M.H., Evans, A.S., and Brooks, G.W. *Drug and Social Therapy in Chronic Schizophrenia*. Springfield: Charles C. Thomas, 1965.

Grinspoon, L., Ewalt, J.R., and Shader, R. "Psychotherapy and Pharmacotherapy in Chronic Schizophrenia." *American Journal of Psychiatry* 124 (1968): 67–74.

Grinspoon, L., Ewalt, J.R., and Shader, R.I. *Schizophrenia: Pharmacotherapy and Psychotherapy.* Baltimore: Williams & Wilkins, 1972.

Growe, G., Crayton, J.W., Klass, D., Evans, H., and Strezich, M. "Lithium in Chronic Schizophrenia." *American Journal of Psychiatry* 136 (1979): 454–462.

Gruen, P.H., Sachar, E.J., Altman, N., Langer, G., Tabrizi, M.A., and Halpern, F.S. "Relation of Plasma Prolactin to Clinical Response in Schizophrenic Patients." *Archives of General Psychiatry* 35 (1978a): 1222–1227.

Gruen, P.H., Sachar, E.J., Langer, G., Altman, N., Leifer, M., Frantz, A., and Halpern, F.S. "Prolactin Responses to Neuroleptics in Normal and Schizophrenic Subjects." *Archives of General Psychiatry* 35 (1978b): 108–116.

Gruzelier, J., Connolly, J., Eves, F., Hirsch, S., Zaki, S., Weller, M., and Yorkston, N. "Effects of Propranolol and Phenothiazines on Electrodermal Orienting and Habituation in Schizophrenia." *Psychological Medicine* 11 (1981): 93–108.

Gunne, L.M., Lindstrom, L., and Terenius, L. "Naloxone-Induced Reversal of Schizophrenic Hallucinations." *Journal of Neural Transmission* 40 (1977): 13–19.

Gunne, L.M., Lindstrom, L., and Widerlov, E. "Possible Role of Endorphins in Schizophrenia and Other Psychiatric Disorders." In *Endorphins in Mental Health Research*, edited by E. Usdin, W.E. Bunney, Jr., and N.S. Kline. New York: Oxford University Press, 1979.

Guy, W., Gross, M., Hogarty, G., and Dennis, H. "A Controlled Evaluation of Day Hospital Effectiveness." *Archives of General Psychiatry* 20 (1969): 329–338.

Hanlon, T.E., Nussbaum, K., Wittig, B., Hanlon, D.D., and Kurland, A. A. "The Comparative Effectiveness of Amitriptyline, Perphenazine, and Their Combination in the Treatment of Chronic Psychotic Female Patients." *Journal of New Drugs* 4 (1964): 52.

Hanlon, T.E., Schoenrich, C., Frenck, W., Turek, I., and Kurland A.A. "Perphenazinebenzotropine Mesylate Treatment of Newly Admitted Psychiatric Patients." *Psychopharmacologia* 9 (1966): 328.

Hanson, L.B., Elley, J., Cristensen, T.R., Larsen, N.E., Naestoft, J., and Hvidderg, E.F. "Plasma Levels of Perphenazine and Its Major Metabolites During Simultaneous Treatment With Anticholinergic Drugs." *British Journal of Clinical Pharmacology* 7 (1979): 75.

Hanssen, T., Heyden, T., Sundberg, L., Wetterberg, L., and Eneroth, P. "Decrease in Serum-Prolactin After Propranolol in Schizophrenia." *Lancet* 1 (1978): 101–102.

Hays, S.E., and Rubin, R.T. "Differential Prolactin Responses to Haloperidol and TRH in Normal Adult Men." *Psychoneuroendocrinology* 6 (1981): 45–52.

Hertz, A., Blasig, J., Emrich, H.M., Cording, C., Piree, S., Kolling, A., and Von Zerssen, D. "Is There Some Indication From Behavioral Effects of Endorphins for Their Involvement in Psychiatric Disorders?" In *Advances in Biochemical Psychopharmacology*, edited by E. Costa, and E. Trabucchi. New York: Raven Press, 1978.

Herz, M.I., Endicott, J., Spitzer, R.L., and Mesnikoff, A. "Day vs. Inpatient Hospitalization: A Controlled Study." *American Journal of Psychiatry* 127 (1971): 1371–1382.

Herz, M.I., Endicott, J., and Spitzer, R.L. "Brief Hospitalization of Patients With Families: Initial Results." *American Journal of Psychiatry* 132 (1975) 413–418.

Herz, M.I., Endicott, J., and Spitzer, R.L. "Brief vs Standard Hospitalization. The Families." *American Journal of Psychiatry* 133 (1976): 795–801.

Herz, M.I., Endicott, J., and Spitzer, R.L. "Brief Hospitalization: A Two-Year Follow-Up." *American Journal of Psychiatry* 134 (1977): 502–507.

Herz, M.I., and Melville, C. "Relapse in Schizophrenia." *American Journal of Psychiatry* 137 (1980): 801–805.

Hirsch, S.R., Gaind, R., Rhode, P.D., Stevens, B.C., and Wing, J.K. "Outpatient Maintenance of Chronic Schizophrenic Patients With Long-Acting Fluphenazine Double-Blind Placebo Trial." *British Medical Journal* 1 (1973): 633.

Hirsch, S.R., Manchanda, R., and Weller, M. "Dextro Propranolol in Schizophrenia." *Progress in Neuro Psychopharmacology* 4 (1981): 633–637.

Hirschowitz, J., Casper, R., Garver, D., and Chang, S. "Lithium Response in Good Prognosis Schizophrenia." *American Journal of Psychiatry* 13 (1980): 916–920.

Hogarty, G.E., and Goldberg, S.C. "Drugs and Social therapy in the Aftercare of Schizophrenic Patients. *Archives of General Psychiatry* 28 (1973): 54.

Hogarty, G.E., Goldberg, S.C., Schooler, N.R., an Ulrich, R.F. "Drugs and Social Therapy in the Aftercare of Schizophrenic Patients: II. Two-Year Relapse Notes." *Archives of General Psychiatry* 31 (1974a): 603–608.

Hogarty, G.E., Goldberg, S.C., and Schooler, N.I. "Drugs and Social Therapy in the Aftercare of Schizophrenic Patients: III. Adjustment of Nor Relapsed Patients." *Archives of General Psychiatry* 31 (1974b): 609–618.

Hogarty, G.E., Schooler, N.R., Ulrich, R., Mussare, I Ferro, P., and Herron, E. "Fluphenazine and Social Therapy in the Aftercare of Schizophrenic Patients *Archives of General Psychiatry* 36 (1979): 128.

Hogarty, G.E., Ulrich, R., Mussare, F., and A istigueta, N. "Drug Discontinuation Among Long Term Successfully Maintained Schizophrenic Ou patients." *Diseases of the Nervous System* 3 (1976): 494.

Honigfeld, G., Rosenblum, M.P., Blumenthal, I. Lambert, H.L., and Roberts, A.J. "Behavioral Improvement in the Older Schizophrenic Patien Drug and Social Therapies." *Journal of the American Geriatric Society* 13 (1965): 57–72.

Horn, A.S., and Snyder, S.H. "Chlorpromazine an Dopamine: Conformational Similarities That Co relate With the Antischizophrenic Activity Phenothiazine Drugs." *Proceedings of the National Academy of Sciences of the United States of America* 65 (1971): 2325.

Horwitz, W.A., Polatin, P., Kolb, L.C., and Hoch, P. "A Study of Cases of Schizophrenia Treated 'Direct Analysis.' " [sic] 114 (1958): 780–783.

Huws, D., and Groom, G.V. "Luteinizing Hormone Releasing Hormone and Thyrotropin Releasing Hormone Stimulation Studies in Patients Given Clomipramine or 'Depot' Neuroleptics." *Postgraduate Medical Journal* Suppl. 4, 53 (1977): 175–181.

Itil, T., Keskiner, A., Heinemann, L., Hatan, T., Gannon, P., and Hsu, W. "Treatment of Resistant Schizophrenics With Extreme High-Dosage Fluphenazine Hydrochloride." *Psychosomatics* 11 (1970a): 456.

Itil, T.M., Polvan, N., and Ucok, A. "Comparison of the Clinical and Electroencephalographical Effects of Molindone and Trifluoperazine in Acute Schizophrenic Patients." *Behavioral Neuropsychiatry* 3 (1970b): 25–32.

Itil, T.M., Saletu, B., Hsu, W., Keremitchi, N., and Keskiner, A. "Clinical and Quantitative EEG Changes at Different Dosage Levels of Fluphenazine Treatment." *Acta Psychiatrica Scandinavica* 47 (1971): 440–451.

Janowsky, D.S., El-Yousef, M.K., Davis, J.M., and Sekerke, H.J. "Provocation of Schizophrenic Symptoms by Intravenous Administration of Methylphenidate." *Archives of General Psychiatry* 28 (1973): 185.

Janowsky, D.S., Judd, L., Huey, L., Roitman, N., Parker, D., and Segal, D. "Naloxone Effects on Manic Symptoms and Growth-Hormone Levels." *Lancet* 2 (1978): 320.

Janowsky, D.S., Segal, D.S., Bloom, F., Abrams, A., and Guillemin, R. "Lack of Effect of Naloxone on Schizophrenic Symptoms." *American Journal of Psychiatry* 134 (1977): 926–927.

Janowsky, D.S., Leichner, P., Parker, D., Judd, L.L. Huey, L., and Clopton, P. "The Effect of Methylphenidate on Serum Growth Hormone." *Archives of General Psychiatry* 35 (1978): 1384–1389.

Jeste, D.V., Neckers, L.M., Wagner, R.L., Wise, C.D., Staub, R.A., Rogol, A., Potkin, S.G., Bridge, T.P., and Wyatt, R.J. "Lymphocyte Monoamine Oxidase and Plasma Prolactin and Growth Hormone in Tardive Dyskinesia." *Journal of Clinical Psychiatry* 42 (1981): 75–77.

Johnson, T. "Differential Response to Lithium Carbonate in Manic Depressive and Schizo-Affective Disorders." *Diseases of the Nervous System* 31 (1970): 613–615.

Johnston, M.H., and Holzman, P. *Assessing Schizophrenic Thinking*. San Francisco: Jossey-Bass, 1979.

Johnstone, E.C., and Ferner, F.N. "Neuroendocrine Markers of CNS Drug Effects." *British Journal of Clinical Pharmacology* 10 (1980): 5–21.

Johnstone, E.C., Crow, T.J., Frith, C.D., Carney, M.W.P., and Price, J.S. "Mechanism of the Antipsychotic Effect in the Treatment of Acute Schizophrenia." *Lancet* 1 (1978): 848.

Judd, L., Janowsky, D., and Segal, D. Naloxone Related Attenuation of Manic Symptoms in Certain Bipolar Depressives." In *Characteristics and Functions of Opioids*, Vol. 4, edited by M. Van Ree. New York: Elsevier, 1978a.

Judd, S.J., Rakoff, J.S., and Yen, S.S.C. "Inhibition of Gonadotropin and Prolactin Release by Dopamine: Effect of Endogenous Estradiol Levels." *Journal of Clinical Endocrinology and Metabolism* 47 (1978): 494–498.

Kanas, N., Rogers, M., Kreth, E., Patterson, L., and Campbell, R. "The Effectiveness of Group Psychotherapy During the First Three Weeks of Hospitalization." *Journal of Nervous Mental Disease* 168 (1980): 487–492.

Kane, J., Cooper, T., Sachar, E., Halpern, F., and Bailine, S. "Clozapine: Plasma Levels and Prolactin Response." *Psychopharmacology* 73 (1981): 184–187.

Kane, J., Quitkin, F., Rifkin, A., and Klein, D.F. "Comparison of the Incidence and Severity of Extrapyramidal Side Effects With Fluphenazine Enanthate and Fluphenazine Decanoate." *American Journal of Psychiatry* 135 (1978): 1539.

Kane, J., Rifkin, A., Quitkin, F., and Klein, D.F. "A Pilot Study of 'Low Dose' Fluphenazine Decanoate in Outpatient Schizophrenics." *Psychopharmacology Bulletin* 15 (1979a): 78.

Kane, J., Rifkin, A., Quitkin, F., and Klein, D.F. "Low Dose Fluphenazine Decanoate in Maintenance Treatment of Schizophrenia." *Journal of Psychiatric Research* 1 (1979b): 341–348.

Kane, J., Woerner, M.G., and Rifkin, A. "Low Dose Neuroleptics in Outpatient Schizophrenics." *Proceedings III World Congress of Biological Psychiatry* S181 (1981).

Karon, B., and O'Grady, P. "Intellectual Test Changes in Schizophrenic Patients in the First Six Months of Treatment." *Psychotherapy: Theory, Research and Practice* 6 (1969): 88–96.

Karon, B.P., and Vandenbos, G.R. "Experience, Medication and the Effectiveness of Psychotherapy With Schizophrenics." *British Journal of Psychiatry* 116 (1970): 427–428.

Karon, B.P., and Vandenbos, G.R. "The Consequences of Psychotherapy to Schizophrenic Patients." *Psychotherapy: Theory, Research and Practice* 9 (1972): 111–119.

Kennedy, P., and Hird, F. "Description and Evaluation of a Short Stay Admission Ward." *British Journal of Psychiatry* 136 (1980): 205–215.

Kiloh, L.G., Williams, S.E., and Grant, D.A. "A Double-Blind Comparative Trial of Loxapine and Trifluoperazine in Acute and Chronic Schizophrenia Patients." *Journal of International Medical Research* 4 (1976): 441–448.

Kirkegaard, C., Bjorum, N., Cohn, D., and Lauridsen, U.B. "Thyrotropin-Releasing Hormone (TRH) Stimulation Test in Manic-Depressive Illness." *Archives of General Psychiatry* 35 (1978): 1017–1021.

Kleinberg, D.L., and Frantz, A.G. "Human Prolactin: Measurement in Plasma by *in vitro* Bioassay." *Journal of Clinical Investigation* 50 (1971): 1557–1567.

Klein, D.F., and Rosen, B. "Premorbid Asocial Adjustment and Response to Phenothiazine Treatment Among Schizophrenic Inpatients." *Archives of General Psychiatry* 29 (1973): 480.

Klett, C.J., and Caffey, E. "Evaluating the Long-Term Need for Antiparkinson Drugs by Chronic Schizophrenics." *Archives of General Psychiatry* 26 (1972): 374.

Knight, A., Hirsch, S., and Platt, S.D. "Clinical Change as a Function of Brief Admission to a Hospital in a Controlled Study Using the Present State Examination." *British Journal of Psychiatry* 137 (1980): 170–180.

Kolakowska, T., Fraser, S., Franklin, M., and Knox, I. "Neuroendocrine Tests During Treatment With Neuroleptic Drugs: I. Plasma Prolactin Response to Chlorpromazine Challenge." *Psychopharmacology* 72 (1981): 283–285.

Kolakowska, T., Orr, M., Gelter, M., Heggie, M., Wiles, D., and Franklin, M. "Clinical Significance of Plasma Drug and Prolactin Levels During Acute Chlorpromazine Treatment: A Replication Study." *British Journal of Psychiatry* 135 (1979): 352–359.

Kurland, A.A., and Richardson, J.M. "A Comparative Study of Two Long-Acting Phenothiazine Preparations, Fluphenazine Enanthate and Fluphenazine Decanoate." *Psychopharmacologia* 4 (1966): 320.

Kurland, A.A., McCabe, O.L., Hanlon, T.E., and Sullivan, D. "The Treatment of Perceptual Disturbances in Schizophrenia With Naloxone Hydrochloride." *American Journal of Psychiatry* 134 (1977): 1408–1410.

Lal, S., and Nair, N.V.P. "Growth Hormone and Prolactin Responses in Neuropsychiatric Research." In *Neuroendocrine Correlates in Neurology and Psychiatry.* New York: Elsevier North Holland Biochemical Press, 1979.

Lamberg, B.A., Linnoila, M., Fogelholm, R., Olkimora, M., Kotilainen, P., and Saarinen, P. "The Effect of Psychotropic Drugs on the TSH-Response to Thyroberin (TRH)." *Neuroendocrinology* 24 (1977): 90–97.

Langer, G. "The Prolactin Model for the Study of the Pharmacodynamics of Neuroleptics in Man." In *Neuroendocrine Correlates in Neurology and Psychiatry,* edited by E.E. Muller and A. Agnoli. New York: Elsevier, 1979.

Langer, G., Sachar, E.J., Gruen, P.H., and Halpern, F.S. "Human Prolactin Responses to Neuroleptic Drugs Correlate With Antischizophrenic Potency." *Nature* 266 (1977a): 639–640.

Langer, G.R., Sachar, E.J., and Halpern, F.S. "Effect of Dopamine and Neuroleptics on Plasma Growth Hormone and Prolactin in Normal Men." *Psychoneuroendocrinology* 3 (1978): 165–169.

Langer, G.R., Sachar, E.J., Halpern, F.S., Gruen, P.H., and Solomon, M. "The Prolactin Response to Neuroleptic Drugs. A Test of Dopaminergic Blockade: Neuroendocrine Studies in Normal Men." *Journal of Clinical Endocrinology and Metabolism* 45 (1977b): 996–1002.

Langsley, D.G., and Kaplan, D.M. *The Treatment of Families in Crisis.* New York: Grune & Stratton, Inc., 1968.

Langsley, D.G., Machotka, P., and Flomenhaft, K. "Avoiding Mental Hospital Admission: A Follow-Up Study." *American Journal of Psychiatry* 127 (1971): 1391–1394.

Lapolla, A., and Nash, L.R. "Treatment of Phenothiazine-Induced Parkinsonism With Biperiden." *Current Therapeutic Research* 7 (1965): 536.

Laughren T.P., Brown, W., and Petruccia, J. "The Effect of Thioridazine on Serum Testosterone." *American Journal of Psychiatry* 135 (1978): 492–494.

Laughren, T.P., Brown, W.A., and Williams, B.W. "Serum Prolactin and Clinical State During Neuroleptic Treatment and Withdrawal." *American Journal of Psychiatry* 136 (1979): 108–110.

LeBlanc, H., Lachelin, G.C.L., Abu-Fadil, S., and Yen, S.S.C. "Effects of Dopamine Infusion on Pituitary Hormone Secretion in Humans." *Journal of Clinical Endocrinology and Metabolism* 43 (1976): 668.

Leff, J.P., and Wing, J.K. "Trial of Maintenance Therapy in Schizophrenia." *British Medical Journal* 3 (1971): 599.

Lehman, H., Nair, N.P.V., and Kline, N.S. "Endorphin and Naloxone in Psychiatric Patients: Clinical and Biological Effects." *American Journal of Psychiatry* 136 (1979): 762–766.

Lemberger, L., and Crabtree, R.E. "Pharmacologic Effects in Man of a Potent, Long-Acting Dopamine Receptor Agonist." *Science* 205 (1979): 1151–1153.

Leppaluoto, J., Mannisto, P., Ranta T., and Linnoila, M. "Inhibition of Mid-Cycle Gonadotropin Release in Healthy Women by Pimozide and Fusaric Acid." *Acta Endocrinologica* 81 (1976): 455–560.

Levin J., Schooler, N., and Cassano, G. "The Role of Depot Neuroleptics in the Treatment of Schizophrenic Patients." *Psychological Medicine* 9 (1978): 383–386.

Levine, J., Schooler, N., Serene, F., Escobar, J., Gelenberg, A., Mandel, H., Somer, R., and Steinbook, R. "Discontinuation of Oral and Depot Fluphenazine in Schizophrenic Patients After One Year of Continuous Medication." In *Long-Term Effects of Neuroleptics,* edited by F. Cattabeni. New York: Raven Press, 1980.

Lindberg, D. "Management of Schizophrenia." *Acta Psychiatrica Scandinavica Suppl 289* 63 (1981): 100–112.

Lindholm, H., Gullberg, B., Ohman, A., and Sedvall, G. "Effects of Perphenazine Enanthate Injections on Prolactin Levels in Plasma for Schizophrenic Women and Men." *Psychopharmacology* 57 (1978): 1–4.

Lindstrom, L.H., and Persson, E. "Propanolol in Chronic Schizophrenia: A Controlled Study in Neuroleptic-Treated Patients." *British Journal of Psychiatry* 137 (1980): 126–130.

Linn, M.W., Caffey, E.M., Klett, C.J., and Hogarty, G. "Hospital vs. Community (Foster) Care for Psychiatric Patients: A Veterans Administration Cooperative Study." *Archives of General Psychiatry* 34 (1977): 78–83.

Linnoila, M., Viokari, M., and Vaisanen, H. "Plasma Neuroleptic and Prolactin Levels in Mentally Retarded Patients." *Acta Pharmacologica et Toxicologica* 46 (1980): 1159–1160.

Lipinski, T., Meyer, R., Kornetsky, C., and Cohen, B.M. "Naloxone in Schizophrenia." *Lancet* 1 (1979): 1292–1293.

Magrini, G., Mean, F., Martin-DuPan, R., Baumann, P., and Feiber, J.P. "Testicular Function During Chronic Neuroleptic Therapy." In *Neuroendocrinology: Biological and Clinical Aspects,* edited by A. Polleri and R.M. MacLeod. New York: Academic Press, 1979.

Mahon, W., and Daniels, E. "A Method for the Assessment of Reports of Drug Trials." *Canadian Medical Association Journal* 90 (1964): 565.

Malih, S.C., and Kumar, K. "Loxapine in Adolescent Schizophrenia." *Current Therapeutic Research* 28 (1980): 432–446.

Mancini, A.M., Guitelman, A., Vargas, C.A., Debeljuk, L., and Aparicio, N.J. "Effect of Sulpiride on Serum Prolactin Levels in Humans." *Journal of Clinical Endocrinology and Metabolism* 42 (1976): 181–184.

Martin-DuPan, R., and Baumann, D. "Neuroendocrine Effects of Chronic Neuroleptic Therapy in Male Psychiatric Patients." *Psychoneuroendocrinology* 3 (1979): 245–252.

Masala, A., Delitala, G., Alagna, S., and Devilla, L. "Effect of Pimozide on Levodopa Induced Growth Hormone Release in Man." *Clinical Endocrinology* 7 (1977): 253–256.

May, P.R.A. "Psychotherapy Research in Schizophrenia—Another View of Present Reality." *Schizophrenia Bulletin* 9 (1974): 126–132.

May, P.R.A. "Schizophrenia: Evaluation of Treatment Methods." In *Comprehensive Textbook of Psychiatry*, edited by A.M. Freedman, H.I. Kaplan, and B.J. Sadock. Baltimore: Williams & Wilkins Co., 1975.

May, P.R.A. *Treatment of Schizophrenia: A Comparative Study of Five Treatment Methods.* New York: Science House, 1968.

May, P.R.A., and Tuma, A.H. "Methodological Problems in Psychotherapy Research: Observations on the Karon-Vandenbos Study of Psychotherapy and Drugs in Schizophrenia." *British Journal of Psychiatry* 117 (1970): 569–570.

May, P.R.A., Tuma, A.H., and Dixon, W. "Schizophrenia—a Follow-Up Study of Results of Treatments: I. Design and Other Problems." *Archives of General Psychiatry* 33 (1976a): 474–480.

May, P.R.A., Tuma, A.H., and Dixon, W.J. "Schizophrenia: A Follow-Up Study of the Results of Five Forms of Treatment." *Archives of General Psychiatry* 38 (1981): 776–784.

May, P.R.A., Tuma, A.H., Yale, C., Potepam, P., and Dixon, W.J. "Schizophrenia—A Follow-Up Study of Results of Treatment. II. Hospital Stay Over Two to Five Years." *Archives of General Psychiatry* 33 (1976b): 481–506.

McClelland, H.A., Farquharson, R.G., Leyburn, P., and Furness, J. "A Very High-Dose Fluphenazine Decanoate: A Controlled Trial in Chronic Schizophrenia." *Archives of General Psychiatry* 33 (1976): 1435.

Meco, G., Casacchia, M., Attenni, M., Iafrate, A., Ecari, U., and Argenta, G. "Haloperidol Decanoate: An Open Study in Acute and Chronic Schizophrenic Outpatients." *Proceedings III World Congress of Biological Psychiatry* p. 300, 1981.

Meltzer, H.Y., and Fang, V.S. "The Effect of Neuroleptics on Serum Prolactin in Schizophrenic Patients." *Archives of General Psychiatry* 33 (1976): 279–286.

Meltzer, H.Y., Goode, D.J., Schyve, P.A., Young. M., and Fang, V.S. "Effect of Clozapine on Human Serum Prolactin Levels." *American Journal of Psychiatry* 136 (1979): 1550–1555.

Meltzer, H.Y., Paul, S.M., and Fang, V.S. "Effect of Flupenthixol and Butaclamol Isomers on Prolactin Secretion in Rats." *Psychopharmacology* 51 (1977): 181–183.

Meltzer, H.Y., Simonovich, M., Fang, V.S., Piyakalamala, S., and Young, M. "A Comparison of the Effects of Antipsychotic Drugs on Pituitary, Striatal and Limbic System Postsynaptic Dopamine Receptors." *Life Sciences* 23 (1978): 605–610.

Meltzoff, J., and Blumenthal, R.K. *The Day Treatment Center: Principles, Application, and Evaluation.* Springfield: Charles C. Thomas, 1966.

Messier, M., Finnerty, R., Botvin, C., and Grinspoon, L. "A Follow-Up Study of Intensively Treated Chronic Schizophrenic Patients." *American Journal of Psychiatry* 125 (1969): 1123–1127.

Michaux, M.H., Chelst, M.R., Foster, S.A., and Pruim, R.J. "Day and Full Psychiatric Treatment: A Controlled Comparison." *Current Therapeutic Research* 14 (1972): 279–292.

Michaux, M.H., Chelst, M.R., Foster, S.A., Pruim, R.J., and Dasinger, E.M. "Postrelease Adjustment of Day and Full-Time Psychiatric Patients." *Archives of General Psychiatry* 29 (1973): 647–651.

Michaux, M.J., Kurland, A.A., and Agallianos, D. "Chlorpromazine-Chlordiazepoxide and Chlorpromazine-Imipramine Treatment of Newly Hospitalized Acutely Ill Psychiatric Patients." *Current Therapeutic Research* Suppl. 8 (1966): 117.

Mielke, D.H., and Gallant, D.M. "An Oral Opiate Antagonist in Chronic Schizophrenia: A Pilot Study." *American Journal of Psychiatry* 134 (1977): 1430–1431.

Mielke, D.H., Gallant, D.M., and Kessler, C. "An Evaluation of a Unique New Antipsychotic Agent, Sulpiride: Effects on Serum Prolactin and Growth Hormone Levels." *American Journal of Psychiatry* 134 (1977): 1371–1375.

Mims, R.B., Scott, C., Modebe, O., and Bethume, J. "Inhibition of L-Dopa Induced Growth Hormone Stimulation by Pyridoxine and Chlorpromazine." *Journal of Clinical Endocrinology and Metabolism* 40 (1975): 256–259.

Moller, H.J., Kissing, W., and Maurach, R. "Relationships Between Serum Levels of Haloperidol and Prolactin, Antipsychotic Effect, and Extrapyramidal Side Effects." *Pharmakopsychiatrie* 14 (1981): 27–34.

Moore, D.F. "Treatment of Acute Schizophrenia With Loxapine Succinate (Loxitane) in a Controlled Study With Chlorpromazine." *Current Therapeutic Research* 18 (1975): 172.

Morgan, R., and Cheadle, J. "Maintenance Treatment of Chronic Schizophrenics With Neuroleptic Drugs." *Acta Psychiatrica Scandinavica* 50 (1974): 78–85.

Moyano, C. "A Double-Blind Comparison of Loxitane Loxapine Succinate and Trifluoperazine Hydrochloride in Chronic Schizophrenic Patients." *Diseases of the Nervous System* 36 (1975): 301.

Muller, E.E., Stefanini, E., Camanni, F., Locatelli, V., Massara, F., Spano, P.F., and Cocchi, D. "Prolactin Releasing Effect of Sulpiride Isomers in Rats and Man." *Journal of Neural Transmission* 46 (1979): 205–214.

Murillo, L., and Exner, J. "The Effects of Regressive ECT With Process Schizophrenics." *American Journal of Psychiatry* 130 (1973): 269–273.

Murray, M.A.F., Brancroft, J.H.J., Anderson, D.C., Tennent, T.G., and Carr, P.J. "Endocrine Changes in Male Sexual Deviants After Treatment With Antiandrogens, Oestrogens or Tranquilizers." *Journal of Endocrinology* 67 (1975): 179–188.

Naber, D., Ackenheil, M., Laakman, G., Fischer, H., and Von Werder, K. "Basal and Stimulated Levels of Prolactin, TSH, and LH in Serum of Chronic Schizophrenic Patients Treated with Long-Term Neuroleptics: Relations to Psychopathology." In *Advances in Biochemistry and Psychopharmacology*, edited by F. Cattaben, G. Racagni, P. Spano, and E. Costa. New York: Raven Press, 1980a.

Naber, D., Ackenheil, M., Laakman, G., Fischer, H., and Von Werder, K. "Basal and Stimulated Levels of Prolactin, TSH and LH in Serum of Chronic Schizophrenic Patients, Long-Term Treated With Neuroleptics." *Pharmakopsychiatrie* 13 (1980): 325–330.

Naber, D., Finkbeiner, C., Fischer, B., Zander, K.J., and Ackenheil, M. "Effect of Long-Term Neuroleptic Treatment on Prolactin and Norepinephrine Levels in Serum of Chronic Schizophrenics: Relations to Psychotherapy and Extrapyramidal Symptoms." *Neuropsychobiology* 6 (1980b): 181–189.

Naber, D., Fischer, F., and Ackenheil, M. "Effect of Long-Term Neuroleptic Treatment on Dopamine Tuberoinfundibular System: Development of Tolerance?" *Communications in Psychopharmacology* 3 (1979): 59–65.

Naber, D., Steinbock, H., and Greil, W. "Effects of Short and Long-Term Neuroleptic Treatment on Thyroid Function." *Progress in Neuro-Psychopharmacology* 4 (1980c): 199–206.

Nair, N.P.V., Yassa, R., Lal, S., Cervantes, P., Guyda, H. "Effect of Clozapine on Apomorphine Induced Growth Hormone Secretion and Serum Prolactin Concentrations in Schizophrenia." *Neuropsychobiology* 5 (1979): 136–142.

Nathan, R.S., Asnis, G.M., Dyrenfurth, I., Halpern, F.S., Halbreich, U., Ostrow, L.C., and Sachar, E.J. "Plasma Prolactin and Testosterone During Penfluridol Treatment." *Lancet* 2 (1980): 94.

National Institute of Mental Health, "Short-Term Improvement in Schizophrenia: The Contribution of Background Factors." *American Journal of Psychiatry* 124 (1968): 900.

Neborsky, R., Janowsky, D., Munson, E., and Depry, D. "Rapid Treatment of Acute Psychotic Symptoms With High and Low Dose Haloperidol." *Archives of General Psychiatry* 38 (1981): 195–199.

Nikitopoulou, G., Thorner, M., Crammer, J., and Ladev, M. "Prolactin and Psychophysiologic Measures After Single Dose of Thioridazine." *Clinical Pharmacology and Therapeutics* 21 (1976): 422–429.

O'Brien, C., Hamm, K., Ray, B., Pierce, J., Luborsky, L., and Mintz J. "Group vs. Individual Psychotherapy With Schizophrenics." *Archives of General Psychiatry* 27 (1972): 474–478.

Ohman, R., and Axelsson, R. "Relationship Between Prolactin Response and Antipsychotic Effect of Thioridazine in Psychiatric Patients." *European Journal of Clinical Pharmacology* 14 (1978): 111–116.

Ohman, R., Forsman, A., and Larsson, M. "Prolactin Response to Haloperidol After A Single Dose and During Prolonged Administration." *Current Therapeutic Research* 27 (1980): 137–143.

Orlov, P., Kasparian, G., DiMascio, A., and Cole, J.O. "Withdrawal of Antiparkinson Drugs." *Archives of General Psychiatry* 25 (1971): 410.

Orr, M., and Oppenheimer, C. "Effects of Naloxone on Auditory Hallucinations." *British Medical Journal* 2 (1978): 481–482.

Orzack, M.H., Bramconnier, R., and Gardos, G. "C.N.S. Effects of Propranolol in Man." *Psychopharmacology* 29 (1973): 299–306.

Paprocki, J., Barcala Peixoto, M.P. and Andrade, N.M. "A Controlled Double-Blind Comparison Between Loxapine and Haloperidol in Acute Newly Hospitalized Schizophrenic Patients." *Psychopharmacology Bulletin* 12 (1976): 32–34.

Paprocki, J., and Versiani, M. "A Double-Blind Comparison Between Loxapine and Haloperidol by Parenteral Route in Acute Schizophrenia." *Current Therapeutic Research* 21 (1977): 80.

Pasamanick, B., Scarpitti, F., and Dinitz, S. *Schizophrenics in the Community: An Experimental Study in the Prevention of Hospitalization.* New York: Appleton-Century Crafts, 1967.

Peckhold, J.C., Ananth, J.V., Ban, T.A., and Lehmann, H.E. "Lack of Indication for Use of Antiparkinson Medication." *Diseases of the Nervous System* 32 (1971): 538.

Peet, M., Middlemiss, D.N., and Yaes, R.A. "Pharmacokinetic Interaction Between Propranolol in Chlorpromazine in Schizophrenic Patients." (ltr. to ed.) *Lancet* 2 (1980): 978.

Penn, H., Racy, J., Lapham, L., Mandel, M., and Sandt, J. "Catatonic Behavior, Viral Encephalopathy and Death." *Archives of General Psychiatry* 27 (1972): 758.

Platt, S., Hirsch, S.R., and Knight, D.C. "Effects of Brief Hospitalization on Psychiatric Patients' Behavior and Social Functioning." *Acta Psychiatrica Scandinavica* 63 (1981): 117–128.

Pourmand, M., Rodriquez-Arnao, M., Weightman, D., Hall, R., Cook, D., Lewis, M., and Scanlon, M. "Domperidone: A Novel Agent for the Investigation of Anterior Pituitary Function and Control in Man." *Clinical Endocrinology* 12 (1980): 211–215.

Prien, R.F., Caffey, E.M., and Klett, C.T. "A Comparison of Lithium Carbonate and Chlorpromazine in the Treatment of Excited Schizoaffectives." *Archives of General Psychiatry* 27 (1972): 182–189.

Prien, R.F., Caffey, E.M., Jr., and Klett C.T. "A Comparison of Lithium Carbonate and Chlorpromazine in the Treatment of Mania." *Archives of General Psychiatry* 26 (1972): 146–153.

Prien, R.F., and Cole, J.O. "High-Dose Chlorpromazine Therapy in Chronic Schizophrenia." *Archives of General Psychiatry* 18 (1968): 482.

Prien, R.F., Levine, J., and Cole, J.O. "High-Dose Trifluoperazine Therapy in Chronic Schizophrenia." *American Journal of Psychiatry* 126 (1969): 305.

Prusoff, B.A., Williams, D.H., Weissman, M.M., and Astrachan, B.M. "A Controlled Clinical Trial of Amitriptyline Added to Perphenazine in the Treatment of Depressed Schizophrenics." *Psychopharmacology Bulletin* 15 (1978): 80.

Prusoff, B.A., Williams, D.H., Weissman, M.M., and Astrachan, B.M. "Treatment of Secondary Depression in Schizophrenia." *Archives of General Psychiatry* 36 (1979): 569.

Quitkin, F., Rifkin, A., Kane, J., Ramos-Loren, J.R., and Klein, D.F. "Long-Acting Oral vs. Injectable Antipsychotic Drugs in Schizophrenia." *Archives of General Psychiatry* 35 (1978): 889.

Quitkin, F., Rifkin, A., and Klein, D.F. "Very High Dose vs. Standard Dosage Fluphenazine in Schizophrenia." *Archives of General Psychiatry* 32 (1975): 1276.

Rackensperger, W., Fritsch, W., Schwarz, D., Stutte, K.H., and von Zerssen, D.V. "Wirkung des Beta-Rezeptoren-Blockers Propranolol auf Manien." *Archiv fuer Psychiatrie und Nervenkrankheiten* 222 (1976): 223–243.

Rackensperger, W., Gaupp, R., Mattke, D.J., Schwartz, D., and Stutte, K.H. "Behandlung von akuten schizophrenen Psychosen mit Beta-Rezeptoren-Blockern." *Archiv fuer Psychiatrie und Nervenkrankheiten* 219 (1974): 29–36.

Ragheb, M., Berney, S., and Ban, T. "Naltrexone in Chronic Schizophrenia." *International Pharmacopsychiatry* 15 (1980): 1–5.

Rama-Rao, V.A., Bailey, J., and Coppen, A. "A Clinical and Pharmacodynamic Evaluation of Sulpiride." *Psychopharmacology* 73 (1981): 77–80.

Rama-Rao, V.A., Bishop, M., and Coppen, A. "Clinical State, Plasma Levels of Haloperidol and Prolactin: A Correlation Study in Chronic Schizophrenia." *British Journal of Psychiatry* 137 (1980): 518–521.

Ramsay, R.A., Ban, T.A., Lehmann, H.E., Saxena, B.M., and Bennett, J. "A Comparative Study of Molindone and Trifluoperazine." *Current Therapeutic Research* 12 (1970): 438–440.

Reibel, S., and Herz, M. "Limitations of Brief Hospital Treatment." *American Journal of Psychiatry* 133 (1976): 518–521.

Rogers, C.R., Gendlin, E.G., Kiesler, D.J., and Traux, C.B. (eds.) *The Therapeutic Relationship and Its Impact: A Study of Psychotherapy With Schizophrenics.* Madison: University of Wisconsin Press, 1967.

Roose, K. "Monthly Haloperidol Decanoate as a Replacement for Maintenance Therapy." *Proceedings from III World Congress of Biological Psychiatry* F410, 1981.

Rosen, J.N. *Direct Analysis: Selected Papers.* New York: Grune & Stratton, Inc., 1953.

Rosen, J.N. "The Treatment of Schizophrenic Psychoses by Direct Analytic Therapy." *Psychiatric Quarterly* 21 (1947): 117–119.

Rosenbaum, A.H., Maruta, T., Jiang, N.S., Avger, R., De La Fuente, J., and Duane, D. "Endocrine Testing in Tardive Dyskinesia: Preliminary Report" *American Journal of Psychiatry* 136 (1979): 102–103.

Rotrosen, J., Angrist, B., Gershon, S., Paquin, J., Branchey, L., Oleshansky, M., Halpern, F., and Sachar, E.J. "Neuroendocrine Effects of Apomorphine: Characterization of Response Patterns and Application to Schizophrenic Research." *British Journal of Psychiatry* 135 (1979): 444–456.

Rubin, R.T. "Plasma Prolactin and Testosterone, Dating Penfluridol Treatment." *Lancet* [sic] (1980): 370.

Rubin, R.T., and Forster, B. "Haloperidol Stimulation of Prolactin Secretion: How Many Blood Samples are Needed to Define the Hormone Response?" *Communication in Psychopharmacology* 4 (1980): 41–47.

Rubin, R.T., and Hays, S.E. "Profiles of Prolactin Response to Antipsychotic Drugs: Some Methodologic Considerations." *Psychopharmacology Bulletin* 14 (1978): 9–11.

Rubin, R.T., and Hays, S.E. "Variability of Prolactin Responses to i.v. and i.m. Haloperidol in Normal Men." *Psychopharmacology* 61 (1979): 17–24.

Rubin, R.T., Poland, R.E., O'Connor, D., Gouin, P.R., and Tower, B.B. "Selective Neuroendocrine Effects of Low-Dose Haloperidol in Normal Adult Men." *Psychopharmacology* 47 (1976): 135–140.

Sachar, E.J., Gruen, P.H., Altman, N., Halpern, F.S., and Frantz, A.G. "Use of Neuroendocrine Techniques in Psychopharmacological Research." In *Hormones, Behavior, and Psychopathology*, edited by E.J. Sachar. New York: Raven Press, 1976.

Sainsbury, P., and Grad, J. "The Effects That Patients Have on Their Families in a Community Care and a Control Psychiatric Service: A Two-Year Follow-up." *British Journal of Psychiatry* 114 (1968): 265–268.

Saldanha, V.F., Havard, C.W.H., Bird, R., and Gardner, R. "The Effect of Chlorpromazine on Pituitary Function." *Clinical Endocrinology* 1 (1972): 173–180.

Salzman, C. "The Use of ECT in the Treatment of Schizophrenia." *American Journal of Psychiatry* 137 (1980): 9.

Schenk, G.K., Enders, P., Engelmeier, M.P., Ewert, T., Herdemerten, S., Kohler, K.H., Lodemann, E., Matz, D., and Pacvk, J. "Application of the Morphine Antagonist Naloxone in Psychic Disorders." *Arzneimittel Forschung* 28 (1978): 1274–1277.

Schiele, B.C. "Loxapine Succinate: A Controlled Double-Blind Study in Chronic Schizophrenia." *Diseases of the Nervous System* 18 (1975): 361.

Schooler, N. "How Generalizable are the Results of Clinical Trials?" *Psychopharmacology Bulletin* 16 (1980): 29–31.

Schooler, N.R., and Levine, J. "Fluphenazine and Fluphenazine HCl in the Treatment of Schizophrenic Patients." In *Proceedings of the Meeting of the Collegium International Neuro-Psychopharmacologicum*, edited by P. Deniker, C. Radouca-Thomas, and A. Villeneuve. Oxford: Pergamon Press, 1978.

Schooler, N.R., Levine, J., and Severe, J.B. "Depot Fluphenazine in the Prevention of Relapse in Schizophrenia: Evaluation of a Treatment Regimen." *Psychopharmacology Bulletin* 15 (1979): 44.

Schwimm, C., Schward, H., McIntosh, C., Milstrey, H.R., Wills, B., and Kobberling, J. "Effect of Dopamine Receptor Blocking Agent Pimozide on the Growth Hormone Response to Arginine and Exercise and the Spontaneous Growth Hormone Fluctuations." *Journal of Clinical Endocrinology and Metabolism* 43 (1976): 1183–1185.

Schyve, D.M., Smithline, F., and Meltzer, H.Y. "Neuroleptic-Induced Prolactin Level Elevation and Breast Cancer: An Emerging Clinical Issue." *Archives of General Psychiatry* 35 (1978): 1291.

Sedvall, G. "Neuroendocrine Correlates in Schizophrenia." In *Neuroendocrine Correlates in Neurology and Psychiatry*, edited by E. Muller and A. Agnoli. Amsterdam: Elsevier Press, 1979.

Seeman, P., Chau-Wong, M., Tedesco, J., and Wong, K. "Brain Receptors for Antipsychotic Drugs and Dopamine: Direct Bindings Assays." *Proceedings of the National Academy of Sciences of the United States of America* 72 (1975): 4376–4380.

Seeman, P., Lee, T., Chau-Wong, M. and Wong, K. "Antipsychotic Drug Doses and Neuroleptic/Dopamine Receptors." *Nature* 261 (1976): 717–719.

Selman, F.B., McClure, R.F., and Elwig, H. "Loxapine Succinate: A Double-Blind Comparison With Haloperidol and Placebo in Acute Schizophrenics." *Current Therapeutic Research* 19 (1976): 645.

Seth, S., Mahal, A.S., and Kumar, K.A. "A Double-Blind Comparative Trial of Loxapine and Trifluoperazine in Chronic Schizophrenia Patients." *Current Therapeutic Research* 25 (1979): 320–329.

Sherman, L., Kim, S., Benjamin, F., and Kolodny, H.D. "Effect of Chlorpromazine on Serum Growth Hormone Concentration in Man." *New England Journal of Medicine* 284 (1971): 72–74.

Shopsin, B., Hirsch, J., and Gershon, S. "Visual Hallucinations and Propranolol." *Biological Psychiatry* 10 (1975): 105–107.

Shopsin, B., Klein, H., Aaronsom, M., and Collora, M. "Clozapine Chlorpromazine and Placebo in Newly Hospitalized Acutely Schizophrenic Patients." *Archives of General Psychiatry* 36 (1979): 657.

Shopsin, B., Pearson, E., Gershon, S., and Collins, P. "A Controlled Double-Blind Comparison Between Loxapine Succinate and Chlorpromazine in Acute Newly Hospitalized Schizophrenic Patients." *Current Therapeutic Research* 14 (1972a): 739.

Shopsin, B., Pearson, E., Gershon, S., and Collins, P. "A Controlled Study of Lithium vs. Chlorpromazine in Acute Schizophrenics." *British Journal of Psychiatry* 119 (1972b): 435–440.

Simon, P., Fermanian, J., Ginestet, D., Goujet, M.A., and Peron-Magnan, P. "Standard and Long-Acting Depot Neuroleptics in Chronic Schizophrenics: An 18-Month Open Multicentric Study." *Archives of General Psychiatry* 35 (1978): 893.

Simpson, G.M., Amin, M., and Edwards, J.G. "A Double-Blind Comparison of Molindone and Trifluoperazine in the Treatment of Acute Schizophrenia." *Journal of Clinical Pharmacology* 11 (1971): 227–236.

Simpson, G.M., Amin, M., Kunz-Bartholini, E., and Laska, E. "Problems in the Evaluation of the Optimal Dose of a Phenothiazine (Butaperazine)." *Diseases of the Nervous System* 29 (1968): 478.

Simpson, G.M., and Cuculic Z. "A Double-Blind Comparison of Loxapine Succinate And Trifluoperazine in Newly Admitted Schizophrenic Patients." *Journal of Clinical Pharmacology* 16 (1976): 60–65.

Simpson, G.M., Branchey, M.H., and Lee, J.H. "A Trial of Naltrexone in Chronic Schizophrenia." *Current Therapeutic Research* 22 (1977): 909–913.

Siris, E.S., Siris, S.G., van Kammen, D., Docherty, J.P., Alexander, P.E., and Bunney, W.E., Jr. "Effects of Dopamine Blockade on Gonadotropins And Testosterone in Men." *American Journal of Psychiatry* 137 (1980): 211–213.

Siris, S.G., van Kammen, D.P., and DeFraites, E.G. "Serum Prolactin and Antipsychotic Responses to Pimozide in Schizophrenia." *Psychopharmacology Bulletin* 14 (1978): 11–14.

Small, J., Kellams, J., Milstein, V., and Moore, J. "A Placebo-Controlled Study of Lithium Combined With Neuroleptics in Chronic Schizophrenic Patients." *American Journal of Psychiatry* 132 (1975): 1315–1317.

Smith, K., Surphlis, W.R.P., Gynther, M.D., and Shimkunas, A.M. "ECT-Chlorpromazine and Chlorpromazine Compared in the Treatment of Schizophrenia." *Journal of Nervous and Mental Disease* 144 (1967): 284.

Smith, R.C., Dekirmenjian, H., Crayton, J., Klass, D., and Davis, J.M. "Blood Levels of Neuroleptic Drugs in Non-Responding Chronic Schizophrenic Patients." *Archives of General Psychiatry* 36 (1979a): 579.

Smith, R.C., Dekirmenjian, H., Davis, J.M., Crayton, J., and Evans, H. "Plasma Butaperazine Levels in Long-Term Chronic Non-Responding Schizophrenics." *Communications in Psychopharmacology* 1 (1977a): 319.

Smith, R.C., Tamminga, C., Crayton, J., and Davis, J. "Relationship of Butaperazine Blood Levels to Plasma Prolactin in Chronic Schizophrenic Patients." *Psychopharmacology* 66 (1979b): 29–33.

Smith, R.C., Tamminga, C.A., and Davis, J.M. "Effect of Apomorphine on Schizophrenic Symptoms." *Journal of Neural Transmission* 40 (1977b): 171–176.

Smith, R.C., Tamminga, C., Haraszti, J., Pandey, G.N., and Davis, J.M. "Effects of Dopamine Agonists in Tardive Dyskinesia." *American Journal of Psychiatry* 134 (1977c): 763.

Snyder, S.H., Cresse, I., and Burt, D.R. "The Brain's Dopamine Receptor: Labelling With ^{3}H-Haloperidol." *Communications in Psychopharmacology* 1 (1975): 663–673.

Sommer, C., and Weinberg, J. "Techniques and Factors Reversing the Trends of Population Growth in Illinois State Hospitals." *American Journal of Psychiatry* 100 (1944): 456–461.

Spohn, H.E., Lacousiere, R., Thompson, K., and Coyne, L. "Phenothiazine Effects on Psychological and Psychophysiological Dysfunction in Chronic Schizophrenics." *Archives of General Psychiatry* 34 (1977): 633.

Stam, F.C. "Enkele Ervarigen mit Propranolol-Behandeling van Schifrenen." *Ned. Tdschrft. Psychiat. voor Psychiat.* (1971): 422–426.

Stein, L., and Test, M. "Alternative to Mental Hospital Treatment I, II, and III." *Archives of General Psychiatry* 37 (1980): 392–411.

Steinbook, R.M., Goldstein, B.J., Banzer, B., Moreno, S.S., and Jacobson, A.F. "Loxapine: A Double-Blind Comparison With Chlorpromazine in Acute Schizophrenic Patients." *Current Therapeutic Research* 15 (1973): 1–7.

Steiner, M., Latz, A., Blum, L., Atsmon, A., and Wijsenbeek, H. "Propranolol vs. Chlorpromazine in the Treatment of Psychoses Associated With Childbearing." *Pyschiatria Neurologia Neurochirurgia* 76 (1973): 421–426.

Sullivan, H.S. *Clinical Studies in Psychiatry.* New York: W.W. Norton & Co., Inc., 1956.

Tamminga, C.A., Schaffer, M.H., Smith, R.C., and Davis, J.M. "Schizophrenic Symptoms Improve With Apomorphine." *Science* 200 (1978): 567–568.

Tamminga, C.A., Smith, R.C., Pandey, G., Frohman, L., and Davis, J.M. "Behavioral and Neuroendocrine Evaluation of Tardive Dyskinesia." *Society for Neuroendocrinology* 6 (1976): 699.

Tamminga, C.A., Smith, R.C., Pandey, G., Frohman, L.A., and Davis, J.M. "A Neuroendocrine Study of Supersensitivity in Tardive Dyskinesia." *Archives of General Psychiatry* 34 (1977): 1199–1203.

Terry, L.C., and Martin, J.B. "Role of Alpha-Adrenergic Mechanisms in the Generation of Episodic Growth Hormone and Prolactin Secretion." *Endocrinology* 108 (1981): 1869–1871.

Toru, M., Shimazono, Y., Miyasaka, M., Kokubo, T., Mori, Y., and Nasu, T. "A Double-Blind Comparison of Sulpiride With Chlorpromazine in Chronic Schizophrenia." *Journal of Clinical Pharmacology* 12 (1972): 221–229.

Tuma, A.H., and May, P.R.A. "Psychotherapy, Drugs, and Therapist Experience in the Treatment of Schizophrenia: A Critique of the Michigan State Project." *Psychotherapy: Theory, Research and Practice* 12 (1975): 138–142.

Tyson, J.E., and Friesen, H.G. "Factors Influencing the Secretion of Human Prolactin and Growth Hormone in Menstrual and Gestational Women." *American Journal of Obstetrics and Gynecology* [sic] (1973): 377–387.

Van Der Velde, C.D., and Kiltie, H. "Effectiveness of Loxapine Succinate in Acute Schizophrenia: A Comparative Study With Tiothixene." *Current Therapeutic Research* 17 (1975): 1–2.

Vannicelli, M., Washburn, S., Scheef, B.J., and Longabaugh, R. "A Comparison of Usual and Experimental Patients in a Psychiatric Day Center." *Journal of Consulting and Clinical Psychology* 46 (1978): 87–93.

Van Praag, H., and Dois, L.C.W. "Fluphenazine Enanthate and Fluphenazine Decanoate: A Comparison of Their Duration of Action and Motor Side Effects." *American Journal of Psychiatry* 130 (1973): 801.

Verhoeven, W., Van Praag, H.M., and de Jong, F. "Use of Naloxone in Schizophrenic Psychoses and Manic Syndrome." *Neuropsychobiology* 7 (1981): 159–168.

Volavka, J., Mallya, A., Baig, S., and Perez-Cruet, J. "Naloxone in Chronic Schizophrenia." *Science* 196 (1977): 1227–1228.

Volk, W., Bier, W., Braun, J.P. Grüter, W., and Spiegelberg, U. "Behandlung von erregten Psychosen mit einem Beta-Rezeptoren-Blocker (Oxprenolol) in hoher Dosierung." *Nervenarzt* 43 (1972): 491–492.

von Zerssen, D. "Beta-Adrenergic Blocking Agents in the Treatment of Psychoses: A Report on 17 Cases." *Advances in Clinical Pharmacology* 12 (1976): 105–114.

Vyas, B.K., and Kalla, V.A. "Six Month Double-Blind Comparison of Loxapine Succinate and Chlorpromazine in Chronic Schizophrenic Patients." *Current Therapeutic Research* 28 (1980): 16–30.

Washburn, S., Vannicelli, M., Longabaugh, R., and Scheef, B.F. "A Controlled Comparison of Psychiatric Day Care and Inpatient Hospitalization." *Journal of Consulting and Clinical Psychology* 44 (1976): 665–675.

Watson, S.J., Berger, P.A., Akil, H., Mills, M.J., and Barchas, J.D. "Effects of Naloxone in Schizophrenia: Reduction in Hallucinations in a Subpopulation of Subjects." *Science* 201 (1978): 73–76.

Wijsenbeek, H., Steiner, M., and Goldberg, S.C. "Trifluoperazine: A Comparison Between Regular and High Doses." *Psychopharmacologia* 36 (1974): 147.

Wilder, J.F., Levin, G., and Zwelling, J. "A Two-Year Follow-up Evaluation of Acute Psychiatric Patients Treated in a Day Hospital." *American Journal of Psychiatry* 122 (1966): 1095–1106.

Wiles, D., Franklin, M., Dencker, S.J., Johansson, R., Lundi, L., and Malm, U. "Plasma Fluphenazine and Prolactin Levels in Schizophrenic Patients During Treatment With Low or High Doses of Fluphenazine Enanthate." *Psychopharmacology* 71 (1980): 131–136.

Williams, B.W., and Brown, W.A. "Psychotropic Drugs Do Not Interfere With Radioligand Assays for Prolactin, Cortisol and Growth Hormone." *Communications in Psychopharmacology* 3 (1979): 359–362.

Willoughby, J.O., Brazeau, P., and Martin, J.B. "Pulsatile Growth Hormone and Prolactin: Effects of (+) Butadamol, a Dopamine Receptor Blocking Agent." *Endocrinology* 101 (1977): 1298–1303.

Wilson, R.G., Hamilton, J.R., Boyd, W.D., Forrest, A.P.M., Cole, E.N., Boyns, A.R., and Griffiths, K. "The Effect of Long-Term Phenothiazine Therapy on Plasma Prolactin." *British Journal of Psychiatry* 127 (1973): 71–74.

Wilson, J.D., King, D.J., and Sheridan, B. "Plasma Prolactin Levels Before and During Propanolol Treatment in Chronic Schizophrenia." *Clinical Pharmacology* 7 (1979): 313.

Wistedt, B. "Withdrawal of Long-Acting Neuroleptics in Schizophrenic Outpatients." *Acta Universities Upsaliensis* (1981): 391–397.

Wode-Helgodt, B., Borg, S., Fyro, B., and Sedvall, G. "Clinical Effects and Drug Concentrations in Plasma and Cerebrospinal Fluid in Psychotic Patients Tested With Fixed Doses of Chlorpromazine." *Acta Psychiatrica Scandinavica* 58 (1978): 149–173.

Wode-Helgodt, B., Eneroth, P., Fyro, B., Gullberg, B., and Sedvall, G. "Effect of Chlorpromazine Treatment on Prolactin Levels in Cerebrospinal Fluid and Plasma of Psychotic Patients." *Acta Psychiatrica Scandinavica* 56 (1977): 280–293.

Yorkston, N.J., Gruzelier, J.H., Zaki, S.A., Hollander, D., Pitcher, D.R., and Sergeant, H.G.S. "Propanolol as an Adjunct to the Treatment of Schizophrenia." In *Propanolol and Schizophrenia*, edited by E. Roberts and P. Amacher. New York: Alan R. Liss, Inc., 1978a.

Yorkston, N.J., Zaki, S.A., Gruzelier, J.H., Hollander, D., and Sergeant, H.G. "Propanolol in Chronic Schizophrenia." *Lancet* 2 (1977): 1082–1083.

Yorkston, N.J., Zaki, S.A., and Havard, C.W.H. "Propranolol in the Treatment of Schizophrenia: An Uncontrolled Study with 55 Adults." In *Propranolol and Schizophrenia*, edited by E. Roberts and P. Amacher. New York: Alan R. Liss, Inc., 1978b.

Yorkston, N.J., Zaki, S.A., Malik, M.K.U., Morrison, R.C., and Havard, C.W.H. "Propanolol in the Control of Schizophrenic Symptoms." *British Medical Journal* 4 (1974): 633–635.

Yorkston, N.J., Zaki, S.A., Themen, J., and Havard, C.W.H. "Propanolol to Control Schizophrenic Symptoms." *Advances in Clinial Pharmacology* 12 (1976a): 91–104.

Yorkston, N.J., Zaki, S.A., Themen, J., and Havard, C.W.H. "Safeguards in the Treatment of Schizophrenia With Propranolol." *Postgraduate Medical Journal* Supplement 4, 52 (1976b): 175–180.

Yorkston, N.J., Zaki, S.A., Weller, M.P., Gruzelier, J.H., and Hirsch, S.R. "DL-Propranolol and Chlorpromazine Following Admission for Schizophrenia." *Acta Psychiatrica Scandinavica* 63 (1981): 13–27.

III

Depression in
Childhood and Adolescence

Part III

Depression in Childhood and Adolescence

Authors for Part III

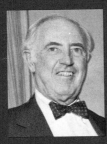

Henry H. Work, M.D., Preceptor

Deputy Medical Director
American Psychiatric Association

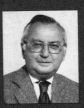

Irving Philips, M.D.
Professor of Psychiatry
    and Director of Child and Adolescent
    Psychiatry
Langley Porter Psychiatric Institute
University of California

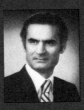

Javad H. Kashani, M.D., F.R.C.P.(C)
Department of Psychiatry
University of Missouri-Columbia
School of Medicine

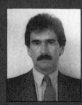

Steven Friedlander, Ph.D.
Assistant Professor of Psychology
   and Psychiatry
Langley Porter Psychiatric Institute
University of California

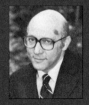

Jules R. Bemporad, M.D.
Director of Children's Services
   and Associate Professor of Psychiatry
Massachusetts Mental Health Center
Harvard Medical School

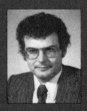

J. Puig-Antich, M.D.
Assistant Professor of Clinical Psychiatry
Columbia University College of
   Physicians and Surgeons
New York State Psychiatric Institute

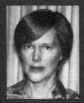

Elva Orlow Poznanski, M.D.
Professor of Psychiatry
Abraham Lincoln School of Medicine
University of Illinois at Medical Center

Depression in Childhood and Adolescence

Introduction
by Henry H. Work, M.D.

Child psychiatry has historically been independent from general psychiatry and has traditionally maintained independent systems for diagnosing and treating its special client population. Whether or not this separation from general psychiatry did itself lead to a comparatively simplistic nosology of psychopathologic disorders in children, the fact remains that the nosology has until very recently suffered from its simplicity.

Before child psychiatry was so labeled and became a discipline in 1934, the effort to define types of psychopathologies in children had begun. In the United States this definition began at the child guidance clinics, which provided most of the available treatment for disturbed children and their parents during the early decades of the century. The result of these early efforts was a terminology which was largely descriptive. A prevailing diagnosis was the so-called adjustment disorder of childhood. So popular was this simple diagnosis that it was for a time extended to adolescents and even to young adults.

Certain disorders of children, however, defied such a classification. Some children were seen as suffering from very severe disorders, disorders to which the moderate and amenable implications of the adjustment disorder concept were hardly applicable. Still, the practitioners who were dealing with such children, including the pediatricians and the members of the new discipline of child psychiatry, had the idea that these children could not actually be as sick as they appeared.

Around 1939 a burgeoning of interest in major disorders of childhood led to a spate of publications that took a different view. As had actually been suggested a hundred years earlier, writers began to assert that children could have major psychoses. A few bold authors, Bradley (1941) and Despert (1938) among them, described these disorders as schizophrenia in childhood. Still, however, a philosophical blackout kept the idea of childhood depression as a diagnostic entity out of the tenets of child psychiatry. Normal grief, sadness, and melancholy, of course, were apparent, and not particularly distressing, to many practitioners. Clinicians were, however, bothered by the pictures of children whose melancholy was continuing, rather than intermittent, and whose sadness was so pervasively manifest in their vegetative, intellectual, and affective functioning. But the concept of major depression was still not a part of the vocabulary in the dominant service setting of the child guidance clinic.

The diagnosis of schizophrenic conditions in children eventually resulted in psychiatric services for children being attached to hospitals associated with academic departments of psychiatry. Thus, by the late 1940's, the concept of major disorders in childhood had become a part of the clinical conversation. Nonetheless, many practitioners continued to avoid labeling even the more long-term and intense forms of childhood grief and sadness as major clinical disorders.

The chapters in this Part in various ways point up the need for and the benefits of a more careful nosological approach to children. The first chapter, by Drs. Irving Philips and Steven Friedlander, describes the continuing evolution of the concept of childhood depression and the current recognition given to it. Their chapter also discusses the advantages and disadvantages of alternative nosological approaches, paving the way for the other chapters.

Putting the concept of child and adolescent depression into a developmental framework, Dr. Jules Bemporad illustrates how development is the major biosocial aspect of life that differentiates the disorders of children from those of adults. He also shows how the major childhood affective disorders, including depression, can be more fully appreciated and, perhaps, better diagnosed within a developmental framework.

Once the profession began to consider depression in childhood a clinical entity, it became possible to explore the phenomenon using an epidemiological approach. Dr. Javad Kashani discusses prevalence in the context of a number of potential contributing factors and points out the need for further studies which could lead to more scientifically designed, and more effective, treatment and prevention strategies.

Scarcely more than a decade ago, a chapter concerning the biological background of depressive disorders in children could not have been written. Both by its content and by its very existence, Dr. Joaquim Puig-Antich's chapter evidences the progress of psychobiology throughout the field of psychiatry in general and within the field of childhood disorders in particular.

Finally, Dr. Elva Poznanski reviews diagnostic criteria and procedures and discusses the differential diagnosis of childhood and adolescent depression in light of other mental disorders, physical illnesses, and normal developmental capacities.

If historically a nosological quandary has created difficulties in the diagnosis and treatment of depression in children, and if, as the chapters reflect, we now have a nosological concept we can apply and use, we are still in somewhat of a quandary. Diagnosis may become more effective, and research may now be able to uncover etiologies and true prevalence. But what modes of therapy are effective remains problematic. Indeed, one must question whether our new diagnostic tools will be as useful to the patient as they will be to the practitioner. Some in our field have even speculated that labeling and diagnosing illnesses may ultimately be more important to case conferences and record librarians than to caring for patients.

Indeed, readers of these chapters will note the apparent omission of a discussion of therapy. Among other reasons for this seeming omission, the fact that the concept of childhood and adolescent depression had not until recently been fully elaborated is paramount. During the last century the continuing uncertainty about the concept was, not surprisingly, accompanied by many variations in the patterns of treatment.

Much of the variation stemmed from a growing recognition of the forces that impel children to act out, to withdraw, to be sad, and so forth. At the beginning of the child guidance movement, Frederick Allen of the Philadelphia Child Guidance Clinic set a rather rigid pattern of therapy for all children. This pattern included psychiatric intervention for the child and casework intervention for the parents, usually the mother. Here the collaborative bond between the parent(s) and the therapist were the focus of supervision and management. Later patterns of therapy focused more on the individual child and incorporated such directive techniques as behavior modification.

More recently, during the last decade, an application of group therapy procedures has led to the emergence of family therapy. Family therapy will, it is hoped, prove to be more than yet another vogue. It promises to be a rational and effective approach to the care of children who are in distress and of the families who are distressed about them. The depressive symptoms of childhood seem ideally suited to a family therapeutic approach, even more so than the acting-out symptomatology which was the focus of early therapeutic intervention with children. The efficacy of family treatment, coupled perhaps with pharmacotherapy, should command the attention of both clinicians and researchers who are concerned about the treatment of children who suffer from depression.

We do help patients when we diagnose them correctly. We are aware, however, in child psychiatry particularly, that our growing interest in chronic diseases, and the subsequent visibility of chronic psychopathology that begins early in chldhood, carries a number of risks both for our patients and for ourselves. In our litigious climate, patients are much more aware of the diagnostic labels affixed to them. A challenge, therefore, in the use of such terms, is to make sure we understand the relationship of the diagnosis to the stage of life of the patient, to the effect that the patient's malady has on others, and, particularly, to the therapeutic process.

This Part updates our knowledge concerning the depressive conditions of childhood. Using and expanding that knowledge should be guided by our concern for therapy and for long-range management with young patients whose affective disorders seem so strikingly manifest, and sometimes so baffling to treatment.

Chapter 16

Conceptual Problems in the Study of Depression in Childhood
by Irving Philips, M.D. and Steven Friedlander, Ph.D.

INTRODUCTION

Recent advances in the study and understanding of adult depression have stimulated renewed interest in childhood depression. Research on adult depression has contributed findings concerning the apparent role of genetics in manic-depressive illness and has led to the formulation of the catecholamine hypothesis. The clarification between endogenous and reactive depression, the effectiveness of anti-depressant medication with adults, and the recognition that ten percent of all hospital admissions to psychiatric facilities are due to depression have also encouraged interest in depression among children (Philips, 1980). While one ultimate goal is preventing depression in adults, this interest also stems from the promise of achieving as much clarity regarding childhood depression itself as we have recently developed in the area of adult depression.

Depression as a clinical phenomenon is still conceptually vague. It refers to an affect, a mood, a specific group of symptoms, as well as to a disorder (Carlson and Cantwell, 1980a), the diagnosis of which can be based on the observation of a group of symptoms or on inference regarding some presumed underlying process. The necessity of considering the added dimension of development when addressing depression in childhood further complicates what is already a very complex concept.

Conceptual problems are not unique to the study of depression in childhood. Grinker outlined some of the difficulties inherent in the study of depression:

> . . . depression is a description of a predominating affect and gives no clue to the underlying processes, the nature of the patient's problems, the predisposing factors, or the precipitating causes. As an affect which may dominate the mood of individual patients, depression may be a symptom of a wide variety of psychological problems and accompany almost any clinical nosological entity.
>
> Furthermore, the mood of depression which leads one to make a diagnosis of this entity is not easy to determine. It may be hidden en masse by a wide variety of behavioral or psychological defenses. Many cover up depressive feelings with smiling, gay, and joking exteriors. Others deny primary sadness, but attribute worry to single symptoms such as insomnia, gastrointestinal distress, headaches, and so forth, or complain of boredom or fatigue. Still others present compulsive doubts or hypochondriacal preoccupation, disassociated states or paranoid delusions (Grinker, 1961, xii).

These difficulties are equally germane, if not more so, to the study of depression in childhood, a concept that has been consistently characterized by confusion and controversy.

The early controversy surrounding childhood depression was, to a great extent, a function of theoretical speculation in the absence of clinical data. The influence of psychoanalytic theory on early thinking about childhood psychopathology resulted in the tendency to dismiss as impossible the occurrence of depression in childhood. Rochlin was most explicit in this regard: "Clinical depression, a superego phenomenon, as we psychoanalytically understand the disorder, does not occur in childhood" (Rochlin, 1959, 299). More recently, systematic study of depression has begun to build on the identification of depressive symptoms and the introduction of the notion of depressive equivalents in prepubertal children (Toolan, 1962; Glaser, 1968; Anthony, 1970; Bowlby, 1973; Cytryn and McKnew, 1972; Poznanski and Zrull, 1970; Malmquist, 1971a, 1971b). Such study brought with it the more rigorous requirements of the scientific method which, at very least, demand precise definition and reliable measurement. Efforts to satisfy these requirements have raised again the fundamental conceptual problems that characterize the study of depression in childhood.

Increasingly systematic study has led to the recognition that although depressive symptoms are readily observable in unselected samples of children (Lefkowitz and Burton, 1978; Friedlander et al., 1981), a reliably manifest depressive constellation is relatively rare in prepubertal children, even in psychiatric clinic samples. Add to these observations the continued vagueness of the depression concept and the complicating factor of developmental considerations in childhood, and it is easy to see why clarity and empirical progress have been so elusive.

The problem of existing studies and data on the prevalence of depression in childhood highlights the issues. There is little agreement in the data regarding the prevalence of depression in childhood, with estimates ranging from less than one percent in both unselected and clinic samples, to thirty percent or more in clinic and school samples (Frommer, 1967; Leon et al., 1980; Seligman, 1980; Weinberg et al., 1973; Rutter et al., 1970; Poznanski and Zrull, 1970).* Furthermore, there are those who argue that the depressive symptoms that are observed in early and middle childhood are transient developmental phenomena and have no particular clinical significance (Lefkowitz and Burton, 1978).

The wide range of variability in the data bearing on such a basic question as the prevalence of depression in childhood seems primarily to reflect the fact that each investigator employed different criteria in defining depression. Clarification of the definition of depression in childhood and refinements in the related matter of its measurement are absolutely fundamental both to understanding the source of the problems that have plagued the study of depression in childhood and to solving those problems.

DEFINITION: THE SEARCH FOR A MODEL

A fundamental issue that arises in constructing a model for the study of depression in childhood is evident in the alternate terminology used to label the study topic. What is being studied, *childhood depression* or *depression in childhood?* Should the model take account of developmental considerations and thus look for a condition or phenomenon unique to childhood, with its own signs, symptoms, and diagnostic criteria? Or, on the other hand, would progress be better served by using a model which incorporates the established group of affective, cognitive, motivational, and vaso-vegetative signs that have become definitive of adult depression? Or is neither of the two models appropriate? This third possibility, originally posed by Lefkowitz and Burton (1978), was reiterated by Cytryn et al. (1980) in their recent discussion of competing conceptualizations of depressive phenomena in children. They assert that both are premature and that childhood depression has not yet been established as a viable clinical entity.

Each of the three positions has advantages and disadvantages, and each investigator in the field must choose among them either explicitly or implicitly. Discussion of these competing viewpoints reveals continuing confusion and controversy.

The argument that empirical data have not yet established the clinical relevance of childhood depression has been most cogently stated by Lefkowitz and Burton in their critique of the concept of childhood depression (see also Costello, 1980; Lefkowitz, 1980):

"Clinical studies of children selected on the basis of psychopathology show that childhood depression is a phenomenon of concern whereas studies of normal children indicate that these same symptoms of depression prevail at a rate too high to be considered statistically deviant. Evidence adduced from the research literature to support the concept of a syndrome of early childhood depression is insufficient and insubstantial" (Lefkowitz and Burton, 1978, 724).

This view in fact emerged from a review of the available data based on

*Preceptor's note: For a review of the prevalence data and studies, see the chapter by Kashani.

the adult model" of depression and describes one of the risks inherent in adopting the established adult model of depression and applying it to children. Although the adult model has the appeal of familiarity and the advantage of addressing phenomena that are known and with which we have some experience, it fails to take account of the wide range of variables encompassed by the notion of developmental phases and does not set the data in the appropriate developmental context. These failures open the door to both the false positive and the false negative diagnostic error. Lefkowitz and Burton (1978) argue that focusing on the constellation of the classic depressive symptoms might lead to false positive errors and the overdiagnosis of depression in childhood. Such symptoms, when absent in children, may represent expected, transitory phenomena and may not be the pathogenic signs of a clinical disorder. The risk of the false negative error might be even more significant, however. Failure to take account of developmental variables, including how the child's age-related cognitive capacities determine the specific means of self-expression, might result in overlooking a number of troubled and depressed children.

The strength of the alternative, developmental viewpoint is, of course, related to the weakness of the adult model. Children are not simply little adults, and based on what is known of children and development, there is no good reason to expect them to behave as such. Theoretical recognition of the importance of developmental considerations in the study of childhood depression (Philips, 1979) has, however, not yet influenced the nature of empirical study in the field.

Similarly, clinically based concepts like masked depression, although inherently respectful of developmental considerations, have not survived the rigors of scientific scrutiny. They have, in fact, contributed to much of the confusion. Some have proposed rather broad definitions of childhood depression, describing depressive equivalents or masking symptoms (Glaser, 1968; Toolan, 1962). From this perspective, depression in childhood has been defined by a variety of symptom clusters, including the familiar symptoms of social withdrawal; weepiness; sleep disturbance; self-depreciation; lack of energy; weight loss; feelings of sadness, helplessness, loneliness, loss, and hopelessness; suicidal ideation; passivity; poor self-concept; and so forth. Also included are less familiar depressive signs, such as poor school performance, school phobia, aggressive behavior, enuresis, encopresis, inhibition, hyperactivity, antisocial behavior, anxiety, and hypochondriasis. The list of the so-called masking symptoms is so long that some believe it could subsume upwards of eighty percent of all childhood psychopathology. Moreover, echoing Grinker's (1961) point, many of these symptoms are actually concomitants of disorders other than depression. Similarly, it has been suggested that the masks are nothing more than presenting complaints at referral or an expression of the type of problems thought to be appropriate to a particular age group by the referring person (Kovacs and Beck, 1977; Carlson and Cantwell, 1980b).

The primary diagnostic risk with the developmental model, as some have advanced it, is the possibility of overdiagnosis. The conceptual risk is even greater. With the diagnostic symptomatology so broadly defined and overinclusive, differential diagnosis becomes difficult, and the meaningfulness of the concept is correspondingly diluted. The diagnostic risk and conceptual problems stemming from over-inclusiveness are not inherent in the developmental model, of course. The overinclusiveness and subsequent problems come from misunderstanding and from the overzealous misapplication of the basic truth that children are different from adults and are likely to express themselves differently.

Convincing arguments remain regarding the need to assume a developmental perspective in the study of childhood psychopathology (Achenbach, 1978), and recent data support the need for such a perspective, especially in the study of childhood depression (Leon et al., 1980).* The field seems nonetheless to have opted for the adult model. For example, Puig-Antich et al. (1978) and McKnew and Cytryn (1979), have assumed that childhood and adult depression have a continuity or at least a common mechanism, and this assumption has led them to seek in children the same biochemical markers associated with depression in adults. Similarly, adapting the language of an adult scale, Kovacs (1977) has designed a self-report scale for measuring in children the severity of the familiar affective, cognitive, motivational, and vaso-vegetative symptoms of adult depression.

Perhaps the most significant index of and contributor to the preferred status of the adult model of depression in childhood is DSM-III. "Because the *essential* features of Affective Disorders . . . are the same in children and adults," DSM-III states, "there are no special categories corresponding to these disorders [in children]" (American Psychiatric Association, 1980, 35). Significantly DSM-III barely acknowledges the potential role of developmental variables. The only example of differences in "age-specific *associated* features" it offers is separation anxiety in the prepubertal child. DSM-III also states, "In a child with a depressive syndrome there may not be complaints of any dysphoric mood, but its existence may be inferred from a persistently sad facial expression" (American Psychiatric Association, 1980, 210).

DSM-III appears then to represent a compromise between the adult and the developmental models of depression in childhood. Its success in regard to depression in childhood will depend, in large measure, on the reliability of the diagnostic categories with children, particularly where the diagnosis is to be based on inference. To what extent might we expect a group of child clinicians, working without benefit of a common set of objective criteria, to be able to agree on what constitutes a "persistently sad facial expression" in a seven-year-old child? Might such a guideline for inference result in the confusion of sadness and depression? Clearly the answers to such questions bear directly on the reliability and validity of the available measures.

MEASUREMENT: ESTABLISHING AN OPERATIONAL DEFINITION

The choice of a model carries with it a particular definition which must in turn be converted into measurement procedures that will provide reliable quantitative indices for diagnosis and study. Available techniques for assessing depression in childhood include the child's self-report, ratings by parents, teachers, and peers, and interviews with a variety of informants. In a recent review, Kazdin (1981) has criticized many of the available techniques. Among other problems with them, a

*Preceptor's note: See the chapter by Bemporad for discussion and evidence of the usefulness of the developmental framework.

significant question is how the data obtained from such procedures are used in making a *diagnosis* of depression.

The study of depression in childhood, particularly when the adult model is used, has often failed to distinguish between identifying the depressive symptoms and conferring a diagnosis of depression. A rating or a measure of the severity of a symptom, or even of a group of symptoms, does not constitute a diagnosis. Diagnosis is the result of a comprehensive clinical evaluation; it is not the summation of numbers on a rating scale. For example, in studying a college student population, Hammen (1980) found that nine percent or 37 of 400 students scored in the moderate depression range of the Beck Depression Inventory (BDI), a self-report scale that provides a measure of the severity of depressive symptoms. In spite of the validity of the BDI (Bumberry et al., 1980), only 13 of 34 students who had scored in the moderate depression range and who were interviewed by a clinician fit the Research Diagnostic Criteria (RDC) for major or minor affective disorder (Spitzer et al., 1978). Thus, more than half of the sample scoring in the moderate depression range of the BDI were not regarded clinically as depressed.

In the study of depression in children, as with adults, the most frequently used measure of depression is a self-report scale. Except as a screening device, the self-report scale is of questionable utility, especially if it supplies the only data used in establishing a diagnosis. Diagnosis of childhood depression must be based on data from multiple sources, including diagnostic interviews of the child and family, psychological testing, school reports, and physical and neurological examinations. The environmental context and recent life events should also be entered into the diagnostic matrix.

Despite these obvious problems and a recent critique underscoring the shortcomings of the available methods for assessing childhood depression (Kazdin, 1981), the prevailing adult model of depression has tended to carry with it a focus on self-report in general, and use of self-report scales in particular. Examples are the Children's Depression Inventory (CDI), a self-report scale for measuring the severity of depression (Kovacs, 1977), and the Kiddie-SADS (Chambers et al., 1978), a structured clinical interview.

The assumption that the self-report provides a reliable index of the child's experience is open to question. Clinicians are particularly aware of the limitations of self-report with children. For example, a child, age eight, was referred to the clinic because of morning abdominal pain, fear of attending school, feeling that his classmates did not like him, thoughts that he would fail in his subjects and not achieve the aspirations of his parents, sleeplessness, a failing appetite, and disinterest in athletic pursuits (a major school recreation). These symptoms had become more severe during the past month-and-a-half following an episode of flu. His parents were concerned and worried. When he was given the self-report CDI, the child's score totaled zero, but the clinician noted a serious depression, based on the parents' report and the interview of the youngster. When asked about his responses to the CDI questionnaire, the child stated that this was the way he felt when he answered the questions.

Further limitations of self-report, symptom-oriented methods for assessing depression in childhood are also evident. Comparable scores or mean levels on a particular scale cannot be taken to mean that the quality or significance of the experience on which those scores are based is comparable. In the Langley Porter Psychiatric Institute study of depression in childhood (Friedlander et al., 1981), the authors have found that children in a psychiatric clinic sample do not differ from children in a healthy pediatric sample on mean CDI score. However, they have observed a number of other differences between these two groups, including levels of parental depression, parental perception of their children, and the child's differential sensitivity to negative life events. This suggests that important differences between these groups are not being measured because there are no questions regarding the level of depressive symptomatology evidenced by the child.

Still another measurement issue intimately related to the choice of a model of depression relates to the reliability of measures of depressive symptoms in children. If depressive symptoms in children are expectable and transitory developmental phenomena, how long are they expected to persist, and when does their continued presence begin to signal developmental deviation and more clinically relevant depression? A DSM-III affective disorder diagnosis requires a symptom duration of two weeks for both adults and children. Yet the National Institute of Mental Health Subcommittee on Clinical Criteria for the Diagnosis of Depression in Children recognized that depressive symptoms in children may be transitory and recommended a minimum symptom duration of four weeks for the diagnosis of childhood depression (Dweck et al., 1977). In the context of the notion that depressive symptoms are expected though transitory in childhood, efforts to establish the reliability of available measures are a real challenge. The psychometric principle that reliability places an upper limit on validity has a parallel in this issue. The depressive symptoms appear to make a transition as they move from the status of transitory developmental phenomena (i.e., unreliable over time) to being considered clinically significant phenomena (i.e., reliable over time). Obviously, symptoms that are unreliable over time can nevertheless be clinically significant. Clarification of this and the many other explicit and implicit questions raised in this discussion will come not from theoretical debate, but rather from empirical studies that are both clinically and methodologically sound.

CONCLUSIONS

There is little question that interest in depression in childhood is on the rise. The number of investigators, research programs, and published papers have increased considerably in recent years. Nevertheless, conflicting data and confusion continue to characterize the field of study. Part of the problem is that there are basically two competing conceptual models of depression in childhood, the developmental model and the adult model, and that each has different implications for study and practice. Recognition of the implications of choosing one model over the other would help significantly to reduce the existing confusion. An integral part of resolving the conceptual difficulties will entail establishing a clear definition of depression in childhood and ensuring that the definition is translated into a viable measure or empirical index of the phenomenon.

For the present, the field in general seems to have opted for the more familiar adult model, as reflected in the DSM-III criteria and in the bulk of the current clinical investigations. In part, this choice represents a reaction to the unwieldy, confusing, overinclusive, and imprecise notions of depressive equivalents and masked depression which have accompanied attempts to apply the developmental model. There is now some indication that the adult model alone is not adequate (Leon et al., 1980; Friedlander et al., 1981) and that we may need to turn once again to the more challenging and complex developmental model. A careful and sophisticated application of the developmental model, an application that is clinically and methodologically sound and buttressed by accumulating clinical data and that thereby avoids the mistakes of previous applications, may ultimately represent the most fruitful conceptual path.

Chapter 17 # Childhood Depression From A Developmental Perspective
by Jules R. Bemporad, M.D.

THE CONCEPT OF CHILDHOOD DEPRESSION

In marked contrast to the paucity of literature on childhood depression prior to the 1970's, a wealth of papers and books on the topic have appeared in the last ten years. In prior years, our way of viewing depression was greatly influenced by orthodox psychoanalytic formulations. Melancholia was seen as the result of an intrapsychic conflict between a stern, primitive superego and a helpless, victimized ego. Since children were believed to lack a fully structured superego until rather late in development, childhood depression was deemed theoretically impossible (Rochlin, 1959). Later formulations of ego psychology conceived of depression as a fall in self-esteem due to a discrepancy between the ego ideal and the actual self. Since, once again, children were thought to lack a stable self-image or ideal, they were thought to be immune from depression (Rie, 1966). Here again the theory argued against the possibility of depression in childhood, since the clinical entity seemed to depend on the presence of internal metapsychological agencies which did not reach full maturity until puberty or later.

This view of depression began to be challenged by the seminal works of Bibring (1953), of Sandler and Joffee (1965), and of Arieti (1978). Bibring (1953) argued that depression is the emotional expression of a fundamental and primary state of the ego when the individual feels hopeless and powerless, unable to obtain gratification or to achieve goals that are important for narcissistic equilibrium. Sandler and Joffee (1965) described depression as a basic negative affect, much like anxiety, which arises whenever an individual has suffered the loss of a former state of well-being. In a manner similar to Bibring, they did not conceive of depression as having to result from object loss but interpreted those depressions that occurred after the loss of a loved one as being caused by the loss of well-being that the object had supplied. Thus, depression could also occur without object loss, if the circumstances forced a loss of well-being.

Sandler and Joffee also made another significant conceptual distinction in their study of depression. They proposed that there are two temporal and clinical forms of depression. The first is a basic psychobiological response to a deprivation and may be seen in all individuals. Most people find ways of dealing with this initial dysphoria. Either they mobilize themselves to find new sources of well-being, or they form defenses against the dysphoria. Other people, who are predisposed by personality structure or prior life events, cannot adequately master the initial dysphoric response and go on to the second form of depression which is the clinical episode. Once the initial response is elaborated into a clinical depression, the individual manifests hopelessness, helplessness, and despair. This distinction is of great significance, for it separates the somewhat ubiquitous and transitory unhappiness following frustration from the less frequent clinical disorder of depression.

Arieti (1978) also believed there is a difference between the initial reaction to deprivation, which he called sadness, and true depression. He further stated that this initial sadness may have a beneficial purpose in alerting the individual that he or she has to make changes in his or her life or readjust ways of obtaining meaning and esteem. The inability to work through this period of mental pain results in true depression. Arieti also classified depression as a basic affect, agreeing with the views of Bibring and of Sandler and Joffee. This simplified formulation obviously would make it easier to accept depression in children, since they are capable of experiencing and expressing basic affects, but Arieti warned that such a conclusion is probably unwarranted. He argued cogently that not all affects are of the same complexity. Rather, through development, affects become less physiological and more reliant on increasing cognitive abilities. For example, fear is an immediate reaction to a negative stimulus which is present, while anxiety presupposes some anticipation of a negative stimulus which is not perceptually available.

Arieti suggested a hierarchy of emotions, in which depression is a higher-order feeling state, requiring a considerable amount of cognitive and social sophistication. The relevance of this line of thinking for our purposes is that it allows us to view depression as a negative emotion that may well be different at various stages of development. As the varying psychological abilities mature, dysphoric states become more complex, possibly more cognitive, and they are produced by different threats to the individual. Depression, just as any feeling or behavior, must be seen from a developmental perspective. In accordance with this formulation, we can appreciate Anthony's (1975a) statement that depression itself undergoes development commensurate with the overall development of the child.

If we adopt this view and consider depression as a primary affect, the experience and expression of which are affected by the increasing maturation of psychological functions, the theoretical problem of childhood depression is transformed. It is no longer a question of whether or not adultlike depression can occur in childhood. It is, rather, a matter of how the child's abilities and limitations, at each developmental stage, impose their characteristic stamp on dysphoric states. With this general framework in mind, we can review the literature on depression in childhood and examine the progressive development of this primary affect from infancy to adolescence.

DEPRESSION AND DEVELOPMENT

Infancy and Early Childhood

The earliest clinical reports of depression in childhood referred specifically to infants. The pioneer studies of René Spitz (1946) on anaclitic depression described six-month-old infants becoming withdrawn and listless following separation from the mother. Unless reunited with the mother within three to five months, these infants became developmentally retarded and unduly prone to infection and higher mortality. Spitz was impressed with the lethargy, withdrawal, and apathy that followed the children's loss of a love object and considered their behavior to be the manifestation of depression.

For many years it was accepted that losing or separating from the mother figure in infancy would produce a depressive episode. In recent years, however, the actual meaning of the infant's response has been reconsidered. Dennis and Najarian (1957) have reported identical behavior in infants who are deprived of cognitive stimulation, and Malmquist (1977) writes about a similar syndrome in malnourished infants. Engel and Reichmann (1956) observed that a deprived infant with a gastric fistula turned away and postulated that this behavior constituted a basic "conservation-withdrawal" reaction. The infant may have been trying to shut out an unpleasant reality in order to conserve himself rather than manifest depression. Poznanski (1979) emphasizes that only 15 percent of Spitz's sample of infants showed the depression-like syndrome, suggests that it is not so ubiquitous, and postulates that the affected children may have been organically damaged. Finally, Rie (1966) points out that the advanced stages of this syndrome do not resemble depression but mental retardation.

This syndrome perhaps should be considered as the infant's reaction to a deprivation of supplies needed for proper development. The fact that infants appear to respond similarly to a lack of mothering, nutrition, or cognitive stimulation may demonstrate the limited repertoire of behavior available at this early stage of development. Their withdrawal and lethargy appear to result from their not having the psychological or physiological nourishment they need for adequate maturation, rather than from a depressive response. There is little doubt that one of the principal developmental tasks of infancy is the formation of an emotional bond with a caretaker. It is questionable, however, to assume that disruption of this bond results in depression at that time or sets a course for later aberrant development.

In contrast to the significant literature on depression in infancy reports on dysphoric states in the toddler period are few. Poznanski and Zrull (1970) reviewed the charts of 1,788 children seen at the child psychiatric hospital at the University of Michigan and found only one child under the age of five who might possibly fit clinical criteria for depression. Other researchers, while not commenting directly on the lack of depressive symptomatology in preschoolers, nevertheless do not mention this disorder in their clinical descriptions of this age group.

This lack of depressive symptoms in the toddler stage may be explained partially by our knowledge of normal development. The toddler is an exuberant, curious, active creature who delights in doing and exploring and who seems impervious to daily repeated falls and hurts. The toddler still uses caretakers as home bases of security but likes to venture forth, intensely attracted to the physical environment

He or she deals with frustration by active, physical, and loud protest or by distraction to more pleasant situations. There is little evidence that the toddler intellectually dwells on experiences. Rather children at this age search unceasingly for fresh stimulation. These developmental characteristics obviously are not fertile soil for the nurturance of depression.

What may be found is an angry response to separation followed by deprivation of well-being. Bowlby (1960) observed that a sequence of protest, despair, and detachment follows maternal separation and may occur as early as the toddler stage. However, Bowlby does not consider that the despair or detachment phases are prototypes of depression but believes they are part of the universal process of mourning an unexpected separation. The duration of this sequence may be contingent on the degree of substitution that is offered the child. The early studies were done on toddlers who, in addition to being separated, were admitted to hospitals where they were in strange surroundings, were not allowed to play, and were the victims of physically painful procedures. If a more benign caretaker is provided and the child is kept in the familiar environment, the extent of the separation sequence is greatly ameliorated and shortened. Poznanski (1979) cites a rigorous study by Heinicke and Westheimer, who followed ten children, ages 15 to thirty months, after they underwent brief separations from their mothers. The immediate reaction to separation was that the child spent about five percent of the total activity time fretting and crying. After two weeks, this fussing had decreased to 0.5 percent of the time. The children also had some sleep and behavioral disturbances, including an increased expression of hostility, but these disappeared after a few days. Five of the children were followed up one year later and showed no obvious or overt effects of the separation.

The studies just cited pertain to the loss of the well-being that the mother figure supplies to the toddler. A less researched but perhaps more important situation is the loss of gratification from normal activities without separation from a love object. Children who experience this loss include those who are so chronically abused or are so physically ill that their existence is one of continuing frustration and pain. Such children, it would be expected, would demonstrate a sense of dysphoria.

Margaret Mahler (1961) has reported on a group of children who do not show any overt signs of depression but who may be at risk for later affective illness. These children have difficulty separating from their mothers, although they appear to derive little pleasure from the maternal relationship. Mahler describes them as whiny and clinging, easily given to surrender and resignation, and showing frequent discontentment and anger. These young children appear overly inhibited, showing none of the exuberance that one expects from a preschooler. They seem to have given up on gratifying satisfaction needs in order to insure security needs, thus laying the groundwork for later depressive episodes. Mahler notes that this behavior is situation specific and seen only in the presence of the mother. Her presence in fact inhibits the child. The child reverts to the usual toddler enthusiasm when away from the mother and with less emotionally confining adults.

In summary, depressive symptoms are exceedingly rare in the preschool period, possibly because of the developmental hallmarks of this stage and the situation-specific nature of the child's moods. When possibly dysphoric symptoms appear, they take the form of angry protest or inhibition in the presence of significant others.

Middle and Late Childhood

It is not until school age that moods become more sustained and less stimulus bound. The child approaches the world more cognitively, and language and symbolic play replace action. Children in this developmental phase have been observed to express prolonged periods of unhappiness. McConville et al. (1973) reported on a group of children, ages six to eight, who displayed an almost pure state of sadness with little or no cognitive content, such as low self-esteem, self-depreciation, or particular reasons for their dysphoria. Bierman, Silverstein, and Finesinger (1958) described a six-year-old boy who exhibited a profound sadness after he had had a lengthy hospitalization for poliomyelitis and had lost the use of his legs. After some weeks of being deprived of gratifying activities because of his paralysis, the boy became despondent, withdrawn, and weepy. He remarked that he did not know how to play anymore and seemed to be totally crushed by his predicament. Fortunately, his dysphoria cleared after he recovered from his primary illness. Despite the enormous magnitude of this boy's deprivation and his appropriately profound response, there was no indication of lowered self-esteem or feelings of guilt. Thus, it would appear, the young school-aged child can become deeply dysphoric, but his or her sadness is not accompanied by the usual depressive cognitions.

This finding is in keeping with Piaget's (1954) description of this developmental stage as "intuitive," meaning that the child, by and large, functions on intuition rather than reasoned logic and accepts experiences at face value. There is little attempt to go beyond the appearance of things, and indeed certain situations which appear totally illogical to us as adults cause no disturbance in the thought of the child.

The symbolic play of young school-age children also reveals their disregard for going beneath surface behavior to search out deeper psychological motives or reasons for events:

> Carol, a six-year-old girl, presented with sadness, withdrawal, and a history of running away. Her great-grandmother brought her to the clinic's attention when Carol loudly announced she would jump out of her third-story window after the great-grandmother had fussed over another child. History revealed that Carol's mother, who was currently in prison for prostitution and drug trafficking, had given birth to her at age 16 and immediately turned over Carol's care to her own mother, who was only 28 at the time. The young grandmother died shortly afterward, and Carol was taken in by her great-grandmother, who was in her fifties. This woman resented having to care for a child at her stage of life and, despite good intentions, left Carol alone a good deal and frequently abused her when drinking. At age four, Carol repeatedly tried to run away to a neighbor's house where she got better care than at home. In her therapy sessions, Carol played out her life situation with a girl doll called Hazel, who was abused, neglected, and ignored. Despite the grim content of her doll play, Carol did not perceive Hazel as bad or unworthy. The only reasons she gave for her mistreatment were superficial, such as that the caretaker was drunk or wanted to be out of the house. She accepted her situation as it presented itself, and this external chronic frustration caused Carol to respond with appropriate unhappiness.

It is significant that Carol continues in therapy and is doing very well after placement in a good foster home.

The child at this age does not appear to form self-evaluations or judgments on any deep basis and responds accurately to environmental rewards or punishments. For example, one child with a severe learning disability was totally unconcerned with her deficiency at age five, since it caused her no immediate discomfort. At age nine, though, she felt very inadequate, blamed herself for her school problems, and had developed symptoms secondary to her basic disability. At a young age the child's gratification comes from a direct apprehension of the environment and is not yet generated from within in the form of deeper evaluations of one's own self and others.

The change toward a more judgmental appreciation of human interaction evolves gradually as the child approaches puberty. The older latency-aged child actively produces reasons, albeit often erroneous ones, for his or her experiences. When there is divorce in a family, for example, a younger child may be appropriately saddened by the loss of emotional closeness or the changes of everyday life. An older child will not only suffer the strains of familial disruption but may also suffer self-blame or blame a particular parent. As a result of these personal evaluations, depression at this stage shows a much greater cognitive component. Poznanski and Zrull (1970) report that the maturing latency child reacts less to unpleasantness in the environment and more to a feeling of disappointment with himself or herself. Similarly, McConville et al. (1973) found that depressed children, ages eight through ten, expressed ideas of low self-esteem, ideas which had been absent in younger dysphoric children.

Now that the sense of dysphoria is truly generated from within as part of intellectual and social advances of development, the evaluations will remain stable across multiple situations. Therefore, older children remain despondent despite an amelioration of their surroundings. Similarly, their dysphoria will affect multiple activities, such as relationships to peers and school work, as well as behavior at home. In addition, the older child begins to crystallize defensive maneuvers that may help avoid pain or humiliation in the short run but may leave him or her vulnerable to increased depressive feelings later on. Quite often these children deal with frustrating situations by avoidance or by clinging to parental figures. Others are forced to become overly responsible at home, to care for inept caretakers who demand parenting from their children. Still others are caught in a depression-filled home atmosphere which will not allow extrafamilial gratification without feelings of guilt.

The common feature of all of these situations is that the child is deprived of an opportunity to master successfully the developmental tasks of latency. The child cannot begin to break away from the familial orbit and find esteem and gratification in socially valued group activities. Sometimes, it is not the family but some self-perceived inferiority that keeps the child from finding avenues of worth outside the home. Children with learning disabilities who find their poor school performance a source of shame and humiliation, for example, may retreat from society back to the security of the family. For a variety of reasons, depressed children at this age do not initiate that first step toward independence from parental values or praise and thereby fail to establish a sound basis for the later true autonomy of adolescence or young adulthood. Therapy with such children often involves implementing activities outside the family to help the child form a new estimation of the self that is based on less demanding, or at least less distorted, expectations.

The disturbed older latency child thus resembles an adult with depression in many ways. Like the adult, the child perpetuates his or her own dysphoria, exhibits low self-esteem and self-blame, magnifies or distorts negative experiences, and shows the rudiments of pathological defenses. However, one important element of adult melancholia is still absent in prepubertal dysphoria—the dread of the future. These children do not despair about the rest of their lives or about having to bear their plight for eternity. They do not, as yet, project their current sense of self on a temporal continuum. They do not deny the future, however; they simply do not think of it. The absence of this future orientation was emphasized by Rie (1966). He argued that since prepubertal children lack the temporal dimension in their thinking, they do not experience the hopelessness and despair so typical of adult depression. In order to experience these two cardinal features of adult depression, Rie maintains, the individual must have an awareness of the relationship of current strivings to long range goals, a sense of infinity, and an understanding of the absolute irrevocability of a loss or disappointment. These observations are congruent with Piaget's (1954) findings that the cognitive ability to handle these types of abstractions is developed during the period of formal operations which begins approximately at the onset of puberty.

Adolescence

The depressive episodes seen in adolescence are infused with a sense of time: the feeling that things can never change, the idea that a trivial frustration or humiliation will have lasting effects, and the dread of the future. A social rebuff means eternal alienation, a disappointment of a date portends perpetual loneliness, or a bad mark on a test insures total academic failure. The particular intensity of adolescent depression may be due to the adolescent's having mastered the adult ability to project the self into the future but not having the moderation of thought and action which comes with the adult's greater life experience. This combination all too often results in the suicidal attempts which are so frequently seen in this age group. Erikson (1959) discusses the grave importance of this sense of time. In his description of severely disturbed youngsters, Erikson writes of their complaints of the missed greatness they will never achieve or their fatal loss of potential for love and intimacy. These adolescents truly believe that things can never be made right and that they will have to endure their current plight for the rest of their existence.

These comments focus on the newly acquired sense of time and the lack of moderation that typify adolescent depression, but they do not reveal the causes. While the adolescent may seek help after a disappointment or a loss, beyond this precipitant emerges a characteristic picture of someone who is ill equipped to deal with the vicissitudes of adolescent life as experienced in our culture. For some, day-to-day existence with the family unit discourages the development of skills that allow for striving on one's own and finding meaning and gratification through one's own activities. These adolescents often feel lost and unable to cope without a powerful other to direct and structure their lives. Some of these adolescents find solace in joining a cult or a group, substituting a charismatic leader for the former parent figure. Others remain pathologically dependent on the parent and return to the security of the family, even though the family environment is no longer satisfying or meaningful for their needs.

Other depressed adolescents are able to separate but carry within themselves unrealistic expectations that were ingrained during earlier periods of development. These youngsters find themselves in a conflict which seems to offer no viable solution. To continue to live according to the old "shoulds" will not bring happiness or fulfillment, yet to go against the internalized rules arouses anxiety and guilt. Anthony (1975b) accurately describes the plight of this type of depressed adolescent by referring to the turbulent youth of John Stuart Mill. As an adolescent, Mill asked himself if he would be happy if he accomplished all that his father had asked of him. Mill was forced to answer no and later wrote about that moment. "At this my heart sank in me, the whole foundation on which my life was constructed fell down . . . I seemed to have nothing to live for" (Anthony, 1975b, 448). Eventually, Mill recovered from his depression as he began to be able to substitute his own ideals for those of his father.

This vignette dramatically portrays the clash of doctrines that occurs at adolescence in our culture. The older familial standards and expectations may differ markedly from those of peers or of new significant adults. At adolescence, the individual is not only able to assess his or her ability to live up to these often conflicting standards, but can also predict where adherence to a code of behavior will lead in the future. These cognitive advances, together with the very real social pressures encountered at adolescence, account for some of the specific forms of depression seen in this developmental stage.

SUMMARY

The foregoing attempt to describe the symptoms and causes of depression at the varying stages of development is summarized in Table 1, which is taken from an earlier work on this topic (Bemporad, 1978). At the extreme right of the table is a list of the stages of ego development as distilled by Jane Loevinger (1976) from various authors and her original research. Each type of dysphoria may be seen as corresponding to a parallel step in the overall development of the child. The concept of stages as stable, permanent entities is a distortion of the reality of the continuous, fluid process of development, but this should be considered an artifact of the method of trying to capture an ongoing process through static concepts. The goal is to further the argument that the quality of affects, positive and negative, changes with the developmental process.

The manifestations and precipitants of dysphoric states in childhood should be considered against a developmental framework which includes: cognitive advances; enlarging social contacts and sources of gratification and esteem; different developmental tasks which may present as sources of frustration and satisfaction; and an increasingly complex repertoire of responses. As the child matures, the dysphoric states become more complex and gradually begin to resemble the depressions of adults, but these episodes are not equal to adult melancholia because of the child's relative cognitive and social immaturity. Similarly, the younger the child, the less structured or internalized is

Table 1. Symptoms and Causes of Depression at Various Stages of Development

Developmental Stage	Symptoms	Major Psychodynamics	Type of Dysphoria	Loevinger Ego Developmental Stages*
Infancy	Withdrawal after crying and protest	Loss of stimulation, security, and well-being supplied by the mother	Deprivation of needed stimulation	Presocial, symbiotic
Early childhood	Inhibition, clinging behavior	Disapproval by parents	Inhibition of gratification of emerging sense of will	Impulsive, self-protective, fear of being caught, externalizing blame, opportunistic
Middle childhood	Sadness as automatically responsive to the immediate situation	Rejection by parents, loss of gratifying activities (i.e., chronic illness)	Sadness, unsustained crying directly related to frustrating or depriving situation	Conformist: conformity to external rules; shame and guilt for breaking rules; superficial niceness
Late childhood	Depression with low self-esteem	Unable to meet parental ideal, unable to sustain threat to parental relationship	Depression with a cognitive component, affect resulting from deduction about circumstances	Conscientious: conformist; differentiation of norms and goals; awareness of self in relation to group; helping
Adolescence	Depression with exaggerated urgency, time distortion, and impulsivity	Unable to fulfill internalized parental ideal, inability to separate from family	Accentuation of depression by cognitive distortions about the finality of events	Conscientious: self-evaluated standards; guilt for consequences; long-term goals and ideals

*Adapted from Loevinger (1976)

the pathology, and the more amenable the person is to environmental changes. As the child grows older, however, the predisposition to become depressed becomes more entrenched and thus the more difficult to alter. In our clinical work with children, we should strive to prevent this stabilization of pathological attitudes toward the self and others. Doing so, within the context of a developmental framework, promises to lead us to a better understanding of childhood psycho-pathology generally and, subsequently, to more effective prevention and treatment.

Chapter 18 Epidemiology of Childhood Depression†
by Javad H. Kashani, M.D., F.R.C.P.(C)

INTRODUCTION

Psychiatric epidemiology involves the study of the various factors which determine the pattern of occurrence of mental disorders, the ecological and human factors that influence those patterns, and the outcome of attempts to alter them. It forms the scientific basis of public health psychiatry and preventative psychiatry (Gruenberg, 1980). Generally, epidemiology is founded on the premise that the distribution of a specific disorder within the general population is not determined completely randomly but that it varies among subgroups defined by age, sex, social background, or other characteristics. The importance of epidemiology stems from the fact that knowledge of the pattern of occurrence of a disorder may eventually suggest causal or contributing factors or strategies for prevention. The hypotheses generated through epidemiologic studies may then be tested by other methods, such as laboratory or clinical investigations. In the past, epidemiologic research has focused on attempts to isolate the single factor that would provide a necessary and sufficient explanation for a given disorder. This approach is being supplanted, especially in psychiatric research, by multifactorial models of causation (Weissman and Klerman, 1978).

Epidemiologic researchers have found a relatively high prevalence of depression among adults (Weissman et al., 1981). Among all psychiatric diagnoses it is the most common, both in regard to point prevalence and lifetime prevalence (Weissman and Myers, 1978). With the recent upsurge of interest in childhood depression, it is appropriate to consider the question of epidemiology, but as yet there are few published reports emphasizing the epidemiological aspects of the topic. This chapter reviews available data on various epidemiologic aspects of childhood depression, such as prevalence, sociodemographic variables, and high risk factors. Based on this review, the chapter concludes with a brief examination of approaches to prevention, emphasizing the limitations of prevention strategies that have incomplete epidemiological bases.

†The author thanks James M.A. Weiss, M.D., M.P.H., Professor and Chairman, Department of Psychiatry, University of Missouri-Columbia, for his critical comments about the manuscript.

PREVALENCE

The reported frequency of childhood depression varies greatly, depending on the sample being studied and the diagnostic criteria which are used. Nissen (1971) found moderately severe and severe depressive states in 1.8 percent of 6,000 children. Meierhofer (1972), in a longitudinal study of institutionalized children, reported that 25 percent had suffered from periods of depression. Ling et al. (1970), using their own diagnostic criteria, found that forty percent of 25 children who presented with headache were diagnosed as depressed. Bauersfeld (1972) found that 13.7 percent of 400 children referred to a child psychiatry setting showed depressed mood or other depressive conditions. Among 10,000 children seen at a psychiatric clinic in Turkey, Cebiroglu et al. (1972) reported a frequency of depression of 0.8 percent. In a psychiatric inpatient population, McConville et al. (1973) found 53 percent of 141 children (ages six to 13 years) to be depressed. Weinberg et al. (1973) reported a prevalence of 58 percent among 72 consecutive, nonhospitalized referrals to an educational diagnostic center. Pearce (1977), using diagnostic criteria similar to those of Weinberg et al. (1973), found depressive symptoms in 23 percent of 547 children (ages one to 17 years) in a child psychiatric setting. Carlson and Cantwell (1980) studied children and adolescents in both inpatient and outpatient settings and made the diagnosis of an affective disorder in 27 percent of 102 cases. Of those diagnosed as having an affective disorder, 43 percent showed primary and 57 percent showed secondary affective disorders. Furthermore, 82 percent of the children diagnosed as having affective disorders were categorized as having major depression. Kuperman and Stewart (1979) used structured interviews with the parents of 175 children (ages eight to 16 years) from both inpatient and outpatient psychiatric services and reported that 13 percent of the girls and five percent of the boys were depressed.

The literature contains only three reports of epidemiological studies of childhood depression in the general population. The first study, performed by Rutter et al. (1970), reported three definite cases of childhood depression from a sample of 2,199 children (1.4 cases per thousand population). This study is important because it reported definite cases of childhood depression within a presumably normal population. Unfortunately, however, the study was completed before current diagnostic instruments were available, and it was not mainly designed to detect depression. Albert and Beck (1975) studied 63 children in a classroom setting. Using the short form of the Beck Depression Inventory, they reported that 33 percent of the children assessed were moderately to severely depressed, but the authors questioned whether their data represented "genuine depression." The only epidemiological study of childhood depression to date which has applied the DSM-III diagnostic criteria for Major Depression to a randomly selected general population of children is that of the author and Simonds (1979). In this study, 103 chidren (ages seven to 12 years) and their parents were interviewed in their homes. The study found that two children (1.9 percent) were suffering from marked depression.

The wide range of frequencies for depression in the aforementioned studies is to be expected for several reasons. First, the populations sampled in the various studies differed. Populations were psychiatric inpatients, psychiatric outpatients, children in residential nurseries or educational diagnostic centers, pediatric patients, or surgical patients. Second, the criteria used to make the diagnosis of childhood depression varied from study to study. Third, the depression among these patients is probably multifactorial in causation, involving interactions of genetic, biochemical, developmental, temperamental, and environmental factors (Klerman, 1980).

Many of the discrepancies and issues could be resolved by studying a large sample drawn from the general population and following it longitudinally. A study of this sort could yield valuable information concerning the prevalence of childhood depression and avoid some of the deficiencies of most of the currently available studies. Samples chosen from a population of psychiatric patients represent only that portion of affected individuals who have sought help for their disorder. It is well known among epidemiologists that the cases seen in clinical care represent only the tip of the iceberg and that below that tip is a large population of persons who are affected but do not seek help (Gruenberg, 1980). It was found in one study, for example, that only about one quarter of adults with major depressive symptoms had sought professional help for their problem during the previous year (Weissman and Myers, 1978). In addition, the Midtown study revealed that only one person in twenty classified as impaired was in treatment at the time of the survey (Srole et al., 1962). In other words, clinical surveys investigate patients, while epidemiological surveys describe patients in relation to the population to which they belong (Barker and Rose, 1976, 35).

A longitudinal study of childhood depression would have the further advantage of yielding information on the *incidence* of the disorder (i.e., the rate of occurrence of new cases) as well as on the *prevalence* of the disorder (i.e., the number of cases that exist at any given time). The importance of obtaining information concerning the incidence stems from the fact that the incidence is not influenced by the duration of the disorder, whereas the prevalence is. With chronic illness, even a low incidence may produce a high prevalence through the buildup of cases. Thus, through continuous follow-up, information on the number of persons who are affected by the disorder during their lifetimes can be obtained.

Another advantage of a longitudinal study is that premorbid data can be collected on persons who later become affected. In this way, adjustment to developmental stages and the relationship of development to childhood depression can be accurately studied.

SOCIODEMOGRAPHIC VARIABLES

Age

Depression in preschool children is reportedly either nonexistent or exceedingly difficult to diagnose, in part because language does not become truly a vehicle of communication until approximately the age of seven years (Kovacs and Beck, 1977). Except for the well-known study by Spitz (1946), there has not been a systematic evaluation of depression in a large number of preschool children. A recent report described anaclitic depression in a three-and-a-half-month-old child who showed sad facies, withdrawal, apathy, absence of pleasure, and psychomotor retardation (Gaensbauer, 1980). Further study of depression and depressive symptoms in preschool children is definitely needed for a better understanding of the condition.

There has been a recent interest in prepubertal depression among clinic and nonclinic samples (Kashani and Simonds, 1979; Philips, 1979; Orvaschel et al., 1980; Puig-Antich, 1980; Petti, 1978; Cytryn et al., 1980; Kashani et al., 1981c). Before puberty depression is reported to be relatively common (Kuperman and Stewart, 1979), but in adolescence it is reported to be more frequent (Rutter et al., 1976; Kashani et al., 1980; Yanchyshyn and Robbins, 1980). Rutter et al. (1976) reported that the frequency of depression was three times higher at age 14 years than at age ten years. The higher frequency of depression reported in adolescents, as compared with younger age groups, could reflect a complex of factors, such as hormonal, developmental, or psychological factors, as well as differences in social expectations. The reported differences could also be the result of the older child's greater skills in verbal communication or of differences in symptomatology at different stages of development.[*]

Sex

Adult depression is reported more frequently in females than in males. For every male diagnosed as depressed, two to six females receive the diagnosis (Penfeld, 1981). Weissman and Klerman (1979) reviewed the literature on sex and depression and favored psychosocial factors as an explanation for the sex differences.

Several clinical studies indicate that childhood depression is more common in males than in females. Weinberg's sample of 42 depressed children included thirty boys and 12 girls (Weinberg, 1973). Other studies which have found a greater frequency of childhood depression in boys than in girls include those by Poznanski and Zrull (1970), Puig-Antich et al. (1978), and Kashani et al. (1981a). Statistical tests for the significance of the sex differences were not done in any of these studies, and the differences reported may reflect the fact that a larger number of prepubertal boys than girls were seen in the clinics (Poznanski and Zrull, 1970). In a study of one hundred physically handicapped children, 14 of the 23 depressed subjects were girls, and nine were boys (Kashani et al., 1981d). Kuperman and Stewart (1979) reported 13 percent of the girls in their sample and five percent of the boys to be depressed. In their sample, however, both children and adolescents were included, and in adolescence a sex distribution similar to that in adulthood emerges.

Ethnic and Socioeconomic Status

Childhood depression has been reported among both black and white children (Puig-Antich et al., 1978; Kashani et al., 1981a), but there are no published data which primarily address the question of childhood depression in different ethnic groups.

The association between social class and the prevalence of adult depression is as yet unsettled, but depression has been considered by some to be greater in higher socioeconomic groups (Ripley, 1977). Bebbington's work, however, indicates that only the circular manic-depressive disorder was more prevalent in higher social classes (Beb-

*Preceptor's note: For further discussion of the likely impact of development, see the chapter by Bemporad.

bington, 1978). He reported that the rate of serious depressive disorders does not vary significantly among different socioeconomic classes. Marsella (1980) reported that the somatic expression of depression is much more common in non-Western cultures, and that within the Western cultures the lower socioeconomic and educationally deprived classes more commonly display somatic expressions of depression.

Environmental Factors

This broad category includes societal, cultural, community, educational, and family influences, as well as specific life events unique to the individual. All of these factors influence the child, but only familial influences and life events are discussed here, and they are discussed briefly, due to limitations of space.

The effect of parental illness on children has been discussed in numerous publications (Philips, 1979; Orvaschel et al., 1980; Poznanski and Zrull, 1979; Orvaschel et al., 1981; Weissman, 1979; Rutter, 1966; McKnew et al., 1979). The onset of depression in a parent may be experienced by the child as a disruption of affectional bonds, and this may lead to the development of symptoms in the child (Weissman, 1979). It has also been shown that depressed children have significantly more depressed parents than do nondepressed children (Gaensbauer, 1980; Poznanski and Zrull, 1970).

As discussed by Lloyd (1980) in a review of life events and depressive disorders, several studies have compared the incidence of childhood bereavement or other childhood loss events among depressed patients and controls and noted an increased incidence of bereavement or loss among the depressed. Although some discrepancies do exist in the data, the risk of depression when a child loses a parent by death is generally two to three times greater than usual. Early loss events may also be related to the severity of subsequent depression and to the frequency of attempted suicide.

A study that compared three distinct groups of children (psychiatric patients, pediatric patients, and normal controls) found no consistent correlations between the number of recent significant life events and the diagnosis of depression (Kashani et al., 1981b). Despite the significant association between childhood loss events and depression, the majority of depressed patients have not experienced an early loss event, so that other factors must be operating as well (Lloyd, 1980). A longitudinal study of the effect of significant life events on the development of childhood depression would help to answer many of the currently unanswered questions about these and other possible contributing factors.

HIGH RISK FACTORS

Children at higher risk of developing depression may include those suffering from parental deprivation due to separation, a parent's psychiatric illness, or parental abuse or neglect. A family history of depression and suicide should also be considered as a risk factor (Weissman, 1979), but genetics may also play a role. Some chronic physical illnesses may also place the child at risk (Kashani et al., 1981a). Losses and the inability to achieve an expected goal, with a consequent loss of self-esteem, are other potential factors (Kashani et al., 1981d).

Parental Factors

A high incidence of parental depression is the most consistent finding in studies of childhood depression, but its etiologic significance is still unclear. Whether parental depression gives rise to childhood depression via psychodynamic mechanisms, such as parental identification, or whether other mechanisms exist, is unknown. Moreover, the occurrence of both childhood and parental depression within the same family may reflect hereditary or genetic vulnerability (Poznanski, 1979). Seven twin studies demonstrated an overall monozygotic twin concordance rate of 76 percent for this disorder, compared with a dizygotic twin rate of 19 percent (Tsuang, 1978). Studies of monozygotic twins reared apart demonstrated a 67 percent concordance rate. Data evaluating genetic influences in the context of adoption are unavailable. Although no subtype of depressive disorders has been shown to be related to a given mode of inheritance, the subtype of parental depression should be considered important and should be studied separately because of the possibility of genetic heterogeneity in affective disorders. An obvious example would involve children of bipolar or unipolar parents (Orvaschel, 1980). Some of the differences between the children of bipolar and unipolar parents have been reported by Conners et al. (1979).

Loss and other Factors

The most common risk factor studied in childhood depression is loss. The term *loss* is, however, very broad and could be used to encompass both real and fantasized loss. A real loss was reported as a possible contributing factor in the physically handicapped children admitted to a surgical hospital (Kashani et al., 1981d). The authors concluded that although each child in the tested sample of one hundred had a severe physical handicap, not all became depressed. This suggests a significant role for other factors, such as acceptance of the handicap by the child, the quality of the parent-child relationship, the temperament of the child, his or her capacity to adapt to the handicap, and cultural factors. However, it remains that over one-fifth of the sample did, in fact, suffer from depression, thus demonstrating that children who become handicapped, with a real not a fantasized loss, are at greater risk than the general population for development of depression.

The child who suffers loss of a parent, parents, or parental surrogates is at risk for becoming depressed (Lucas, 1977). It is not a simple sequence of losing a parent and then developing depression, but hinges rather on the ability to substitute other figures for the lost parent and on the sex of the parent as well. Rutter (1966) stated, "Children who lose a parent of the same sex are most likely to have a psychiatric disorder, which suggests that the same-sexed parent plays a special role in the child's development, perhaps by providing a model."

The child with a learning disability, especially if the family is highly educated and expects high scholastic achievement, often loses self-esteem and feels inadequate. The learning disability may exemplify the child's failure to achieve parental expectations, leading to feelings of helplessness and inadequacy with a resultant loss of self-esteem. This represents an overlap between two conceptual models of depression, the learned helplessness model (Seligman, 1975), and Bibring's idea that when the ego is aware of its goal and is yet unable to attain it, depression occurs (Robertson, 1979).

PREVENTION

The scope of prevention, it has been written, extends to "information and education programs, to anticipatory guidance before life crisis, and to providing extra community support systems during ordinary life crises. That concept of prevention is based on the theory that [such services] will reduce the frequency with which certain forms of deterioration arise" (Gruenberg, 1980, 546). Traditionally, prevention has been divided into three parts, primary, secondary, and tertiary (Spiro, 1980).

Primary prevention has been defined as the elimination of factors that cause the disease. In the case of childhood depression, primary prevention should ultimately include efforts to eliminate causes of the disorder, but the causes are unclear. In the meantime, based on what we do know, treating the depressed and psychiatrically disturbed parents might be an example of primary prevention in children. In children who have suffered loss, the substitution for any possible losses and in learning disabled children the provision of tutorial services may be primary prevention measures. As greater knowledge about childhood depression accumulates, we will be better able to delineate primary prevention measures.

Secondary prevention has been defined as early detection and treatment of the disease, clearly indicating the importance of early diagnosis. Secondary prevention in childhood depression may involve not only the psychiatrist and other mental health professionals, but also the many other professionals who are working with children and their families. Because of its many and varied physical symptoms and signs, several studies indicate, depression is the psychiatric disorder most commonly encountered in the practices of family physicians, in prepaid health plans, and in the nonpsychiatric wards of general hospitals. Unfortunately, however, depression frequently remains underdiagnosed. For example, one study showed that primary physicians failed to diagnose about fifty percent of both depressed and otherwise psychiatrically impaired patients (Nielsen and Williams, 1980). Somatic complaints in depressed children have been reported in numerous studies (Kashani et al., in press).

The parents of children who suffer from depression and somatic complaints are likely to take them to pediatricians or family doctors rather than to mental health professionals. This highlights the early detection role of nonpsychiatric professionals, i.e., pediatricians, general practitioners, family doctors, and others, such as teachers. It is our responsibility as psychiatrists to educate these professionals, as well as the general public, to increase their knowledge of the symptomatology of depression. Identifying and treating a depressed mother at an early stage would not only be a means of secondary prevention for the mother, but perhaps more importantly could be considered primary prevention for the child. In the not too distant future, an instrument may be available for the early detection of depression. Such instruments have been developed by Birleson (1981) and by Kashani, McKnew, and Cytryn based on DSM-III diagnostic criteria (Kashani et al., 1980).

Tertiary prevention refers to rehabilitation, eliminating disability following the acute phase of a disorder, and helping the patient achieve maximal functioning. For most patients, a return to the premorbid state is the tertiary prevention goal. Tertiary prevention has been the most successful kind of prevention in the rehabilitation of seriously mentally ill patients (Spiro, 1980). In the case of childhood depression, tertiary prevention could aim to keep the condition from deteriorating and to help the patient to return to his or her previous level of functioning. By treating the child's primary depression, we might also avoid extensive medical procedures, such as upper and lower GI X-rays. Depression has been shown to be significantly higher among children with GI disorders (Kashani et al., 1981a). Treatment could also prevent other disabilities from developing: poor performance at school, poor social skills, withdrawal, somatic complaints, and even suicide could be prevented.

In general, specific methods of preventing childhood depression can hardly be applied and evaluated until the diagnosis can be made with greater conviction and precision and until the contributing and causative factors are better recognized.

CONCLUSION

The results of epidemiological studies of childhood depression will remain inconclusive until there is general agreement about an acceptable set of criteria for diagnosis (Anthony, 1977). Achieving agreement is complicated by the recognition that several subtypes of depression exist, i.e., major, atypical, and dysthymic, as well as primary, secondary, endogenous, reactive, and so forth. Obviously, simply lumping these subtypes together would not clarify the issue. Preferably, one would seek to identify and study different variables within each subtype. If each subtype were studied separately, a more homogeneous group could eventually emerge. Recent biological validation of childhood depression (Puig-Antich, 1979; 1980) and availability of a set of criteria for diagnosis such as DSM-III are a good start.

Based on present data, however, we cannot identify any single causative factor. A combination of interacting factors—environmental, familial, physical, and other factors—is most likely contributory. Therefore, a comprehensive evaluation which approached the problem from a multidimensional perspective, and which studied it in different developmental stages, would help to give us a better grasp of the subject. Since answers to the many questions regarding childhood depression are not only of importance to psychiatrists but are also crucial to other professionals who are dealing with families and children, childhood depression will undoubtedly be an area of active investigation in the 1980's.

Chapter 19
Psychobiological Correlates of Major Depressive Disorder in Children and Adolescents†
by Joaquim Puig-Antich, M.D.

INTRODUCTION

Part III
Psychiatry
1982
288

The concept of childhood depression, which has gained so much credence in the last few years, started its life in the 1950's (Campbell,

†This chapter is based in part on research supported by Grant Nos. MH 30838 and MH 30839 from the National Institute of Mental Health.

1952; 1955), but did not make an impact until the early 1970's (Poznanski et al., 1970; Cytryn et al., 1972). At birth, the concept of child and adolescent depression appeared as a full-fledged counterpart to the well-known adult depressive syndrome. By the 1970's there was much confusion about it. Not accepted by most child psychiatrists at the time, depression in children was also foreign to adult psychiatrists. People held widely divergent points of view about its prevalence, from thinking it nonexistent (Rie, 1966), to believing it remarkably ubiquitous (Glesser, 1967). Such a phenomenon occurs frequently in science when scarce data are matched only by proliferating untested theories.

A key development to lead us out of this confusion, in the author's opinion, was the discovery that Research Diagnostic Criteria (RDC) for major depression in adults (Feighner et al., 1972; Spitzer et al., 1978) could be used successfully with children and adolescents, either unmodified (Puig-Antich et al., 1978), or with some modifications (Weinberg et al., 1973; Ling et al., 1970). During the last few years there has emerged in the U.S. a consensus that adult criteria for the diagnosis of major depression may be used with children and adolescents (Carlson et al., 1979; 1980; Carlson, 1980; Cytryn et al., 1980; Kupferman et al., 1979; Puig-Antich et al., 1978; Weinberg et al., 1973; Welner et al., 1977). This consensus is reflected in the DSM-III classification of mental disorders, where the same major criteria for depressive disorders are used for all age groups*

While the new consensus is data based to some degree, it should be clear that the research data are only feasibility data. Using either unstructured or semistructured clinical interview protocols, several investigators have assessed all the symptoms included as systematic criteria of major depression and have determined that some children fit the criteria for the disorder. But this does not define the limits of depressive illness in children. Rather it does suggest that the children identified are likely to be the most severely affected, since they fit the same criteria (endogenous subtype) as the most severely depressed adults (Puig-Antich et al., 1978; Carlson et al., 1978; Strober et al., 1980). Thus, the lower diagnostic limit of the disorder in youngsters has not yet been identified.

Contrary to this general observation, one little known clinical study used a superior strategy to investigate the existence of depressive illness in children as it is known in adults. In that study, Pearce (1977) used the symptomatic records of 547 psychiatric patients ages one to 17 years and divided them into two groups according to the presence (25 percent of the sample) or absence (75 percent of the sample) of dysphoric mood. Discriminant function analysis showed that the symptoms of the depressive syndrome clustered with depressed mood. This finding provides strong support for the hypothesis that the diagnosis of depressive disorder is not simply superimposed on youngsters by child psychiatric researchers using adult criteria. Instead it indicates that depressive disorders may be real entities in youngsters. And this is the issue this chapter addresses.

The main questions to be answered at present are: what is the nature of depressive illness in youngsters, and what are the relationships between prepubertal, adolescent, adult, and geriatric major depressive

*Preceptor's note: The consensus around this view, it should be noted, does not mean that alternate or complementary views are either nonexistent or invalid. See the chapters by Philips and Friedlander and by Bemporad.

disorders? Both questions can be answered through validation studies.

If an adult-type depressive syndrome can be identified in children, we can then attempt to validate the finding by studying in these children and appropriate controls all the psychological and biological characteristics which have been found associated with adult major depression. Such validation studies can further define the multi-dimensional nature of the disorder and eventually may yield guidelines and tests for diagnosis. Fortunately, the number and type of characteristics which can be used for validation are larger and more diverse than is usual in psychiatric research. During the last twenty years a variety of biological correlates have been found to accompany adult major depressions. These include:

(1) family history;
(2) response to imipramine and other antidepressants;
(3) neuroendocrine correlates:
   growth hormone (GH) hyporesponsivity to insulin-induced hypoglycemia (Gregoire et al., 1977; Gruen et al., 1975);
   cortisol hypersecretion (Carroll et al., 1976a; 1976b; Sachar, 1975; Sachar et al., 1973);
   hyporesponsivity to desmethylimipramine (Laakman, 1979) and to D-amphetamine (Langer et al., 1976); and
   blunting of thyrotropin (TSH) response to infusion of thyrotropin-releasing hormone (TRH) (Kirkegaard et al., 1975; Prange, 1977; Takahasi et al., 1974);
(4) polysomnographic correlates:
   increased REM density (Coble et al., 1980; Gillin et al., 1979; Vogel et al., 1980);
   shortened REMP latency (Gillin et al., 1979; Kupfer, 1976; Vogel et al., 1980);
   decreased delta sleep (Coble et al., 1980; Kupfer et al., 1979);
   decreased sleep efficiency (Gillin et al., 1979; Kupfer et al., 1979); and abnormal temporal distribution of REM sleep (Vogel et al., 1980); and
(5) long-term follow-up.

At this time data have been reported for categories (1), (2), (3), and (4) in prepubertal major depression, and for (1) in adolescent major depression. In the interest of brevity, the author reviews the highlights of these reports and of his ongoing studies. Long-term follow-up reports, category (5), when they become available, will be of great importance to our understanding of the psychobiology of childhood and adolescent depression.

FAMILY HISTORY

In an ongoing, blind, family history study of prepubertal major depressive disorders, the author and his colleagues have used the family history RDC method (Andreasen et al., 1977). Midpoint analysis indicates that the lifetime morbidity risk for prepubertal major depressive disorder in first-degree biological relatives over 16 years of age is 0.42. The morbidity risk for alcoholism is 0.29, for antisocial personality 0.18, and for mania 0.04. Schizophrenia is found at the same rate as in the general population. When these figures are eventually corrected for age, the rates for depression and alcoholism will increase, given the youth of these relatives (late 20's to early 30's). In contrast, the lifetime morbidity risk for major depression in first-degree biological relatives (over 16 years of age) of adult major depressives is 0.30 (Theodore Reich, personal communication, 1980). The data suggest that prepubertal major depressives are likely to be a highly genetically loaded group, and this may, at least partially, account for such an early onset.

Strober et al. (unpublished) have recently completed a similar study in sixty adolescent inpatient major depressives. Seventy-seven percent of the probands had at least one first- or second-degree relative with a lifetime diagnosis of major depressive disorder. The joint morbidity risk for first- and second-degree relatives for affective disorder could be calculated to be 0.21. It can be considered likely that it would be much higher if only first-degree relatives were considered.

In summary, data from family history studies of prepubertal and adolescent major depressive disorder support the validity of the diagnosis in these age groups. They also suggest that the early onset of illness may be related to high genetic loading. The likelihood of this is underlined by the high proportion of bipolarity (Achenbach, 1978) reported by Strober, Green, and Carlson (1980) on the follow-up of their sample of adolescent major depressives.[*]

RESPONSE TO IMIPRAMINE

During the last 12 years there have been reports of a variety of open studies in which antidepressant drugs were used to treat children diagnosed as depressed (Connell, 1972; Frommer, 1968; Kuhn and Kuhn, 1972; Lelord et al., 1972; Ling et al., 1970; Polvan and Cebiroglu, 1972; Stack, 1972). In practically all, about 75 percent of the children were reported to have responded. Nevertheless, making conclusions from the studies cited is difficult for a variety of reasons. All of the studies were uncontrolled, the diagnosis was made in clinical fashion, no structured interview protocols were used, no diagnostic criteria were specified, there were no indications of what specific symptoms had been observed, the length of the therapeutic trials was highly variable (from a few weeks to several months), and dosages were by and large too low.

Three different open studies, however, had better designs and assessment methods (Weinberg, 1973; Frommer, 1967; Puig-Antich et al., 1978). In these studies, too, about 75 percent of the children responded. Taken as a whole, the studies do suggest that the drugs are effective with depressed children and justify our undertaking properly controlled studies.

Recently the author and his colleagues completed work on the possible effectiveness of imipramine in prepubertal children with major depressive disorder. They simultaneously conducted two studies in the same sample of children who fit the criteria for this diagnosis: (1) a five-week double-blind, placebo-controlled study of imipramine up to 5.0 mg/kg/day; and (2) a study of the relationship between steady-state plasma levels of imipramine plus desmethylimipramine and clinical response in children randomly assigned to the drug. Imipramine was administered in three daily doses, divided roughly equally. Dosage was increased to 5.0 mg/kg/day over a 12-day period. The dose was raised every third day in stepwise fashion from 0 to 1.5, 3.0, 4.0, and 5.0 mg/kg/day. Before each dose increase, electrocardiographic (EKG), blood pressure, and other clinical side effects were measured. If any of the following occurred, the dose either was not increased any further

[*]Preceptor's note: See also the discussion of parental, family, and genetic factors in Kashani's chapter.

or was slightly decreased: (1) EKG changes induced by imipramine reached predetermined safety criteria, (resting heart rate $\geq$ 130 per minute, PR interval $\geq$ 0.18, or QRS $\geq$ 130 percent of baseline); and/or (2) systolic blood pressure $\geq$ 145 or diastolic blood pressure $\geq$ 95 mm Hg; and/or (3) unacceptable clinical side effects developed.

In a preliminary paper on the plasma level study, the author and his colleagues reported that six responders had significantly higher plasma levels than seven nonresponders (mean = 231 ng/ml vs. 128 ng/ml; $p < 0.05$, two-tailed) (Puig-Antich et al., 1979). Analysis of results for thirty subjects at the end of the study confirms the initial results (Puig-Antich et al., submitted[a]). Responders have significantly higher plasma levels than nonresponders ($p < 0.007$). Plasma levels over 155 ng/ml are associated with clinical response, and most optimal responses were obtained at plasma levels over 200 ng/ml.

The double-blind study, just completed, shows a sixty percent response rate for the group receiving placebo and a sixty percent response rate for the group receiving imipramine. Therefore it indicates that imipramine, administered up to 5.0 mg/kg/day, with the current safety criteria, does no better than placebo in inducing clinical response. However, when the group receiving imipramine is subdivided according to steady-state plasma level above and below 155 ng/ml, the response rate in the high plasma level subgroup is one hundred percent, while in the low plasma level subgroup it is only 33 percent. Weller and Preskorn (1981) have studied plasma level and clinical response in depressed inpatient children and recently reported findings which basically confirm these initial findings.

In summary, the effectiveness of imipramine in the treatment of prepubertal major depressive disorder does not receive final support from the studies. The data do suggest that plasma level may be a key variable in determining clinical response. As in adults, dose does not generally predict plasma level. The exception to this generalization is that, in a given individual, higher dosages, administered in the same fashion, will produce higher steady-state plasma levels. Based on these data the author and his co-workers have hypothesized that if plasma levels could be systematically measured, and adjustments in dose were made to produce a steady-state plasma level of 200 ng/ml, the rate of clinical response of the depressive syndrome in prepuberty could be maximized to nearly óne hundred percent.

NEUROENDOCRINE CORRELATES

Growth Hormone (GH) Hyporesponsivity to Insulin-Induced Hypoglycemia

The author and his team have recently studied GH response to insulin-induced hypoglycemia in prepubertal children (Tabrizi et al., 1979). They have measured and analyzed the response in ten children with endogenous depression, ten children with nonendogenous depression, and seven nondepressed children with neurotic emotional disorder. Based on plasma samples obtained every 15 minutes after injection of insulin, they found highly significant differences between the groups in plasma concentrations of GH at 30, 45, and 60 minutes after injection. Most of the differences were accounted for by hyposecretion of GH in the group with endogenous depression. Ninety percent of the endogenous group had a peak GH concentration in the first hour below 4.0

ng/ml, while fifty percent of the nonendogenous group and one hundred percent of the neurotic group had peak values above 4.0 ng/ml. All subjects included in the analysis had drops in blood glucose level of at least fifty percent of baseline values.

Correlational analyses within each experimental group showed no evidence of a relationship between the speed and magnitude of the drop in glucose level, on the one hand, and GH response on the other. To the author's knowledge no other test of GH secretion has been studied in youngsters with endogenous depressions.

Although not much psychoendocrine research has been carried out in prepubertal psychiatric disorders, hyposecretion of GH in response to hypoglycemia has been reported in psychosocial dwarfism (Brown, 1976; Money et al., 1976). Actually, it was this work on psychosocial dwarfism which prompted Sachar to hypothesize that adult depressives may also secrete less GH in reponse to the same stimulus (Sachar et al., 1971). Sachar based his hypothesis on the fact that some clinical features of psychosocial dwarfs appeared similar to what Spitz described as anaclitic depression in maternally deprived infants (Spitz, 1945).

Despite the similarities, however, several clinical characteristics of psychosocial dwarfism and prepubertal major depression, as well as their respective GH hyporesponses to hypoglycemia, indicate that these are different and easily differentiated disorders, although they may conceivably coexist. Children with psychosocial dwarfism by definition present abnormally short stature and severe sleeplessness (Wolf et al., 1973). Their sleep and growth disorders, as well as their GH hyporesponse to insulin-induced hypoglycemia, quickly reverse when they are placed outside the home, be it in a hospital or in a residential center. In contrast, in the sample of the author and his colleagues, prepubertal children with major depression are not shorter than controls, polysomnographic studies do not show any major differences from controls (Puig-Antich et al., 1978), and preliminary data indicate that the endogenous group may continue to hyposecrete GH in response to hypoglycemia months after clinical recovery while in a nondepressed state.

Cortisol Hypersecretion

In a preliminary paper the author and his colleagues reported the presence of cortisol hypersecretion in two out of four prepubertal, medically healthy children, who fit unmodified RDC for major depressive disorder, endogenous subtype (Spitzer et al., 1978). They analyzed the cortisol curves of a nine-year-old male patient before treatment and when he was drug free and had fully recovered. A full 24-hour study with sampling every twenty minutes revealed that during illness the boy had an almost threefold increase in mean 24-hour cortisol, 8.45 micrograms per deciliter (mcg/dl). During illness the number of secretory episodes almost doubled, peak values and minimal values were both higher, and a greater amount of time was spent secreting. The "decay" curve slopes did not change during or after illness, indicating no differences in half-life of plasma cortisol secretion. This hypersecretory pattern resembled the pattern which had been described in adult endogenous depressives (Sachar et al., 1973). Fifteen days after the boy experienced the onset of a depressive recurrence six months later, the author and his co-workers studied him again. His mean 24-hour cortisol level was already almost twice as great (5.7 mcg/dl) as the one found when he was fully recovered (3.0 mcg/dl).

The study of the 24-hour pattern of cortisol secretion has now been completed. Between ten percent and fifteen percent of prepubertal major depressives present the hypersecretory pattern. The others do not. Moreover, group comparisons do not turn up significant differences between depressives and controls, even if specific periods during the day are considered. Thus, although cortisol hypersecretion does exist in about ten percent of prepubertal major depressives when studied during and after their depressive episode, the phenomenon has no value in discriminating between depressed and nondepressed children.

The low prevalence of the phenomenon in prepuberty may be due to a maturational or age factor. In his adult depressive sample of 26, Sachar found an interaction between age and cortisol hypersecretion. The older the depressive the more likely was he or she to hypersecrete cortisol (Asnis et al., 1981). Prepubertal children may lie on the left side of the regression line. No 24-hour cortisol studies have been done in depressive adolescents. Data on this age group could help to clarify the relationship between age and cortisol hypersecretion in depressives.

The lack of group differences with 24-hour studies does not necessarily indicate that cortisol secretion in prepubertal depression is normal. It is clear now that the low-dose dexamethasone suppression test (DST) identifies more adult endogenous depressives than the 24-hour studies. At present at least two studies are ongoing investigating the DST in major depressive youngsters (Poznanski; Puig-Antich). Conceivably dexamethasone suppression and cortisol hypersecretion are mediated by different mechanisms.

Overall, the neuroendocrine results so far tend to validate both the existence of prepubertal major depression and its similarity to adult major depression. Future work in this area promises to validate the disorder further, to lead to diagnostic tests for the condition, and perhaps to provide guidelines to clinicians regarding the solidity of apparent clinical recoveries and the appropriate timing for discontinuation of treatment.

POLYSOMNOGRAPHIC CORRELATES

Kane et al. (1977) reported on prepubertal depression in an 11-year-old girl who presented a shortened first REMP latency as compared to published age norms (Williams et al., 1974), disturbed continuity of sleep, and low sleep efficiency. The same group of investigators published a report (Kupfer et al., 1979) on the effect of antidepressant medication on polysomnographic patterns in a group of 12 early adolescent and prepubertal depressives. Before treatment, they found, neither the depressives nor the normal controls were significantly different from published norms (Williams et al., 1974) as to sleep architecture, sleep continuity, or REM latency. Findings from these open studies are difficult to interpret because the clinical diagnosis was made using the criteria of Weinberg et al. (1973). These have been shown to be less specific than DSM-III criteria for Major Depression (Carlson et al., 1980).

The author and his team have completed a controlled study of polysomnographic patterns that four groups of drug-free prepubertal subjects exhibit during illness (Puig-Antich et al., 1981). Results fail to indicate any significant differences between RDC endogenous major depressives, nonendogenous major depressives, nondepressed neurotic emotional disorders, and normals. The few significant differences (total sleep period and total sleep time) that occurred during the first night could be entirely attributed to adaptation effects in the neurotic group, and these differences had disappeared by the second night.

First REMP latencies were quite stable between 130 and 170 minutes in all four groups. Their percentages of stages 1, 2, 3, 4, and REM sleep showed no significant differences and no trends. Similarly, no differences appeared in sleep efficiency, number of minutes of body movement, number of awakenings, sleep latency, or REM density.

These findings on the sleep architecture of prepubertal depressives do not support the hypothesis that major depressive disorders are identical in prepuberty and in adulthood. Nevertheless, the negative findings in prepuberty do seem to be consistent with age effects on sleep architecture in both normals and depressives. Normative data across age groups indicate a progressive decrease with age in the percentage of delta sleep, REM latency, and sleep efficiency (Williams et al., 1974). Coble et al. (1980) have shown that the sleep architecture of middle-aged primary endogenous depressives differed from that of young adults with the same diagnosis on four variables. The older group presented higher REM density, lower first REMP latency, lower sleep efficiency, and lower number of minutes of delta sleep. Ulrich et al. (in press) have also reported a high negative correlation between age and first REMP latency during illness in adult primary endogenous depressives. It is conceivable that differences in the sleep patterns of adult depressives as compared with younger populations derive from an interaction between depressive illness and age. The lack of sleep findings in prepubertal major depressives could thus be due to maturational differences.

SUMMARY

Psychobiological studies are generating a substantial body of data to support validation of the diagnosis of major depressive disorder in prepuberty and adolescence. Family aggregation studies and GH response to insulin-induced hypoglycemia very strongly favor the hypothesis that the essential nature of the illness remains the same across ages. The positive relationship between plasma level of imipramine plus desmethylimipramine and clinical response of the depressive syndrome provides indirect, weaker evidence in the same direction. Sleep studies and cortisol hypersecretion studies do not support the identity of the disorders. The lack of differences in both of these types of studies, however, can be explained in light of age influences. The weight of the evidence, in the author's opinion, supports the validity of the diagnosis of major depression in youngsters and also indicates that age is a very important factor affecting most markers of depression. Normative data across age groups would facilitate validation.

As well as helping to validate the diagnosis, the studies are providing a substantial amount of information which will help the practicing child psychiatrist to diagnose and treat child and adolescent depressive conditions. Markers used in the studies can also be used as diagnostic tests to help with the diagnosis, to monitor treatment effectiveness, and to predict relapse. In the coming years, therefore, the practice of child psychiatry may be deeply influenced by knowledge generated with the aid of psychobiological approaches to depressive disorders.

Chapter 20 # The Clinical Characteristics of Childhood Depression†
by Elva Orlow Poznanski, M.D.

Through the ages, physicians have attempted to identify a common cluster of symptoms and have then looked for this cluster in other patients. Their goal has been to relate treatment, outcome, and etiological factors to that particular cluster of symptoms which they have finally designated a syndrome. As it is in adults, depressive affect in children is frequently accompanied by a common cluster of behavioral symptoms. The symptom cluster accompanying depressive affect in children is remarkably similar, whether it is seen in pediatric units, psychiatric outpatient clinics, or residential institutions. Some have argued that the symptom cluster of depressive affect indicates a depressive syndrome only when the symptoms are severe. To some extent, this is valid, and it is reflected in those depression rating scales that correlate an increasing degree of depressive affect with an increasing number and severity of behavioral symptoms. Nevertheless, the depressive syndrome does occur in children, and a variety of diagnostic criteria are now available to assist the clinician.

DIAGNOSTIC CRITERIA
The most commonly used diagnostic criteria for childhood depression have subtle differences, but these are of more interest to researchers than to clinicians. Two currently used sets of criteria were designed for adults and have not been modified for children—Research Diagnostic Criteria (RDC) (Spitzer et al., 1977) and DSM-III (American Psychiatric Association, 1980). Two others were modified for use with children—the author's (Poznanski's) (Poznanski et al., 1981b) and Weinberg's (Weinberg et al., 1973; Petti, 1978). All four sets of criteria are strikingly similar.

All require the presence of dysphoric mood. DSM-III allows pervasive anhedonia to substitute for depressed mood, but pervasive anhedonia without dysphoria is very uncommon. Both sets of adult criteria for dysphoria require a verbal description. Poznanski's criteria and Weinberg's criteria, however, both permit using nonverbal manifestations of depressive affect, as rated by an experienced clinician. Poznanski requires two such observations, two weeks apart. Weinberg's criteria also require low self-esteem. Each set of criteria has different requirements for the duration of dysphoria—one week, two weeks, or one month. This difference is rarely clinically significant, though, since the parents of most depressed children wait months or sometimes years before seeking psychiatric help.

The symptomatic behaviors to be associated with a diagnosis of depression are almost identical in RDC, DSM-III, and Poznanski's cri-

†This chapter is based in part on research supported by Public Health Service Grant No. PHS: MH 34196 01-02.

teria. All require the presence of four or more of several behaviors. These behaviors are anorexia and/or weight loss (social withdrawal is substituted in Poznanski's criteria); anhedonia; sleep disturbance; decreased concentration (or a change in school performance); excessive fatigue; hypoactivity (RDC and DSM-III allow agitation with or without hypoactivity); and low self-esteem (or self-reproach in DSM-III and RDC).

Weinberg's criteria require the presence of two of the following eight behaviors: aggressive behavior, change in attitude towards school, somatic complaints, diminished socialization, change in appetite or weight loss, loss of usual energy, sleep disturbance, or change in school performance. The first three behaviors differ from those in RDC, DSM-III, and Poznanski's criteria, and the first four differ from RDC and DSM-III criteria. Overall, the Weinberg criteria are the least exclusive. Under them some children would be diagnosed depressed who would not be so diagnosed under any of the other three sets of criteria.

CLINICAL SIGNS AND SYMPTOMS

Depressed Affect

Depressed affect is the sine qua non of the clinical diagnosis of depression, and masked depression or depressive equivalents are no longer felt to be children's primary mode of expressing depression (Carlson and Cantwell, 1980; Cytryn et al., 1980). Children can express a depressed mood verbally or nonverbally or may manifest it in both nonverbal and verbal communication.

The clinical observer of nonverbal depressed affect in a child must attend carefully to the child's face. Since children have no facial lines as adults do, the characteristic sagging eyelids of the depressed adult are not present, but downcast eyes and sagging lips are evident even in young children. A depressed child looks distinctly unhappy. The fleeting smiles that may occur disappear rapidly. It is easier to discern depression when the child portrays sadness with obvious psychic pain, exhibiting a state of affect arousal, than it is to identify depression in the child with affect suppression. The bland, frozen look of diffuse and pervasive affect suppression can be far more difficult to identify.

Children often become anxious and lose their spontaneity when talking with a stranger for the first time. The distinction between this anxiety and depression must be made on the basis of the overall quality of the child's affect during an in-depth evaluative interview. Anxiety in response to the stranger diminishes when the parent joins the child in the interview. Depressive affect itself may vary with the area under discussion during the interview, but the presence of the parents will not relieve it. In some cases, a second interview on another day may be necessary.

Young children vary enormously in their ability to perceive their own depressions. To some extent, the child's ability to label his or her mood as depressed, blue, or down varies with the setting. Depressed children on medical wards are rarely able to identify these feelings. Depressed children in outpatient psychiatric clinics are variable in this ability: some can label their depressed moods, and others cannot. Adolescents usually have little difficulty in identifying depressive feelings in themselves, although some very depressed adolescents may be guarded in their answers. In the latter situation the depressed ado-

Table 1. Diagnostic Criteria for Childhood Depression

RDC (Spitzer et al., 1977)	DSM-III (A.P.A., 1980)	POZNANSKI (Poznanski et al., 1981b)	WEINBERG (Weinberg et al., 1973)
Dysphoria *and/or*	Dysphoric mood *and/or*	Depressed mood, behavior, or appearance	Dysphoric mood (melancholy) *and* Self-deprecatory ideation
Pervasive loss of pleasure	Loss of interest in almost all usual activities and pleasure		
AND four (probable) or five (definite) of the following:	*AND* four or more of the following:	*AND* four (probable) or five (definite) of the following:	*AND* two of the following:
• Poor appetite or weight loss or increased appetite or weight gain	• Poor appetite or weight loss increased appetite or weight gain		• Unusual change in appetite and/or weight
		• Social withdrawal	• Diminished socialization
• Sleep difficulty or sleeps too much	• Insomnia or hypersomnia	• Difficulty with sleep	• Sleep disturbance
• Loss of energy, fatigability, or tiredness	• Loss of energy, fatigue	• Complaints of fatigue	• Loss of usual energy

• Psychomotor agitation or retardation

• Loss of interest in pleasure

• Self-reproach or excessive guilt

• Decreased ability to think or concentrate

• Recurrent thoughts of death or suicide

DURATION:
1 week, probable
2 weeks, definite

• Hypoactivity

• Anhedonia

• Lowered self-esteem or pathological guilt

• Difficulty with schoolwork

• Psychomotor agitation or retardation

• Loss of pleasure in usual activities

• Feelings of worthlessness or guilt

• Decreased ability to think

• Morbid ideation, suicidal ideation

• Recurrent thoughts of death or suicide

DURATION:
2 weeks or more

DURATION:
1 month

• Change in school performance

• Change in attitude toward school

• Somatic complaints

• Aggressive behavior (agitation)

DURATION:
1 month

lescents are usually trying to hide their feelings from themselves as much as or more than they are trying to withhold information from the psychiatrist.

Anhedonia

One of the most characteristic affective features of depression in children, and the one with the strongest correlation to depression, is anhedonia. Anhedonia is particularly striking in a child. Having fun is an integral part of a child's life and a necessary ingredient for learning and playing. Adults can look serious and still derive pleasure, but a child's pleasure is rarely hidden.

Bored, unhappy, or apathetic children and adolescents openly communicate their misery to the world frequently enough that most clinical observers will recognize this affective state. Some of the most severely and pervasively anhedonic children and adolescents, however, are difficult to recognize, and considerable probing is needed to assess the anhedonia. When asked about what they do for fun, they may respond in the wintertime that they play baseball outdoors and in the summertime that they throw snowballs. One depressed child described a single past family event as his favorite way to have fun. Other children dodge the question by focusing on their efforts to get out of the house. The mother of one such child said he was "too busy" to come in for lunch. Actually, once he or she is out of the house, such a child may sit on the curb, ramble up and down the streets, or sit in the park. Fun is not an everyday reality.

Sometimes children say they are bored when they are actually anhedonic. Although being bored is an occasional fact of life, a child who describes being bored half or nearly all the time probably has few interests. Very depressed children simply stare at television programs, unaware of the program that is on. Viewing television can be either active or passive for anyone, but for severely depressed children, it is nearly always passive.

Morbid Ideation, Suicidal Ideation, or Suicide Attempts

Depressed children, particularly moderately and severely depressed children, often have morbid or suicidal thoughts or both. Since they frequently do not coexist (Poznanski et al., 1981b), it is best to inquire about morbid and suicidal thoughts separately. A depressed child may center morbid ideation around some real event, such as the death of a grandparent or a pet. There is, of course, both a quantitative and a qualitative difference between a normal grief reaction and morbid ideation. In some children the theme of death occurs spontaneously and without a precipitating event. When there is a real precipitating event, the child may add elaborate fantasies to it.

In today's television-educated world, almost all young children know the word *suicide*. They may comment on it by saying, "Oh, you mean like running in front of a car." Children themselves are rarely upset when the clinician asks about suicide. Some clinicians are more anxious about discussing it than are the children. When children are upset by questions about suicide, it may be that they are in fact having suicidal ideation. And when they deny their suicidal ideas, moderately depressed children are at risk for suicide, just as depressed adults who deny them are.

Reported suicide attempts in prepubertal children are rare. We know, however, that in adolescence suicide ranks third as a cause of death. Even this group is underreported, though, since the coroners' offices are vigorously protective (Finch and Poznanski, 1971).

Assessment of suicide risk should be a part of every psychiatric evaluation. Although not all suicidal children are depressed, about eighty percent of adolescent suicide attempts are made by depressed adolescents, a percentage similar to that among adults (Crumley, 1979). Reliable statistics for younger children are not available, and it is important to recognize that a youngster can be suicidal and not be depressed.

Prepubertal children, it is now evident, do think about suicide prior to the act. They do not simply act impulsively. Many depressed children actively plan their suicide attempts and think about them for some time. It is an absolute necessity to inquire about suicidal thoughts with every depressed child. In the author's experience, the parents of children who have suicidal ideation or who have made a suicide attempt do not want to recognize that the child is thinking of suicide or has made an attempt. Tightly denying the meaning of an attempt, they say, "It was just an accident," or, "He didn't really mean it; it was just for attention." The parents' denial is a major hurdle in the clinical management of these children. Unfortunately, the courts and social agencies frequently support the parents' denial out of ignorance and financial considerations. The physician owes it to the patient to pursue the issue as forcefully as is necessary in order to secure the treatment the patient needs.

Lowered Self-Esteem

Depressed children often have low opinions of themselves. This symptom is difficult to explore, particularly with young children. Children do not develop the abstract idea of a self-concept until they are between the ages of six and nine. Younger children can talk about the concrete aspects of self-image, such as how they look, whether their friends like them, and whether they would want to change something about themselves.

Adding difficulty to the challenge of assessing self-esteem in children is the fact that they are more sensitive about this area than about many others, and they may consciously try to hide the intensity of their emotions. Answers to questions about self-esteem may be hesitant or evasive, but often the feelings will come out regardless. Children will describe themselves with negatively tinged words, like "stupid" or "not popular." Or they will admit that their friends call them derogatory nicknames, such as Fat Lips, Fag, Moldmouth, or Big Ears. Derogatory nicknames are very hard on children. They dislike repeating them to adults almost as if the name itself had the magical ability to come true simply by virtue of its being uttered. Depressed children disproportionately collect these nicknames, and this further lowers their self-esteem.

Some children and adolescents present the opposite picture. They brag about how great they are with such obvious effort that their thin facade is unconvincing and easy to recognize. They rarely succeed in convincing themselves either, and these children are not hard to distinguish from those with healthy narcissism.

Pathological Guilt

Children can feel overwhelmingly guilty, but, as with self-esteem, getting consistent and reliable information about guilt feelings is difficult. Parents may be helpful here, if they are emotionally in tune with the child. Lack of evidence, moreover, does not mean that the young child does not feel guilty. The problem may be that the child does not have the developmental ability to discuss the feelings. Or it may be that the child is making a conscientious effort to make a good impression or simply has difficulty admitting these feelings to himself or herself. Children and adolescents who give little verbal evidence of guilt may demonstrate guilt through their behavior, when they deliberately elicit punishment, for instance, or destroy their favorite possessions (Robbins et al., in press).

Social Withdrawal

Social withdrawal is frequently seen in childhood depression, but poor peer relationships are, of course, characteristic of many other emotional problems as well. Unlike children with other disorders, however, the child with an acute depression has usually developed the capacity for interpersonal relationships and has been able to socialize prior to the onset of the illness. For example, one boy commented in the interview that the teacher last year had said he was one of the most popular kids in the classroom, but he showed little current interest in interacting with his peers. Depressed children may directly state that they do not have any friends or say, "I like them [children], . . . but they don't like me." These children so frequently turn down opportunities to play with others that the neighborhood youngsters gradually cease to ring their doorbells.

In another variant of the disturbed social behavior of depressed children, the child repeatedly sets himself or herself up to be rejected by other children. For example, a child who is usually aware of the feelings of other children may begin insisting on imposing his or her own rules to such an extent that he or she loses friends.

Chronically depressed children and adolescents often have poorly developed social skills. Since an improvement in mood is a necessary prerequisite to improved social relationships, the painful wish for more friends is not immediately alleviated. Developing social skills takes many hours of psychotherapy, a fact easily appreciated by most therapists. The depressed child may turn to the family dog or cat for a substitute friend. One depressed child, desperate for friends, built a doghouse in hopes of getting a dog, despite his family's great reluctance to acquire a dog. Another depressed child was so upset that a family dog was put to sleep that, several months later, the child cried four or five times a week thinking about the dog. A more severely depressed child no longer cares about having friends, even dogs.

Impairment of Schoolwork

An abrupt decline in a child's schoolwork may indicate the onset of depression. The depressed child is different from the learning disabled child in that the depressed child has been able to perform in school prior to his or her depression. The learning disabled child, on the other hand, has usually had difficulty with academic functioning from the first grade onward. A depressed child's school performance will often vary with the mood of the day.

The poor school performance stems both from a lack of interest in any activity and, more importantly, from difficulty in concentrating. Although the attention span of the depressed child is poor like that of a hyperactive child, the source of the difficulty is different. The hyperactive child's attention is distracted by external stimuli, while the depressed child's attention is turned inward. Preoccupied with his or her own worries and thoughts, the depressed child tunes out the exterior world. Nonetheless, a combination of both sources of attentional difficulty is sometimes seen. The depressed child may be distracted by both internal and external stimuli.

Most depressed teenagers do poorly in school, often fluctuating unduly on the basis of their personal feelings towards a particular teacher. Occasionally, though, a strong student will continue to do well academically, studying compulsively with little pleasure and foregoing peer interaction. It is the latter type of student, such a "good" boy or girl, who surprises the community if he or she commits suicide. Depression, of course, occurs in students who get A's as well as in dropouts.

Psychomotor Retardation

Depressed children and adolescents often manifest psychomotor retardation. They walk slowly, speak slowly, and move very little once settled into a chair. Psychomotor retardation in children does not appear very different from adult psychomotor retardation. A severely depressed child may just sit in a slumped posture, staring at the floor throughout the interview.

Hypoactivity can be particularly outstanding on the pediatric wards in children with potentially fatal illnesses. These children, with their secondary depressions, lie in bed all day, barely moving in their beds, not because of the physical illness, but because of the depression. Many physicians and parents find it emotionally easier to attribute the inactivity of these children to the physical illness. Experienced nurses, however, often make note of a hypoactive state that is distinctly disproportionate to a child's physical illness.

Agitated depressions do occur in children, and distinguishing them from hyperactivity can be difficult (Cytryn et al., 1980). Hyperactivity per se does not appear to be a depressive equivalent, and agitation is more variable, and more directly related to anxiety, than hyperactivity.

Retardation of speech and language is common among depressed children. They tend to answer questions in one or two words and in a monotone voice. Since clinicians also hear short answers from children who are simply oppositional or from those children who have a distinct cultural barrier from themselves, retardation of speech has to be considered within the context of the entire clinical assessment. Because of this characteristic decrease in verbalization, it is difficult to obtain fantasy material. Contrary to the experience of others (Cytryn and McKnew, 1974), the fantasy material is so reduced that it would often be difficult to form a diagnostic impression on the basis of the child's fantasies.

Complaints of Fatigue

Adults envy and frequently remark on children's seemingly endless amount of energy. Even so, it has taken child psychiatrists a long time to ask if a youngster gets tired during the day or feels so tired that he or she voluntarily takes an afternoon nap. A depressed child who is asked such questions often responds by saying, "I feel tired in the afternoon." Or the child may report feeling too tired to engage in the activities children normally enjoy. Complaints of excessive fatigue are common with depressed children.

Difficulty with Vegetative Functions

Many depressed children have difficulty sleeping, but this difficulty appears clinically to be related more to anxiety than to depression. They report difficulty going to sleep and, more rarely, speak of middle insomnia or early morning awakening. Generally, a child is far more aware of a sleep disturbance than the parents, who may assume the child immediately goes to sleep. Children describe their sleeping problems with convincing accuracy. But because they will rarely cite the problems spontaneously, they do need to be asked, "Do you have trouble sleeping?" Prepubertal children do not often report middle or terminal insomnia. When they do, they will usually be found to have other features of endogenous depression.

Weight loss frequently goes unnoticed in children, and the author and her colleagues found that a psychiatrically depressed group of children were ten pounds lighter than their nondepressed counterparts at an equivalent chronological age (Poznanski et al., 1981a). Children are poor reporters of the common symptom of appetite reduction, particularly if they are mildly depressed. Usually, if a child has not been eating well, the mother has urged the child to eat and has effectively conveyed the idea that not eating will result in parental disapproval. Hence, it is not surprising that a depressed child glosses over the issue of appetite reduction. In a hospital setting, the child pushes away the tray of food, frustrating the medical personnel who do not recognize the behavior as a symptom of depression. Thus, even this obvious physical symptom of depression may be difficult to observe, whether the child is at home or in the hospital.

Associated Symptoms

The affective and behavioral symptoms discussed above are the most commonly used as criteria for a clinical diagnosis of a depressive syndrome in a child, but there are some additional behaviors which are so frequent as to deserve mention.

Irritability in depressed children is commonly described by their parents and teachers. This irritability, rather than the underlying depression, may actually be the initial focus of the adults' concern. Depressed children may display some of their irritability during the evaluation, but they are a somewhat less reliable source of information about the degree of their irritability than the parents or the teacher.

Excessive weeping, or the feeling of wanting to cry, is another symptom seen in childhood depression, and some children cannot admit to crying.

Somatic complaints, without organic cause, particularly stomachaches and headaches, are frequent afflictions of depressed children. Children with somatic complaints tend to gravitate to pediatric clinics rather than to psychiatric clinics. The somatic complaints of the depressed child are not equivalent to such complaints in adult masked depression. In the latter, the adult focuses all affect on a somatic symptom and denies depressive feelings. Depressed children with the frequent somatic symptoms of headaches and stomachaches will usually verbalize their depressed feelings, and the link between these complaints and depression is not difficult for the clinician to ascertain (Poznanski et al., 1981b).

DIFFERENTIAL DIAGNOSIS

A depressed affect may be present in a variety of psychiatric illnesses other than depression. A primary depressive disorder can and must be distinguished from psychiatric and other conditions which may have a dysphoric component. Several of the more commonly confused conditions are discussed below.

Adjustment Disorder with Depressed Mood

The diagnosis of *Adjustment Disorder with Depressed Mood* is frequently misused. The crucial factor in the differential diagnosis between the adjustment reaction and a primary diagnosis of depression is the presence or absence of the symptomatology required by the various diagnostic criteria for childhood depression. Child psychiatrists tend to use the Adjustment Disorder category because it implies the least severe psychopathology in the child, but this is a disservice when, in the long run, the removal of the stressful agent does not change the child's behavior. Since there are multiple life stresses in all children who come to a psychiatric clinic, whether they are depressed or not depressed, the severity of the psychosocial stressor itself is rarely helpful in distinguishing an adjustment disorder from depression.

Grief Reaction

A loss of a parent, a sibling, or other important person can precipitate a *grief reaction* in a child. If the reaction endures, it may become a depression. Even in adults, the line between grief and depression is not always easy to make. Freud, in his classic 1917 paper, "Mourning and Melancholia," stressed the differential importance of self-esteem (Freud, 1959). Low self-esteem occurs in depression and is absent in grief. Spitzer et al. (1977) include in RDC a "quality of mood" item as a criterion for depression. The criterion requires asking the patient if he or she feels the same way or different when feeling grief as opposed to depression. Such a distinction cannot be made by all adults and is difficult to impossible for a young child.

The normal reactions of children to bereavement are described less clearly in the literature than are normal adult reactions. Grieving children can have a disturbance in their behavior for very long periods of time, but the affective component was not recognized in the earlier literature. Such children were thought to have depressive equivalents rather than depressive affect. The current focus is on overt depressions in children, and while the concept of depressive equivalents, which stemmed from studies of bereavement in children, may still be valid, it requires a tighter definition than the original.

Despite the distinction between a grief reaction and depression in children, we should be aware that children often date the onset of their depression two to four years back to the time when an important other died. Some of them, when asked to draw a picture of the family, will include the dead member in the drawing. The author has never seen this behavior in a nondepressed child.

Separation Anxiety Disorder

Children with a *Separation Anxiety Disorder* may appear to be depressed when they are away from their parents, particularly the mother. The mother's presence or absence influences not only the child's mood but many other behaviors as well. The clinician should observe a child in question both with and without the parent and note whether the presence of the parent relieves all or just part of the child's depressive affect. While somewhat older children can themselves distinguish separation anxiety from depression, direct observation is still more reliable.

Learning Disabilities

With some young children it is very difficult to sort out whether the child's *learning disabilities* have precipitated a secondary depression or whether a primary depression has interfered with learning at school. Generally a young child's sense of time is too poor for the clinician to be able to make the distinction through an interview with the child. Psychological testing can aid in both identifying developmental lags and in observing the child's learning attitude during testing, since, psychologically, testing is more like school than an unstructured interview. Where a parent can give a good history, this may help to separate which condition, the learning problems or the depression, occurred first in the child's life. In one sense, of course, the question is academic. An improvement in the child's depression, whether it is primary or secondary, will generally lead to improved school performance.

Psychosis with Depressive Affect

A *psychotic child with depressive affect* presents a difficult diagnostic problem. Psychosis with depressive features may be caused in children by one or more of several conditions: (1) a reaction to severe stress, such as physical abuse; (2) a reaction to street or prescription drugs; (3) childhood schizophrenia; (4) a psychotic depression with mood-congruent auditory hallucinations and delusions; or (5) an early expression of manic-depressive illness. Assuming that a careful history has first been done, the distinction must then be made between psychotic features and fantasies that are developmentally appropriate. The next step is to assess whether the child's hallucinations and delusions are mood-congruent or incongruent. It may still be difficult to differentiate psychosis if reality testing is minimal and the presence of auditory hallucinations is questionable. Some children may need to be followed over time to arrive at a proper differential diagnosis.

Physical Illness with Dysphoric Mood

Diagnosing children who have a *physical illness with dysphoric mood* requires the psychiatrist to distinguish between the apathy associated with physical illness and a truly depressive affect. The apathy and fatigue of the medically ill child have a different flavor from the depressive mood of the child with primary depressive disease. Relatives and referring physicians may be eager for a psychiatric diagnosis, particularly if there has been difficulty establishing a medical diagnosis. The diagnosis of depression should be made only on the basis of the clinical characteristics of depression, however. It should not be a diagnosis of last resort, one that is made because all medical tests have proven negative. The author has had children referred as possibly depressed who ultimately proved to have Crohn's Disease, Schilder's Disease, or leukemia.

TREATMENT CONSIDERATIONS

The recognition and diagnosis of prolonged depression in a child usually indicates the need for treatment. In the author's experience, getting families to follow through is one of the first treatment issues. Whether the child should be referred to an inpatient psychiatric facility or for outpatient treatment is a second issue. Generally the choice depends on the overall psychiatric evaluation of the child. Actively suicidal children, of course, should be referred to a psychiatric inpatient unit. A pediatric unit is not a good substitute, since life-preserving precautions are impossible in a general medical hospital.

A third issue is selecting the appropriate type and mix of treatments. A wide number of the available therapeutic approaches have been used with depressed children, including individual psychotherapy, group psychotherapy, family therapy, cognitive therapy, and therapy with psychopharmacological agents. Unfortunately, few of these therapies have been evaluated through controlled studies, with the exception of recent work on the effectiveness of imipramine with depressed children (Puig-Antich et al., 1979; Weller et al., 1981). Within the next few years the effectiveness and clinical role of psychopharmacological agents should become clearer.

A final treatment consideration concerns the therapist's role. While psychotherapy with these children is not substantially different from psychotherapy with other emotionally disturbed children, the therapist must play an unusually active role, and this can be fatiguing. If the pharmacotherapies prove to be effective co-therapies, therapists will have greater stamina for the long-term, active treatment that depressed children most often require.

Bibliographies to Part III

Bibliography for the Introduction

Bradley, C. *Schizophrenia in Childhood.* New York: MacMillan, 1941.

Despert, J.L. "Schizophrenia in Children." *Psychiatric Quarterly* 12 (1938): 366-371.

Bibliography for Chapter 16

American Psychiatric Association, *Diagnostic and Statistical Manual of Mental Disorders, 3d ed.,* Washington, D.C.: American Psychiatric Association, 1980.

Anthony, E.J. "Behavior Disorders." In *Carmichael's Manual of Child Psychology, 3d ed.,* vol. 2, edited by P.H. Mussen. New York: Wiley & Sons, 1970.

Achenbach, T.M. "Psychopathology of Childhood: Research Problems and Issues." *Journal of Consulting and Clinical Psychology* 46 (1978): 759–776.

Bowlby, J. *Attachment and Loss,* vol. 2, *Separation,* New York: Basic Books, 1973.

Bumberry, W., Oliver, J.M., and McClure, J.N. "Validation of the Beck Depression Inventory in a University Population Using Psychiatric Estimates as the Criterion." *Journal of Consulting and Clinical Psychology* 46 (1980): 150–155.

Carlson, G.A., and Cantwell, D.P. "A Survey of Depressive Symptoms, Syndrome and Disorder in a Child Psychiatric Population. *Journal of Child Psychology and Psychiatry* 21 (1980a): 19–25.

Carlson, G.A., and Cantwell, D.P. "Unmasking Masked Depression in Children and Adolescents." *American Journal of Psychiatry* 137 (1980b): 445–449.

Chambers, W., Puig-Antich, J., and Tabrizi, M.A. "The Ongoing Development of the Kiddie-SADS (Schedule for Affective Disorders and Schizophrenia for School-age Children)." Read at the Annual Meeting of the *American Academy of Child Psychiatry,* San Diego, California, 1978.

Costello, C.G. "Childhood Depression: Three Basic but Questionable Assumptions in the Lefkowitz and Burton Critique." *Psychological Bulletin* 87 (1980): 185–190.

Cytryn, L. and McKnew, D.H. "Proposed Classification of Childhood Depression." *American Journal of Psychiatry* 129 (1972): 149–155.

Cytryn, L., McKnew, D.H. and Bunney, W.E. "Diagnosis of Depression in Children: A Reassessment." *American Journal of Psychiatry* 137 (1980): 22–25.

Dweck, C.S., Gittelman-Klein, R., McKinney, W.T., and Watson, J.S. "Summary of the Subcommittee on Clinical Criteria for Diagnosis of Depression in Children." In: *Depression in Childhood: Diagnosis, Treatment, and Conceptual Models,* edited by J.G. Schulterbrandt, and A. Raskin. New York: Raven Press, 1977.

Friedlander, S., Philips, I., Morrison, D., and Traylor, J. "Depression in Childhood: An Exploratory Study." Paper presented at the annual convention of the *American Psychological Association,* Los Angeles, California, 1981.

Frommer, E. "Depressive Illness in Childhood." *British Journal of Psychiatry* Special Publ. 2 (1968): 117–123.

Glaser, K. "Masked Depression in Children and Adolescents." *American Journal of Psychotherapy* 21 (1967): 565–574.

Grinker, R.R. *Phenomena of Depression.* New York: Paul B. Hoeber, Inc., 1961.

Hammen, C.L. "Depression in College Students: Beyond the Beck Depression Inventory." *Journal of Consulting and Clinical Psychology* 48 (1980): 126–128.

Kazdin, A.E. "Assessment Techniques for Child Depression." *Journal of the American Academy of Child Psychiatry* 20 (1981): 358–375.

Kovacs, M. *Child Depression Inventory,* 1977. (Available from M. Kovacs, Western Psychological Institute and Clinic, 3811 O'Hara St., Pittsburgh, PA., 15261.)

Kovacs, M., and Beck, A.T. "An Empirical Clinical Approach Towards a Definition of Childhood Depression." In *Depression in Children: Diagnosis, Treatment and Conceptual Models,* edited by J.G. Schulterbrandt, and A. Raskin. New York: Raven Press, 1977.

Lefkowitz, M.M. "Childhood Depression: A Reply to Costello." *Psychological Bulletin* 87 (1980): 191–194.

Lefkowitz, M.M., and Burton, N. "Childhood Depression: A Critique of the Concept." *Psychological Bulletin* 85 (1978): 716–726.

Leon, G.R., Kendall, P.C., and Garber, J. "Depression in Children: Parent, Teacher and Child Perspectives." *Journal of Abnormal Child Psychology* 8 (1980): 221–235.

Malmquist, C. "Depression in Childhood and Adolescence, I." *New England Journal of Medicine* 284 (1971): 887–893.

Malmquist, C. "Depression in Childhood and Adolescence, II." *New England Journal of Medicine* 284 (1971): 955–961.

McKnew, D.H., and Cytryn, L. "Urinary Metabolites in Chronically Depressed Children." *Journal of the American Academy of Child Psychiatry* 18 (1979): 608–615.

Philips, I. "Childhood Depression: Interpersonal Interactions and Depressive Phenomena." *American Journal of Psychiatry* 136 (1979): 511–515.

Philips, I. "Research Directions in Child Psychiatry." *American Journal of Psychiatry* 137 (1980): 1436–1438.

Poznanski, E., and Zrull, J.P. "Childhood Depression: Clinical Characteristics of Overtly Depressed Children." *Archives of General Psychiatry* 23 (1970): 8–15.

Puig-Antich, J., Blau, S., Marx, N., Greenhill, L.L., and Chambers, W. "Prepubertal Major Depressive Disorder." *Journal of the American Academy of Child Psychiatry* 17 (1978): 695–707.

Puig-Antich, J., Chambers, W., Halpern, F., Hanlon, C., and Sachar, E.J. "Cortisol Hypersecretion in Prepubertal Depressive Illness." *Psychoneuro-endocrinology* 4 (1979): 191–197.

Rochlin, G. "The Loss Complex." *Journal of the American Psychoanalytic Association* 7 (1959): 299–316.

Rutter, M., Tizard, J., and Whitmore, K. *Education in Health and Behavior.* London: Longman, 1970.

Seligman, M. Personal Communication, 1980.

Spitzer, R.L., Endicott, J., and Robbins, E. "Research diagnostic Criteria." *Archives of General Psychiatry* 35 (1978): 773–782.

Toolan, J.M. "Depression in Children and Adolescents." *American Journal of Orthopsychiatry* 32 (1962): 404–414.

Weinberg, W., Rutman, J., Sullivan, L., Penick, E.C., and Dietz, S.G. "Depression in Children Referred to an Educational Diagnostic Center: Diagnosis and Treatment." *Journal of Pediatrics* 83 (1973): 1065–1072.

Bibliography for Chapter 17

Anthony, E.J., "Childhood Depression." In *Depression and Human Existence,* edited by E.J. Anthony and T. Benedek. Boston: Little, Brown, and Co., 1975a.

Anthony, E.J. "Two Contrasting Types of Adolescent Depression and Their Treatment." In *Depression and Human Existence,* edited by E.J. Anthony and T. Benedek. Boston: Little, Brown, and Co., 1975b.

Arieti, S. "The Psychobiology of Sadness." In *Severe and Mild Depression,* edited by S. Arieti and J. Bemporad. New York: Basic Books, 1978.

Bemporad, J. "Psychodynamics of Depression and Suicide in Children and Adolescents." In *Severe and Mild Depression,* edited by S. Arieti and J. Bemporad. New York, Basic Books, 1978.

Bibring, E. "The Mechanism of Depression." In *Affective Disorders,* edited by P. Greenacre. New York: International Universities Press, 1953.

Bierman, J.S., Silverstein, A.B., and Finesinger, J.E. "A Depression in a Six-Year-Old Boy with Acute Poliomyelitis." *Psychoanalytic Study of the Child* 13 (1958): 430–450.

Bowlby, J. "Separation Anxiety." *International Journal of Psychoanalysis* 41 (1960): 89–113.

Dennis, W., and Najarian J. "Infant Development Under Environmental Handicap." *Psychological Monographs* 71 (1957): 1–13.

Engel, G.L., and Reichmann, F. "Spontaneous and Experimentally Induced Depression in an Infant With a Gastric Fistula." *Journal of the American Psychoanalytic Association* 4 (1956): 428–452.

Erikson, E.H. *Identity and the Life Cycle.* (Psychological Issues, Vol. 1). New York: International Universities Press, 1959.

Loevinger, J. *Ego Development.* San Francisco: Jossey-Bass, 1976.

McConville, B.J., Boag, L.C., and Puromit, A.P. "Three Types of Childhood Depression." *Canadian Psychiatric Association Journal,* 18 (1973): 133–138.

Mahler, M.G. "Sadness and Grief in Childhood." *Psychoanalytic Study of the Child* 16 (1961): 332–351.

Malmquist, C. "Childhood Depression: A Clinical and Behavioral Perspective." In *Depression in Childhood,* edited by J.G. Schulterbrandt and A. Raskin. New York: Raven Press, 1977.

Piaget, J. *The Construction of Reality in the Child.* New York: Basic Books, 1954.

Poznanski, E.O. "Childhood Depression: A Psychodynamic Approach to the Etiology and Treatment of Depression in Children." In *Depression in Children and Adolescents,* edited by A. French and I. Berlin. New York: Human Sciences Press, 1979.

Poznanski, E.O., and Zrull, J.P. "Childhood Depression." *Archives of General Psychiatry* 239 (1970): 8–15.

Rie, H.E. "Depression in Childhood: A Survey of Some Pertinent Contributions." *Journal of the American Academy of Child Psychiatry* 5 (1966): 653–685.

Rochlin, G. "The Loss Complex." *Journal of the American Psychoanalytic Association* 7 (1959): 299–316.

Sandler, J. and Joffee, W.G. "Notes on Childhood Depression." *International Journal of Psychoanalysis* 46 (1965): 88–96.

Spitz, R. "Anaclitic Depression." *Psychoanalytic Study of the Child* 2 (1946): 113–117.

Bibliography for Chapter 18

Albert, N., and Beck, A.T. "Incidence of Depression in Early Adolescence: A Preliminary Study." *Journal of Youth and Adolescence* 4 (1975): 301–307.

Anthony, E.J. "Depression and Children." In *Handbook of Studies on Depression,* edited by G.D. Burrows. Excerpta Medica (1977): 105–120.

Barker, D.J.P., and Rose, G. *Epidemiology in Medical Practice.* London, New York: Churchill Livingstone, 1976.

Bauersfeld, K.H. "Diagnosis and Treatment of Depressive Conditions at a School Psychiatric Center." In *Depressive States in Childhood and Adolescence,* edited by A.L. Annell. Stockholm: Almquist & Wiksell, 1972.

Bebbington, P.E. "The Epidemiology of Depressive Disorder." *Culture, Medicine and Psychiatry* 2 (1978): 297–341.

Birleson, P. "The Validity of Depressive Disorder in Childhood and the Development of a Self-Rating Scale: A Research Report." *Journal of Child Psychology and Psychiatry* 22 (1981): 73–88.

Caplan, G. "An Approach to Preventive Intervention in Child Psychiatry." *Canadian Journal of Psychiatry* 25 (1980): 671–682.

Carlson, G.A., and Cantwell, D.P. "Unmasking Masked Depression in Children and Adolescents." *American Journal of Psychiatry* 137 (1980): 445–449.

Cebiroglu, R., Sumer, E., and Polvan, O. "Etiology and Pathogenesis of Depression in Turkish Children." In *Depressive States in Childhood and Adolescence,* edited by A.L. Annell. Stockholm: Almquist & Wiksell, 1972.

Conners, C.K., Himmelhoch, J., Goyette, C.H., Ulrich, R., and Neil, J.F. "Children of Parents With Affective Illness." *Journal of the American Academy of Child Psychiatry* 18 (1979): 600–607.

Cytryn, L., McKnew, D.H., Jr., and Bunney, W.E., Jr. "Diagnosis of Depression in Children: A Reassessment." *American Journal of Psychiatry* 137 (1980): 22–25.

Gaensbauer, T.J. "Anaclitic Depression in a Three-And-One-Half Month-Old Child." *American Journal of Psychiatry* 137 (1980): 841–842.

Gruenberg, E.M. "Epidemiology." In *Comprehensive Textbook of Psychiatry*, edited by H.I. Kaplan, A.M. Freedman, and B.J. Sadock. Baltimore: Williams & Wilkins, 1980.

Kashani, J., and Simonds, J.F. "The Incidence of Depression in Children." *American Journal of Psychiatry* 136 (1979): 1203–1205.

Kashani, J., Manning, G.W., McKnew, D.H., Cytryn, L., Simonds, J.F., and Wooderson, P.C. "Depression Among Incarcerated Delinquents." *Psychiatry Research* 3 (1980): 185–191.

Kashani, J., Barbero, G.J., and Bolander, F. "Depression in Hospitalized Pediatric Patients." *Journal of the American Academy of Child Psychiatry* 20 (1981a): 123–134.

Kashani, J., Hodges, K.K., Simonds, J.F., and Hilderbrand, E. "Life Events and Hospitalization in Children: A Comparison With a General Population." *British Journal of Psychiatry* 139 (1981b): 221–225.

Kashani, J., Husain, A., Shekim, W.O., Hodges, K.K., Cytryn, L., and McKnew, D.H. "Current Perspectives on Childhood Depression: An Overview." *American Journal of Psychiatry* 138 (1981c): 143–153.

Kashani, J., Venzki, R., and Miller, E.A. "Depression in Children Admitted to Hospital for Orthopedic Procedures." *British Journal of Psychiatry* 138 (1981d): 21–25.

Kashani, J., Lababidi, Z., and Jones, R.S. "Depression in Children and Adolescents With Cardiovascular Symptomatology: The Significance of Chest Pain." *Journal of the American Academy of Child Psychiatry* in press.

Klerman, G.L. "Overview of Affective Disorders." In *Comprehensive Textbook of Psychiatry, 3d ed.,* edited by H.I. Kaplan, A.M. Freedman, and B.J. Sadock. Baltimore: Williams & Wilkins, 1980.

Kovacs, M., and Beck, A.T. "An Empirical-Clinical Approach Toward a Definition of Childhood Depression." In *Depression in Childhood: Diagnosis, Treatment, and Conceptual Models*, edited by J.G. Schulterbrandt and A. Raskin. New York: Raven Press, 1977.

Kuperman, S., and Stewart, M.A. "The Diagnosis of Depression in Children." *Journal of Affective Disorders* 1 (1979): 213–217.

Langsley, D.G. "Community Psychiatry." In *Comprehensive Textbook of Psychiatry, 3d ed.,* edited by H.I. Kaplan, A.M. Freedman, and B.J. Sadock. Baltimore: Williams & Wilkins, 1980.

Ling, W., Oftedal, G., and Weinberg, W. "Depressive Illness in Childhood Presenting as Severe Headache." *American Journal of Diseases of Children* 120 (1970): 122–124.

Lloyd, C. "Life Events and Depressive Disorders Reviewed. I. Events as Predisposing Factors." *Archives of General Psychiatry* 37 (1980): 529–535.

Lucas, A.R. "Treatment of Depressive States." In *Psychopharmacology in Childhood and Adolescence,* edited by J. M. Wiener. New York: Basic Books, Inc., 1975.

Marsella, A.J. "Depressive Experience and Disorder Across Culture." In *Handbook of Cross-Cultural Psychology, Vol. 6, Psychopathology,* edited by H. Triandis, and Draguns. Boston: Allyn & Bacon, 1980.

McConville, B.J., Boag, L.C., and Purohit, A.P. "Three Types of Childhood Depression." *Canadian Psychiatric Association* 18 (1973): 133–138.

McKnew, D.H., Cytryn, L., Efron, A.M., Gershon, E.S., and Bunney, W.E. "Offspring of Patients With Affective Disorders." *British Journal of Psychiatry* 134 (1979): 148–152.

Meierhofer, M. *Depressive Verstimmungen im frueben Kindesalter.* In *Depressive States in Childhood and Adolescence,* edited by A.L. Annell. Stockholm: Almquist & Wiksell, 1972.

Nielsen, A.C., and Williams, T.A. "Depression in Ambulatory Medical Patients." *Archives of General Psychiatry* 37 (1980): 999–1004.

Nissen, G. *Depressive Syndrome im Kindes und Jugendalter.* Berlin: Springer Verlag, 1971.

Orvaschel, H., Weissman, M.M., and Kidd, K.K. "Children and Depression." *Journal of Affective Disorders* 2 (1980): 1–16.

Orvaschel, H., Weissman, M.M., Padian, N., and Lowe, T.L. "Assessing Psychopathology in Children of Psychiatrically Disturbed Parents." *Journal of the American Academy of Child Psychiatry* 20 (1981): 112–122.

Pearce, J. "Depressive Disorder in Childhood." *Journal of Child Psychology and Psychiatry* 18 (1977): 79–82.

Penfeld, P.S. "Women and Depression." *Canadian Journal of Psychiatry* 26 (1981): 24–31.

Petti, T.A. "Depression in Hospitalized Child Psychiatry Patients." *Journal of the American Academy of Child Psychiatry* 17 (1978): 49–58.

Philips, I. "Childhood Depression: Interpersonal Interactions and Depressive Phenomena." *American Journal of Psychiatry* 136 (1979): 511–515.

Poznanski, E., and Zrull, J.P. "Childhood Depression: Clinical Characteristics of Overtly Depressed Children." *Archives of General Psychiatry* 23 (1970): 8–15.

Poznanski, E. "Childhood Depression: A Psychodynamic Approach to the Etiology of Depression in Children." In *Depression in Children and Adolescents,* edited by A. French, and I. Berlin. New York and London: Human Sciences Press, 1979.

Puig-Antich, J., Blau, S., Marx, N., Greenhill, L.L., and Chambers, W. "Prepubertal Major Depressive Disorder: A Pilot Study." *Journal of the American Academy of Child Psychiatry* 17 (1978): 695–707.

Puig-Antich, J., Chambers, W., Halpern, F., et al. "Cortisone Hypersecretion in Prepubertal Depressive Illness: A Preliminary Report." *Psychoendocrinology* 4 (1979): 191–197.

Puig-Antich, J. "Affective Disorders in Chilhood: A Review and Perspective." *Psychiatric Clinic of North America* 3 (1980): 403–424.

Ripley, H.S. "Depression and the Life Span: Epidemiology in Depression." In *Clinical Biological and Psychological Perspectives,* edited by G. Usdin. New York: Brunner/Mazel, 1977.

Robertson, B.M. "The Psychoanalytic Theory of Depression, I. The Major Contributors." *Canadian Journal of Psychiatry* 24 (1979): 341–352.

Rutter, M.L. "Children of Sick Parents: An Environmental and Psychiatric Study." *Maudsley Monograph 16.* London, New York, Toronto: Oxford University Press, 1966.

Rutter, M.L., Tizard, J., and Whitmore, K. *Education, Health, and Behavior.* London: Longman, 1970.

Rutter, M.L., Graham, P., Chadwick, O.F.D., and Yule, W. "Adolescent Turmoil: Fact or Fiction?" *Journal of Child Psychology and Psychiatry* 17 (1976): 35–56.

Seligman, M.E.P. *Helplessness: On Depression, Development, and Death.* San Francisco: W.H. Freeman & Co., 1975.

Spiro, H.R. "Prevention in Psychiatry: Primary, Secondary and Tertiary." In *Comprehensive Textbook of Psychiatry, 3d ed,* edited by H.I. Kaplan, A.M. Freedman, and B.J. Sadock. Baltimore: Williams & Wilkins, 1980.

Spitz, R. "Anaclitic Depression." *Psychoanalytic Study of the Child* 2 (1946): 113–117.

Srole, L., Langner, T., Michael, S.T., Opler, M.K., and Rennie, T.A.C. *Mental Health in the Metropolis.* New York: McGraw-Hill, 1962.

Tsuang, M.T. "Genetic Counseling for Psychiatric Patients and Their Families." *American Journal of Psychiatry* 135 (1978): 1465–1475.

Weinberg, W.A., Rutman, J., Sullivan, L., Penick, E.C., and Dietz, S.G. "Depression in Children Referred to an Educational Diagnostic Center: Diagnosis and Treatment." *Journal of Pediatrics* 83 (1973): 1065–1072.

Weissman, M.M., and Klerman, G.L. "Epidemiology of Mental Disorder. Emerging Trends in the U.S." *Archives of General Psychiatry* 35 (1978): 705–712.

Weissman, M.M., and Myers, J.K. "Affective Disorders in a U.S. Urban Community." *Archives of General Psychiatry* 35 (1978): 1304–1311.

Weissman, M.M., and Klerman, G.L. "Sex Differences and the Epidemiology of Depression." In *Gender and Disordered Behavior: Sex Differences in Psychopathology,* edited by E.S. Gomberg, and V. Franks. New York: Brunner/Mazel, 1979.

Weissman, M.M. "Depressed Parents and Their Children: Implications for Prevention." In *Basic Handbook of Child Psychiatry, 4th ed,* edited by I.N. Berlin, and L.A. Stone. New York: Basic Books, 1979.

Weissman, M.M., Meyers, J.K., and Thompson, W.D. "Depression and Its Treatment in a U.S. Urban Community—1975–1976." *Archives of General Psychiatry* 38 (1981): 417–421.

Yanchyshyn, G.W., and Robbins, D.R. "The Assessment of Depression in Normal Adolescents: A Comparison Study." Paper presented at the 27th *Annual Meeting of the American Academy of Child Psychiatry,* Chicago, 1980.

Bibliography for Chapter 19

Achenbach, T.M. "DSM-III in Light of Empirical Research on the Classification of Child Psychopathology." *Journal of the American Academy of Child Psychiatry* 19 (1980): 395–412.

Achenbach, T.M. *Research in Developmental Psychology.* New York: Free Press, 1978.

Andreasen, N.C., Endicott, J., Spitzer, R.L., et al. "Family History Method Using Diagnostic Criteria." *Archives of General Psychiatry,* 34 (1977): 1229–1233.

Asnis, G.M., Sachar, E.J., Halbreich, U., Nathan, R.S., Novacenko, H., and Ostrow, L. "Cortisol Secretion in Relation to Age in Major Depression." *Psychosomatic Medicine* 3 (1981): 235–242.

Brown, G.M. "Endocrine Aspects of Psychosocial Dwarfism." In *Hormones, Behavior and Psychopathology,* edited by E.J. Sachar. New York, Raven Press, 1976.

Campbell, J.C. "Manic-Depressive Disease in Children." *JAMA* 158 (1955): 154–157.

Campbell, J.C. "Manic-Depressive Psychoses in Children. Report of 18 Cases." *Journal of Nervous and Mental Disease* 116 (1952): 424–439.

Carlson, G.A., and Cantwell, D.P. "A Survey of Depressive Symptoms in a Child and Adolescent Psychiatric Population." *Journal of the American Academy of Child Psychiatry* 18 (1979): 587–599.

Carlson, G.A., and Cantwell, D.P. "Diagnosis of Childhood Depression: A Comparison of Weinberg and DSM-III Criteria." Paper presented at the *American Psychiatric Association,* Annual Meeting, San Francisco, California 1980.

Carlson, G.A., and Cantwell, D.P. "Unmasking Masked Depression in Children and Adolescents." *American Journal of Psychiatry* 137 (1980): 445–449.

Carlson, G., and Strober, M. "Manic Depressive Illness in Early Adolescence." *Journal of the American Academy of Child Psychiatry* 17 (1978): 138–153.

Carroll, B.J., Curtis, G.C., and Mendels, J. "Neuroendocrine Regulation in Depression: I. Limbic System-Adrenocortisol Dysfunctions." *Archives of General Psychiatry* 33 (1976a): 1039–1044.

Carroll, B.J., Curtis, G.C., and Mendels, J. "Neuroendocrine Regulation in Depression: II. Discrimination of Depressed from Nondepressed Patients." *Archives of General Psychiatry* 33 (1976b): 1051–1058.

Coble, P., Kupfer, D.J., Spiker, D.G., et al: "EEG Sleep and Clinical Characteristics in Young Primary Depressives." Presented at the Annual Meeting of *the Association for the Psychophysiological Study of Sleep.* Mexico City, 1980.

Connell, H.M. "Depression in Childhood." *Child Psychiatry and Human Development* 4 (1972): 71–85.

Cytryn, L., and McKnew, D.J. "Proposed Classification of Childhood Depressions." *American Journal of Psychiatry* 129 (1972): 149–155.

Cytryn, L., McKnew, D., and Bunney, W. "Diagnosis of Depression in Children: Reassessment." *American Journal of Psychiatry* 137 (1980): 22–25.

Feighner, J.P., Robins, E., Guze, S.B., et al. "Diagnostic Criteria for Use in Psychiatric Research." *Archives of General Psychiatry* 26 (1972): 57–61.

Frommer, E.A. "Treatment of Childhood Depression With Antidepressant Drugs." *British Medical Journal* 1 (1967): 729–732.

Gillin, C., Duncan, W., Pettigrew, K.D., et al. "Successful Separation of Depressed, Normal and Insomniac Subjects by EEG Sleep Data." *Archives of General Psychiatry* 36 (1979): 85–90.

Glaser, K. "Masked Depression in Children and Adolescents." *American Journal of Psychotherapy* 21 (1967): 565–574.

Gregoire, F., Branman, G., DeBuck, R., et al. "Hormone Release in Depressed Patients Before and After Recovery." *Psychoneuroendocrinology* 2 (1977): 303–312.

Gruen, P.H., Sachar, E.J., Altman, N., et al. "Growth Hormone Responses to Hypoglycemia in Postmenopausal Depressed Women." *Archives of General Psychiatry* 32 (1975): 31–33.

Kane, J., Coble, P., Conners, C.K., et al. "EEG Sleep in a Child With Severe Depression." *American Journal of Psychiatry* 134 (1977): 813–814.

Kirkegaard, C., Norlem, N., Lauridsen, U.B., et al. "Protirelin Stimulation Test and Thyroid Function During Treatment of Depression." *Archives of General Psychiatry* 32 (1975): 1115–1118.

Kuhn, B., and Kuhn, R. "Drug Therapy for Depression in Children." In *Depressive States in Childhood and Adolescence,* edited by A.L. Annell. New York: John Wiley and Sons, 1972.

Kupfer, D. "REM Latency: A Psychobiological Marker for Primary Depressive Disease." *Biological Psychiatry* 11 (1976): 159–174.

Kupfer, D.J., Coble, P., Kane, J., et al. "Imipramine and EEG Sleep in Children With Depressive Symptoms." *Psychopharmacology* (Berlin), 60 (1979): 117–123.

Kupfer, D., and Foster, F.G. "EEG Sleep and Depression." In [sic], edited by R.L. Williams, and I. Karacan. New York: J. Wiley and Sons, 1979.

Kupferman, S., and Stewart, M.A. "The Diagnosis of Depression in Children." *Journal of Affective Disorders* 1 (1979): 213–217.

Laakman, G. "Neuroendocrine Differences Between Endogenous and Neurotic Depression as seen in Stimulation of Growth Hormone Secretion." *Neuroendocrine Correlates in Neurology and Psychiatry,* edited by E.E. Muller and A. Agnoli. Amsterdam: Elsevier, 1979.

Langer, G., Heinze, G., Reim, B., et al. "Reduced Growth Hormone Responses to Amphetamine in Endogenous Depressive Patients." *Archives of General Psychiatry* 33 (1976): 1471–1475.

LeLord, G., Etieene, T., and Veauuy, N. "Action de l'opripramol (G33.040) dans les syndromes depressifs de l'enfance et de l'adolescence." In *Depressive States in Childhood and Adolescence,* edited by A.L. Annel. New York: John Wiley and Sons, 1972.

Ling, W., Oftedal, G., and Weinberg, W.A. "Depressive Illness in Children Presenting a Severe Headache." *American Journal of Diseases of Children* 120 (1970): 122–124.

Money, J., Annecillo, C., and Werlwas, J. "Hormonal and Behavioral Reversals in Hyposomatotropic Dwarfism." In *Hormones, Behavior and Psychopathology,* edited by E.J. Sachar. New York: Raven Press, 1976.

Polvan, O., and Cebiroglu, R. "Treatment With Psychopharmacologic Agents in Childhood Depression." In *Depressive States in Childhood and Adolescence,* edited by A.L. Annell. New York: John Wiley and Sons, 1972.

Poznanski, E.O., and Zrull, J.P. "Childhood Depression." *Archives of General Psychiatry,* 23 (1970): 8–15.

Prange, A.J. "Patterns of Pituitary Responses to TRH in Depressed Patients." In *Phenomenology and Treatment of Depression,* edited by W. Fann, I. Karacan, A.D. Pokorny, and R.L. Williams. New York: Spectrum Publ., 1977.

Puig-Antich, J., Blau, S., Marx, N., et al. "Prepubertal Major Depressive Disorder: Pilot Study." *Journal of the American Academy of Child Psychiatry,* 17 (1978): 695–707.

Puig-Antich, J., Chambers, W., Halpern, F., et al. "Cortisol Hypersecretion in Prepubertal Depressive Illness." *Psychoneuroendocrinology,* 4 (1979): 191–197.

Puig-Antich, J., Hanlon, C., Goetz, R., Davies, M., Bianca, J., Chambers, W.J., Tabrizi, M.A., and Weitzman, E. "Polysomnography in Prepubertal Major Depressive Disorders and Controls." Paper presented at *APSS Annual Meeting,* Hyannis, Mass. June, 1981.

Puig-Antich, J., Perel, J.M., Lupatkin, W., et al. "Plasma Levels of Imipramine (IMI) and Desmethylimipramine (DMI) in Clinical Response to Prepubertal Major Depressive Disorder." *Journal of the American Academy of Child Psychiatry* 18 (1979): 616–627.

Puig-Antich, J., Perel, J., Lupatkin, W., Chambers, W.J., Tabrizi, M.A., Davies, M., King, J., Johnson, R., and Stiller, R.R. "Imipramine Effectiveness in Prepubertal Major Depression, I. Relationship of Plasma Levels to Clinical Response of the Depressive Syndrome." Submitted manuscript[a].

Puig-Antich, J., Tabrizi, M.A., Chambers, W.J., Lupatkin, W., Davies, M., Goetz, R., King, J., and Nuccitelli, V. "Imipramine Effectiveness in Prepubertal Major Depression, II. A Double-Blind Placebo Controlled Study." Submitted[b].

Rie, H.E. "Depression in Childhood: A Survey of Pertinent Contributions." *Journal of the American Academy of Child Psychiatry* 4 (1966): 653–686.

Sachar, E.J. "Neuroendocrine Abnormalities in Depressive Illness." In *Topics in Psychoneuroendocrinology,* edited by E.J. Sachar. New York: Grune and Stratton, 1975.

Sachar, E.J., Finkelstein, J., Hellman, L. "Growth Hormone Responses in Depressive Illness: Response to Insulin Tolerance Test." *Archives of General Psychiatry* 25 (1971): 263–269.

Sachar, E.J., Hellman, L., Roffwarg, H.P., et al. "Disrupted 24 Hour Pattern of Cortisol Secretion in Psychotic Depression." *Archives of General Psychiatry* 28 (1973): 19–25.

Spitz, R.A. "Hospitalism." *Psychoanalytic Study of the Child* 1 (1945): 53–74.

Spitzer, R.L., Endicott, J., and Robins, E. "Research Diagnostic Criteria: Rationale and Reliability." *Archives of General Psychiatry* 35 (1978): 773–782.

Stack, J.J. "Chemotherapy in Childhood Depression." In *Depressive States in Childhood and Adolescence,* edited by A.L. Annell. New York: John Wiley and Sons, 1972.

Strober, M., and Carlson, G. "Clinical, Genetic and Psychopharmacological Predictors of Bipolar Illness in Adolescents With Major Depression." Unpublished.

Strober, M., Green, J., and Carlson, G. "Phenomenology and Subtype of Major Depressive Disorder in Early Adolescence." Paper presented at the *American Psychiatric Association, Annual Meeting,* San Francisco, California, 1980.

Tabrizi, M.A., Puig-Antich, J., Chambers, W.J., et al. "Growth Hormone Hyposecretion to Insulin-Induced Hypoglycemia in Prepubertal Major Depressive Disorder." Read at the *Annual Meeting of the American Academy of Child Psychiatry,* Atlanta, Georgia, 1979.

Takahasi, S., Kondo, H., Yoshimura, M., et al. "Thyrotropin Response to TRH in Depressive Illness." *Folia Psychiatrica et Neurologica Japonica* 28 (1974): 355–365.

Ulrich, R., Shaw, D.H., and Kupfer, D.J. "The Effects of Aging on Sleep." *Sleep,* in press.

Vogel, G.W., Vogel, F., McAlbee, R.S., et al. "Improvement of Depression by REM Sleep Deprivation." *Archives of General Psychiatry* 37 (1980): 247–253.

Weinberg, W.A., Rutman, J., Sullivan, L., et al. "Depression in Children Referred to an Educational Diagnostic Center: Diagnosis and Treatment." *Journal of Pediatrics* 83 (1973): 1065–1072.

Weller, E., and Preskorn, S. "Imipramine Plasma Levels in Depressed Children." Presented at the *American Psychiatric Association Annual Meeting,* New Orleans, Louisiana, May, 1981.

Welner, Z., Welner, A., McCray, M.D., et al. "Psychopathology in Children of Inpatients With Depression: A Controlled Study." *Journal of Nervous and Mental Disease* 164 (1977): 408–413.

Williams, R.L., Karacan, I., and Hursch, C. *EEG of Human Sleep: Clinical Applications.* New York: John Wiley and Sons, 1974.

Wolf, G., and Money, J. "Relationship Between Sleep and Growth in Patients With Reversible Somatotropin Deficiency (Psychosocial Dwarfism)." *Psychological Medicine* 3 (1973): 18–27.

Cytryn, L., McKnew, D., and Bunney, W. "The Diagnosis of Depression in Children: A Reassessment." *American Journal of Psychiatry* 137 (1980): 22–25.

Cytryn, L., and McKnew, D. "Factors Influencing the Changing Clinical Expression of the Depressive Process in Children." *American Journal of Psychiatry* 131 (1974): 879–881.

Finch, S.M., and Poznanski, E.O. *Adolescent Suicide,* Springfield, IL.: C.C. Thomas, Publisher, 1971.

Freud, S. "Mourning and Melancholia (1917)." *Collected Papers IV.* New York: Basic Books, 1959.

Petti, T.A. "Depression in Hospitalized Child Psychiatry Patients: Approaches to Measuring Depression." *Journal of the American Academy of Child Psychiatry* 18 (1978): 49–59.

Poznanski, E., Cook, S.C., Carroll, B.J., and Corzo, H. "The Children's Depression Rating Scale: Its Performance in a Residential Psychiatric Population." Unpublished Manuscript.

Poznanski, E., Carroll, B.J., Banegas, M., Cook, S., and York, J. "The Dexamethasone Suppression Test in Prepubertal Depressed Children." Presented at the *American Psychiatric Association Annual Meeting,* New Orleans, 1981a.

Poznanski, E., Grossman, J., Banegas, M., Nitzberg, Y., and Gibbons, R. "The Children's Depression Rating Scale: An Update." Paper given at the *American Academy of Child Psychiatry,* Dallas, 1981b.

Poznanski, E., and Zrull, J. "Childhood Depression: Clinical Characteristics of Overtly Depressed Children." Archives of General Psychiatry 23 (1970): 8–15.

Puig-Antich, J., Perel, J.M., and Lupatkin, W. "Plasma Levels of Imipramine and Desmethylimipramine and Clinical Response in Prepubertal Major Disorders." *Journal of the American Academy of Child Psychiatry* 18 (1979): 616–627.

Robbins, D., Alessi, M., Cook, S., Poznanski, E., and Yanschyshyn, G.W. "The Systematic Assessment of Depression in Adolescent Psychiatric Inpatients." *Journal of the American Academy of Child Psychiatry,* in press.

Spitzer, R.L., Endicott, J., and Robins, E. *Research Diagnostic Criteria (RDC) for a Selected Group of Functional Disorders, 3d ed.* New York: New York State Psychiatric Institute, 1977.

Weinberg, W.A., Rutman, J., and Sullivan, L. "Depression in Children Referred to an Educational Diagnostic Center." *Journal of Pediatrics* 83 (1973): 1064–1072.

Weller, E., Weller, R., Preskorn, H., and Glotzbach, R.A. "Plasma Imipramine Levels in Prepubertal Children." Presented at the *American Psychiatric Association Annual Meeting,* New Orleans, 1981.

Zrull, J., McDermott, J.F., and Poznanski, E. "Hyperkinetic Syndrome: The Role of Depression." *Child Psychiatry and Human Development* 1 (1970): 1.

Bibliography for Chapter 20

American Psychiatric Association. *Diagnostic and Statistical Manual of Mental Disorders, 3d ed.* Washington: American Psychiatric Association, 1980.

Carlson, G., and Cantwell, D. "Unmasking Masked Depression in Children and Adolescents." *American Journal of Psychiatry* 137 (1980): 445–449.

Crumley, F. "Adolescent Suicide Attempts." *JAMA* 241 (1979): 2404–2407.

IV

Law and Psychiatry

Part IV
Law and Psychiatry

Authors for Part IV

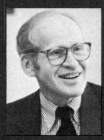

**Alan A. Stone, M.D.,
Preceptor**

Professor of Law and
  Psychiatry in the Faculty of
  Law and the Faculty of
  Medicine
Harvard University

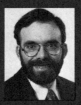

Paul S. Appelbaum, M.D.
Assistant Professor of Psychiatry
Program in Law and Psychiatry
University of Pittsburgh School of
  Medicine and
  Assistant Professor of Law
University of Pittsburgh School of
  Law
Western Psychiatric Institute and
  Clinic

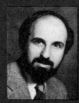

Joel I. Klein, J.D.
Partner
Onek, Klein and Farr

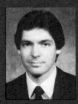

Clifford D. Stromberg, J.D.
Arnold and Porter

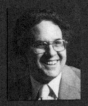

Loren H. Roth, M.D., M.P.H.
Associate Professor of Psychiatry
Director, Law and Psychiatry Program
Western Psychiatric Institute and
    Clinic
University of Pittsburgh School of
    Medicine

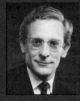

Mark J. Mills, J.D., M.D.
Commissioner Department of
    Mental Health
and
Assistant Professor (on leave)
Department of Psychiatry
Harvard Medical School

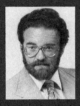

Thomas G. Gutheil, M.D.
Associate Professor of Psychiatry
    and Director of the Program in
    Psychiatry and Law
Harvard Medical School
Massachusetts Mental Health
    Center

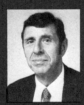

Seymour L. Halleck, M.D.
Professor of Psychiatry, School of
    Medicine and Adjunct Professor,
    School of Law
University of North Carolina

Law
and
Psychiatry

Introduction
by Alan A. Stone, MD.

Any valid historical account of American psychiatry in the second half of the twentieth century will need to contain at least one long chapter on legal developments. That chapter will describe a number of historical firsts—the first time the Supreme Court of the United States dealt with the rights of mental patients involuntarily confined in state hospitals *(Donaldson* v. *O'Connor,* 1975); the first time the Bill of Rights was invoked to assert that mental patients had a right to treatment *(Wyatt* v. *Stickney,* 1971) and a right to refuse treatment *(Rennie* v. *Klein,* 1979); the first time that psychiatrists were accused of violating their patients' constitutional rights *(Donaldson* v. *O'Connor,* 1975); and the first time that a federal judge ordered that the control of a state mental hospital be removed from state officials and handed over to a master appointed by the court.[1] All these firsts are the result of constitutional litigation brought by so-called public interest lawyers on behalf of mental patients (see the chapter by Klein). The success of this litigation has transformed public-sector psychiatry.

Typically these lawsuits assert alleged violations of constitutional rights, asking for example that various state laws controlling civil commitment be struck down as a deprivation of liberty without due process of law.[2] Although the legal theory of this litigation involves technical constitutional law, many of the actual decisions require judges to fashion mental health policy. Justice Potter Stewart of the Supreme Court made this point explicit. Writing in *Parham* v. *J.R.* he clearly stated the problem: "[I]ssues concerning mental illness are among the most difficult that courts have to face, involving as they often do serious problems of policy disguised as questions of constitutional law" *(Parham* v. *J.R.,* 1979, 2515).

A review of the landmark federal court decision will certainly confirm Justice Stewart's opinion. Imagine the extraordinary difficulties a judge confronts in making mental health policy. Not only is the discipline itself filled with controversy, conflict, and uncertainty, it is also a subject about which all of us, judges included, are apt to have charged feelings as a result of some personal or family experience. A further handicap to dealing with these serious problems of policy is that courts must resolve the legal issues before them, issues which, in accord with the tradition of appellate review, typically get narrower and narrower as they move up the appellate ladder. This narrowing of issues makes cases more decidable, but it also wrenches them out of their social context and reality, so that the court often must struggle with broad policy problems while exercising judicial tunnel vision.

The *Parham* case itself was a most striking example of this process. The lower court's decision *(J.L.* v. *Parham,* 1976) had adopted as its own the policy recommendations of a commission which had evalu-

---

[1] Courts have now so ordered in a number of cases, among them *Wyatt* v. *Stickney* (1971) and *Davis* v. *Watkins* (1974).
[2] See, for example, *Lessard* v. *Schmidt* (1972).

ated Georgia's inpatient services for children and found them wanting. The three-judge court in essence copied the recommendations of the commission into its decision. It made no effort to disguise the serious policy problems as constitutional issues. That happened only in the Supreme Court, where the question of the quality of institutions for children fell outside the Court's tunnel vision, and the Court narrowed the issue to consider only the constitutional requirements of due process for the admission of children to mental health facilities.

But despite its narrowness, the Supreme Court's decision in *Parham* represented a moral victory for American psychiatry. Even the most objective historian would have to conclude that the constitutional decisions prior to *Parham,* indeed all through the late 1960's and the 1970's, demonstrated an obvious antipathy to psychiatry.[3] One federal judge, reviewing with approval earlier decisions which struck down state statutes allowing psychiatric discretion in civil commitment, offered a typical opinion. The decisions to hold state statutes unconstitutional rested, he said, primarily on constitutional guarantees of personal liberty, but "a close second consideration has been that the diagnosis of mental illness leaves too much to subjective choice by less than neutral individuals" (King, in *Suzuki* v. *Quisenberry,* 1976).

This impugning of psychiatric decision making is a theme sounded again and again in important constitutional decisions. This is true not only in decisions setting new objective standards and procedural safeguards for civil commitment, but also in rulings on such issues as the right to refuse treatment. Even the right to treatment has brought with it a legal slogan—"the least restrictive alternative"—which is meant to limit the psychiatrist's discretion in decision making (see the chapter on this topic by Klein). In the fifteen years that led up to *Parham,* the lower federal courts in their constitutional rulings often fashioned mental health policy that had as a premise the courts' distrust of the psychiatrist's ability and neutrality.

One of the most important reasons for this trend is a product of the litigation process itself, a process which may be unfamiliar to most psychiatrists. When judges write opinions, they depend on the evidence and the briefs supplied by the legal advocates. No judge, even with the assistance of clerks, can do independent research on all the many subjects which come before him or her each term. But the information the parties' lawyers supply to the court is adversarial. Each side argues its strongest case, rather than presenting an entirely balanced and impartial interpretation of the facts. The legal advocates representing the mentally ill in these cases did just that—they represented the patient's side of the case. Their adversarial presentation to the courts brought together all of the radical criticism of psychiatry in a most forceful fashion. The advocates on the other side, usually state assistant attorneys general, were typically much less zealous. Certainly they made little if any effort to defend psychiatry or to describe the benefits of good psychiatric practice. The result of this imbalance in advocacy was not only a sweeping series of new constitutional holdings. The collection of decisions also reflected and even cited as authority the viewpoints of persons who were critical of if not hostile to psychiatry.[4] Moreover, the imbalance contributed to a proliferation of

[3]See Stone (1979).
[4]For a more detailed discussion of this point, see Stone (1981).

legal standards and procedures which removed discretion from psychiatrists and placed it in the hands of judges.

In *Parham* Chief Justice Warren Burger repudiated this trend, writing, "Although we acknowledge the fallibility of medical and psychiatric diagnosis [citations omitted], we do not accept the notion that the shortcomings of specialists can always be avoided by shifting the decision from a trained specialist using the traditional tools of medical science to an untrained judge or administrative hearing officer after a judicial-type hearing" (*Parham* v. *J.R.,* 1979, 2507). Justice Burger's decision is itself an example of the point just made. In reaching his decision he specifically acknowledges his reliance on the *amicus* brief of the American Psychiatric Association (*Parham* v. *J.R.,* 1979, 2506). But if the *Parham* decision was a moral victory for psychiatry, it is certainly no more than that. Not only did the court's majority fail to consider the quality of institutions for children, it also failed to address the problem of parents and states "dumping" mentally ill children in institutions when they might better be cared for elsewhere.[5] Nor did the *Parham* decision extend this deference to psychiatric expertise beyond the commitment stage. It did not, for example, control lower federal courts addressing such other aspects of psychiatric decision making as the treatment of those properly confined (see the chapter by Gutheil). Nor did it prevent state legislatures from imposing procedural safeguards by law. The state legislatures can do more than the Constitution requires, but they cannot do less. The court in *Parham* held that states need not hold a formal adversary hearing before a judge before committing a juvenile to a mental institution, but it did not prohibit states from requiring such a judicial hearing.

Many of the radical reforms sought in constitutional litigation have in fact been enacted by state legislatures. During this same fifteen-year period of litigation, most state legislatures enacted new mental health laws, and all of them have moved in the direction advocated by legal activists seeking to set limits on psychiatric discretion[6] (see the chapter by Stromberg). The most extraordinary psychological paradox of these years of legal ferment and change is that the reformers saw psychiatrists as possessing enormous power and needing to be restrained by law, and the psychiatrists viewed themselves as relatively powerless from the start and almost helpless by the end. One reason for the great success of this legal reform is undoubtedly that it was packaged and presented to the courts and legislatures as an extension of the civil rights movement.[7] Some of this civil libertarian reform could be accomplished without fiscal consequences, but the right to treatment is another matter. It does not fit neatly into the legal precedents of civil liberties, procedural due process, and equal protection. Nor can it be granted to the mentally ill without great expense to the states (see the chapter by Mills).

The historian will find the task of explaining these momentous legal developments no simple matter. Consideration will have to be given to the special role of the federal courts. In those courts, activist judges apparently became convinced that neither Congress nor the state legislatures were willing to remedy the terrible conditions in many

[5]Justice Brennan, concurring in part and dissenting in part, showed greater sensitivity to these problems. See *Parham* v. *J.R.* (1979), 2515–2522.
[6]See generally, the *Harvard Law Review* (1974).
[7]See Stone (1981), note 4, *supra.*

prisons, jails, juvenile facilities, state mental hospitals, and institutions for the mentally retarded.[8] These judges were consequently receptive to class action suits, the extraordinary new litigation which has pitted the courts against the legislative and executive branches of government. There is now evidence that the Supreme Court is not entirely in sympathy with this judicial activism,[9] and the fiscal constraints of the coming decade suggest that there will be increasing state resistance to these court-ordered reforms.

Many federal judges were acutely aware that in their attempts to remedy obvious abuses in state mental institutions they would have to fashion mental health policy.[10] They therefore encouraged the two disputing sides in the case to resolve policy questions on their own through a negotiated settlement. Judges then simply gave their imprimatur to the "consent decrees," the settlements which state officials and the attorneys representing the patients had agreed upon. The judges thus spared themselves the difficulties involved in detailing policy guidelines for the operation of mental institutions (see the discussion of this issue in Mills' chapter on the right to treatment). The consent decrees were an important element in the chronicle of deinstitutionalization. Many decrees required mass deinstitutionalization, which after all was not incompatible with what was then the dominant ideology in psychiatry—community mental health.[11]

When legal advocates negotiate a consent decree for the entire "class" of patients confined in a state's mental hospitals, there is no way they can realistically take into account the actual needs of all the members of this variegated group. Legal advocates who speak for patients understandably emphasize liberty interests, and where the need for treatment conflicts with liberty, treatment may get slighted. The negotiation of a consent decree typically takes place in the glare of adverse media publicity, adverse not only to the public-sector psychiatrist but also to elected state officials. When fiscal constraints were not so great as they seem today, state officials were more willing to make sometimes unrealistic concessions and thereby avoid the adverse publicity. Given these and other influences on the decrees, many have proved difficult if not impossible to fulfill. We can now expect more resistance to this kind of negotiated settlement and more legal resistance to judicial activism through appeals to higher courts and to the Supreme Court. That scenario is already developing at this writing.

The crusade is over. Most of the major constitutional battles over the rights of the mentally ill have already been fought. During the coming decade, as the courts, the legislatures, and the public realize that the pendulum has swung too far, it may well be possible to make at least small accommodations with clinical realities. Fiscal constraints may make this process difficult, but the crucial legal issue in these accommodations will very likely be competency/incompetency (see the chapter by Roth on this latter issue).

The historian who focuses only on the rights of the mentally ill will not do justice to all the remarkable developments in law and psychiatry

---

[8]On this general judicial trend, see Eisenberg and Yeazell (1980).
[9]See, for example, the recent decision in *Pennhurst State School and Hospital* v. *Halderman* (1981).
[10]See, for example, Judge Orrin Judd's opinion in *New York State Association for Retarded Children, Inc.* v. *Rockefeller* (1973).
[11]See Stone (1981), note 4, *supra*.

over the past decade and a half. Medicine is in the process of becoming a regulated industry, and although the present administration in Washington is intent on deregulation, regulation is too advanced and too entrenched to be excised completely. Furthermore, much of the regulation of medicine and psychiatry comes not from government but through the system of third-party payment. Insurance-company payment formulas create incentives to provide certain varieties of health care rather than others. Unfortunately those incentives favor technical procedures and the maximum number of patient contacts rather than the kind of care traditional in psychiatry. Third-party payment not only establishes these incentives. In the effort to achieve accountability and to police fraudulent claims, it also intrudes on the privacy of the patient-doctor relationship. Psychiatric confidentiality has never had so great a challenge as it now confronts (see the chapter by Appelbaum).

Even though third-party payment has, with rare exceptions, not been generous in providing psychiatric coverage, it has been a crucial inducement for nonmedical mental health professionals to seek independent licensure, provider status, and compensation from third-party payers. This struggle to participate in the provider market has already led to antitrust litigation,[12] and more is in the offing. Whatever the merits of this dispute, one possible consequence is an economic solution. To offset the increase in the volume of claims, payers and regulators could reduce the allowable benefits to each patient.

For this and other reasons legislative action and litigation will certainly be necessary to extend existing coverage of psychiatric care, and perhaps even to maintain what now exists. Thus, the future private-sector psychiatrist may well not only lobby the legislatures but also appear in the courts as plaintiff rather than as defendant.[13]

State and federal regulation of medicine by statute and by administrative agencies, like the Department of Health and Human Services, the Federal Trade Commission, and the Food and Drug Administration, and *de facto* regulation by third-party payment do not exhaust the catalogue of regulatory influences on the psychiatrist. Every department of mental health, like every hospital, now has its own lawyers spinning out regulations on an almost daily basis. Some of this regulation is a response to the constitutional litigation already described, to other court decisions, and to the demands of various accrediting bodies, like the Joint Commission on Accreditation of Hospitals, which also regulate the practice of psychiatry. As this web of regulation tightens around psychiatry, the clinician's discretion is inevitably constrained.

Recently J.J. Paris (1981) surveyed New York's latest court decisions on incompetent dying patients. His analysis was clear, critical, and damning. He urged the medical profession to ignore the courts and to continue to do what is right. But his urging is misplaced. He should have directed his plea to the lawyers who now advise and issue regulations for hospitals. Their job is to protect the hospitals from legal risks, or at least to minimize those risks. How can the doctors continue to do what is right when the hospitals' lawyers are no doubt already drafting regulations to comply with the decisions Paris urges the doctors to ignore?

[12]See *Virginia Academy of Clinical Psychologists* v. *Blue Shield of Virginia* (1979).
[13]There have already been serious challenges to statutory provisions excluding psychiatric care from Medicaid coverage.

Psychiatrists are not alone in this web of regulation, for the entire medical profession is similarly involved. Although claims against psychiatrists for malpractice are still infrequent, compared with the rest of the medical profession, each new malpractice precedent, e.g., the *Tarasoff* case, has a regulatory impact.[14] So-called defensive medicine is the regulatory consequence of rising malpractice liability. Still further regulatory constraints are coming from state boards of licensure, which have become increasingly active in recent years.

The reader will note that nothing has yet been mentioned about the traditional areas of forensic psychiatry—the insanity defense, competency to stand trial, testamentary capacity, and the psychiatrist as an expert witness in the courtroom. But this does not mean that forensic psychiatry has remained unchanged. Indeed, the historian would have to report that at every juncture where the criminal justice system relies on psychiatry, there have been legal reforms and legislative changes akin to those already described in the laws dealing with civilly committed patients (see the chapter on these topics by Halleck). Forensic psychiatry has also had its historic firsts, e.g., *Jackson* v. *Indiana* (1972). The traditional forensic psychiatrist now in effect practices a subspeciality within the much larger domain of law and psychiatry. Stimulated by the remarkable legal ferment, the subspecialty is flourishing. Many forensic psychiatrists have drawn on their legal backgrounds to make themselves familiar with these broader legal developments and have joined with the other psychiatrists and lawyers who are experts in the growing common domain of law and psychiatry.

The new interdisciplinary specialty of law and psychiatry is well represented in the chapters that follow. The Part includes contributions from two lawyers who have immersed themselves in the field—Joel Klein, counsel for the American Psychiatric Association, and Clifford Stromberg, consultant to the Association's Council on Government Policy and Law. Dr. Mark Mills is not only commissioner of mental health for Massachusetts; he also holds degrees in both law and medicine. Dr. Loren Roth is distinguished both by great expertise and by the fact that he conducts empirical research in a field dominated by legal argument. Dr. Paul Appelbaum is one of the most promising of the younger generation of psychiatrists drawn to law and psychiatry. Dr. Thomas Gutheil has emerged as an eloquent spokesman for the clinician's perspective in the face of legal intervention. Dr. Seymour Halleck is one of the outstanding leaders in law and psychiatry and has received the Isaac Ray Award.

Since each of these authorities is specially qualified to write on the subject of his chapter, the Preceptor has taken no liberties with their ideas even where he disagrees (rarely) or where they disagree with each other (even more rarely). He has, rather, moderated the scope, size, and clarity of the chapters so that the whole is a thorough but balanced presentation of the knowledge and issues in a complex and growing field.

Appelbaum (on confidentiality), Stromberg (on standards of civil commitment), Roth (on competency), and Mills (on the right to treatment) have written chapters that may be of continuing value as reference works. Klein's chapter on the least restrictive alternative should provide those unfamiliar with law a special insight into the

[14]See Stone (1976).

litigating strategy of legal reformers. Gutheil raises many of the crucial clinical considerations which the courts have ignored in fashioning the right to refuse treatment and suggests the reasons for what he regards as their misguided decisions. Halleck has surveyed the growth within the subspecialty of forensic psychiatry, emphasizing both what we can contribute and the special ethical problems we confront.

This collection cannot cover all of the many new and important intersections of law and psychiatry—that would require a massive volume. But it should give the reader an excellent opportunity to understand some of the most important issues in an interdisciplinary field that is of increasing importance for our profession.

Chapter 21 # Confidentiality in Psychiatric Treatment
by Paul S. Appelbaum, M.D.

The growing interest in using legal mechanisms to define and regulate the nature and extent of confidentiality in the physician-patient relationship would have struck most of our medical forebears as odd, indeed. From the days of Hippocrates, physicians have acknowledged their obligation to protect sensitive information obtained in the course of their daily rounds. "[W]hatsoever I shall see or hear in the course of my profession," reads the Hippocratic Oath, "as well as outside my profession in my intercourse with men, if it be what should not be published abroad, I will never divulge, holding such things to be holy secrets" (Reiser et al., 1977). But the self-assumed obligation of the Hippocratics was not based on a fear of lawsuits or the threat of licensure revocation; it was rooted instead in the recognition of an ethical principle intrinsic to all therapeutic relationships.

That ethical principle remains valid today. The individual in the role of patient acts differently than he or she does in almost any other context. Shedding the protective mantle of privacy which ordinarily hides from public view the personal fears, fantasies, antipathies, past errors, and current excesses, the patient appears to the physician as a naked, and therefore dependent and vulnerable, fellow human being. No individual could assume such a role without the trust that the physician will not take advantage of this helplessness. Although the physician is already bound by the principle of nonmaleficence, the maxim to do no harm, he or she is here doubly so enjoined. Having persuaded the patient to enter this dependent state (even if only implicitly), the physician has thereby induced a situation from which harm could result. As a consequence, the physician must guard even more carefully against the possibility that his or her acts may rebound to the detriment of the patient. While some may challenge the accuracy of this description of the current, typically impersonal and mechanistic doctor-patient relationship (Wigmore, 1961), no one can gainsay its relevance to the dyadic interplay of patient and psychiatrist.

Yet the inescapable fact is that this ethical reasoning no longer solely determines the shape of psychiatrists' actions in regard to confidentiality. The law, via judicial decision, statute, and administrative regulation, has moved into the area energetically. Two factors, opposite in vector, account for the law's interest in the issue. First, despite the ethical maxim, physicians and others have not always been scrupulous about protecting patients' confidentiality. The law has responded by providing redress for the victims of such breaches and establishing mechanisms to deter and to punish the malefactors. Here the law weighs in on the side of the ethical principle.

The second factor, however, reflects less legal devotion to the preservation of confidence. As society has become increasingly complex and interdependent, the value of confidentiality has come into conflict with other important ends, including the rights of defendants to secure justice, the needs of insurers to guarantee equity and prevent fraud, and the desire of society to protect itself from future violent acts. Here, in its role as conciliator of conflicting values, the law often acts to limit the domain of psychiatrist-patient confidentiality.

This chapter reviews both of these functions of the law and in doing so enters into the complex and often confusing world of legal reasoning. The chapter concludes that despite the prominence of recent legal approaches to the issue of confidentiality, confidentiality in practice is more influential as an ethical precept than as a legal rule.

LEGAL SUPPORT FOR CONFIDENTIALITY

Tort Remedies

The most frequently discussed legal buttresses for physician-patient confidentiality are among the least commonly invoked. These are the remedies which the law of torts (civil wrongs) provides for harms suffered as a result of improper disclosure of information. The courts (for innovations in tort law are usually fashioned by judges in their decisions, not by legislators in their statutes) have come to consider breaches of confidentiality under a number of legal theories which include (1) invasion of privacy, (2) breach of contract, (3) breach of fiduciary duty, (4) malpractice, and (5) violation of licensing statutes (*American Law Reports,* 1968; Cooper, 1978; Eger, 1976). Each of these will be discussed, but it should be noted that reported cases of physicians being sued under any of these legal theories are rare and that instances of psychiatrists being defendants are even rarer. Thus, any attempt to define precisely the impact of these causes of action on medicine and psychiatry is laden with ambiguity.

Invasion of privacy, the first of these theories, is a relative newcomer to the law of torts, having first been suggested in a classic paper by Warren and Brandeis in 1890 (Warren and Brandeis, 1890). The Warren-Brandeis doctrine recognized a common law right to privacy and argued that the pain, distress, and pecuniary damages caused by an invasion of privacy warranted compensation. The doctrine has recently been accepted in several courts, and in some cases the right to privacy has been elevated to constitutional status (*Griswold* v. *Connecticut,* 1965; *Roe* v. *Wade,* 1973). One of the few reported cases of invasion of privacy involving a psychiatrist was *Doe* v. *Roe* (1977), in which damages were awarded to a patient after her psychiatrist published a book detailing, with inadequate disguise of those involved, the patient's experiences in psychoanalysis.

Doe v. *Roe* was also grounded on the second of the legal theories allowing recovery for unauthorized disclosure, breach of contract. Although the patient involved in this case had never signed a formal agreement with the psychiatrist that her communications would be kept confidential, the court found "that a physician, who enters into a contract with a patient to provide medical attention, impliedly covenants to keep in confidence all disclosures made by the patient. . . This is particularly and necessarily true of the psychiatric relationship. . . ." (*Doe* v. *Roe*, 1977).

Breach of fiduciary duty, the third basis for legal action, relates to the trust that is seen as underlying every doctor-patient relationship. A fiduciary is an individual, usually possessed of superior knowledge, who promises, even if only implicitly, to place another individual's best interests above his or her own. When a physician violates that duty, liability may ensue. For example, in *Horne* v. *Patton* (1973) the defendant physician revealed the existence of psychiatric problems to his patient's employer.

Malpractice is a closely related ground for suit, in which the physician is held not to the standard of the ideal fiduciary, but to the standard of care prevalent among professional colleagues. The reasoning is that if colleagues do not generally disclose confidences, neither should an individual practitioner. The American Psychiatric Association's *Principles of Medical Ethics with Annotations Especially Applicable to Psychiatry* may be taken as one indication of the standard of care for psychiatrists. All psychiatrists should be familiar with it (American Psychiatric Association, 1981).

Licensing statutes, the last of the bases for an action in tort, often require maintenance of confidentiality, thereby providing, in addition to the administrative remedies discussed below, a supporting basis for a patient's legal action.

While these five grounds for tort liability of the psychiatrist may appear to afford considerable protection to confidentiality, the reality is probably otherwise. Lawsuits cannot be brought unless the patient is aware of the violation of confidentiality and, usually, unless he or she suffers some clear-cut damage as a result. One suspects that in the majority of cases of unauthorized disclosure one or both of these elements are lacking. Suits are expensive and time-consuming and provide, if successful, only *post facto* compensation for what are essentially irremediable breaches of privacy. The awkwardness of the tort law as a tool for guarding patients' confidences is reflected in the small number of claims for damages that have reached the appellate courts.

Administrative Law

In part because of the deficiencies in tort law protections of confidentiality, state statutes and regulations directed at providers of medical and psychiatric care are being used with increasing momentum (American Medical Association, 1981). Statutes vary greatly from state to state. Some limit protections to state-licensed facilities, while others cover treatment that takes place in private offices as well. Psychiatric records may be covered separately from other medical documents. The laws may, like the Pennsylvania statute and regulations, define the conditions under which patients may consent to release information, how patients themselves may gain access to their records, and what circumstances warrant release of information without patients' consent (*Pennsylvania Statutes Annotated,* 1978; *Pennsylvania Code,* 1979). Auxiliary provisions, as in the Massachusetts Patients' Bill of Rights (*Massachusetts Acts of 1979*), may require that patients be informed of their rights concerning confidentiality and access. These bills may also specify penalties for violations of their provisions. The American Psychiatric Association has drafted a model law designed to aid legislators grappling with these issues (American Psychiatric Association, 1979). On the federal level, strict rules have been adopted governing confidentiality of records in federally funded drug and alcohol treatment programs (*Code of Federal Regulations,* 1976). Given the wide variation in what the statutes cover and the frequent amendments they undergo, psychiatrists would do well to keep themselves apprised of the latest developments in their states.

Licensing statutes are the other administrative mechanism available to encourage adherence to the ethic of confidentiality. Many states permit proceedings against physicians for revocation of licensure in the event of a breach of confidentiality (Privacy Protection Study Commission, 1977, 284). The effectiveness of such provisions is questionable. Revocation proceedings can drag on over a considerable period of time and offer no financial benefit to the aggrieved patient. Confidentiality provisions in licensing statutes may be of greater use, as noted above, in establishing grounds for actions for damages in tort.

Testimonial Privilege

The final major area of protection the law provides for patients' confidences is limited to the courtroom setting. To counteract the common-law principle that anyone (except an attorney or a spouse) who has information relevant to a judicial proceeding may be compelled to testify, a majority of states have passed laws exempting certain classes of relationships from this obligation (Woodman, 1979). Technically, the statutes confer *testimonial privilege,* in which an individual has the right to prevent a third party from revealing in court information obtained in confidence (Gutheil and Appelbaum, 1982). Information revealed to psychiatrists may be protected under statutes granting privilege to all physicians' patients or under legislation aimed at the patients of a narrowly defined class of psychotherapists.

Several salient points about privilege must be stressed. First, with the notable exception of Illinois, state laws almost always confer the privilege on the patient, not the psychiatrist (Beigler, 1972; *Illinois Laws,* 1979). If the patient desires the psychiatrist's testimony, the latter may be compelled to testify. Second, the statutes are often so laden with exceptions, such as when the patient has raised the issue of his or her mental state in court, as to render them inapplicable in a large number of instances. Third, even when the statutes seem to be applicable, courts have generally found ways to circumvent them in order to obtain information they truly desired (Slovenko, 1975).

A recent series of cases may hold some promise for enhancing the scope of psychiatrist-patient privilege, even without new legislation (Appelbaum and Roth, 1981). Two California cases have recognized that a patient's constitutional right to privacy may limit the admissability of unconsented psychiatric testimony to information directly relevant to the case at hand (*In re Lifshutz,* 1970; *Caesar* v.

Mountanos, 1976). A Pennsylvania court extended that reasoning to find an absolute constitutional privilege for psychiatric patients, although that precedent has yet to be adopted elsewhere (*In re B.,* 1978). The Alaska Supreme Court had reached a similar conclusion on a common-law basis some years earlier (*Allred* v. *State,* 1976). Most recently, the Pennsylvania Supreme Court again broke new ground by finding a common-law basis to extend a modified privilege to rape counselors who were previously unprotected by any privilege statute (*In re Pittsburgh Action Against Rape,* 1981).

LEGAL IMPEDIMENTS TO CONFIDENTIALITY

The Duty to Protect Third Parties

When asked to balance patients' rights to confidentiality against other societal values, the courts do not always favor the former. The most controversial example of this was *Tarasoff* v. *Regents of University of California* (1976). In this California case it was held that a psychotherapist who knows or ought to know of the danger his or her patient presents to an identifiable third party has an obligation to take steps to protect that party. Psychiatrists have vigorously protested that such a requirement means the end of trust in psychotherapy and that it is, furthermore, unlikely to achieve the desired result (Gurevitz, 1977; Stone, 1976). Nonetheless, courts in New Jersey (*McIntosh* v. *Milano,* 1979) and Nebraska (*Lipari* v. *Sears,* 1980) have accepted the *Tarasoff* doctrine, and therapists nationwide are concerned about its implications.

Despite the uproar, many of the most feared effects of *Tarasoff* have failed to develop (Appelbaum, 1981). Although *Tarasoff*-like situations are likely to arise infrequently, psychiatrists have devised techniques for managing them without breaching patients' confidentiality (Roth and Meisel, 1977). Indeed, there is evidence that many therapists recognized their obligation to protect third parties well before *Tarasoff* and have thus changed their actual practices little (Wise, 1978). The courts themselves have displayed ambivalence about *Tarasoff* and its implications, rejecting it altogether in two states (in Maryland *Shaw* v. *Glickman,* 1980, and in Pennsylvania *H.* v. *A.,* 1981), and even restricting it somewhat in California (*Bellah* v. *Greenson,* 1977). In most jurisdictions, however, there is no precedent to guide clinicians, who must decide for themselves when, if ever, a patient's threat warrants disclosure to a third party.

Reports to Insurers

Less dramatic than *Tarasoff,* but of far greater frequency and significance, are the legally sanctioned breaches of confidentiality that occur when third-party payers demand information about patients' care (American Psychiatric Association, 1975). Although some information must be communicated to insurers in order for them to validate requests for reimbursement, the current system often encourages abuse (Grossman, 1971). Information requested may be excessive (Shwed et al., 1979); it may be processed in such a manner (for example, through the patient's employer) as to guarantee leakage (American Psychiatric Association, 1975); and it may subsequently be redisclosed to others, including to massive data banks, without the patient's knowledge or consent (Privacy Protection Study Commission,

1977). Similar problems may arise as a result of the scrutiny of Professional Standards Review Organizations or other peer-review procedures (Sullivan, 1977).

Concern about these matters in the middle 1970's led to a number of conferences cosponsored by the American Psychiatric Association (Aldrich and Turner, 1978; Spingarn, 1975) and even to some statutes restricting redisclosure to third parties (National Commission on Confidentiality of Health Records, 1978), but much of the momentum to address the problem appears now to have faded. Many psychiatrists are taking measures on their own to limit or distort the information that insurers receive in order to protect patients' privacy (Sharfstein et al., 1980). These measures, though often commendable, may sometimes border on fraud, and, in the extreme, they may result in denial of coverage for patients' care. A recent Hawaii case suggests that the courts may be willing to limit some third-party access to records on constitutional privacy grounds, in this case access by the state's Medicaid program (*Hawaii Psychiatric Society* v. *Ariyoshi,* 1979). The only definitive solution, however, would be legislation regulating third-party payers' demands for information and their subsequent use of it.

Mandatory Reporting

Society has long demanded that physicians report to the police or health authorities certain patients whose conditions raise issues of social concern. Historically, this group of patients was primarily composed of individuals with communicable diseases or of those who suffered certain kinds of trauma, such as gunshot wounds. More recently, some states have required reporting of individuals with epidemiologically important diseases, most notably cancer.

Of greater significance to psychiatrists than these is the requirement to report victims of child abuse. The problems with this requirement are manifold. What constitutes child abuse has resisted clear definition and may be highly susceptible to cultural influences (Taylor and Newberger, 1979). The response of child protective agencies, which is often to remove the child from the home, may irreparably damage the psychiatrist-patient relationship, thus limiting the possibility that the causes of the abuse can be effectively identified and dealt with. On the other hand, failure to report when suspecting abuse can, in many states, leave the physician open to considerable liability (Curran, 1977). Similar issues arise in states that require reporting of medical or psychiatric illnesses that may impair patients' abilities to drive motor vehicles.

Other Legal Impediments to Confidentiality

This is by no means an exhaustive accounting of ways in which the law diminishes confidentiality. The opportunity to diminish or to protect it arises each time society decides to use the information gathered in the psychiatrist-patient relationship to further some other end. An interesting example of its protection occurred in California. A 1976 statute designed to limit use of electroconvulsive therapy required that, prior to its use, a patient's relatives be informed of the proposed treatment, including the nature and seriousness of the disorder to be treated (*Mental Disability Law Reporter,* 1977). A California court declared that these requirements violated both the patients' right to privacy and the statutes which guaranteed confidentiality (*Aden* v. *Younger,* 1976). Despite examples such as this, efforts to use psychiatric information for other ends are likely to continue.

IMPLICATIONS OF THE CURRENT LEGAL STATUS OF CONFIDENTIALITY

Two conclusions should be evident from this rapid survey of the impact of current law on confidentiality in psychiatry. First, to the extent that the law seeks to protect patients' communications from those not involved in their care, it does so inadequately and usually by means of *post facto* remedies of dubious effectiveness. Second, to the extent that the law permits or requires disclosure of information about patients, it creates the opportunity for widespread dissemination of potentially damaging material, and in doing so it often hampers the establishment of the trusting relationship that is essential to good psychiatric care. As a result, if patients' confidences are to be guarded, whether for ethical reasons or for more practical ones, the burden of their protection falls upon the individual psychiatrist.

Most authorities agree, and many state confidentiality statutes require, that patients' informed consent must be obtained prior to any disclosure of identifiable information. While appealing in its simplicity, such a rule immediately suggests complications (Gutheil and Appelbaum, 1982). Many statutes, for example, require disclosure in certain instances regardless of a patient's wishes. There will be occasions when patients are not available to give consent or are incompetent to do so. Even when they are not legally incompetent, patients who are severely disturbed may oppose release of information when disclosure would clearly be in their best interests. And, most important of all, many patients who do give consent may be acting under the coercive pressures of an employer or an insurer, or patients may not be fully aware of the nature of the material to be released or the potential ramifications of its disclosure or redisclosure.

A variety of methods have been suggested to deal with these difficulties. When disclosure is legally required, some propose, the patient should be informed in advance about the fact and extent of the planned revelation. In some cases, this may permit the patient to correct erroneous data or to challenge the basis for the request. In all cases, others suggest, patients should be informed as fully as possible about the nature of the material that will be disclosed. And some have even suggested informing patients at the beginning of a therapeutic relationship of the potentially applicable limitations on confidentiality (Noll, 1976).

Nonetheless, rules can be multiplied endlessly without either providing for all foreseeable circumstances or offering guidance when unique situations arise. Only a return to the underlying ethical principle promises to help here. If the psychiatrist's primary obligation, as suggested earlier, is to protect the patient from the harm that may result from breached confidences, the psychiatrist's behavior ought always to be focused on that obligation. Psychiatrists who successfully internalize it will usually act, even in ambiguous circumstances, to sustain it.

Thus, the psychiatrist who appreciates the ethical underpinnings of confidentiality will avoid mentioning a patient's name in casual conversation or discussing identifiable information in settings such as elevators, where uninvolved third parties are present. Written reports or oral presentations based on case material will be appropriately disguised to protect the patient. When patients have given consent to information disclosure, only the data that are immediately relevant to the purpose for which disclosure is requested will be released. When the patient is unavailable or incompetent to give consent, information will be disclosed only to protect the patient from harm or to advance the patient's clear-cut interests.

It would be foolish to pretend that merely stating this ethical principle will resolve all conflicts concerning confidentiality. Most philosophers and legal scholars today would probably agree that the psychiatrist's obligation to protect the patient, which involves injunctions both to act and to refrain from acting, is subordinate to the patient's right to exercise personal autonomy. In such a view, the psychiatrist has no right to withhold information that a patient desires to have disclosed. Yet there are psychiatrists who feel strongly otherwise, particularly when the patient's decision may be influenced by the intense emotional atmosphere of a psychotherapeutic relationship.

Further, ethical and legal principles are not always congruent. "When the psychiatrist is ordered by the court to reveal the confidences entrusted to him/her by patients . . . he/she may ethically hold the right to dissent within the framework of the law" (American Psychiatric Association, 1981). Psychiatrists have chosen in the past, and may again choose in the future, to suffer legal penalties rather than to reveal patients' communications (*In re Lifshutz,* 1970; *Caesar* v. *Mountanos,* 1976; *In re B.,* 1978). Not every psychiatrist may want to take such a step, nor would every psychiatrist arrive at the same result when balancing societal and individual needs, but these cases are exemplars of passionate concern about confidentiality. In the end, it is with just such concern that the future of confidentiality rests.

Chapter 22 # Developments Concerning The Legal Criteria For Civil Commitment: Who Are We Looking For?
by Clifford D. Stromberg, J.D.

THE PROBLEM

In recent years, civil commitment of the mentally ill increasingly has come to resemble the criminal justice process. Civil commitment now looms as a concatenation of legal petitions, hearings, cross-examinations, rulings, and appeals. To civil liberties lawyers, this is a dream come true. To many psychiatrists, it is a nightmare in which civil commitment's basic goal—providing care and treatment to those who need it—is virtually forgotten.

An overarching problem, however, is that this interprofessional debate has often focused on whether civil commitment procedures are too little or too much like criminal procedures. This has obscured critical differences in the substantive decisions which the two systems seek to make. The difference is not simply that the criminal justice system seeks to punish and deter, while the civil commitment system seeks to care for and treat. It is, rather, that in the criminal system we share a consensus on who we are looking for, while in civil commitment, we do not.

Criminal trials seek to determine whether persons have committed physical acts statutorily defined as crimes. In most cases, any intent or mental state which is an element of the offense is quickly inferred from the acts constituting the crime. Thus, while there are animated debates over what ought to be defined as criminal behavior in the first place, and over what sentences are appropriate after conviction, everyone in the courtroom is likely to agree on what is meant by *guilty. Guilty* means "he did it."

In civil commitment, we share no such consensus. Instead, there is confusion and contention as to the meanings of *mentally ill, dangerous to himself or others,* and *gravely disabled.* Despite the much vaunted outpouring of judicial decisions concerning the mentally ill during the 1970's, the criteria for civil commitment were sharpened little on the anvil of this legal strife. Most of the leading court decisions dealt with either procedural issues or the right to treatment, and not with the criteria for commitment.[1] Until recently, the legislatures also devoted their efforts primarily to devising more rigorous (or cumbersome) commitment procedures, while abiding in the commitment criteria a vast uncertainty which engulfed the whole system.

This very problem was at the root of much of the confusion, acrimony, and legal struggles which beset the mental health system during the 1970's. While civil commitment historically has been premised on several quite distinct rationales,[2] few state laws clearly differentiated them, or required judges to state the rationale they acted under in committing a person or the precise criteria which had been satisfied. The ambiguous basis of many commitments bedevilled later efforts to decide issues such as how long confinement could properly continue, whether and how far involuntary treatment should be pursued, and what must be shown to justify release.[3] What was needed was

---

[1]*See, e.g., Vitek* v. *Jones,* 445 U.S. 480 (1980) (procedures for transfer of person from prison to mental hospital); *Addington* v. *Texas,* 441 U.S. 418 (1979) (standard of proof in civil commitment hearings); *Parham* v. *J.R.,* 442 U.S. 584 (1978) (whether an adversary hearing is required in commitment of a minor); *Jackson* v. *Indiana,* 406 U.S. 715 (1972) (relationship of purposes of confinement to duration); *Welsch* v. *Likins,* 550 F.2d 1122 (8th Cir. 1977) (and prior decisions in the case) (civil commitment procedures); *Wyatt* v. *Aderholt,* 503 F.2d 1305 (5th Cir. 1974) (and prior decisions in the case) (right to treatment); *Eckerhart* v. *Hensley,* 475 F. Supp. 908 (W.D. Mo. 1979) (institutional conditions); *Eubanks* v. *Clarke,* 434 F. Supp. 1022 (E.D. Pa. 1977) (rights concerning transfer from one facility to another); *Davis* v. *Watkins,* 384 F. Supp. 119 (N.D. Ohio 1974) (right to treatment).

[2]Commitment has generally been thought to be justified (1) under the state's police power if the person is dangerous to others; (2) under the state's *parens patriae* power if the person is mentally ill and in need of treatment; and (3) under either the police or the *parens patriae* power if the person is likely to harm himself, either by direct action or by inability to provide for his basic needs.

[3]For example, the difficult issue in the *Rogers* and *Rennie* cases, of whether an involuntarily committed patient has a right to refuse treatment, arose in part because neither the Massachusetts nor the New Jersey statute required that persons be committed only if they lacked capacity to make a reasoned decision concerning treatment. *See Rogers* v. *Okin,* 478 F. Supp. 1342 (D. Mass. 1979), *aff'd in part* and *rev'd in part,* 634 F.2d 650 (1st Cir. 1980), *cert. granted,* No. 80–1417 (U.S. April 20, 1981); *Rennie* v. *Klein,* 462 F. Supp. 1131 (D.N.J. 1978).

far more rigorous consideration by legislatures and courts of the criteria for commitment. To an extent, this is now occurring.

Therefore, in reviewing the most recent legal developments concerning civil commitment, this chapter focuses not upon the procedures, but exclusively on the criteria for commitment.[4] What is perhaps most clear is that, increasingly, legislatures and courts are taking a more sophisticated look at the statutory criteria for commitment. It is now recognized that the precise wording of the statutes is in fact critical to the real-world workings of the civil commitment process.

This last observation may be viewed skeptically by some, because of the current corrosive cynicism among both lawyers and psychiatrists about civil commitment statutes. Many lawyers assume that psychiatrists recommend commitment of people they believe should be institutionalized regardless of the statutory criteria. The view of psychiatry purveyed so effectively during the 1960's and 1970's was that "psychiatric diagnoses are stigmatizing labels phrased to resemble medical diagnoses and applied to persons whose behavior offends or annoys others" (Szasz, 1974). Many psychiatrists, for their part, believe that no matter how the statutes are crafted, they will always be phrased in legally rather than diagnostically meaningful terms. Accordingly, they are unconcerned with efforts to revise statutes, believing that the adversary process will distort what they have to say in any event.

Neither group should abandon the battle yet, for it can still be won. Recent legal decisions demonstrate that while certain statutory criteria for commitment are so irrelevant to clinical realities as to invite confusion and abuse in practice and invalidation in court, others are precise enough to make civil commitment far better than a pseudolegalistic charade.

---

[4] I discuss primarily the criteria for indefinite or medium-term (*e.g.,* 30 day) commitment; many states have slightly different criteria for emergency confinement and for long-term recommitment.

For those who are especially concerned with commitment procedures, the following sampling of cases may be of interest: *In re Hop,* 623 P.2d 282 (Cal. 1981) (procedural rights in commitment of developmentally disabled persons); *Ex parte Ullmann,* 616 S.W. 2d 278 (Tex. Civ. App. 1981) (right to counsel); *Warren* v. *Harvey,* 632 F.2d 925 (2d Cir. 1980) (procedural and evidentiary rights of insanity acquittees vs. persons civilly committed); *Benham* v. *Edwards,* 501 F. Supp. 1050 (N.D. Ga. 1980) (same); *Interest of Henderson,* 610 P.2d 1350 (Colo. Ct. App. 1980) (voluntary patient absent without authorization may be involuntarily committed); *Sisneros* v. *District Court,* 606 P.2d 55 (Colo. 1980) (involuntary commitment only proper if voluntary commitment is refused); *State ex rel. Doe* v. *Madonna,* 295 N.W. 2d 356 (Minn. 1980) (rights concerning pre-hearing confinement); *In re Field,* 412 A. 2d 1032 (N.H. 1980) (various evidentiary and procedural rights); *Matter of Dean,* 607 P.2d 132 (N. Mex. Ct. App. 1980) (live testimony as to dangerousness not required); *In re Hutchinson,* 421 A.2d 261 (Pa. Super. Ct. 1980) (admissibility of hearsay); *Jones* v. *Texas,* 610 S.W.2d 535 (Tex. Civ. App. 1980) (privilege does not bar testimony as to psychiatric examination); *Matter of Mathews,* 613 P.2d 80 (Ore. 1980) (fifth amendment privilege does not apply); *Heap* v.*Roulet,* 590 P.2d 1 (Cal. 1979) (right to jury trial before appointment of conservator); *In re Ottolini,* 392 N.E. 2d 736 (Ill. App. Ct. 1979) (use of hearsay evidence); *Markey* v. *Wachtel,* 264 S.E.2d 437 (W.Va. 1979) (no jury right in civil commitment, and other issues); *Matter of Farrow,* 255 S.E.2d 777 (N.C. Ct. App. 1979) (privilege; due process in change from voluntary to involuntary status); *Pennsylvania ex rel. Platt* v. *Platt,* 404 A2d 410 (Pa. Super. Ct. 1979) (spousal privilege does not apply); *Von Luch* v. *Rankin,* 558 S.W.2d 445 (Ark. 1979) (voluntary patient must be released on request or given full due process hearing); *Matter of Wagstaff,* 287 N.W.2d 339 (Mich. Ct. App. 1979) (right to jury trial on need for continued confinement); *In re Watson,* 154 Cal. Rptr. 151 (Cal. Ct. App. 1979) (right to be present at commitment hearing).

The following discussion of developments concerning each of the criteria for civil commitment highlights the prospects for a civil commitment system that is both clinically and legally functional.

THE CRITERIA FOR COMMITMENT

The Criterion of Mental Illness

Under current state statutes, the threshold criterion for civil commitment is, of course, that the person is *mentally ill.* But psychiatrists and lawyers should be aware that this criterion does not entail a single, binary judgment, i.e., mental illness or no mental illness. Instead, in most states mental illness has come to be defined further by reference to other specific conditions. These are enumerated sometimes fairly precisely (e.g., "a psychiatric disorder which substantially disturbs a person's thinking, feeling, or behavior or impairs the person's ability to function")[5] and sometimes so imprecisely as to expand the concept of mental illness seemingly beyond the bounds of medicine.[6] Next, some statutes specifically include within *mental illness,* while an increasing number exclude conditions such as mental retardation, epilepsy, alcoholism, and addiction to or use of narcotic drugs.[7] Finally, the statutes usually require that the condition evidencing a person's mental illness be one which impairs his or her functions "to a degree sufficient to require protection, supervision, treatment, [or] confinement."[8]

These laws, if conscientiously applied, require the psychiatrist and the court to make not a single judgment, but a series of judgments. Is there mental illness? Of the kinds enumerated? Not due solely to excluded conditions? Of a nature such as to seriously impair the person's capacity? Despite the recent efforts by states to move toward more nuanced definitions of mental illness, the courts have continued to rule that civil commitment cannot be justified by a finding of mental illness and need for treatment alone (the *parens patriae* rationale).

In the middle 1970's, several courts seemed to suggest that proof of dangerousness was an absolute precondition to commitment.[9] But the argument for pure *parens patriae* commitments never received an entirely fair hearing. In most of the landmark cases, the commitment statutes were vague, were construed elastically, and were used to commit persons, some of whom were not treatable, for periods of time which were indefinite and to institutions in which conditions were execrable and treatment was minimal. Not surprisingly, the courts balked. For example, in *O'Connor* v. *Donaldson* (1975), the Supreme

[5]Ind. Code Ann. § 16-14-9.1.1 (1980). *See also* N.D. Cent. Code. § 25-03.1-02 (1979).
[6]*See, e.g.,* Mich. Stat. Ann. § 14.800 (400a) (1980) (any kind of "disorder of thought or mood which significantly impairs . . . ability to cope with the ordinary demands of life"); Colo. Rev. Stat. § 27-9402 (1980) (any "person afflicted with disease, infirmity, old age or disorder").
[7]*Compare, e.g.,* Hawaii Rev. Stat. § 334-53 (1980) (mental illness refers to "any person mentally ill or habituated to the excessive use of drugs or alcohol, to an extent requiring hospitalization"), *with* N.D. Cent. Code § 25-03.1-02 (1979) (mental illness does not refer to mental retardation, drug abuse or alcoholism).
[8]Colo. Rev. Stat. § 27-9402 (1980). *See also* Alaska Stat. § 47.30.340.ii (1978); Ohio Rev. Code Ann. § 5122.01 (1980).
[9]*See, e.g., O'Connor* v. *Donaldson,* 442 U.S. 563 (1975); *Lessard* v. *Schmidt,* 349 F. Supp. 1078 (E.D. Wis. 1972), *vacated and remanded on other grounds,* 414 U.S. 472 (1974), *judgment reinstated,* 413 F. Supp. 1318 (E.D. Wis. 1976); *Doremus* v. *Farrell,* 407 F. Supp. 509 (D. Neb. 1975); *Bell* v. *Wayne Co. Gen. Hosp. at Eloise,* 384 F. Supp. 1085 (E.D. Mich. 1974); *cf. Humphrey* v. *Cady,* 405 U.S. 504 (1972).

Court declared that "[a] finding of 'mental illness' alone cannot justify a State's locking up a person against his will and keeping him indefinitely in simple custodial confinement." The Court, however, had no occasion to decide whether commitment could be justified for a person who suffers from a serious mental disorder, lacks capacity to make a reasoned decision concerning treatment, and is to be committed for a finite period, to a genuinely therapeutic facility.

Nevertheless, many courts continue to construe *Donaldson* as dictating that "standards for commitment to mental institutions are constitutional *only if they require a finding of dangerousness to others or to self.*"[10] Statutes have repeatedly been struck down as unconstitutional when they permitted involuntary commitment merely because the person was mentally ill and "in need of treatment," or the commitment was "in the best interests" of the person.[11] Occasionally, statutes survived challenge when they appeared to incorporate a prediction of harm, however murky, such as in commitment of a patient "for his own welfare and protection" (see, e.g., *Reynolds* v. *Sheldon,* 1975).

There are, however, some signs of progress in the courts' ability to deal with mental illness as an element in commitment.

The courts are now more prone to look behind the diagnostic labels[12] in order to ascertain the facts on which they are based. For example, in *In re D.W.H.* (1980),[13] a psychiatrist testified that the patient suffered from "dissociative reaction." When asked if this was a psychiatric disorder, he replied that it was, "but only when it creates symptoms or dysfunction or when it is maladapted." The court examined the patient's behavior, was not convinced "that the dissociative reaction is a psychiatric disorder in D.W.H.'s case," and therefore discharged him. Other courts have also reversed commitments when psychiatric opinions were very equivocal or seemed to lack a solid factual basis.[14]

In a related trend, the courts are examining more closely than before each element of a compound criterion. They are recognizing that committing a person "for his own welfare and protection and the protection of others" (e.g., *Lodge* v. *State,* 1980), or because he or she is "mentally ill . . . and is in need of further treatment" (e.g., *In the Matter of Hiatt,* 1980) entails more than one determination. Interestingly, several courts have concluded that it is an implicit requirement of a proper *parens patriae* commitment that the person, in addition to

[10]*Doe* v. *Gallinot,* 486 F. Supp. 983, 991 (C.D. Cal. 1979). (Emphasis supplied.) *See also Suzuki* v. *Yuen,* 617 F.2d 173 (9th Cir. 1980); *Benham* v. *Edwards,* 501 F. Supp. 1050 (N.D. Ga. 1980); *Colyar* v. *Third Judicial District Court,* 469 F. Supp. 424 (D. Utah 1979); *Bension* v. *Meredith,* 455 F. Supp. 662 (D.D.C. 1978); *Bethany* v. *Stubbs,* 393 So. 2d 1351 (Miss. 1981); *cf. Lodge* v. *State,* 597 S.W.2d 773 (Tex. Civ. App. 1980).

[11]*See, e.g., Johnson* v. *Solomon,* 484 F. Supp. 278 (D. Md. 1979); *Goldy* v. *Beal,* 429 F. Supp. 640 (M.D. Pa. 1976); *Stamus* v. *Leonhardt,* 414 F. Supp. 439 (S.D. Iowa 1976); *Kinner* v. *State,* 382 So. 2d 756 (Fla. Dist. Ct. App. 1980); *Commonwealth ex rel. Finken* v. *Roop,* 339 A.2d 764 (Pa. 1975).

[12]*See, e.g., Hill* v. *County Bd. of Mental Health,* 279 N.W.2d 838 (Neb. 1979); *Gross* v. *Pomerleau,* 465 F. Supp. 1167 (D. Md. 1979); *Estate of Chambers,* 131 Cal. Rptr. 357 (Cal. 1977); Utah Code Ann. § 64-7-28(1) (1979) (since amended); Md. Code Art. 59 § 22 (a)(4) (1980).

[13]411 N.W.2d 721 (Ind. Ct. App. 1980). *See also Matter of Torsney,* 394 N.E.2d 262 (N.Y. 1979) ("personality disorder" might warrant continued confinement for dangerousness, but did not in this case); *In re Hatley,* 231 S.E.2d 633 (N.C. 1977).

[14]*See, e.g., Wege* v. *Texas,* 593 S.W.2d 145 (Tex. Civ. App. 1980); *In re Hogan,* 232 S.E.2d 492 (N.C. 1977).

being mentally ill, also lacks capacity to make a reasoned decision concerning his or her need for treatment.[15]

The Criterion of Dangerousness

Civil commitment is now beset by a major paradox. Just when legislatures and courts have declared that all commitments must turn on the pivot of whether the person is *dangerous to himself or others,* psychiatrists are asserting that they cannot reliably predict dangerousness! *Dangerousness* has thus become an interdisciplinary hot potato. For many years, psychiatrists were called upon to give, and unselfconsciously gave, their predictions as to whether individuals would be dangerous.[16] Then, as the abuses of civil commitment became apparent, and the antipsychiatry movement mounted, an opposite trend developed. Civil liberties lawyers who had insisted on a standard that involved dangerousness charged that psychiatry, in claiming it could predict dangerous conduct, had "promised more than it can deliver." They "found no evidence that psychiatrists can predict dangerous behavior . . . with substantially more reliability and accuracy than laymen." And they asserted that the "mentally ill, as a class, are even less dangerous than other members of society"[17] (Ennis, 1978). Therefore, it was argued, in helping to commit the mentally ill based on predictions of dangerous conduct, psychiatrists were perpetrating a pseudoscientific hoax.

Stung by such criticisms, psychiatrists acknowledged that "the state of the art regarding predictions of violence is very unsatisfactory," and that "the ability of psychiatrists or other professionals to reliably predict future violence is unproved"[18] (American Psychiatric Association, 1975). In essence, the psychiatrists threw the issue back to the lawyers. This has placed the courts in an ambiguous and difficult situation. While in theory they make independent judgments as to dangerousness, in practice they often rely upon psychiatrists to give them the answers.[19]

In recent years, several courts have flatly declared that "the condition of dangerousness is not a medical concept but rather a legal one," about which the judge must reach an independent judgment (*State v.*

---

[15]*See e.g., Kinner* v. *State,* 382 So. 2d 756 (Fla. Dist. Ct. App. 1980); *In re Beverly,* 342 So. 2d 481 (Fla. 1977); *Commonwealth ex rel. Finken* v. *Roop,* 339 A.2d 764 (Pa. 1975).

[16]In a sense, "dangerous" is a crude locution, since it suggests an unchanging, ontological status of the person. One court was thus led to conclude that "An individual is not committed because of his conduct or actions, but rather because of his *status as a mentally ill and dangerous person.* The overt act or behavior is merely evidence of this status." *Matter of F.B.,* 615 P.2d 867 (Mont. 1980) (emphasis supplied). This is contrary to the theory embodied in DSM-III, which refers to current disorders (*e.g.,* "a person suffering from schizophrenia") rather than to classes of individuals (*e.g.,* "a schizophrenic"). *See* American Psychiatric Association, (1980), p. 6.

Instead of referring to "dangerousness," about ten states refer to whether the person is "likely to harm himself or others," which is preferable in that it candidly places predictions of harm in the realm of probabilities, and invites inquiry into not only the dangerous "character" of the person, but also the contingencies in which his particular dangerousness may become expressed. *But see Holiday* v. *Florida,* 386 So. 2d 316 (Fla. Ct. App. 1980).

[17]Ennis, B.J., (1974). *See also* Ennis, B.J., and Litwack, T.R. (1974).

[18]American Psychiatric Association (1975), p.v. *See also* Stone, A. (with Stromberg, C.) (1975), pp. 25-27.

[19]*See Matter of Collins,* 271 S.E.2d 72 (N.C. Ct. App. 1980); *Buzzell* v. *Commissioner,* 423 A.2d 246 (Me. 1980); *Application of Noel,* 601 P.2d 1252 (Kan. 1979).

Hudson, 1979).[20] The corollary that "a finding of dangerousness [need not] be founded only on psychiatric or other expert medical testimony" has also been quickly embraced (*State* v. *Hudson,* 1979). Nonexpert testimony alone may suffice (*Moore* v. *Duckworth,* 1979), and at least one court has found a person dangerous based on lay testimony, even though two psychiatrists testified that she was not (*Haber* v. *People,* 1979).

Because of the unmistakable trend among the states toward making dangerousness the linchpin of all commitments and defining it in more complex ways,[21] it is important to consider precisely how the lawmakers and courts are now thinking about dangerousness.

Dangerous to Others

The first issue, of course, is exactly what kind of predicted harm justifies commitment. Likely physical violence to another person is clearly sufficient. So are likely nonviolent acts which would harm others.[22] The more difficult question arises where the predicted behavior would do less than cause violence or injury, but would do more than merely annoy a person. For example, what of the patient who is not violently assaultive, but who touches, kisses, or pinches women he encounters on the street? Still more problematic is the patient who is predicted likely to commit acts which do not physically touch others, but which cause emotional harm, such as exposing himself, peering through the windows of his former spouse's home, or making threatening phone calls. In some cases, the theoretical issue can be avoided because the potential victim will suffer not only emotional harm, but also physical sequelae, such as insomnia, anxiety disorders, and so forth. But such cases beg the question.

Many state laws appear to require that the harm anticipated be "serious physical injury" or "serious bodily harm."[23] However, several refer more broadly to the threat of "substantial physical or emotional injury" or simply "substantial harm."[24] Where the law is unclear, several courts have stated that mere emotional harm might be sufficient to warrant commitment,[25] but few of the reported cases involve only such harm.

The still more difficult issue is whether the threat of harm to property, rather than to persons, justifies commitment. Property crimes which may also seriously harm people, e.g., arson, clearly are sufficient.

[20]409 A.2d 1349, 1351 (N.H. 1979). *See also Matter of Newsome,* 424 A.2d 222, 225 (N.J. Super. Ct. 1980); *State* v. *Krol,* 344 A.2d 289, 305 (N.J. 1975).

[21]*See, e.g.,* N.C. Gen. Stat. § 122-58.2 (1980) (1979 Sess. Laws Ch. 915). *See also* State of New Mexico Department of Hospitals and Institutions, (1977).

[22]*See Matter of Snowden,* 423 A.2d 188 (D.C. App. 1980). One court has said that any anticipated felony, even one involving no injury to others, would suffice. *In re Patterson,* 579 P.2d 1335 (Wash, 1978) (en banc). This seems a curious view, however, since felonies include such things as auto theft, which is a leading crime among teenagers who are not mentally ill.

[23]Mich. Stat. Ann. 14.800 (401)(1980); N.C. Gen. Stat. § 122.58.2 (1980). *See also* Ill. Stat. Ann. Art. 91 1/2 § 119 (1980); Ga. Code Ann. § 88-501 (v) (1980); Ark. Stat. Ann. § 59-1401 (1980).

[24]Hawaii Rev. Stat. § 334-1 (1980); Ala. Code Tit. 22 § 52-10 (1980). *See also* Iowa Code § 229.1 (2) ("serious emotional injury").

[25]*See, e.g., Lynch* v. *Baxley,* 386 F. Supp. 378, 391 (M.D. Ala. 1974) (the "threat of harm comprehends the positive infliction of injury, ordinarily physical but possibly emotional as well").

But what of the mentally ill person who threatens to "trash" his hotel room, or to pour blood on the steps of a corporation's headquarters?

An interesting case is *Suzuki* v. *Yuen* (1980), which held unconstitutional a Hawaii statute providing that commitment could be based on the threat of damage to "any property." The court insisted that some higher standard such as "substantial property damage" be employed. Further, several states have recently amended their laws to delete danger to property alone as a basis for commitment.[26]

As suggested above, the issue of what type of harm should justify commitment is a complex one. But still more difficult than defining the type of harm is the question of how one proves that harm is in fact likely to occur.

One way that lawyers deal with this issue is by defining the overall standard of proof which applies in civil commitment hearings. After being hotly contested for many years, this issue was partly resolved in *Addington* v. *Texas* (1979), in which the Supreme Court held that persons could be committed for indefinite periods only on the basis of at least "clear and convincing" evidence. This standard of proof is intermediate between the "preponderance of evidence" standard used in civil trials, and the "beyond a reasonable doubt" standard used in criminal trials.[27] The Court stressed that the choice of a standard of proof was more than an "empty semantic exercise" because "[i]ncreasing the burden of proof is one way to impress the fact finder with the importance of the decision and thereby perhaps to reduce the chances that inappropriate commitments will be ordered." However, it frankly conceded that "there are no directly relevant empirical studies" comparing the three standards of proof "to determine how juries, real or mock, apply them."[28]

While the jury or court must decide whether there is *clear and convincing* proof overall as to the criteria for commitment, the testifying psychiatrist is asked to describe the degree of likelihood that the person will in fact commit dangerous acts. Most statutes do not define the degree of likelihood which is required, though some adopt specific standards varying from *substantial risk* to *substantial probability.*[29] And some courts have developed their own standards, such as whether there is "an extreme likelihood that if the person is not confined, he will do immediate harm."[30]

Thus, commitments for dangerousness are really based upon a two-step probability equation. There must be (1) something like 75 percent *clear and convincing* proof that (2) there is an x percent likelihood that the person will in fact commit the harm. The x may be 25 percent

---

[26]*See, e.g.,* Kansas Stat. Ann. § 59-2902 (1980). *Cf. Matter of Gatson,* 593 P.2d 423 (Kan. 1979).

[27]"Preponderance of evidence" is generally understood to mean a degree of certainty of at least 51%; "clear and convincing" means a degree of certainty of perhaps 75%; and "beyond a reasonable doubt" means a degree of certainty on the range of 95-99%. Before *Addington* was decided, about 25 states already used the "clear and convincing" standard, and others used still higher standards such as "beyond a reasonable doubt," which continue to be acceptable under *Addington.*

[28]441 U.S. at 427 & n.3.

[29]Wash. Rev. Code Ann. § 71.05.020(B) (1979); Wis. Stat. Ann. § 51.20 (1980). North Dakota uses the particularly cryptic standard of "reasonable expectation of substantial likelihood." N.D. Cent. Code § 25-03.1-02 (1980).

[30]*Lessard* v. *Schmidt,* 349 F. Supp. 1078, 1093 (E.D. Wis. 1972). *See also Suzuki* v. *Alba,* 438 F. Supp. 1106, 1110 (D. Hawaii 1977) ("imminent and substantial danger").

in some states (*substantial risk*) and sixty percent in others (*substantial probability*). And whatever the statutory standard, it cannot be applied woodenly. While probability may be an appropriate threshold where the harm anticipated is punching someone in the nose, a lesser degree of certainty should suffice if the person threatens to set off a bomb in Times Square. Although the statutes do not provide a sliding scale of risks and probabilities, the courts have generally considered the seriousness of the potential harm as they evaluate the likelihood of its occurring.

Recently, much legal debate has centered on whether it should be an absolute prerequisite to commitment for dangerousness that there be a "recent overt act, attempt or threat."[31] Several statutes so require.[32] Courts have differed on the matter:

OVERT ACT REQUIRED: *Lessard* v. *Schmidt* (1972) (1974) (1976) held that because "attempts to predict future [dangerous] conduct are always difficult," a commitment on this ground is justified only if it "is based on a finding of a recent overt act, attempt or threat to do substantial harm to oneself or others."[33]

OVERT ACT NOT REQUIRED: (1) *Colyar* v. *Third Judicial District Court* (1979) held that due process does not always require proof of an "overt act." It conceded that the "science of psychiatry is at times imprecise and subjective," but found that "there is no scientific evidence that the requirement [of a recent overt act] decreases the chance of error in predicting dangerousness."[34]

(2) *U.S. ex rel. Mathews* v. *Nelson* (1978) rejected the argument that a "reasonable expectation" of harm could never be reached in the absence of an "overt act." It concluded that "there are instances in which a psychiatrist can determine from a psychiatric clinical examination [alone] that a mentally ill person is reasonably likely to injure himself or another," although it conceded that "these cases may be relatively few."

Overall, recent court decisions tend to the view that an overt act or threat is not always necessary,[35] and several state legislatures, including

---

[31]The use of the phrase "overt act" is somewhat confusing. It is borrowed from the law of criminal conspiracy, where it means not only attempts or threats, but "virtually any act," however innocuous (*e.g.*, a telephone call or traveling to a city) which is done to advance the purposes of the conspiracy. Lefave, W.R., and Scott, A.W. Jr., (1972), pp. 477-78. *See also Braverman* v. *United States*, 317 U.S. 99 (1942). In the civil commitment cases, however, the courts seem to use "overt act" differently. They distinguish it from attempts or threats, and sometimes seem to mean an act which itself places a person in danger.

[32]*See, e.g.*, Ala. Code Tit. 22 § 52-1 (1980); Ark. Stat. Ann. § 59-1401 (1979); Ga. Code Ann. § 88-501 (b) (1979); Hawaii Rev. Stat. § 334-1 (1980); Ohio Rev. Code § 5122.01 (1980); Wis. Stat. Ann. § 51.20 (1980).

[33]349 F. Supp. 1078, 1093 (E.D. Wis. 1972), *vacated and remanded on other grounds*, 414 U.S. 472 (1974), *judgment reinstated*, 413 F. Supp. 1318 (E.D. Wis. 1976). *See also Suzuki* v. *Alba*, 438 F. Supp. 1106 (D. Hawaii 1977); *Stamus* v. *Leonhardt*, 414 F. Supp. 439 (S.D. Iowa 1976); *Doremus* v. *Farrell*, 407 F. Supp. 509 (D. Neb. 1975); *Lynch* v. *Baxley*, 386 F. Supp. 378 (M.D. Ala. 1974).

[34]469 F. Supp. 424, 434-35 (D. Utah 1979). This statement may be somewhat unfair to the scientific literature.

[35]*See, e.g.*, *Matter of Hernandez*, 264 S.E.2d 780 (N.C. Ct. App. 1980), and cases cited therein; *Matter of Snowden*, 423 A.2d 188 (D.C. App. 1980); *People* v. *Howell*, 586 P.2d 27 (Colo. 1978) (en banc); *In re Sonsteng*, 573 P.2d 1149 (Mont. 1977); *Scopes* v. *Shah*, 398 N.Y.S.2d 911 (1977); *Matter of Salem*, 228 S.E.2d 649 (N.C. Ct. App. 1976); *People* v. *Sansone*, 309 N.E.2d 733 (Ill. App. Ct. 1974); *cf. Bell* v. *Wayne County Gen. Hosp. at Eloise*, 384 F. Supp. 1085 (E.D. Mich. 1974).

Illinois, have recently rejected proposals to require proof of a "recent overt act" in all cases. However, a number of states have recently amended their statutes to require an overt act, attempt, or threat.[36]

It surely remains true that "a showing of present dangerousness *will normally require* evidence of a recent act, attempt, threat or omission [to care for oneself]."[37] And, as the Montana Supreme Court has observed, "while not every threat can be considered an overt act, the testimony and circumstances in this case" showed that "a threat to kill is a verbal act that falls within the definition of an 'overt act.' "[38] Other courts have agreed.[39] And in *Lux* v. *Mental Health Board of Polk Co.* (1979), the Nebraska Supreme Court concluded that a person described as suffering from a "paranoid state, assaultive and homicidal ideation,"[40] who had once assaulted his father, met the statutory requirement for "recent violent acts." To "read the statute as requiring evidence of more than one violent act or threat," it said, "would be ridiculous."

Finally, some courts continue to commit persons they truly believe to be dangerous, even where the overt act is hard to define.

> *In the Matter of Powell* (1980). An Illinois court affirmed the commitment of a 27-year-old man who had never been in a mental institution, but was picked up by police when he blocked the door to the office of a clothing manufacturer who, he angrily claimed, owed him one million dollars for designing various clothes. At the commitment hearing, Powell insisted that "Everybody is God. Everybody got sense. God has sense. Be productive. . .I'm being productive, making the book of designs for clothes for everybody in the world, in the universe." The examining psychiatrist concluded that he was a paranoid schizophrenic. The court decided that he might be dangerous, because of the "possibility" that "if he returned in order to obtain the money that he thought was owed him," he "might be harmed by an irate employee" or he "might harm someone."

Other courts, however, have gone to extremes in demanding that there be copious overt acts demonstrating dangerousness. Two examples:

> (1) *In the Matter of Barker* (1979). Barker became convinced that a woman he had lived with for ten years (referred to as his "wife") was having an affair with a neighbor. Four events, all occurring within a few months of the hearing, were adduced to show dangerousness. The first was an incident in which Barker tried to punch the neighbor but missed, and the neighbor successfully knocked him down. The second was when Barker, who had been drinking, argued with his wife, fired shots from a revolver through an open door, and then feigned an attempt at suicide by firing a blank shell at his head. The third event was when he appeared at his sister's house brandishing a gun, said he was looking for his wife, but then left peaceably. The fourth event was when he broke beer bottles and waved the jagged shards at his wife. The event triggering the commitment was a midnight phone call by Barker in which he charged that the neighbor and his wife were then engaged in sodomy. No specific threats were made, and Barker had previously given his guns to his father.

[36]*See* statutes cited in footnote 32.

[37]*Matter of Gatson,* 593 P.2d 423, 426 (Kan. 1979). (Emphasis supplied.)

[38]*Matter of Goedert,* 591 P.2d 272 (Mont. 1979). *See also Matter of F.B.,* 615 P.2d 867 (Mont. 1980).

[39]*See, e.g., Hill* v. *Bd. of Mental Health,* 279 N.W.2d 838 (Neb. 1979); *Matter of Oseing,* 296 N.W.2d 797 (Iowa 1980).

[40]A judicial opinion is not a very reliable guide to the clinical facts about a patient; nevertheless, it is worth noting how the court at least understood the problem.

The two examining psychiatrists agreed that Barker suffered from paranoid psychosis characterized by paranoid jealousy delusions, but disagreed about whether he would be dangerous. The court clearly thought that there might be something to Barker's belief that his neighbor was engaged in an affair with his wife. It concluded that "[e]ven if we assume that the defendant was in fact delusional, we must recognize that the delusion did not produce at the time it happened any violent or dangerous conduct." Therefore, even after considering all Barker's actions together, the court reversed the commitment![41]

(2) *In the Matter of O'Brien* (1980). O'Brien's mother came home one day to find that her son had trashed their basement, removed the electric fuses, and broken things in his father's room. He angrily demanded that she give him matches and a lighter so he could "finish the job I started to do," namely, "burn the house down." The police were called and took O'Brien to a mental health center. A physician later testified that O'Brien had persecutory and other delusions. He believed that his father manipulated him by means of a watch and electric wires; that God and Mother Nature guided him; that he could use his penknife on his father, but did not only because he "is my father." The court concluded that these facts did not present any "overt act" which itself threatened harm, and that "it would be mere speculation at best to conclude that [he] intended to actually burn the house down and thereby cause harm to anyone." The court discharged O'Brien.

The question also arises whether commitment for dangerousness is justified if there is neither an overt act nor any specific threat. Might it not be enough grounds to commit a person if he or she suffers from a serious mental disorder, e.g., psychotic depression or certain impulse disorders, in which suicide or mutilating acts are generally known to be common? The Arkansas law appears to permit this,[42] and guidelines for psychiatrists distributed by the New Mexico Department of Hospitals and Institutions suggest that it would be sufficient.[43] However, some courts are not hospitable to this rationale. Several have ruled that commitment is not warranted simply because the patient "might be dangerous if this pattern of thinking continued as it seemed to be developing" (*In the Matter of Conrad,* 1978), or because "possibly" he "could become dangerous," since his mental illness could lend him to "misinterpret" situations.[44] In sum, commitment for dangerousness requires either proof of prior dangerous overt acts or an explicit medical prediction of dangerous conduct based on clinical facts which the court finds persuasive.[45]

Where there is an overt act, the next question is how recent it must be to justify commitment. In *Hill* v. *County Bd. of Mental Health* (1979), the court found that suicidal and self-abusive acts which occurred nine months, four months, and six weeks prior to the hearing did constitute "recent violent acts or threats of violence." In addition, several years before, Hill had set fire to the vehicle of a person with whom he had an argument, had threatened various people, and had

---

[41]The same court took a similar view, though in a less extreme case, in *Matter of Nelson,* 580 P.2d 590 (Ore. Ct. App. 1978).

[42]Ark Stat. Ann. § 59-1401 (1980) ("suicidal" refers not only to threats or attempts, but also to "thoughts that create a grave and imminent risk").

[43]*See* "Guidelines for Clinical Determination of 'Dangerousness' Related to Mental Disorder" (1977).

[44]*Matter of Christofferson,* 615 P.2d 1152 (Ore. Ct. App. 1980). *But see Matter of Olson,* 596 P.2d 620 (Ore. Ct. App. 1979).

[45]*See Matter of Chapman,* 385 N.E.2d 56 (Ill. App. Ct. 1978).

apparently pleaded not guilty by reason of insanity to a rape and murder. The court refused to "blindly disregard [these] other incidents more remote in time which give some insight into the man's mental state." Interestingly, a few states now specify the time periods within which the acts triggering commitment must have been performed.[46]

Another timing issue is how near in the future the predicted harm is likely to occur. Some state statutes require that the anticipated harm be "imminent,"[47] or "real and present,"[48] while others use less definite terms such as "in the near future,"[49] and many others do not state any necessary standard of proximity.[50]

The requirement that harm be predicted to occur in the reasonably near future helps to assure that a prediction is based on facts. One would rightly be skeptical of a psychiatrist who was unsure whether a person would attempt to commit murder in the next six months, but was certain he would do so in the next five years. On the other hand, the definition of *near future* depends on the context. If a deranged man makes a credible threat to assault the President the next time he comes to New York, the harm may lie in the near future, even though the President's next visit is six months hence. Likewise, the time period encompassed by *near future* may properly be shorter when the threatened harm is small, and longer when the harm is greater.[51]

Recent legal developments on this issue do not establish a pattern. In *Suzuki* v. *Yuen* (1980), the court struck down a Hawaii law because it failed to require that persons to be committed be "imminently" dangerous, and in *Colyar* v. *Third Judicial District Court* (1979), a Utah court set a standard of "imminent danger" to self. On the other hand, North Carolina recently deleted from its civil commitment statute the requirement that danger be "imminent."[52] And in *Hatcher* v. *Wachtel* (1980), the West Virginia Supreme Court rejected the view that harm must be imminent.

Dangerous to Self or Gravely Disabled

The other type of dangerousness is, of course, *dangerousness to self.* Under several court decisions and statutes,[53] this can be shown not only by physical self-abuse or suicidal acting out, but also by extreme neglect of one's basic needs. Some state laws make this criterion a bit less diaphanous by requiring that the alleged self-neglect be so extreme "that such failure threatens the person's life."[54] However, most are not so stringent or clear.

In some states, danger to self by passive neglect has evolved into a basis for commitment entirely separate from *dangerous to self,* usually called *gravely disabled. Gravely disabled* means that the individual, "as

[46]*See, e.g.,* Pa. Stat. Ann. tit. 50 § 7301 (1980) (within 30 days); N.C. Gen. Stat. § 122-58.2 (1980) ("within the recent past"); Ariz. Rev. Stat. Ann. § 36-501 (1980) (within 30 days for threats, and 180 days for assaults).
[47]*See, e.g.,* Mont. Rev. Code Ann. § 53-21-102 (14) (1980); Cal. Welf. & Inst. Code. § § 5260, 5300; Ga. Code 88-501 (v) (1980).
[48]*See, e.g.,* Ala. Code tit. 22 § 52-01 (1980).
[49]*See, e.g.,* Ill. Rev. Stat. Ch. 91-1/2, § 1-119 (1980); Mich. Stat. Ann. 14.800 (401) (1980).
[50]*See, e.g.,* Conn. Gen. Stat. § 17-176 (1979); Idaho Code § 66-317 (1980).
[51]*See State* v. *Krol,* 344 A.2d 289, 302 (N.J. Sup. Ct. 1975).
[52]*See* N.C. Gen Stat. § 122-58.2 (1980) (1979 Sess. Laws Ch. 915).
[53]*See Lynch* v. *Baxley,* 386 F. Supp. 378, 391 (M.D. Ala. 1974); *Doremus* v. *Farrell,* 407 F. Supp. 509, 515 (D. Neb. 1975); *Matter of Evans,* 408 N.E.2d 33 (Ill. App. Ct. 1980); Hawaii Rev. Stat. § 334-1 (1980).
[54]Kan. Stat. Ann. § 59-2902 (1980).

a result of a mental disorder, is unable to provide for his basic physical needs such as food, clothing and shelter."[55] When proposed, the *gravely disabled* statutes gave rise to concern that they could be used to effect the commitment of people on the basis merely of different life-styles or of eccentricities (e.g., college students or aged persons whose reproving families believe that they are living in subhuman conditions). In fact, under the statutes, the inability to provide for one's needs must be caused by mental disease. Recently, several courts have concluded that such statutes are not unconstitutionally vague, while conceding that "there could be some difference in interpretation of what constitutes basic need," and that there is a "significant risk of erroneous application of the standard."[56] And some courts recently have sought to reduce this risk by reading into *gravely disabled* a tacit requirement that the person lack capacity to make an informed decision concerning his or her need for treatment.[57]

In evaluating danger to self and grave disability, courts appear to be ever more energetic in pressing beyond the surface eccentricities. Nevertheless, the recent cases are far from consistent, as even a brief sampling will show. First, there are many cases in which commitments seem to have been approved without very convincing evidence of an inability to cope with basic needs. For example:

> In *Estate of Roulet* (1979), a California jury found a woman gravely disabled based on a petition which simply alleged that "[s]he is so confused and disorganized that she is unable to make clear living plans. If she has some funds, she will waste [them] on cigarettes and drinking."

Other examples of this type include: *Interest of Paiz* (1979), *In the Matter of Evans* (1980), *Walker* v. *Dancer* (1980), *In the Matter of Gregorovich* (1980), *In re Janovitz* (1980), and *In re Frick* (1980).

Nevertheless, in a larger number of reported cases,[58] courts have reviewed the evidence of dangerous to self or grave disability with a very critical eye—and reversed commitments.

For example:

> In *County Atty., Pima Co.* v. *Kaplan* (1980), an Arizona court found that there was not sufficient proof that the patient was gravely disabled even though he was "schizophrenic and had a long history of mental illness;" he "gave away most of his clothes, squandered his money, took long purposeless trips, had difficulty finding a place to live because of his improper behavior, and refused treatment;" and two psychiatrists testified that he could not meet his needs (though a psychiatric resident disagreed). Despite "the likelihood that he will decompensate, give away his money, and become dependent on social agencies," the court concluded that if he "can provide himself with adequate food, clothing and shelter, he does not come within 'gravely disabled,' " merely because he

---

[55]Cal. Welf. & Inst. Code § 5008 (h)(1)(1980). *See also* Neb. Rev. Stat. § 83-1009 (1980) ("Inability to provide for his basic human needs, including food, clothing, shelter, essential medical care or personal safety.")

[56]*Doe* v. *Gallinot*, 486 F. Supp. 983, 991 (C.D. Cal. 1979). *See also Colorado* v. *Taylor*, 618 P.2d 1127 (Colo. 1980).

[57]*See, e.g., Northern* v. *State Dept. of Human Serv.*, 575 S.W.2d 946 (Tenn. 1978); *Colorado* v. *Taylor*, 618 P.2d 1127 (Colo. 1980); *Walker* v. *Dancer*, 386 So. 2d 475 (Ala. Civ. App. 1980).

[58]A statistical comparison would not itself be very meaningful; judges may well be more likely to publish those opinions in which the result is the less common one of reversing a commitment on legal grounds.

chose "to live under conditions that most society would conclude to be substandard."

Similar cases include *In the Matter of Fields* (1978), *State ex rel. Pifer* v. *Pifer* (1980), *Sheffel* v. *Sulikowski* (1980), and *In the Matter of Linderman* (1981).

These cases represent a collage of many colors, and the rulings may be less revealing than the trends in the reasoning process itself. One such trend is that our courts are becoming more willing to examine and more confident in questioning the factual bases for allegations of dangerousness and grave disability.

OTHER CRITERIA

Refuses Voluntary Admission

Several states now specifically authorize involuntary commitment only if the person has been advised of and has refused the opportunity for voluntary admission.[59] In other states this may also be the practice, even though it is not required by law. The preference for voluntary admission reflects both a wise economy in the exercise of state power and a recognition of the clinical experience that treatment is often more effective when the patient receives it voluntarily.

While some believe that the threat of involuntary commitment makes voluntary admission essentially a charade, the courts have generally taken the opposite view. They hold that voluntary admission is a meaningful right of the patient. In recent cases, courts have generally held that unless a person threatens to become dangerous, or voluntary admission clearly is a ruse, the person may not be committed involuntarily if he or she is willing to be admitted voluntarily.[60] For example, the Supreme Court of Colorado, in reversing an involuntary commitment because the person had not been advised of the opportunity for voluntary admission, said the "civil commitment statutes must be liberally construed to promote the legislative purpose of encouraging the use of voluntary rather than coercive measures to secure treatment and care for mental illness."[61]

Is Treatable

Several states require as a criterion of commitment that the person be "likely to benefit from treatment."[62] This is perhaps premised on the reasoning that "without some form of treatment, the state justification for acting as *parens patriae* becomes a nullity" (*In re Ballay, 1973*). But what of police power commitments based solely on the grounds that the person is mentally ill and dangerous? Some would say that if a dangerous person cannot be treated, the mental health system has nothing to offer but preventive confinement. Society, they would say, should then do what it does in the case of persons who are not mentally ill but are dangerous. It should wait for them to commit an illegal act

---

[59]*See, e.g.,* Md. Code Ann. Art. 59 § 12 (a) (iii) (1980); Cal. Welf. & Inst. Code § § 5250, 5260 (1980); Ore. Rev. Stat. § 426. 130 (1980); Colo. Rev. Stat. § 27-10-107 (1980).

[60]*See, e.g., In re Henderson,* 610 P.2d 1350 (Colo. Ct. App. 1980); *Illinois* v. *Hill,* 391 N.E.2d 51 (Ill. App. Ct. 1979); *In re Farrow,* 255 S.E.2d 777 (N.C. Ct. App. 1979); *Matter of Byrd,* 386 N.E. 2d 385 (Ill. App. Ct. 1979).

[61]*Sisneros* v. *District Court,* 606 P.2d 55, 57 (Colo. 1980). *See also Goedecke* v. *State Department of Institutions,* 603 P.2d 123 (Colo. 1979).

[62]*See, e.g.,* N. Mex. Rev. Stat. § 43-1-11 (1980); Ohio Code § 5122.01 (1980).

(hopefully an attempt that does no harm), and then it should confine them.

Few courts have examined the difficult theoretical issue of the dangerous but untreatable, noncriminal person. At least one court has recently held that a dangerous person need not be demonstrably treatable to be committed, [63] and, of course, courts routinely commit persons who may not be treatable under statutes requiring proof only of mental illness and dangerousness.

Lacks Capacity to Make a Reasoned Decision Concerning Treatment

A number of years ago, courts began to recognize that mental illness did not always entail an incapacity to make a reasoned decision concerning treatment.[64] Several courts declared that properly to commit a person under the *parens patriae* power requires that the person lacks "the capacity to weigh for himself the risks of freedom and the benefits of hospitalization" (*Lynch* v. *Baxley,* 1974), or is "incapable of making a rational choice regarding the acceptance of care or treatment."[65]

Despite such judicial pronouncements, until recently few state statutes required a finding of incapacity for persons who are dangerous to themselves or others, and fewer than half required such incapacity for persons who are nondangerous but mentally ill.[66] Some courts have recently read such a requirement into the statutory meaning of *mentally ill,*[67] but this is far from a trend. A number of recently revised state statutes, however, do make lack of capacity an integral requirement for at least some commitments.[68] The Association of State Mental Health Program Directors has continued to believe, however, that requiring proof of lack of capacity as a condition of commitment, at least for dangerous persons, represents "a travesty of justice and common sense."[69]

Least Restrictive Alternative*

A final criterion for commitment in an increasing number of states, now over twenty, is the statutory requirement that hospitalization is the

[63]*See, e.g., Matter of Oseing,* 296 N.W.2d 797 (Iowa 1980).
[64]The proper assessment is of whether a person has the capacity to make a reasoned, not a reasonable decision. While not every "reasoning" process, however bizarre, will establish capacity, nor should psychiatrists or courts simply decide whether a person's decisions were appropriate or correct in their view, and on this basis alone decide whether he should be deemed to have capacity to make a reasoned decision. *See Colyar* v. *Third Judicial District Court,* 469 F. Supp. 424, 434 (D. Utah 1979).
[65]*Colyar* v. *Third Judicial District Court,* 469 F. Supp. 424, 434 (D. Utah 1979). *See also In re Ballay,* 482 F.2d 648 (D.C. Cir. 1973); *Doremus* v. *Farrell,* 407 F. Supp. 509 (D. Neb. 1975); *Lessard* v. *Schmidt,* 349 F. Supp. 1078 (E.D. Wis. 1972).
[66]*See* the 1974 data presented in "Developments in the Law; Civil Commitment of the Mentally Ill." Harvard Law Review (1974), 1212.
[67]*See, e.g., Kinner* v. *State,* 382 So.2d 756 (Fla. Ct. App. 1980); *In re Beverly,* 342 So. 2d 481 (Fla. 1977); *Commonwealth ex rel. Finken* v. *Roop,* 339 A.2d 764 (Pa. 1975).
[68]*See, e.g.,* Wyo. Stat. § 25-3-101 (ix) (1980) (mentally ill person is one who, *inter alia,* "cannot comprehend the need for or purposes of treatment"); Colo. Rev. Stat. § 27-10-102 (1980) (gravely disabled means "unable to take care of his basic needs" and "lacks the capacity to understand that this is so"); Hawaii Rev. Stat. § 334-1 (1980) (dangerous to self means likely to injure oneself "together with incompetence to determine whether treatment . . . is appropriate").
[69]*See Mental Disability Law Reporter* (1978), 527.
*Preceptor's note: For a full description of the least restrictive alternative see the chapter by Klein.

least restrictive alternative for the individual.[70] In about 15 other states, the statute urges the court to consider the alternatives, but in some less precise way. And where the statutes do not so provide, some courts have nevertheless required that this criterion be met, as a sort of quasi-constitutional right.[71]

Neither the statutes nor the court decisions define the continuum on which the restrictiveness is to be measured, or what are the appropriate trade-offs among physical restrictions, treatment efficacy, and protection from harm. The legal analysis, in short, has not progressed much beyond the declaration that "due process requires that the state place individuals in the least restrictive setting consistent with legitimate safety, care and treatment objectives" (*Eubanks* v. *Clarke*, 1977).

In a semiempirical study of how judges interpret the *least restrictive alternative*, Hoffman and Foust summed up their findings thus: "erratic interpretation between jurisdictions and inconsistent application within jurisdictions" (Hoffman and Foust, 1977). As one judge observed, "The least restrictive alternative is a nice phrase— unfortunately, few if any exist" (quoted in Hoffman and Foust, 1977). Such a statement, although not universally applicable, could be used to characterize the reality within which many judges must apply the criterion of the least restrictive alternative.

CONCLUSION

For good or ill, the mental health system is locked in a close and uneasy embrace with the law. The feverish legal activity in the mental health field continues apace. New statutes and court decisions flood forth. In many states, the legislatures have revised their civil commitment laws virtually every year since 1975. Likewise, whereas in 1970 about three hundred new judicial decisions concerning mental health appeared in the West Publishing Company's National Reporter System, by 1980 the annual number of new decisions had doubled.

Until recently, most of this legal effort was focused on reforming civil commitment procedures. The procedures presented legal issues far more familiar to legislators and judges than did the diagnostic and behavioral criteria for commitment. In the last few years, however, increasing attention has been given to the criteria themselves.

Several trends are now clear:

The statutory definitions of mental illness are becoming more sophisticated in conception and more precise in language. The courts are more inclined to look behind diagnostic labels to the facts and judgments supporting them.

Proof of dangerousness to self or others is increasingly being made the fulcrum of all commitments. The possible justification for pure *parens patriae* commitments is still not seriously examined by the courts. Commitments based on dangerousness require more and more proof of specific overt acts or threats, or in rare cases, a very persuasive clinical prediction of harm.

---

[70]*See, e.g.,* Ala. Code Tit. 22 § 52-10 (1980): N. Mex. Code § 42-1.11, 43.1.3 (1980); Md. Code Art. 59 § 12 (a) (iii) (1980); N.D. Cent. Code § 25-03.1-21 (1980). *See also* Hoffman and Foust (1977), 1112–1113.

[71]*See, e.g., Eubanks* v. *Clarke,* 434 F. Supp. 1022 (E.D. Pa. 1977); *Stamus* v. *Leonhardt,* 413 F. Supp. 439 (S.D. Iowa); *Lynch* v. *Baxley,* 386 F. Supp. 378 (M.D. Ala. 1974); *Davis* v. *Watkins,* 384 F. Supp. 1196 (N.D. Ohio 1974); *Welsch* v. *Likins,* 373 F. Supp. 487 (D. Minn. 1974); *Lessard* v. *Schmidt,* 349 F. Supp. 1078 (E.D. Wis. 1972).

Commitments based on grave disability appear to be increasing. However, the courts are requiring that the disability be manifested by far more than the routine problems of living.

Finally, lack of capacity to make a reasoned decision concerning treatment is more often recognized as a proper criterion, at least for commitments due to grave disability, and possibly for some commitments due to dangerousness as well.

As suggested at the outset, the precise language of the statutes is a critical issue for all concerned with the workings of the mental health system. The Chief Counsel to the California Department of Mental Health reached the same conclusion. After reviewing a decade of experience under California's commitment law, landmark legislation considered to be particularly well conceived, he nevertheless "concluded that our major problems are actually problems resulting from our current statutory language and our [consequent] misconceptualization of several significant issues in mental health care" (Chell, 1981).

Some may argue that no matter how well the commitment statutes are written, they will remain a fertile field for dispute and litigation, and this may be so. But recent legal developments suggest that thoughtful and precise commitment statutes can be fashioned and that they can work reasonably well in practice. They may yet help the civil commitment system to achieve the public legitimacy which its therapeutic goals warrant.

Chapter 23

Competency to Consent to or Refuse Treatment†
by Loren H. Roth, M.D., M.P.H

INTRODUCTION

"Every human being of adult years and sound mind has a right to determine what shall be done with his own body . . . ." (*Schloendorff* v. *Society of New York Hospitals*, 1914).

These well-known words of Mr. Justice Cardozo are a concise introduction to the subject of patient competency to consent to or refuse treatment. The Cardozo dictum, however, bespeaks its own exceptions (those of unsound mind or not of adult years) to the traditional law of consent which holds that patients, not doctors or others, must consent to their own medical treatment (Meisel et al., 1977; Meisel, 1979). While the law is clear that most persons with sound minds have the right to consent to or refuse medical treatment and that some persons without sound minds do not, many questions remain about the exceptions. What does the law mean by a *sound mind*? Who determines whether minds are sound or not? Using what medical and/or legal definitions? Through what set of procedures? With what consequences resulting for the patient and for others? Also, why is it that some persons

†Supported in part by the Foundations Fund for Research in Psychiatry and by PHS Research Grant No. MH 27553, NIMH Center for Studies of Crime and Delinquency and Mental Health Services Development Branch.

with sound minds, e.g., children or adolescents, do not have the right to consent and are considered to be *de jure* (as a matter of law, if not fact) incompetent to consent or refuse? This chapter briefly touches upon these questions, and it aims to demonstrate their practical and procedural significance for the psychiatric clinician.

Since the late 1950's the law of informed consent has mushroomed (Meisel et al., 1977; Meisel, 1977). According to legal doctrine, for an informed consent to be valid, three things are necessary: the consent must be voluntary, it must be knowing or informed, and it must be competently given (Mills et al., 1980). Competent persons possess both the right and the ability to give informed consent; incompetent persons have neither the requisite ability nor the right. These issues are by no means academic. Psychiatrists enhance their therapeutic alliance with patients (and they avoid liability) by ensuring that patients' consents to medical treatment are both competent and valid (Appelbaum and Roth, 1981; Gutheil and Appelbaum, in press). Similarly, when patients refuse treatment, psychiatrists may be compelled, ethically and practically, if not legally, to consider whether the patient's refusal of treatment is competent and valid (Roth et al., 1977; Appelbaum and Roth, 1981).

It is difficult to discuss the subject of competency or to offer definitions of competency within a value-free context. While in a general way it may be asserted that from the legal perspective a competent person is one who possesses or manifests the ability to do a requisite action or task, in this case to give informed consent to treatment, such an approach to defining competency does not take us too far. Upon close scrutiny, the approach may even be tautological. In practice, establishing substantive criteria and a proper procedural approach for assessing patient competency is extremely complicated. While the construct of competency is primarily and perhaps exclusively legal, the practice of determining competency does not involve legal dimensions alone. Medical, social, and even moral dimensions are also involved. (Roth et al., 1977; Freedman, in press; Michels, in press).

The legal construct of competency operates similarly to other legal constructs, in that determinations of competency serve to validate or set aside individual rights. With the boundary between competency and incompetency, the law sets apart some persons from others, demarcating some who may be treated more nearly as objects, and who may have things done to them rather than with them (Toulmin, 1980). Thus the concept of competency is not neutral. Because of this, determinations of patient competency are susceptible to abuse, and some leading scholars even propose that they should be abolished (Goldstein, 1978; Alexander and Szasz, 1973). This, however, is not possible. So long as controversies persist as to whether psychiatric or other medical patients have sufficient ability to decide for themselves whether to accept or consent to or refuse treatment, the concept of competency must be addressed (Stone, 1981). Unfortunately, only a few empirical or conceptual studies exist to help illuminate the path. Those which have been done are briefly mentioned in this chapter.

DE JURE AND DE FACTO COMPETENCY

At the outset some legal points must be made about the distinction between *de jure* and *de facto* competency (Meisel, 1979). *De jure* competency relates to a person's status under the law. Under the common law, all persons of adult age are presumed to be competent to make medical treatment decisions until they are shown to be otherwise at a court hearing or through some other means (Stone, 1981).

Children and adolescents are, however, *de jure* incompetent. As such, they cannot, under most circumstances, make legal contracts, marry, or decide about their medical care. Others must do these things for them, if in fact children and adolescents are permitted to do these things at all. Historically, the age of consent has varied. It was once fixed at age 13, then at age 19, then at age 21, and then at age 18 (*Medical World News*, 1971). More recently, there has been a trend towards lowering the age of consent at which minors may make medical and related decisions, especially where the minor's reproductive rights are involved (*Children's Rights Report*, 1978).

Establishing the age of consent to make medical decisions is usually a matter of state law, though sometimes constitutional issues come into play. For example, in 1976 the Pennsylvania Legislature passed a new mental health act lowering to age 14 the age when adolescents are permitted to give informed consent to psychiatric hospitalization (Pennsylvania Mental Health Procedures Act, 1976). Setting the age of consent is both complicated and arbitrary. It involves a legislative judgment (1) that the best interests of minors require that they receive certain medical procedures; (2) that the law should not discourage such procedures by requiring parental consent when such consent may not be forthcoming (e.g., in instances of treatment for venereal diseases or counseling for drug or alcohol problems); (3) that minors, not only adults, have a right to make decisions about medical procedures, and that this includes a right to refuse them; and, usually, (4) that the age of consent comports with what is generally known about the developmental capacity of children and adolescents and their reasoning power, judgment, and maturity to make such decisions (Grisso and Vierling, 1978).

Once the age of consent is fixed, all persons who achieve that age are subsequently presumed by the law to be competent to consent to or refuse medical care. They are thus *de jure* competent. In this way, many institutionalized, mentally retarded adults, who most probably cannot understand proposed medical treatments, are nevertheless *de jure*, if not clearly *de facto*, competent (see below). Similarly, adults who refuse medical procedures, e.g., amputation of gangrenous legs or biopsies of breast lumps, cannot be forced, in nonemergency circumstances, to undergo these procedures, unless there is first a court hearing and a declaration of incompetency by a court. Furthermore, consent for the procedure must be obtained from a substitute decision maker, usually, but not always, the patient's appointed guardian (*Lane* v. *Candura*, 1978; *Matter of Quackenbush*, 1978; *In re Yetter*, 1973).

The consent of a *de jure* incompetent person is no consent at all. Under such circumstances, the consent of someone other than the patient must always be secured in order for the physician to be immunized from legal liability for any bad result or harm to the patient.

Complicating the issue, the law also distinguishes between *de facto* competency and the already complex idea of *de jure* competency (Meisel, 1979). This is where the greatest problem lies for psychiatry. Even if the legal presumption for adults is one of competency, the consent of a person who was in fact incompetent, i.e., *de facto* incompetent, at the time of consent to medical treatment may later be set aside as invalid. Thus, it may be alleged that when the patient consented to or refused medical treatment, a condition of mental illness, mental retardation, or severe mental disability was present and prevented the person from understanding what was proposed (Meisel, 1979). Because the person did not or could not understand what was being proposed, his or her consent or refusal was not valid. The person was *de facto* incompetent.

There has, over the last few years, been considerable discussion of this issue in relationship to the legal regulation of psychiatric practice. Some have questioned, for example, whether institutionalized, mentally disabled persons are *de facto* competent, even if they are *de jure* competent, to consent to participate in psychiatric research. Rather, it is argued, the consents of such mentally disabled persons should be checked by others before their consents are honored (The National Commission for the Protection of Human Subjects of Biomedical and Behavioral Research, 1978). Similarly, under the influence of an anti-electroconvulsive-treatment lobby, the California Legislature passed a bill requiring that before electroconvulsive treatment could be given, even to voluntary consenting patients, a second medical opinion must document the patient's *de facto* competency to consent to the treatment (Amendments to California Welfare and Institutions Code, 1976).

Psychiatrists, of course, have also been quick to argue that some, if not all, committed patients, even if they have not been clearly shown to be legally incompetent at the time of the commitment hearings, probably do not have the capacity to consent to or refuse treatment. Therefore, it is argued, refusals of committed psychiatric patients should be overridden by their physicians (*Rogers* v. *Okin,* 1979). Questions concerning the *de facto* and *de jure* competency of committed psychiatric patients are among those that have fueled the right-to-refuse treatment controversy (see also the chapter by Gutheil).

Finally, the issue of *de facto* incompetency often confronts the psychiatric consultant who is asked to evaluate medical patients concerning their competency to accept or refuse medical procedures such as limb amputations, blood transfusions, sterilization, renal dialysis, and even heroic procedures such as transplants. Court hearings to adjudicate and thus establish *de jure* competency are expensive, time-consuming, and impractical, and the mental status of some medical and psychiatric patients is frequently changing even as a result of treatment. Psychiatrists are therefore asked to give opinions about a patient's *de facto* competency as a prelude to, or instead of, a formal legal review of the matter, even if the psychiatrist's opinion lacks a legal imprimatur. Because of the widespread applicability of the competency construct, few psychiatrists are able to avoid thinking about or dealing with problems of patient competency even though, ultimately, legal as well as medical values and procedures are involved in making determinations.

STANDARDS FOR COMPETENCY

Given the centrality of the idea of competency-for-consent law, it is disheartening to note that Anglo-Saxon law provides no generally accepted guidelines for establishing patient competency to consent to or refuse treatment (Roth et al., 1977; Meisel, 1979). Lacking such guidelines, courts have in the past often adjudicated patients as generally or globally incompetent or competent to manage their affairs and/or persons, rather than focusing in depth upon the more relevant issue of the patient's limited specific competency to make medical decisions. Broad rather than narrow criteria have historically been used to establish the patient's general incompetency, such that the patient had a guardian appointed to make all relevant decisions about the person, not only decisions about medical matters. While the National Conference of Commissioners on Uniform State Laws is drafting a "Uniform Health Care Consent Act" for promulgation to the states, the law of patient competency to decide about treatment is now in flux.

In 1977, the author and his colleagues reviewed the relevant literature on competency and their own experiences, noting that there appeared to be five prevalent types of tests or standards for competency to make medical decisions. These five tests involve a determination of whether (1) *the patient evidences a choice about treatment* (under this test, the competent patient is one who manifests, behaviorally or verbally, a clear preference for or against a treatment); (2) *the patient's choice is deemed reasonable* (this test entails evaluating the patient's capacity to reach the reasonable, right, or responsible decision); (3) *the patient's choice is based on rational reasons* (this test considers whether the patient's decision to consent or refuse is a direct consequence of delusional thinking); (4) *the patient manifests the ability to understand* (this test, probably the test most consistent with the informed consent law, looks to the patient's ability to understand the risks and benefits of and the alternatives to treatment, including the consequences of no treatment); and (5) *the patient manifests actual understanding of the information relevant to consent or refusal*.

In a more recent paper, Appelbaum and the author (Appelbaum and Roth, in press) amplify and reclassify these tests or standards for competency, noting that they focus on four aspects of patient decision making, aspects which are potentially relevant to the assessment of competency. The four aspects—choosing, understanding, reasoning, and appreciating—may also be ranked hierarchically to furnish a progressively more stringent standard whereby patient competency is evaluated. Appreciation, the fourth standard, is particularly problematic for psychiatry. According to this standard, the only patients deemed competent would be those who could grasp the relevance to their own condition of information presented about treatment. This standard for competency addresses both cognitive and affective aspects of patient decision making, including the problem of patient denial of illness (see also Roth et al., in press).

Appelbaum and the author have also discussed the many aspects of the patient's mental status that may affect competency under each of the four standards (Appelbaum and Roth, in press). For example, psychiatric conditions compromising the patient's *ability to manifest a choice* about treatment include mutism as a result of catatonic stupor or severe depression; catatonic excitement; mania; profound psychotic thought disorder that renders communication unintelligible to others; and marked ambivalence as in schizophrenia or severe obsessive states.

Assuming that attempts have been made to inform the patient about treatment, the patient's *ability to understand* the risks and benefits of or alternatives to treatment may also be compromised by a patient's low intelligence, poor education, deficient language skills, poor attention, disorientation, and poor recall and recent memory.

The patient's *ability to reason* about treatment may be compromised not only by delusions and hallucinations, or other manifestations of thought disorder, but also by extreme degrees of phobia, panic, anxiety, euphoria, depression, anger, agitation, or obsessive preoccupation (Michels, in press). For the patient to be evaluated as incompetent, it should be stressed, however, that the mere presence of delusional thinking manifested by the patient, or some other sign of psychosis, is insufficient. Instead, it must be shown that the patient's disordered or delusional thinking makes him or her unable to weigh rationally the risks and benefits of the proposed treatment.

Finally, concerning the *appreciation* standard, denial is the clinical condition most likely to affect the patient's appreciation of both the facts and the severity of his or her illness. The patient refuses treatment because he or she does not evaluate the physician's proposal of treatment as having relevance for him or her, even if the patient otherwise understands what is proposed (Roth et al., in press).

While the above recitation of elements of the patient's mental status as they pertain to competency will be familiar to the clinician, it should be emphasized that choosing a standard for competency, and in particular setting the threshold for competency, involves issues that lie beyond psychiatric expertise. Setting the standard for competency to consent to or refuse treatment is a matter for social policy and law, not psychiatry (Appelbaum and Roth, in press). Thus, the application of any of the four standards promotes certain values at the expense of others. Discussing these issues is beyond the scope of this review. It should be obvious without further discussion, however, that applying differing standards for competency will act to promote or diminish patient autonomy, to assure or prevent patients from having their treatment needs met, or to protect or fail to protect the patient from receiving potentially risky treatments whose rationale the patient does not fully grasp. Freedman has recently formulated what he believes is a more value-free approach to assessing patient competency: the patient's reason for consent or refusal must be recognizable, if not rational, in order to be competent (Freedman, in press). Despite the desirability of such an apparently neutral standard, there remains considerable doubt as to how one would implement such a value-free approach to competency.

PROCEDURAL MATTERS

McGarry et al., in their study of mental health commitment, show that at the law-psychiatry interface, it is the procedures followed as much as the substantive criteria used that affect the outcome for the patient (1981). The same is true for competency assessments. Clinicians need to consider not only which test or standard should be used in assessing patient competency but also what steps should be followed in making these determinations. Appelbaum and the author have recently formulated some helpful guidelines (Appelbaum and Roth, 1981). The legal presumption is one of competency. Before a patient should be considered to be possibly incompetent to make medical decisions, a number of steps should be followed. The evaluation of competency requires that a thorough clinical approach be pursued.

First, the psychiatrist should consider the psychodynamic aspects of patient consent or refusal. What fears or anxieties does the patient have about proposed procedures? What psychological defenses have been mobilized by the physician's proposal of treatment? Do these fears or defenses compromise the patient's understanding of treatment? These issues should be addressed therapeutically where possible.

Second, studies show that one reason patients may not seem to understand is that they may not have been told (Ashley et al., 1980). Before he or she reaches conclusions about the patient's capacity to consent or refuse, the psychiatrist should ensure that information has been clearly presented to the patient about the proposed treatment (see also Freedman, in press). When the psychiatrist is asked to assess a patient's competency to decide about a medical procedure with which he or she is not very familiar, the psychiatrist should join with the patient's primary physician to explain to the patient the proposed treatment and its risks and benefits. Then the psychiatrist can properly assess the patient's capacity to handle that information most relevant to treatment decision making.

Third, the psychiatrist should assess the stability of the patient's choice and the patient's ability to understand over time. The patient's mental status may be changing daily or even hourly, perhaps as a result of ongoing treatment. When the patient's incompetency has been induced by the patient's medical condition or management, e.g., by encephalopathy, metabolic disorders, or drug toxicity or withdrawal, decisions as to competency should be deferred until medical status is more stable.

Fourth, it is important to note that the patient may be a less than reliable informant about the facts that relate to competency assessment. The psychiatrist should obtain historical data about the patient from others as well as from the patient. To the extent that patients deny illness or fail to appreciate why treatment has been recommended for them, they may be unable or unwilling to give an accurate picture of their illness, thus also failing to understand what are the psychosocial, if not the technical-medical, risks and benefits of treatment. Obtaining histories from others allows comparison of the patient's beliefs with what is objectively known.

Fifth, the psychiatrist should approach a patient's competency not so much as an isolated characteristic of the patient but within a social and even interactive framework. Patients are sometimes better able to understand about treatment when they are informed by persons able to "talk their language" or by persons whom the patient does not distrust because of disparity of class or race. Attempts should therefore be made to include more than one clinician or even the patient's family or friends in the patient's education. Only after such conscientious efforts are made should it be concluded that the patient is unable to choose, understand, reason, or appreciate (Appelbaum and Roth, 1981).

The value of the above clinical approach toward competency assessment is evident. Avoiding hasty one-shot determinations permits many instances of questionably valid consents or refusals to be clarified over time. As medical care progresses, the necessity for patient consent for some procedures may even disappear as these procedures turn out not to have been medically necessary. By pursuing the issues of competency over time, second opinions can be obtained and documented to show that the clinician has gone about the task of assessing patient competency reasonably. Eventually, however, where treatments offer potential risks for the patient or are controversial or both, and where questions of patient competency persist, more formal mechanisms, such as court hearings, may be required.

EMPIRICAL STUDIES

Relatively few empirical studies have been performed in the area of competency, and some of those which do exist fall short in their conceptualization of the issues. In a recent review, for instance, of published studies that examine how informed consent doctrine actually works, Meisel and the author (in press) found that such a problem compromises the value of many of these studies, as well as studies of competency. While investigators did study the important issue of patients' understanding of treatment, they failed to inquire into, examine, or document the prior issue of attempts to inform patients about treatment or research. Thus, the studies' findings of poor understanding of treatment and research on the part of both medical and psychiatric patients do not necessarily mean that patients lack the capacity to make medical decisions.

Whatever their conceptual problems, the available studies do offer some empirical data worth reviewing. But the data do not give rise to optimism. Appelbaum et al., in a study of fifty patients voluntarily admitted to a psychiatric hospital, found that the majority appeared to have severely impaired competency to consent to hospitalization, regardless of the standard used to assess competency (Appelbaum et al., 1981). Other studies of patient understanding of admission to the psychiatric hospital, of their status as voluntary or involuntary patients, and of their rights as patients have similar findings (Palmer and Wohl, 1972; Olin and Olin, 1975).

Soskis's 1978 study of hospitalized schizophrenic patients receiving antipsychotic medication is particularly interesting. Soskis found that while the schizophrenic patients, as compared with medical patients, did not have defective understanding of the side effects and risks of medication, the schizophrenic patients were less knowledgeable about how their medication related to the nature of their problem (Soskis, 1978). To the extent that schizophrenic patients fail to understand the nature of their problem, it may be anticipated that they will also fail to understand the risks and benefits of treatment or to weigh risks and benefits in deciding whether to accept treatment (see also Roth et al., in press).

Grossman and Summers' study of schizophrenic patients' understanding of the risks and benefits of medication also showed poor patient understanding (1980). Other experienced psychiatric clinicians claim, based on no systematic data, that stabilized schizophrenic outpatients do have the ability to understand about important medication issues, such as the issue of tardive dyskinesia (Grossman and Summers, 1980; Sovner et al., 1978). In what appears to be the first systematic study of this issue, Munetz et al. (1981) found that even after having been carefully informed, most of the schizophrenic outpatients treated in a cognitive disorder clinic did not absorb or understand information about tardive dyskinesia.

Another ongoing set of studies by the author and his colleagues (Roth et al., 1980) focuses on consent to electroconvulsive treatment on the part of hospitalized, depressed patients. These studies have shown that the majority of such patients (more than 75 percent) were able to understand the information the consent forms gave about electroconvulsive treatment. In videotaped studies the majority of these patients were also deemed by two lawyers and two psychiatrists to be competent to consent to or refuse treatment. Patients deemed likely to be incompetent to consent to or refuse treatment were those judged clinically psychotic and were patients with lower educational backgrounds. The incompetent patients also performed more poorly on another measure of illness, whether they were willing or motivated to be educated about treatment. Consenting patients, the studies found, understood more than refusing patients. The competency of refusing patients was particularly difficult to evaluate reliably, however, because such patients are often unwilling or unable to undergo a meaningful exchange of information with their physician about treatment.

In the area of consent to research, one study concluded that a high proportion (sixty percent) of hospitalized schizophrenic patients could not understand what was involved in research (Pryce, 1978). This study is problematic, however, because no definition for competency is given. By contrast, Stanley et al. (1981), in a study of psychiatric patients' willingness to participate in hypothetical research studies, reported that psychiatric patients make decisions similar to those of other medical patients.

Recently initiated empirical studies have begun to examine how psychiatrists and attorneys go about evaluating competency (Kaufmann and Roth, 1981; Kaufmann et al., unpublished). Psychiatrists, they found, were more likely to relate judgments about competency to their perception of the severity of the patient's illness, in other words, the patient's general competency, than were attorneys. Attorneys were more inclined to assess the patient's understanding of risks, benefits, and alternatives of treatment, in other words, the patient's specific competency.

Empirical studies of competency are just beginning, and they continue to confront the crucial questions of the field itself. Like practitioners, researchers must relate the medical and psychological findings about patient understanding to the legal doctrine. They, too, must address the fundamental questions: where should the legal threshold be set? how much ability to choose, understand, reason, or appreciate must the competent patient manifest?

WHO DECIDES

Medical professionals with front-line responsibility for patient care are usually the ones who raise questions about patient competency. Historically, however, once the physician suspected incompetency, it was the responsibility of the court, not the physician, to conduct hearings and adjudicate competency. But the law of competency is in flux. The issue of who decides about competency, as well as the related issue of who subsequently consents or refuses for the patient, has become more complex. Legal scholars recommend, for example, and some institutions have created, special interdisciplinary committees, often called human rights committees, to rule on the factual competency of patient decisions about invasive treatment such as aversive conditioning. Such committees also decide whether it is in the patient's best interest to receive such treatment (Friedman, 1975).

More recently, in attempting to fashion a workable system for assessing the competency of committed psychiatric patients who refuse treatment, judges have permitted so-called independent psychiatrists,

psychiatrists who are not members of the patient's treatment team, to make competency determinations. Thus, in *Rennie* v. *Klein* (1979), a federal district court ruled that when a patient refuses treatment and when that patient's physician still wishes to treat the patient with medication, an independent psychiatrist must review the propriety of the patient's refusal. Among other matters the independent psychiatrist decides whether the patient lacks the capacity to make a treatment decision.

Also moving away from the courtroom, in *Rogers* v. *Okin* (1980), the first circuit court of appeals ruled that "in situations where any delay [in treating refusing patients] could result in significant deterioration of the patient's mental health," competency determinations could be made by means other than a court hearing. Clinicians should follow these legal developments, since future formal competency determinations will probably more frequently be made by psychiatrists, members of institutional committees, patient advocates, and others. Judges and courts will continue to be involved in some instances, but the trend is toward more independent clinical authority.

THE CONSEQUENCES OF INCOMPETENCY

In the past when patients were adjudicated incompetent, courts appointed guardians to make medical decisions on behalf of the patient. Family members or others were often appointed guardians to give proxy consent for the patient or what has come to be called proxy permission for treatment (Meisel, 1979). While this approach still applies in most jurisdictions, there are new developments of great legal complexity in this arena. Of these the chapter takes note, although an adequate review is beyond its scope.

A developing legal trend is to separate the issue of the propriety of forced treatment for the patient from the issue of patient competency to make treatment decisions. Historically, the law's working assumption was that once determined incompetent, patients would be treated in their best interests. This state of affairs, however, may not persist. Some writers, for example, have proposed that even the apparently irrational decisions of patients to refuse electroconvulsive treatment should be honored, unless it can be shown that without treatment the patient's life is clearly endangered (Culver et al., 1980). Others suggest that even though patients who manifest denial might reasonably be deemed incompetent to make treatment decisions, courts may still need to consider carefully, on an individual basis, the risks and benefits of involuntary treatment for such apparently incompetent patients before permitting it (Roth et al., in press). Conversely, the law may also wish to declare more explicitly than has formerly been the case that patient consents to psychiatric hospitalization are valid, even though, when scrutinized, these consents may be *de facto* incompetent (Appelbaum et al., in press).

The growing legal trend to separate the social policy decision of whether the patient should be treated over his or her objection from the competency decision itself finds its most extreme exposition in a recent case from the Massachusetts Supreme Court, *In the Matter of the Guardianship of Richard Roe III* (1981). In *Roe* the Massachusetts court elaborated a position it had developed in several prior cases, ruling that a schizophrenic patient's guardian, in this case the patient's father, did not have the right to authorize psychotropic drug treatment for his ward, even though the patient had correctly been declared legally incompetent and the father had been appointed his guardian. Because of the potential harm from the psychotropic drugs, the court ruled that only a judge was empowered to determine whether it was in the patient's best interest to receive the medicine. The basis of the judge's decision, in accord with a tantalizing and complicated theory of substituted consent, should be his or her assessment of whether the patient, if competent, would have decided to receive the medication (see also *In re Boyd,* 1979). Meanwhile, contrary to *Roe,* the Federal District Court of Appeals in *Rogers* v. *Okin* (1980) ruled that once involuntarily committed psychiatric patients are determined to be incompetent, then physicians, perhaps monitored through peer review, can medicate them without having to have a guardian appointed to make the treatment decision for the patient.

This necessarily brief review indicates the growing legal complexity as to what treatments, if any, patients may receive subsequent to a declaration of incompetency and who, if anyone, has the power to consent for the patient. Clinicians should keep current with case and statutory law in their localities so that they know the practical consequences of a finding of incompetency.

A FINAL WORD

Approaching the problem of competency requires common sense. Adult patients, it should be remembered, are competent to consent to or refuse treatment until proven otherwise. Thus, the author and his colleagues have written, "Competency is presumed as long as the patient modulates his or her behavior, talks in a comprehensible way, remembers what he or she is told, dresses and acts so as to appear to be in meaningful communication with the environment, and has not been declared legally incompetent" (Roth et al., 1977). Assuming patients appear generally competent, neither clinicians nor courts should usually determine to the contrary, absent convincing evidence. Repeated conscientious attempts must be made to educate the patient about treatment before determining that the patient cannot choose, understand, reason, or appreciate what is involved. If this rule is followed, then patients who are generally competent to conduct their affairs will, only in rare instances, be found specifically incompetent to consent to or refuse medical care.

It cannot so easily be assumed, however, that patients who are mentally retarded, brain damaged, intoxicated, or psychotic are competent *de facto,* if not *de jure,* to make treatment decisions. While many and even a majority of such persons may be competent to consent, in these circumstances a greater burden is placed on the clinician to demonstrate and document that the patient is *de facto* or specifically competent and that his or her consents or refusals to treatment are valid. Taking steps to help such severely disordered patients to become more competent provides rewards not only for the patient but also for the clinician.

Chapter 24

The Right to Treatment:
Little Law but Much Impact†
by Mark J. Mills, J.D., M.D.

INTRODUCTION

To deprive any citizen of his or her liberty upon the altruistic theory that the confinement is for humane therapeutic reasons and then fail to provide adequate treatment violates the very fundamental of due process (*Wyatt* v. *Stickney, 1971a*).

It is now the settled doctrine of this Court that the Due Process Clause embodies a system of rights based on moral principles so deeply embedded in the traditions and feelings of our people as to be deemed fundamental to a civilized society as conceived by our whole history (Frankfurter dissenting, *Solesbee* v. *Balkcom*, 1950).

[T]here can be little doubt that in the exercise of its police power a State may confine individuals solely to protect society from the dangers of significant antisocial acts (Burger concurring, *O'Connor* v. *Donaldson*, 1975).

The chapter's title and the three epigraphs underscore the author's thesis that although judicial holdings[1] on the right to treatment are few, the clinical impact has been profound. During the past two decades, the right-to-treatment doctrine has enlarged in status. At first considered a "radical innovation in . . . legal thinking," it became the predominant rationale for a series of significant consent decrees affecting mentally ill and mentally retarded patients (Powell, 1980). In two important respects, the right to treatment stands in contrast to its counterpart, the right to refuse treatment. The legal precedent for the latter can be precisely outlined,[2] but it has had relatively little nationwide clinical impact (Powell, 1980).[3] On the other hand, the right to treatment is difficult to articulate in legal precedent, but it has literally transformed the care of thousands. This chapter explores that anomaly by presenting an overview of the history, legal theory, and implementation of the right to treatment. It concludes with a critique and some speculation about how this right may evolve.

HISTORY

Morton Birnbaum, a physician and lawyer, is the acknowledged originator of the doctrine of the right to treatment (Powell, 1980; Halleck, 1980), although earlier court decisions had begun to suggest such a right (Powell, 1980). Essentially, Birnbaum argued that state-funded institutions provided inadequate treatment, that this occurred because

---

†The author acknowledges Ms. Lee Rubin, Research Associate, Department of Mental Health, for her editorial assistance, and Ms. Patricia Murphy and Ms. Joan Mitchell for their aid in the preparation of this manuscript.

[1]A holding is the legal term that denotes the points of law which a case determines, i.e., the points which are decided by the court.

[2]See, for example, Appelbaum and Gutheil (1979), Cocozza and Melick (1977), Hoffman (1976), Mills (1981), and Stone (1981).

[3]Only six states have recognized what one might characterize as a meaningful right to refuse treatment (Colorado, Massachusetts, New Jersey, Oklahoma, Pennsylvania, and Utah). The implementation and enforcement of that right varies greatly (Mills, 1980).

insufficient funds were appropriated, and that this situation, if un-challenged, would continue indefinitely. He next observed that tra-ditional legal objections to civil commitment on procedural grounds were inadequate to correct the situation. Finally, he proffered his remedy—the judicial recognition of a new, constitutionally based right. And he predicted correctly that if such a right were enforced, the states might often choose to release the patient rather than to provide the type of expensive care which a meaningful right to treatment man-dated. Left vague, however, was the constitutional basis for this right. Quoting Frankfurter (the second epigraph), Birnbaum suggested that due process provided the necessary constitutional underpinning, but he did not spell out the legal details.

Rouse v. *Cameron*, first heard in 1966, was the first case to recognize the nascent right to treatment, but it did so on statutory, not con-stitutional, grounds.[4] That case involved a *habeas corpus* proceeding against a criminal defendant who had been found not guilty by reason of insanity. The defendant, Rouse, was committed to St. Elizabeth's Hos-pital, where he had remained for more than three years; had he been found guilty of the crime for which he had been charged, the maximum sentence would have been one year. Perhaps moved by these cir-cumstances, Chief Judge Bazelon found a newly enacted civil com-mitment statute that conferred a right to treatment.[5] In *dicta* (non-binding judicial opinion) he went further. Citing Birnbaum's article, he opined that all involuntarily committed patients might have this same right. He then observed that three theories could support such a right: due process, equal protection, and the prohibition against cruel and unusual punishment. He also noted that the hospital need not show that the treatment was ameliorative, but only "adequate in light of the present knowledge" (*Rouse* v. *Cameron*, 1966). The case was re-manded to the district court for a determination of the adequacy of treatment with the admonition that continued confinement had to be grounded in the defendant's mental disability.

Nason v. *Superintendent of Bridgewater State Hospital* (1968) was the first state court case to find a constitutional right to treatment. As did *Rouse*, this case involved a criminally committed patient. The case held that due process and equal protection rights required clinically appropriate treatment. Though it relied primarily on the due process right, the court unfortunately did little more than state its legal con-clusion. It did not provide a legal analysis to explain the basis for its reliance on due process.

Wyatt v. *Stickney* constitutes the watershed case in the right to treatment. Properly, *Wyatt* is a series of cases that spanned nearly a decade and resulted in the Alabama mental health system's being placed in receivership.[6] Before that happened, however, the litigation produced both a clearly articulated, constitutionally based right-to-treatment doctrine and a comprehensive set of minimum clinical standards.

---

[4]See "Note" (1967), *Rouse* v. *Cameron* (1966), and *Rouse* v. *Cameron* (1967).
[5]The right to treatment may be grounded on either a constitutional or a statutory foundation. However, a statutory basis is generally seen as merely precatory, and not regarded as an enforceable source of this right.
[6]Cases in the *Wyatt* series include *Wyatt* v. *Stickney* (1971a); *Wyatt* v. *Stickney* (1971b); *Wyatt* v. *Stickney* (1972a); *Wyatt* v. *Stickney* (1972b); *Wyatt* v. *Aderholt* (1972); *Wyatt* v. *Aderholt* (1974); *Wyatt* v. *Hardin* (1975); and *Wyatt* v. *Ireland* (1979).

Unlike earlier cases, *Wyatt* arose in the context of civil commitment. It started as a class action suit against Alabama officials to improve conditions at two state hospitals and a state school. The judge, Frank Johnson, issued four opinions,[7] the first of which articulated the constitutional reasoning, and which is quoted in the first epigraph (*Wyatt* v. *Stickney,* 1971a). By then, the constitutional arguments had been presaged, but the detail of Johnson's order was revolutionary ("Note," 1975). Starting with the second opinion, Judge Johnson charted new territory by particularizing the constitutionally mandated components of minimally adequate treatment. With the help of several *amici* the court found that those standards included "(1) a humane psychological and physical environment, (2) qualified staff in numbers sufficient to administer adequate treatment and, (3) individualized treatment plans" (*Wyatt* v. *Stickney,* 1971a). When the defendants failed to implement these standards, the court provided its detailed order, specifying, inter alia, staff-patient ratios for all personnel, size and temperature standards for patient wards, and nutritional standards (*Wyatt* v. *Stickney,* 1972a). On appeal, the Fifth Circuit, relying on its holding in *Donaldson* v. *O'Connor,* affirmed the constitutional right to treatment and Judge Johnson's order (*Wyatt* v. *Aderholt,* 1974). The court also defined concretely the legal underpinning of its decision: "[O]ur holding in *Donaldson* and here rests on the *quid pro quo* concept of 'rehabilitative treatment . . . and care beyond the subsistence level custodial care that would be provided in a penitentiary'" (*Wyatt* v. *Aderholt,* 1974).

Donaldson was the first right-to-treatment case to reach the Supreme Court (*O'Connor* v. *Donaldson,* 1975). It posed the legal issue in a somewhat confused fashion. One reading of the case was that Donaldson was suing for damages because he had been deprived of his newly created right to treatment. Another more narrow reading was that, absent treatment and absent any danger to the community, he was suing for damages because he had been deprived of his right to liberty. If the account in *The Brethren* is accurate, the resulting opinion was a compromise between Chief Justice Burger, who wanted the Court to extinguish explicitly the right to treatment, and the majority, who wanted to decide the case on the latter narrower grounds (Woodward and Armstrong, 1979).

The Court apparently also went out of its way to deprive the lower court opinion of any precedential effect. Setting aside the right-to-treatment issue, the Court instead decided that civil liability[8] could arise when the state held without treatment a nondangerous individual who had others in the community willing to provide for his needs (Lottman, 1977). In short, the Court addressed almost exclusively the liberty interest of the patient. The Fifth Circuit, in contrast, had opined broadly about the right to treatment, finding two constitutional theories supporting that right (*Donaldson* v. *O'Connor,* 1974; 1975).

Perhaps the most striking aspect of the case, however, is Chief Justice Burger's concurring opinion. In it he pointedly criticized the Circuit's *quid pro quo* theory, asserting that if the theory were correct, pro-

[7]Johnson's opinions were issued in *Wyatt* v. *Stickney* (1971a); *Wyatt* v. *Stickney* (1971b); *Wyatt* v. *Stickney* (1972a); and *Wyatt* v. *Stickney* (1972b).
[8]The hospital superintendent was being sued for damages (money) based on the theory that he had illegally confined the plaintiff patient against his will.

cedural guarantees could be overlooked if treatment were provided (*O'Connor* v. *Donaldson,* 1975). Thus, his opinion is generally read as a sharp disapproval of both the procedural and the substantive right to treatment, though formally the issue has still not been read before the Court.[9] Since 1975, then, the existence of both the right to treatment and any constitutional theories supporting it have been quite uncertain.

Within the last two years several opinions have suggested that some district and appellate courts may not consider Burger's concurrence determinative. *Eckerhart* v. *Hensley* (1979), the first of these cases, held that the right to treatment exists constitutionally and that the right extends even to patients hospitalized because of their dangerousness. The court relied on previous cases,[10] but its reasoning in doing so appears suspect at best, given the Supreme Court's pointed disavowal in *Donaldson.* More recently, the Supreme Court has decided *Pennhurst State School and Hospital* v. *Halderman* (1981). Though nominally faced with determining whether the language of a federal statute conferred a right-to-treatment enforcement power, the court again faced the issue of the constitutional basis of the right to treatment (Boston University Center for Law and Health Sciences, 1981). Once more, it chose to decide the case on as narrow a basis as possible, confining its decision strictly to one of statutory interpretation. Holding that the language of the statute was hortatory, the court deemed that the statute encouraged but did not confer rights.

Finally, two cases from the Third Circuit have significantly extended, at the federal appellate level, the right to treatment by invoking the least restrictive alternative as part of that right (*Romeo* v. *Youngberg,* 1980; *Scott* v. *Plante,* 1976). (See the chapter by Klein concerning the least restrictive alternative).

Even without considering the impact of the many additional cases which have affected the right to treatment, one might well ask what, in aggregate, all these cases mean.[11] This analysis should have suggested several points. First, as a legal doctrine, the constitutionally derived right to treatment is still evolving. Second, the Supreme Court has so far avoided direct consideration of this right, but lower federal courts have not. Third, at least at present, it is probably safe to say that there is no settled constitutionally based right to treatment. In sum, there is little law supporting the right to treatment.

[9]See Powell (1980), "Comment" (1975), "Comment" (1979), Grant (1976), and Levine (1980).

[10]*Rouse* v. *Cameron* (1966); *Rouse* v. *Cameron* (1967); *Wyatt* v. *Stickney* (1971b); *Donaldson* v. *O'Connor* (1975); *Welsch* v. *Likins* (1977); and *Davis* v. *Watkins* (1974).

[11]Additional cases include: *Bell* v. *Wolfish* (1979); *Bowring* v. *Godwin* (1977); *Burnham* v. *Department of Public Health* (1972); *Creek* v. *Stone* (1967); *Davis* v. *Balson* (1978); *Davy* v. *Sullivan* (1973); *Director of Patuxent Inst.* v. *Daniels* (1966); *Dixon* v. *Weinberger* (1975); *French* v. *Blackburn* (1979); *Harper* v. *Cserr* (1976); *Holt* v. *Sarver* (1971); *Inmates of Boys' Training School* v. *Affleck* (1972); *In the Matter of Spring* (1979); *In re Wilson* (1970), *Lora* v. *Board of Education* (1978); *Lynch* v. *Baxley* (1974); *Martarella* v. *Kelley* (1972); *Morales* v. *Turman* (1977a); *Morales* v. *Turman* (1977b); *Morales* v. *Turman* (1977c); *Naughton* v. *Bevilacqua* (1978); *Nelson* v. *Heyne* (1974); *Parisi* v. *Rockefeller* (1973); *Pugh* v. *Locke* (1976); *Ragsdale* v. *Overholser* (1950); *Rogers* v. *Okin* (1979); *Sas* v. *Maryland* (1964); *Saville* v. *Treadway* (1974); *Schever* v. *Rhodes* (1974); *Stachulak* v. *Coughlin* (1973); *Stamus* v. *Leonhardt* (1976); *Suzuki* v. *Quisenberry* (1976); *Tippet* v. *Maryland* (1971); *U.S.* v. *Pardue* (1973); *Vitek* v. *Jones* (1980); and *Wood* v. *Strickland* (1975).

CONSENT DECREES

To consider the holdings of the right-to-treatment cases alone would be to miss the most essential point. The action of the cases has not been in their holdings, but in their remedies. Most right-to-treatment cases have been settled by consent decree, without formal adjudication ("Notes," 1977; Lottman, 1976b).

When a group of patients from a state mental institution brings suit against that institution, it has two options. The group may seek a formal trial and adjudication, or it may settle the dispute through an agreement with the state. The product of the latter process is a consent decree, in effect a contract between the patients and the state (represented by the governor and the mental health commissoner), subsequently implemented and enforced by a court. Such an agreement avoids the problems of finding a constitutional right to treatment, since the decree is settled without judicial ruling on the facts or the law. Hence, the plaintiffs give up the chance of finding a constitutionally enforceable right to treatment, and the defendants give up the chance of finding that there is no such right.

When reform, rather than the enforcement of an individual's rights, is the primary objective, consent decrees hold some advantages over adjudication. The consent-decree process tends to be free from the delays of trial and appeal. Decrees can be very specific, issuing such detailed provisions as staff-patient ratios, guidelines for bathroom privacy, and recreational facilities (*Mills* v. *Board of Education of the District of Columbia,* 1975). In contrast, trial litigation usually deals with only one practice of the institution and mandates restitution without wide reform. The consent decree also has the advantage of being less adversarial than adjudication, not bounded by the rules of trials and judicial decorum; thus, the consent-decree process gives the two parties an opportunity to cooperate in reaching a mutual agreement.

But the use of consent decrees in right-to-treatment cases poses problems as well. Reform is always difficult to accomplish, as institutions often move slowly. Patient advocates, however, are eager for immediate change. The problems raised by the use of the consent decrees may be classified as jurisdictional, implemental, and substantive. An examination of each type of problem will clarify the strengths and weaknesses of consent decrees.

Traditionally, the judiciary's powers have been limited to the adjudication of disputes between parties, leaving the courts rather insulated from the political and administrative arenas ("Notes," 1977). The consent-decree procedure, however, draws the judiciary into both of these arenas, without the benefit of full evidentiary hearings, findings of law and fact, and appellate review. The implementation of consent decrees often requires judges to oversee the administration of large institutions; to evaluate on a day-to-day basis their compliance with or violation of detailed procedural and substantive requirements; and, in effect, to appropriate funds. In so doing, the judiciary assumes authority traditionally reserved for the executive and legislative branches of the government.

Both the separation-of-powers doctrine and Article III of the Constitution appear to militate against this widening of the judiciary's powers (*U.S. Constitution,* Art. III, Sec.2) particularly in the absence of a clearly established, underlying constitutional right. There is little legal justification for the mixing of roles, though some policy-based rationales have been offered. The courts have entered decrees regarding other bureaucratic institutions, such as public schools and prisons (*Swann* v. *Charlotte-Mecklenberg Board of Education,* 1971; *Cruz* v. *Beto,* 1972). However, such action has been questioned by legal observers and has not been accepted without debate. Another policy argument is that the legislature has failed to implement policies to remedy the problems of institutional care and that, in view of this inaction, the courts are justified in attempting to rectify any violations of civil rights. Although this power of rectification is limited, since the judiciary is not constitutionally empowered to appropriate money for remedial changes, the courts have *de facto* managed to circumvent this restriction. Hundreds of millions of state dollars have been spent complying with judicial decrees (Memorandum, 1972).

A further difficulty with consent decrees is that judges may not possess the expertise necessary to examine their provisions critically. Institutional administration is complex, and the psychiatric and medical aspects of the right to treatment are difficult to master. A court may not be able to make a reasoned judgment in these matters, especially when it must assess whether an institution has fulfilled the terms of its agreement to a reasonable extent. Others have argued that courts regularly rule on subjects (economics and medicine, for example) in which they hold no special expertise (Stone, 1975). But in the case of consent decrees, the court's authority extends far beyond its usual scope, and its technical knowledge must extend similarly.

Furthermore, conditions of mental institutions change rapidly as financial and social currents shift in the community. Given their specificity, the consent decrees lack flexibility. The mechanisms for amendment are slow and may leave institutions attempting to meet standards that are, within the period of a few years, outdated. This was the case in *Welsch* v. *Likins* (1974), where the hospital was faced with renovating a facility it had previously planned to close. Departments of mental health, at first pleased by the prospect of increased funding that consent decrees promised, are now disenchanted with the restrictions they have placed on their operations.

To be effective, the provisions of a consent decree must be implemented. Implementation is quite problematic, as many psychiatric and legal observers have noted.[12] Consent decrees are often lengthy. Separate provisions may number in the hundreds and may be difficult to incorporate into the hospital's administrative procedure. Among the problems faced in the implementation stage are: complexity of the regulated institution ("Notes," 1977); the institution's resistance to change (Harvard Law Review, 1977); lack of finances (*Wyatt* v. *Stickney,* 1971b; "Note," 1975); dependence on the legislature for funding (Stone, 1977); inefficient use of available resources (Harvard Law Review, 1977); labor union resistance in the case of deinstitutionalization ("Notes," 1977); and the lack of effective punitive sanctions in the event of noncompliance (Lottman, 1976a). Due to these and other problems, some commentators have noted that "the implementation record in mental heath litigation has not been impres-

[12]See, for example, Halleck (1980); "Note" (1975); "Notes" (1977); Lottman (1976a); and Lottman (1976b).

sive" and have recommended expanded judicial authority to implement the consent decrees ("Notes," 1977).

Some remedies for these problems with the implementation of consent decrees do exist. Most decrees empower monitors, review panels, or special masters to oversee the in-hospital implementation.[13] Their success has been limited.[14] Critics note that review committees in some cases have lacked mental health experts (*Wyatt* v. *Stickney*, 1972a) and in others have had neither guidelines for their responsibilities nor authority to enforce their recommendations (*New York State Association for Retarded Citizens and Parisi* v. *Carey*, 1975). Institutions and monitors are often required to submit compliance reports, but the collection of accurate information is difficult.[15] The court usually retains jurisdiction over the case, but in the event that it discovers violation of the decree, its enforcement power is limited. Some sanctions are too drastic, e.g., citations for contempt, while others are largely ineffective, e.g., special masters ("Notes," 1977).

In summary, the implementation of consent decrees is difficult, ridden with institutional, financial, and judicial impediments.

Impact

Despite their problems, consent decrees have had a significant impact. Institutions, which had previously been insulated from public scrutiny, now find they must meet much needed minimum standards of quality in their facilities and treatment programs (*Eckerhart* v. *Hensley*, 1979; *Welsch* v. *Likins*, 1977). Improvements in mental health care are important, and consent decrees may be necessary where legislative initiative has failed. Unfortunately, the means used to implement these changes have been highly intrusive. Psychiatrists and other mental health workers are burdened by legal supervision; departments of mental health are torn by financial requirements; and the entire process is cumbersome to implement and to enforce.[16] An examination of the consequences of recent consent decrees reveals that they may produce some unanticipated negative outcomes, effects that may be unfortunate for patients and doctors alike.

The problem begins with the formation of a decree. In many cases, the attorneys for the plaintiffs are far more vigorous in their pursuit of the case than are the attorneys for the state, for whom right-to-treatment cases are of low priority (Stone, 1977). As a result, the provisions of the decree may not reflect the state's true interests, and may be a rather one-sided attempt at reform. Typically decrees drastically curtail the state's ability to set its own mental health priorities because they drastically curtail fiscal flexibility. Since the consent decree need not rely formally on constitutional or statutory provisions,

[13]See *Wyatt* v. *Stickney* (1972a); *Welsch* v. *Likins* (1974); *Davis* v. *Watkins* (1974); *New York State Association for Retarded Citizens and Parisi* v. *Carey* (1975); *Horacek* v. *Exon* (1975); and *Pennsylvania Association for Retarded Children* v. *Pennsylvania* (1972).

[14]For discussion see Levine (1980); "Notes" (1977); Lottman (1976a); and Lottman (1976b).

[15]See *Wyatt* v. *Aderholt* (1972); "Notes" (1977); Lottman (1976a); Lottman (1976b); and *New York State Association for Retarded Citizens and Parisi* v. *Carey* (1975).

[16]For example, the Massachusetts Department of Mental Health was called to confer on the implementation of its consent decrees more than seven times during one recent month.

it may overstep the required standards for the right to treatment.[17] As noted earlier, the right to treatment may not rest on a constitutional foundation; unfortunately, the absence of such a foundation leaves consent decrees without clear, reasonable boundaries for their massive reforms.

Another potential problem with consent decrees is the amount of money required to carry them out. The sums can be enormous. Four consent decrees in Massachusetts have cost the Commonwealth over $317 million through 1981, with total expenditures projected over $530 million by 1983.[18] Nationwide, these figures climb into the billions. Appropriating these funds from the state is burdensome ("Notes," 1977; Stone, 1977), but the lack of funds may at least curtail some inappropriate and unnecessary reconstructions of mental health institutions. On the other hand, decrees themselves sometimes give priority to cosmetic changes in the physical plant, changes that ought to be subordinate to substantive issues of treatment.[19] In other cases, the decrees are so rights oriented that they actually overlook the importance of patients' treatment (Appelbaum and Gutheil, 1979).

Another serious untoward effect of the fiscal demands of the decrees is that some institutions, rather than gather the necessary large sums of new money, may instead reduce their patient populations. They release large numbers of patients and restrict their admissions ("Note," 1975; Stone, 1977). It is sadly ironic that decrees intended to improve the treatment of the mentally ill may instead be denying treatment to many of those who need it.

Court-appointed monitors are often thought essential to the implementation of judicial decrees, but their presence in the institutions has created some adverse effects (Stone, 1975). Psychiatrists and other mental health professionals often bear the burden of the monitoring. They have to comply with new legal restrictions on their therapeutic activities, and they may be forced to spend time documenting compliance or reporting directly to the court. In two cases, psychiatrists have been called as defendants in suits for noncompliance (*Davis* v. *Watkins,* 1974; *Parisi* v. *Rockefeller,* 1973). Recruiting competent psychiatrists to serve in the public sector is already an onerous task. The pay is low, and the conditions are often inferior to those in private hospitals. These additional legal restrictions and requirements may both compel some psychiatrists to leave state institutions and also deter the recruitment of new psychiatrists. This result poses great problems, for many consent decrees require increased numbers of doctors to meet predetermined staff-patient ratios. On the other hand, hospitals, perhaps constrained by limited finances, have sometimes failed to implement necessary improvements on their own. Burdensome moni-

---

[17]As noted previously, with the constitutional standards so vague and arguably nonexistent, and with statutory rights often unenforceable, there may be few "required" standards.

[18]See Memorandum (1981); *Gauthier* v. *Benson* (1975); *Mass. Association for Retarded Citizens* v. *Dukakis* (1975); *McEvoy* v. *Mahoney* (1974); and *Ricci* v. *Greenblatt* (1972). Some portion of the costs, however, may be attributed to the state's decision to meet Title XIX standards in order to receive Medicaid reimbursements at the state schools for the mentally retarded. However, the specific percentage cannot be determined.

[19]See, for instance, *Wyatt* v. *Aderholt* (1972) and *Mass. Association for Retarded Citizens* v. *Dukakis* (1975).

toring may be the price psychiatrists must pay during the transition to higher quality patient care.

The formalistic requirements of consent decrees may have a negative impact on psychiatrists, who find their medical autonomy compromised. They may affect patients negatively by causing premature releases or refusals of admission. A further negative consequence for patients is the inequity with which only patients included in the defined class receive the decreed benefits. A class of patients is usually defined at a particular period in time. Those who fall outside the definition at that time are left without aid. And since funds are scarce, there is little impetus for the institution to extend the costly decreed benefits to patients not in the class.

Consent decrees can initiate institutional reform. For reform to be implemented, however, decrees should avoid formalistic requirements not easily adapted to the hospitals' usual practices. Lacking provisions for reasonable adjustment by each institution, consent decrees to date have tended to favor the patients' claims to the point where the state is sometimes unable to meet the requirements. As a result, both doctors and patients lose. This problem can be remedied to some extent by increasing institutions' participation in the formation of the consent decree, helping to insure that the decree's provisions are reasonable and without oppressive costs (Stone, 1977).

DISCUSSION

Consent decrees have resolved some problems and brought some new problems to the psychiatric-legal arena. Despite the difficulties, however, consent decrees, and not formal law, constitute the essence of the right to treatment. More than 29 consent decrees have been issued in 15 states since 1972.[20] They have had a profound impact: minimum treatment standards have been enforced in many institutions, and billions of dollars have been appropriated to fulfill those requirements. The right to treatment, as it has been enforced through the consent decrees, remains one of the most controversial doctrines on the boundary of law and psychiatry.

Humane psychiatric treatment, cognizant of patients' rights, must be implemented with proper legal means, with measures that neither violate jurisdictional boundaries nor burden psychiatrists and the state. The makers of consent decrees have attempted to devise reasonable measures, but jurisdictional, implemental, and substantive problems have undercut their efforts. Institutional reform is necessary, but consent decrees have thus far had trouble striking the proper balance among the interests. Balancing among all the interests is a delicate

[20]*Wyatt* v. *Aderholt* (1972); *Wyatt* v. *Aderholt* (1974); *Wyatt* v. *Hardin* (1975); *Wyatt* v. *Ireland* (1979); *Scott* v. *Plante* (1976); *Mills* v. *Board of Education of the District of Columbia* (1975); *New York State Association for Retarded Citizens and Parisi* v. *Carey* (1975); *Horacek* v. *Exon* (1975); *Pennsylvania Association for Retarded Children* v. *Pennsylvania* (1972); *Gauthier* v. *Benson* (1975); *Mass. Association for Retarded Citizens* v. *Dukakis* (1975); *McEvoy* v. *Mahoney* (1974); *Ricci* v. *Greenblatt* (1972); *Abraham* v. *Winters* (1981); *Brewster* v. *Dukakis* (1978); *Colorado Association for Retarded Citizens* v. *Colorado* (1978); *Community Psychiatric Centers of Oregon, Inc.* v. *Grant* (1980); *Davis* v. *Baylor* (1976); *Dixon* v. *Harris* (1980); *Doe* v. *Klein* (1977); *Evans* v. *Washington* (1978); *Garrity* v. *Thomson* (1978); *Halderman* v. *Pennhurst State School* (1978); *In re Lee* (1972); *In re Shepard* (1979); *New man* v. *State of Alabama* (1972); *Romeo* v. *Youngberg* (1979); *Sidles* v. *Delaney* (1976); *States* v. *Collier* (1973); and *Wuori* v. *Zitnay* (1978).

process, and mistakes are inevitable. But with a careful consideration of the interests at stake, and with attention to standards that can be implemented, the right to treatment may rise to fulfill its promise.

The right to treatment remains without a constitutional foundation, although it has been expounded and expanded implicitly in numerous consent decrees and explicitly in some lower court decisions. The Supreme Court again has an opportunity to rule on the right to treatment in the case *Romeo* v. *Youngberg* (1981). Since the Court is likely to avoid the right-to-treatment issue and rule instead on a narrower ground or on other constitutional grounds, consent decrees may continue to be the primary forum for right-to-treatment cases. As the right to treatment has grown in impact through this judicially sanctioned, consensual process, executive and legislative branches of the government have taken increasing notice. With the fiscal difficulties facing many states, legislatures are becoming more reluctant to allocate funds for decreed reforms. The executive branch, too, has become chary of the judiciary's expansion into administrative matters and in the future will scrutinize and may eschew the quasi-contractual obligations of the consent-decree process.

In spite of the problems of the consent decrees, they have had the beneficial effect of shifting much needed resources into patient care. In that respect, the underlying doctrine of the right to treatment has been, is, and will continue to be worthwhile. With reasonable qualifications, that right can continue to be the agent of constructive reform.

Chapter 25 **The Least Restrictive Alternative: More About Less**
by Joel I. Klein, J.D.

INTRODUCTION

The legal concept of the least restrictive alternative is more often invoked than understood. This chapter examines the history of the legal concept and how it has been applied to the legal situations of mentally ill and retarded persons. Following a general legal introduction to the doctrine of the least restrictive alternative and its origins, the chapter reviews how the activist mental health bar used the doctrine in its strategy for accomplishing certain results in mental health and mental retardation litigation. An analysis of the judicial and legislative response to this litigation effort reveals a number of legal problems with the doctrine. In an era when courts are more conservative and economic constraints more pressing, the legal problems that remain are likely to become even more problematic in the ongoing quest for adequate treatment.

As the chapter develops, the author demonstrates how words and concepts have influenced the development of substantive doctrine.[1] Through the process of critical examination, the author also aims to demonstrate how and why the doctrine has had destructive effects on mental health care.

[1] For a more complete consideration of this influence, see Bachrach (1980).

HISTORICAL BACKGROUND

Like most legal doctrines, the doctrine of the least restrictive alternative did not spring full-blown from the head of any particular lawyer. It developed gradually, over a period of years. Its clearest statement came in 1960 in *Shelton* v. *Tucker*, a case that had nothing at all to do with mental health. *Shelton* involved an Arkansas statute which required teachers to identify all their political affiliations and memberships in organizations. The plaintiffs in *Shelton* argued that the statute infringed upon their First Amendment rights to freedom of association. The Supreme Court held that schools have an interest in assuring the loyalty of teachers, and in promoting a democratic, constitutional system of government. But the Court went on to declare that "even though the government purpose be legitimate and substantial, that purpose cannot be pursued by means that broadly stifle fundamental personal liberties when the end can be more narrowly achieved. The breadth of legislative abridgment must be viewed in the light of less drastic means for achieving the same basic purpose" (*Shelton* v. *Tucker*, 1960, 488). This declaration is the classic modern formulation of the least-restrictive-alternative doctrine.[2]

This doctrine has been applied in a number of different legal contexts, but its basic import is that the state may not use a sledgehammer when a scalpel will do. Thus, in one case, Mr. Justice Frankfurter wrote of a Michigan statute that banned all distribution of sexual literature on the ground that it was unsuitable reading matter for children, "Surely, this is to burn the house to roast the pig" (*Butler* v. *Michigan*, 1957, 383). The court applied the least-restrictive-alternative doctrine and instructed the state to tailor carefully the means it employed to meet the specific end it sought and to ensure that the means did not impinge upon other protected interests. If the state wished to keep certain materials from children, it must take care that the statute not reach so far as to keep those materials from adults as well.

Before examining how this doctrine became a central element in mental health litigation, a brief review of that litigation itself will be helpful. Between the time that Congress passed the Community Mental Health Centers Act in 1963 (P.L. 88–164, 77 *Stat.* 282) and the early 1970's, few of the hopes the Act reflected were actually fulfilled. A number of other developments seem to have distracted attention from deinstitutionalization and the mental health movement, among them President Kennedy's death, the civil rights movement generally, and, most important, the Vietnam war.

Whatever else history will ultimately show, the civil rights and Vietnam eras left at least one clear legacy—an activist judiciary, one less patient with the slow pace of legislative reform and less willing to await the formation of political consensus. In the mental health area, the earliest of these activist judges, along with Judge David Bazelon, was Frank Johnson of Alabama. Johnson, in *Wyatt* v. *Stickney*, was first to declare a constitutional right to treatment (*Wyatt* v. *Stickney*, 1971). *Wyatt* was in some ways a remarkable decision. It spawned a decade of

---

[2]The doctrine's roots go back as far as an 1821 case, *Anderson* v. *Dunn*, which concerned persons held in contempt of Congress for refusal to testify. The Supreme Court there ruled that, though Congress must have the power to assure witness compliance and respect for its procedures, it could only do so in the way that least affects individual liberties.

successful litigation by mental health lawyers. No other area of public interest law—except, perhaps, civil rights—has had such success. The reason for this success, from a doctrinal point of view, is quite interesting.

A legal right, as distinguished from a moral or ethical right, is one that is enforceable in court. Regrettably, there is no general legal right to services in our society. There is no right to good housing; there is no right to adequate food. Indeed, despite many legal challenges in the late 1960's, it now appears to be generally accepted that there is no federal constitutional right to any form of government largesse. The Constitution guarantees liberties, which the government may not restrict. By contrast, welfare benefits, housing, and food stamps are statutory, not constitutional, entitlements. Since the legislature created them, it may also restrict or eliminate them.

This right to treatment for the mentally ill, on the other hand, is a constitutional right. Judge Johnson reached this conclusion by reasoning that the state, in committing a person to an institution, deprives him or her of at least some personal liberty. But if the state deprives a person of liberty, it is obligated to fulfill its half of the bargain by providing treatment. Since liberty is protected by the Constitution, treatment becomes a constitutional imperative on the state once it has chosen to take a person's liberty away. When a person enters an institution voluntarily, however, he or she does not have a right to treatment from the state, because it was not the state that made the choice. Thus, though the distinction between "voluntary" and "involuntary" patients is often in fact illusory, it is a distinction that has had great significance in the legal arena.

THE LAWYERS' STRATEGIES

The *Wyatt* decision, declaring the constitutional right to treatment for involuntarily confined mental patients, led to court-ordered improvements in state mental hospitals. But these improvements left many people unsatisfied, especially the idealistic young lawyers who felt that existing mental hospitals could never be good enough. To them, the right-to-treatment decisions looked like judicial approbation of a system they thought should be scrapped altogether. But few of these people had any clinical experience, and no one came forward with a better proposal for caring for the mentally ill. Still, for many of the mental health lawyers of the early and middle 1970's, the right to treatment remained an "Uncle Tom" approach to mental health law.

The Mental Health Law Project, the public interest law firm that spearheaded the lawyers' movement, began in the middle 1970's to search for a new legal approach that would allow the courts to shift the locus of care from the hospital to the community. Here strategy became important: the movement had a cause, but it had no effective way to achieve its goals. After casting about for some time, lawyers finally seized on the doctrine of the least restrictive alternative.

Several factors motivated this decision. First, the Project relied upon some language from an opinion by Judge Bazelon of the United States Court of Appeals for the District of Columbia, in a 1966 case, *Lake* v. *Cameron*. An elderly woman had been committed to St. Elizabeth's Hospital not because she was mentally ill, but because she needed some form of custodial care and there was nowhere else for her to go. This troubled Judge Bazelon, who wrote in his opinion that the trial judge should at least have explored other alternatives before sending the woman to St. Elizabeth's. Bazelon's opinion is often misunderstood, but it is clear that he did not find a right to any alternative form of care. Rather, he directed trial judges to be more careful about committing persons to mental hospitals and more sensitive to available alternative resources. Chief Justice Warren Burger, then a judge on the Court of Appeals, wrote a blistering dissent declaring that the business of canvassing alternatives was for clinicians, not for courts (*Lake* v. *Cameron*, 1966, 663). It may turn out that Judge Burger, years after *Lake* v. *Cameron*, will, as Chief Justice, have the final word on the issue.

A second factor which led the Project to adopt the least-restrictive-alternative doctrine was the Ervin Act, a District of Columbia law which contained a broad declaration of patients' rights (Hospitalization of the Mentally Ill Act). Lawyers felt that, for an initial judicial foray, it might be better to test the claim under a statutory provision, rather than directly under the Constitution. Courts are always more receptive to basing new rights on statutory grounds; it looks more conservative, more judgelike. Project lawyers hoped that by winning a statutory decision they would build great momentum for a later suit seeking a constitutional ruling. In addition, a statutory decision would be insulated from Supreme Court review. At that time, the Burger Court was in full gear, and the lawyers feared that it would quickly overturn a radical ruling by a lower court. But statutory rulings involving state law (the District of Columbia is considered a state for these purposes) are not subject to Supreme Court review. Thus, if the Project won its case in the trial court, the only appeal would be to the Court of Appeals for the District of Columbia. That court, with Judge Bazelon, Judge Wright, and others, and minus Warren Burger, was quite liberal. It had already decided the *Lake* case, and had even expanded the doctrine in *Covington* v. *Harris*, a 1969 case challenging, under the least-restrictive-alternative doctrine, the placement of patients in a maximum security hospital.

The third factor the lawyers considered was that St. Elizabeth's Hospital in Washington had already indicated that at least half the 3,000 people there could properly be treated in the community and were being kept at St. Elizabeth's only because there were no places for them in the community. Thus, the Project could avoid the "clinical issue." They would not have to argue that a court should overrule the treatment staff's decision on appropriate placement. That argument could await another day. In this case, the goal, plain and simple, was to win a court order directing that 1,500 patients from St. Elizabeth's be discharged and given appropriate care in the community. Because St. Elizabeth's was a federal facility, there was some chance that federal money would help pay for the relief. No other general mental hospital is run by the federal government.

Finally, the best legal theory for linking these other factors together appeared to be the least-restrictive-alternative doctrine. The analogy to other cases involving the doctrine was simple, perhaps even a bit simplistic. Building on *Wyatt*, the lawyers argued that, though the government's purpose is treatment, commitment nonetheless infringes on liberty. But just as in other cases of state action, the government is obligated to accomplish its goal in the way that least interferes with liberty. Community placements were less restrictive because they kept patients in a more traditional setting. So the argument ran. The litigation took two years, but finally the Federal District Court accepted the argument and ordered both the District of Columbia and the United States to provide community placements for the 1,500 people (*Dixon* v. *Weinberger*, 1975).

The St. Elizabeth's decision was important in terms of a judicial "marketing strategy." Much in the law, like much in marketing, is done with mirrors. The repeated reflection of a single idea lends the idea an aura of legitimacy. Judges, in general, are conservative by instinct; Judge Johnson is an exception. But once a lawyer wins a ruling, he has a precedent to ask the next judge to follow. And judges find it much easier to follow precedent than to make it.

Legal strategies are not always implemented with great precision. The law is too complex, and there are too many lawyers, for anyone to control a complicated course of litigation as carefully as he or she might wish. But in the mental health arena, the lawyers planned their strategy carefully, and implemented it exceptionally well.

EXTENSIONS OF THE DOCTRINE

The earliest and easiest extension of the doctrine after the St. Elizabeth's case came in cases involving individual persons. In essence, the claim in each of those cases was that a named individual should not be in a hospital, but was there because there was no alternative. Such suits had the virtue of compelling only limited relief; solving the problem in any individual case required designing community placement for only one person. Unlike a large class action, the cost of compliance in such individual suits was relatively small. Thus, such cases rarely generated much controversy. They did, however, provide opportunities to expand the scope of the least-restrictive-alternative doctrine. Single patient lawsuits were fairly easy to manage, so several could be brought. And though such suits had fewer immediate ramifications than a successful class action suit would have had, they nevertheless enabled lawyers to build a formidable body of precedent. Moreover, individual suits were fairly easy to win, because the lawyer could choose a sympathetic plaintiff, someone for whom community care was clearly appropriate, and sue on his or her behalf. Not surprisingly, then, the lawyers won several such cases in the middle 1970's.

For all these reasons, the single-patient lawsuit was the ideal vehicle for the shift from a statutory to a constitutional claim of rights for the mentally ill. Only by accomplishing this shift, moreover, could lawyers get the least-restrictive-alternative doctrine applied nationwide. A federal constitutional right extends to the people of every state, whereas rights under a state statute extend only to the inhabitants of the particular state. To improve the treatment of the mentally ill without a constitutional claim of right would have required lawyers to bring—and win—separate statutory lawsuits in every state. And many state statutes gave the mentally ill fewer rights than the Ervin Act gave the mentally ill of the District of Columbia. Moreover, state courts generally are fiscally more conservative than the federal courts which hear constitutional claims, and so are less likely to look favorably on claims that will cost the state money. Thus, real progress could come about only after a successful federal lawsuit claiming constitutional rights for the mentally ill. This shift from statutory to constitutional rights was accomplished in the single-patient lawsuits of the middle 1970's.

Since a revolution cannot be won by shooting at one member of the enemy every six months, class action litigation was eventually necessary. Strategy again became crucial. In the middle 1970's there was a strong push toward "normalization" for the mentally retarded. At the same time, there was already some growing discontent with de-institutionalization of the mentally ill. Community care was at best a mixed blessing. Often it had proven to be little more than a euphemism for abandonment. Thus, the lawyers decided to seek expansion of the least-restrictive-alternative doctrine from individuals to classes of persons in the mental retardation area. Abandonment there was less likely to occur. At least some people believe that the mentally ill should be left alone, but there is universal agreement that the retarded need some form of care. And despite the differences in clinical needs, the legal principles governing the care of the retarded are quite similar to those governing the mentally ill.

Once again, the lawyers looked for target institutions, like Willowbrook in New York, which would disturb, if not disgust, the federal judges to whose attention they were brought. During the middle 1970's lawyers brought three or four such suits. Amazingly, in almost all of them the states refused to fight. Instead, they agreed to consent decrees which in effect provided for mass deinstitutionalization of the retarded. Living with those decrees has proven to be extremely difficult, and cases that started in the middle 1970's are still in dispute today. But from a political point of view, the initial acceptance of consent decrees provided tremendous momentum.

This background set the stage for what is, in the author's opinion, the most remarkable decision in this area—*Pennhurst*. The case involved a challenge to a mental retardation facility outside Philadelphia which housed over a thousand people and which had deteriorated in many ways and become outmoded. Four years after the suit commenced, the trial court held that the federal Constitution gave the same right to a least restrictive alternative which the court in the St. Elizabeth's case had found in the District of Columbia statute (*Halderman* v. *Pennhurst State School and Hospital*, 1977). As a result of this holding, and because most of the experts who testified considered normalization to be preferable to continued institutionalization, the 1,040 people living in Pennhurst were ordered discharged into community facilities. The hospital was to be phased out of operation and shut down. In addition, the court ruled that many other retarded people who were not confined to Pennhurst were entitled to community facilities as well. Though the decision had far-reaching implications, the judge made it look as though he was applying well-settled principles, citing case after case as precedent for the principle that the mentally ill had a constitutional right to the least restrictive alternative.

The decision was appealed to the Third Circuit Court of Appeals. (*Halderman* v. *Pennhurst State School and Hospital*, 1979). The court declined to rule on the constitutional question, but reached the same result as the lower court by relying on the Developmentally Disabled Assistance Act, which contains language providing that the developmentally disabled are entitled to treatment "in the setting that is least restrictive of the person's personal liberty" (The Developmentally Disabled Assistance Act, 42 *U.S. Code* §1060).

The court ordered quasi-judicial hearings for each of the 1,040 patients of Pennhurst to determine whether the community alternative was better or worse for them than hospitalization. Expressing a preference for the community, the court put the burden of proof on the parents to show that Pennhurst was better than the particular community placement which had been prepared but which remained untested. This decision was appealed to the Supreme Court, which in April 1981 reversed the Court of Appeals on its statutory finding of a right to the least restrictive alternative.[3] The case is now back in the Court of Appeals, which will have to address the issue it earlier declined to consider—whether there is a *constitutional* right to the least restrictive alternative.

The Doctrine Applied to the Form of Treatment: A Critique

Legal doctrines have a life of their own. Once the least restrictive alternative became widely accepted as a doctrine applicable in the mental health area, courts readily adapted it to new situations. Thus, in several recent cases, the doctrine has been used to challenge not the setting for treatment, but the form of treatment, e.g., is electroshock more or less restrictive than psychotropic medication? The virtue of this approach in practical terms, as a lawyer views it, is that the relief is not costly. The court need not order new facilities. It only need limit the use of certain medical practices.

No doubt some forms of treatment are misused in state hospitals, and the consequences are grave. Still, applying the least-restrictive-doctrine seems less sensible in this context than in that of selecting an appropriate facility. For whatever its merits, the doctrine is simply unworkable in this context. Take this purely hypothetical example. Assume that thirty days on medication is equivalent to fifty days of psychotherapy in a state hospital. Which is more restrictive? How does one even make those kinds of judgments? Such a hypothetical case is much less complicated than the real-world problems the courts face in this area. At best, courts will end up, despite their lack of training in the field, making clinical decisions about treatment for the mentally ill. Aside from the costs of such an approach, in terms of attendance at court hearings by both lawyers and mental health professionals, the devastating effect on clinical morale cannot be overstated. Still, if the doctrine of the least restrictive alternative applies in the mental health arena—as is now widely accepted—this result appears inevitable.

The Court of Appeals for the Third Circuit has just rendered a major decision, *Romeo* v. *Youngberg* (1980), upholding the application of the doctrine to the treatment setting. The nine judges who decided the *Romeo* case disagreed sharply on whether the doctrine of the least restrictive alternative should be extended from the initial decisions about confinement to subsequent decisions about treatment. The court's majority held that treatment decisions, like confinement decisions, were subject to the least-restrictive-alternative requirement. But four judges disagreed,[4] disputing the wisdom of extending what

[3]*Pennhurst State School and Hospital* v. *Halderman* (1981). The statutory finding had been based not on a state statute but on the federal statute and was therefore applicable to all the states.
[4]See *Romeo* v. *Youngberg* (1980) at 173 (Seitz, Chief Judge, concurring), at 182 (Aldisert, Circuit Judge, concurring), and at 186 (Garth, Circuit Judge, concurring).

was originally a First Amendment doctrine still further into the province of mental health.

First, they argued, it is hardly meaningful to speak of most forms of treatment as "restrictive". One form of treatment may be more or less "intensive" than another, but it only confuses the issue to speak of treatment decisions in terms that properly apply only to the threshold decision about whether to confine a person. Second, the initial decision to confine a mentally ill or retarded person has already been made on least-restrictive-alternative grounds. Thereafter, the issue should be which form of treatment is most appropriate and beneficial, not which form least "restricts" the patient. Third, they argued, though courts have a role to play in assuring that the state does not confine persons unnecessarily, they are hardly equipped to decide what form of treatment is acceptable in each, indeed any, case. When the courts try to make such decisions, they end up shackling mental health professionals in legal standards which are both too general to respond to the needs of individual patients and inappropriate as a basis for making what are properly medical decisions. Finally, even if the Constitution does require the least restrictive or intrusive form of treatment, how does anyone, least of all the courts, decide whether one medical procedure is less restrictive than another? Despite these objections, the majority fashioned complicated constitutional standards regulating the care and treatment of the institutionalized mentally retarded. The ultimate disposition of the issues in *Romeo* awaits the decision of the Supreme Court, which in May 1981 agreed to hear the case during its next term (*Youngberg* v. *Romeo,* 1981).

Thus, the circle is now complete. Twenty years ago the least-restrictive-alternative doctrine was unheard of in the mental health area. Now it is the fundamental judicial guidepost. Indeed, it has become so well accepted that Congress routinely writes it into major statutes, such as the Developmental Disabilities Assistance Act and the Mental Health Systems Act. State legislatures, too, have often adopted the doctrine in their commitment laws. Despite this universal acceptance, the greatest number of congressmen and state legislators likely could not say what the phrase "least restrictive alternative" means, and those who tried to define it probably could not agree among themselves on its meaning. Surely few would guess that it means what the records of the district court in *Pennhurst* or of the court of appeals in *Romeo* say it means.

In the author's opinion the doctrine is simply inappropriate for extension into the treatment area. At best, it is valuable as a symbol. Courts should, as Judge Bazelon instructed, remain alert to the possibility of alternative, more appropriate facilities. Likewise, clinicians should remain sensitive to the power of the treatments they use and to the possibility that moderation may in the end prove more helpful. Beyond that, however, the doctrine is ineffective at best and counterproductive at worst. Although it has been a painful lesson to learn, courts cannot in fact call forth the money necessary to provide alternative care systems. While courts make life easy and provide a sense of achievement for lawyers, in our society only legislatures can back up rights with funds. In the St. Elizabeth's case, for example, though the decision was handed down in 1975, almost no one has been placed in community programs. The District of Columbia and the federal government continue to refuse to pay the bill.

On a conceptual level, the premise of the least-restrictive-alternative doctrine is fundamentally flawed. Treatment and liberty cannot be viewed as independent variables, with one—treatment—kept constant, while the other—liberty—is titrated along a continuum of restrictiveness. The provision of treatment is ultimately a clinical matter. Where resources are available, we can assume that in most cases clinicians will use the most effective form of care. Despite the rhetoric, there is no sound basis for suggesting that psychiatrists needlessly confine people, or keep them in the hospital when available community facilities would do as well. Although the courts do lend legitimacy and propriety to the process by intervening, they also deflect resources from treatment into increased transactions costs. When applied to choice of treatment, moreover, the least-restrictive-alternative doctrine places a premium on safety, that is, on the least intrusive form of treatment, at the expense of efficacy. Though safety is always an important factor, it is never the only factor to be considered in treating serious illnesses. We should not conscript the mentally ill into an inferior form of treatment simply because they are involuntary patients. If they are committed, they should get the best available treatment, not merely the safest.

In the end, moreover, when courts use a doctrine that views treatment and liberty as independent variables, liberty will surely prosper to the detriment of treatment. For courts, like other social institutions, like to be effective. When it comes to protecting liberty, they do very well, because that is their constitutional role, and because protecting liberty does not cost money. When it comes to assuring treatment, on the other hand, courts are outside their depth. As a result, the least-restrictive-alternative doctrine has been most useful in limiting hospitalization, and it has left very needy people without any meaningful assistance.

FUTURE PROSPECTS

Until this year, the Supreme Court has largely stayed out of this area. In the one major case the Court heard, *O'Connor* v. *Donaldson* (1975), it sidestepped all the hard issues. Perhaps the Court, having realized that state hospitals and facilities for the mentally retarded were often shameful, consciously decided to leave the lower courts to attempt to deal with the problem themselves. Perhaps the Court has now decided that it has seen enough. Last term's *Pennhurst* decision, though decided on narrow statutory grounds, evidences the Court's clear disfavor with continuing judicial activism in this area.

This term the Court has already agreed to hear the *Romeo* case, concerning the least restrictive form of treatment, and the *Rogers* case, involving the right to refuse medication (*Okin* v. *Rogers*, 1981). The Court has an opportunity to use these cases to restore civil commitment to its place as a meaningful form of intervention aimed at providing treatment. Though the Court alone cannot provide the requisite funds, it could at least remove the needless impediments to effective treatment. Indeed, the *Romeo* case might provide an opportunity to establish a minimum set of requirements for the states. Now that the Court has adopted such an approach with respect to prisons, it could address the even greater need for minimum standards for civil commitment of the mentally ill. With the sanction of the Supreme

Court, adequate mental facilities might eventually rise to a higher rank among state and federal spending priorities.

Moving beyond those minimum requirements will not be easy. Even though the shortcut of judicial intervention may no longer be available, the victories in legislatures and in the arena of public opinion, though difficult to win, would be more meaningful and more enduring. Progress does always appear to come too slowly. Even after two hundred years, we are a young and impatient society. We will mature when we come to realize that a house—unlike a revolution—must be built one brick at a time. The goal for each of us should be to move at least one brick.

Chapter 26 The Right to Refuse Treatment
by Thomas G. Gutheil, M.D.

INTRODUCTION

The newest right detected within the shadows (*penumbrae*) of the Constitution is the right to refuse treatment. Usually equating medications with treatment, this right seems the most problematic for clinicians on several grounds. First, it represents a swing in the legal pendulum. Not long ago (*Whitree* v. *State,* 1968), a New York court held that the proper standard of care for hospitalized psychiatric patients required physicians to override refusals of treatment. Second, the right to *treatment,* a concept which most clinicians support, may be totally vitiated by the right to *refuse* treatment. When right thus contends against right, the clinician is understandably bewildered. Third, many clinicians feel it violates basic ethical and clinical principles when a patient is hospitalized involuntarily for an illness which later manifests itself symptomatically in treatment refusal, thwarting its own treatment (Appelbaum and Gutheil, 1980). The result is that the patient is hospitalized indefinitely, "rotting with his rights on" (Appelbaum and Gutheil, 1979).

Most serious clinicians and legal scholars would probably agree that rights are properly balanced in two types of scenarios. In the first, the patient is voluntary, nondangerous, and competent. This patient, of course, has every right to accept or reject treatment and, in turn, when he or she rejects proffered treatment, the patient may safely be discharged or referred elsewhere. The second scenario entails an acute, danger-producing emergency. In this case, involuntary interventions, such as medication or seclusion, may or must be performed for the protection of all concerned, regardless of the status or competence of the patient at the moment of emergency.

The controversy over the right to refuse treatment focuses pragmatically on a third scenario—when the nondangerous patient, who is not producing an acute emergency, refuses treatment on incompetent, e.g., delusional, grounds and is too ill to be humanely discharged. Examples include the raving psychotic, but nondangerous, patient; the profoundly yet quietly depressed patient who feels delusionally unworthy of treatment; or the paranoid patient whose subtle delusional incompetence may require a keen critical assessment to detect. These are the patients about whom the controversy swirls. Even greater controversies have arisen about the proper legal procedures for implementing the right to refuse treatment and for carrying forth its exceptions. But before this latter topic can be reviewed, it is important to consider the probable parentage of this newborn right.

The Covert Issue

It is likely that a covert issue confounding the right to refuse treatment is quality of care (Appelbaum and Gutheil, in press).[1] Since quality of care often does not lend itself readily to direct judicial remedies,* the issue is now being thrashed out in the arena of rights litigation simply because that arena appears most accessible to the courts. It is, metaphorically, as if there were a drought on the land, and the courts, being unable to make it rain, were attempting a remedy within their compass by forbidding the drinking of water. The thirst of the citizenry, of course, is not alleviated.

More literally, since money cannot readily be extracted from legislatures to raise the quality of care in state hospitals, the issue of quality is wrenched into the shape of constitutional questions to bring the matter within the possible scope of judicial remedy. To avert some of the abuses so often found in state hospitals, the courts attempt to protect some patients, under some circumstances, from having medication forced upon them. The need of most state patients for good treatment, like the metaphoric thirst of the citizenry, is not alleviated (Appelbaum and Gutheil, in press).

Support for this hypothesis about the parentage of the right to refuse treatment may be drawn from the curious and extravagant way several courts acted and from the fact that legal and judicial discussions of the right so rapidly shift to arguments over the actual delivery of care above certain minimum standards. Ironically, by using this right to try to solve the problem, the courts risk obliterating the very good for which they strive. An examination of issues and cases in point reveals why this is so.

COMMITMENT, COMPETENCE, AND TREATMENT REFUSAL

While historically a committed patient was considered *de facto* incompetent to make many life decisions, the thrust of most modern legislation and litigation is to presume the committed patient competent unless there is evidence to the contrary. Simultaneously, the legal view of standards for commitment has shifted more and more to the issue of dangerousness and away from the issue of need for care. Thus, the committed patient is mentally ill, dangerous, and competent by law unless proven otherwise.

If a person is found incompetent to make a certain decision, of course, e.g., to consent to treatment, a substitute decision maker must be found. In the past, a number of persons have filled that role, from kings to next of kin, to physicians, to guardians, to courts (Gutheil and Appelbaum, 1980).

---

[1]While some authorities propose an abstract and universal right to refuse treatment, independent of *any* factual circumstances, it is even then unclear whether knowledge of the notoriously terrible conditions in some hospitals does not color, even unconsciously, the reasoning about this right.

*Preceptor's note: For a contrary opinion see Mills' chapter, "The Right to Treatment," in this Part.

In reality, while they are often associated, the issues of voluntariness, illness, dangerousness, need for treatment, competence, and acceptance of treatment are not simply superimposable, but have numerous points of nonalignment as well as overlap. Failing to grasp this reality, however, the courts treat voluntary patients, for example, as if they were automatically not dangerous simply because they are not committed. Actually, many voluntary patients cannot safely leave the hospital.

Another legal distinction is drawn between hospitalization and treatment, usually medication, in the hospital. In 1974, an important law review article noted that an intent for a patient to be treated was inherent in the concept of commitment and that commitment without treatment was, in essence, jailing without a crime ("Developments in the Law," 1974). Recently, however, the right to privacy has come into ascendance (Gutheil and Appelbaum, 1982), synthesized from several amendments to the Constitution via certain landmark cases.[2] As one consequence, while clinicians see hospitalization and medication merely as individual elements of a total treatment plan for a suffering patient, the judiciary has separated these elements and even caused them to conflict. The courts see involuntary medication as an infringement on the rights to bodily privacy and involuntary hospitalization as a "quarantine"[3] inspired by the dangerousness of mentally ill persons. Thus, on the one hand, the courts send patients involuntarily to hospitals and, on the other, allow them to refuse the very treatment which is not only their sole justification for being there, but often their only hope of getting well enough to leave. Clinicians are understandably dismayed.

Judicial Fantasies About Medication

An important but often neglected dimension of this controversy is the manner in which certain courts conceptualize medication. Lacking any medical training and apparently strongly influenced by the negative press of certain members of the mental health bar, judges appear to lose sight of the beneficial, restitutive, and normalizing effects of medications. They treat medications as invaders, intruders, transformers, or preventers of free thought and speech (*Rogers* v. *Okin,* 1979). The drugs are, in short, a necessary evil, grudgingly allowed to slip through the bars of judicial restraint to assault the patient at the physician's behest. This view of medications explains, though may not excuse, the strange remarks often found in opinions in cases relevant to the right to refuse treatment. From *Rogers* v. *Okin* (1979) come two such remarks:

> Because the drug's purpose is to reduce the level of psychotic thinking, it is virtually undisputed that they are mind-altering...

> Whatever powers the Constitution has granted our government, involuntary mind control is not one of them. The fact that mind control takes place in a mental institution in the form of medically sound

---

[2]See *Griswold* v. *Connecticut* (1965); *Doe* v. *Bolton* (1973); and *Mackey* v. *Procunier* (1973).

[3]This term was employed by federal judge Joseph Tauro in one of the most problematic of all cases in this area, *Rogers* v. *Okin* (1979): "The involuntary patient was committed *primarily* to quarantine that patient from the outside world, hopefully going to be able to be treated and cured" (emphasis added). Note the view of treatment as quite secondary to confinement.

treatment of mental disease is not, in itself, an extraordinary circumstance warranting an unsanctioned intrusion on the integrity of a human being.

Two other examples come from *In the Matter of Guardianship of Richard Roe III* (1981):

... the impact of the chemicals upon the brain is sufficient to undermine the foundations of personality.

Although ... the intended effects of antipsychotic drugs are extreme, their unintended effects are frequently devastating and often irreversible.

THE SIGNIFICANT CASES

While many legal cases in recent years have dealt with the right to refuse treatment, we must here relinquish exhaustive review in favor of digests outlined for heuristic purposes. Four cases illustrating legal approaches to the right to refuse treatment are presented in order of increasing clinically based reasonableness rather than according to other possible criteria. In all cases, we must regrettably give short shrift to the actual plaintiffs, defendants, and details in order to highlight the basic principles and assumptions of greatest importance to the subject.

In the Matter of Guardianship of Richard Roe III (1981), a case decided by the Massachusetts Supreme Judicial Court, continues a series of rulings by that court through which runs a single thematic thread, namely, the arrogation of psychiatric and general medical decision making to the courts and away from physicians or even legal guardians.[4] Though it presents many extremely problematic issues, the *Roe* decision is particularly noteworthy for establishing two major points on the way to its ultimate ruling that only the courts may decide whether an incompetent outpatient who is refusing medication may receive the antipsychotic drugs involuntarily. Aside from the rulings, the opinion first is noteworthy for drawing so heavily on the negative concepts about medication noted above and for virtually ignoring sound medical information in favor of a hopelessly biased legal source (Plotkin, 1977). Second, it is noted for demanding that the judge use a so-called substitute judgment, in which the judge assesses what the incompetent person would decide about medication if he or she were competent. The six elaborated factors it supplies as guidelines would, in actual practice with real patients and real judges, in all likelihood be quite unworkable. Like other courts, moreover, the Massachusetts court fails to address some important implications. While the question is, "What would the incompetent person choose if competent?" the choice—medication—is more likely than not to be the agent of restoring the very competence lost through mental illness in the first place (Appelbaum and Gutheil, 1979).

Another Massachusetts case, *Rogers* v. *Okin* (1979), exhaustively reviewed elsewhere,[5] is a right-to-refuse-medication class action suit by patients in an unusual situation. While the patients came from a state

[4]See, for example, *Superintendent of Belchertown State School* v. *Saikewicz* (1977); *Doe* v. *Doe* (1979); and *In the Matter of Spring* (1980).
[5]See Appelbaum and Gutheil (1979); Gutheil and Appelbaum (1982); Appelbaum and Gutheil (1980); Gutheil and Appelbaum (1980); Gutheil (1980); Ford (1980); Mills (1980); and Mills (1981).

hospital that was typical in its dilapidation, poor condition, and bureaucratically strangled funding, hiring, and operation, the hospital was most atypical in that its medical staff were residents and faculty from leading local medical schools, backed by formidable consultative resources. The case is, for present purposes, noteworthy on four grounds: (1) the curious distortions of psychopharmacology noted in the previous section; (2) built upon these distortions, a right to refuse drawn not only from the right of privacy but also from First Amendment freedom of speech;[6] (3) the use of guardians as decision makers for incompetent patients; and (4) a significant narrowing of the definition of emergency. The definition narrowed the situation permitting involuntary treatment regardless of competence to acute dangerousness in persons and excluded suffering, deterioration, and other clinically based grounds for treatment. Again, the distorted view of the use of medications appears to lead to a police-powers level of protection for the patient (for further discussion, see Stone, 1981).

The opinion on appeal challenged a number of holdings of *Rogers,* including the use of guardians and the narrow definition of emergency (*Rogers* v. *Okin,* 1980). The case was remanded, however, and the final ruling had not appeared at the time of this writing. The Supreme Court has granted *certiorari* on this case, moreover, and it is possible that it will be heard together with the next case example. The next example was of this writing still awaiting decision by the Third Circuit Court of Appeals.

Rennie v. *Klein* (1979) is a New Jersey case in which the quality of care issue noted at the outset served as the obvious mainspring of the matter (Appelbaum and Gutheil, in press). The case has several noteworthy facets. First, the issue of the inpatient's competence is addressed at a quasi-judicial procedure by an independent psychiatrist outside the line of clinical responsibility. Second, the psychiatrist is assigned four guidelines on which to make formal determinations. In essence, these are (1) how dangerous the patient is, (2) whether, in effect, the patient is competent to decide about treatment, (3) whether the treatment proposed is the least restrictive alternative, and (4) how severe are the risks of permanent side effects. A third component of the case was invisible but crucial—Judge Brotman's exhaustive pretrial exploration, fact-finding, consultation, and amassing of expert opinion. A fourth facet was the ironic dilemma posed by the ruling that compliant patients will get what treatment there is, while patients who refuse will have their medication regimens reviewed by an independent expert. Thus, it might be plausibly argued that for patients in New Jersey state hospitals, the only way to obtain good treatment, or at least have its quality reviewed, is to refuse it! This case best highlights the problem noted earlier of seizing a quality of care issue by a constitutional handle: the compliant majority of patients remain unaided (see Appelbaum and Gutheil, in press). Above all of these facets, however, the case's paramount significance lies in its return of medical decisions to medicine, a theme elaborated in the fourth case example.

<hr/>

[6]This is the "involuntary mind control" conceit earlier noted. Somehow, Judge Tauro managed to ignore the role of medications in restoring, liberating and even permitting that normal mentation which has been blocked by illness—a point clear in the psychiatric literature. Compare, for example, Meadow (1975); Hymowitz and Spohn (1980); and Spohn et al. (1975).

A Utah case, *A.E. and R.R.* v. *Mitchell* (1980), represents inter alia an exception to the current trend in law separating committability and competence. A newly amended Utah statute included a specific determination of competency to consent to treatment as one of a list of criteria for committability. This novel approach is readily distinguishable from and superior to the old legal view that commitment implies incompetence. A separate judicial ruling serves as the due process permitting involuntary treatment, a determination made even before commitment occurs.[7] The opinion in question entailed a legal test that affirmed the constitutionality of the statute. It held that since the incompetence of the committed patient had already been judicially determined, the treating psychiatrist could decide on the treatment according to the usual medical criteria, and additional decisions or procedures would be redundant.

This ruling evinces the greatest faith in psychiatry and appropriately justifies commitment by coupling it with treatment. However, the patient who was either dangerous or sorely in need of treatment, yet competent to consent to medication, could not be committed in that jurisdiction. The outcome of such an instance and the actual effects on social policy are unclear.

SUMMARY AND CONCLUSIONS

The foregoing review must be viewed as a still snapshot of a rapidly and actively evolving process. As the law evolves and as reviews are written, we can simultaneously see caring as well as abusive psychiatric treatment, personnel, and settings. The understanding of disease and its treatment itself is evolving. We see the arbitrary capriciousness of some courts juxtaposed with the objective realism of others. But first and foremost stands out the need of vast numbers of our patients for good care. As clinicians we must keep our eyes ever on the suffering patient before us, a person whom no amount of "legalizing" will succor. The right to refuse treatment is, at base, a clinical rather than a legal question.[8] Through research that gets the facts, through education that spreads the facts, and through advocates to fight with those facts in the determinative arenas (Stone, 1979), we may return the entire matter of the right to refuse treatment to its actual base—the needs of the patient.

Chapter 27 **The Role Of The Psychiatrist In The Criminal Justice System**
by Seymour L. Halleck, M.D.

Psychiatrists play diverse and important roles in the criminal justice system. This chapter examines the practice of forensic psychiatry and how psychiatrists work with police officers, provide services to defendants in jail, advise in the determination of defendants' competency

[7]In many respects, the Utah criteria are reminiscent of Stone's "thank you" theory of commitment, *q.v.* Stone (1976, chapter 4).
[8]See *Whitree* v. *State* (1968); Appelbaum and Gutheil (1980); Appelbaum and Gutheil; (1979); Gutheil and Appelbaum (1982); Rachlin (1975); and Rachlin (1974).

or insanity, assist in the sentencing process, and work both with the criminally insane and with imprisoned criminals. In the course of this examination, the chapter reviews two legal concepts which are fundamental to forensic psychiatry—incompetency to stand trial and the insanity defense.

PSYCHIATRISTS AND THE POLICE

Psychiatrists frequently play educational roles in their work with police officers. In their responsibility for maintaining an orderly and peaceful community, police officers work to prevent crime and disruption as well as to apprehend offenders. These responsibilities require that they encounter many emotionally disturbed individuals. Where disturbed individuals have no close family ties, the policeman is often the person called to help. Officers deal with many people who may not have done anything illegal but who are behaving strangely. Moreover, when a citizen is doing something illegal and also appears to be emotionally disturbed, the officer must quickly decide whether to arrest that person or to bring the person to a hospital. It is often the police officer who initiates a civil commitment. Officers also intervene in many domestic conflicts. They may have the opportunity to resolve highly charged conflicts through on-the-scene counseling and crisis management. Since they are at high risk of being injured in the course of dealing with domestic conflict, they have good reason to be interested in improving their psychological skills (Teplin et al., 1980).

Psychiatrists who have educated police to interact more effectively with mentally ill people or to improve their skills in family counseling have found a friendly and receptive audience. Police officers respond positively to a range of educational techniques, including lectures, group discussions, films, and even consciousness-raising sessions, i.e., a small group meeting with a group of gays. Almost all psychiatrists who have worked with police in these ways have reported surprisingly little difficulty in establishing rapport. Indeed, they have discovered much in common. Both psychiatrists and police officers have to learn to manage the substantial power which society entrusts to them and to deal with public misperceptions of their professional roles (Symonds, 1972).

A second role psychiatrists play in police departments is diagnosing and treating disturbed officers. The incidence of depression and alcoholism is high among police officers, whose work is unusually stressful and often goes unappreciated. Psychiatrists who do this kind of work must have a clear understanding about what they may be expected to reveal to the department. The officer who is examined must also have an accurate understanding as to how much confidentiality he has. Similar considerations apply to therapy. Before any therapeutic interaction begins, both the officer and the psychiatrist must be aware of any circumstances in which confidentiality will be compromised.

In a third role, psychiatrists are employed by police departments to screen people who apply for work. Departments want to screen out those whose emotional disturbances might lead to erratic responses or might impair their capacity to adapt to the daily stresses of police work. While public safety needs make it difficult to do controlled studies as to the efficacy of such screening, behavioral scientists who have provided this service and police administrators who have used it view it as highly desirable and useful.

Finally, a few psychiatrists have involved themselves in the process of crime detection by trying to develop psychological profiles of the kind of individual who is likely to have committed a certain type of crime. This is a highly speculative art. While a few may have some special talent for it, generally it falls outside the area of psychiatric expertise.

PSYCHIATRY IN JAILS

A person who has just been booked and locked up in a local jail obviously experiences a crisis. Abruptly taken from a situation of freedom and relative comfort to one of massive restraint and deprivation, a person has no clear sense of when this ordeal will end. The prisoner may anticipate an early release on bail but sometimes fears or knows that bail is impossible. A person in jail may also face a long prison sentence. Many of those who are brought to jail were emotionally disturbed long before the arrest. Some arrive intoxicated with alcohol or other drugs. If they are dependent on these agents, their withdrawal is abrupt. The incidence of depression, massive anxiety, psychosis, and suicide in jails is very high. All of this is, of course, made worse by the dismal, oppressive, and unsafe atmosphere of most jails.

Those few psychiatrists who work in jails are in an ideal position to provide considerable help to people in crisis. Many recently apprehended inmates need detoxification. Others need medication for anxiety or depression, as well as treatment for physical disorders. The psychiatrist in such situations can provide treatment without facing many of the cumbersome ethical problems which arise in other psychiatric interventions in the criminal justice process. However, even in these therapeutic efforts it is essential for the psychiatrist to be aware of the patient-defendant's Fifth Amendment privilege against self-incrimination.

INCOMPETENCY TO STAND TRIAL

Psychiatrists have a part to play in judicial determinations of accused persons' competency to plea bargain, to be sentenced or executed, or, most often, to stand trial. According to the common law, an accused person is incompetent when he or she is so emotionally disturbed as to be mentally "absent" from the courtroom and unable properly to assume the role of defendant. This concept reflects the court's fundamental concern for fairness. An offender, because of mental illness, may be compromised in the ability to recall events, to produce evidence, to testify in his or her own defense, or to confront hostile witnesses. Disturbance may prevent the offender from projecting a proper demeanor to the court and maintaining an effective psychological presence. The Supreme Court has consistently ruled that the conviction of a legally incompetent defendant violates that person's right to due process (*Pate* v. *Robinson,* 1966; *Drope* v. *Missouri,* 1975).

Once the court determines that an individual charged with a crime cannot be tried, it must find some legal resolution. The alternatives are to drop the charges, to treat the person as an outpatient until competency is regained, or, particularly if an offender is believed to be dangerous, to restrain the person while treatment is attempted. In practice, most defendants found incompetent to stand trial used to be confined indefinitely until their competency was restored. Recent constitutional and statutory changes have produced radical reforms in many states.

The judge, the defense attorney, or the prosecuting attorney may request an examination for competency. Judges make such requests in the interest of fairness and to avoid being overruled on appeal. Some judges also view the competency examination as a means of getting additional psychiatric information about the defendant.

The defense attorney may be convinced that the client is incompetent and should not be tried at the scheduled time. Or the attorney may ask for a competency examination simply to obtain a psychiatric examination to use later as a basis for a plea of not guilty by reason of insanity. The defense attorney may also view the incompetency plea as a means of helping the client "beat the rap" by being civilly committed or released or by doing "easier time" in a hospital rather than in a prison. Often the defense attorney requests the competency examination as a means of delaying the trial until the vengeful emotions of prosecution witnesses dissipate so that the defendant may incur a less severe penalty.

The prosecuting attorney may ask for a competency examination to avoid having a conviction overruled on a later appeal, or to realize a genuine wish not to convict an incompetent defendant of a crime. The prosecuting attorney, like the defense attorney, however, may also wish to postpone the trial. When a prosecuting attorney's case is weak, having the defendant temporarily institutionalized while competency is determined at least reassures the public that an allegedly dangerous person is being kept off the streets.

In many jurisdictions a request for a competency examination still results in the patient being sent to a hospital for the criminally insane, where the examination procedure may last from two to three months. During this time the patient is deprived of the opportunity to plea bargain and usually of bail as well. At their discretion courts may allow examinations for competency to take place in outpatient settings, but this is not the customary practice.

Once the defendant's examination is completed, he or she returns to court, where psychiatric reports are used to determine whether the person is competent to stand trial. In the majority of instances, the defendant is found competent. If a determination of incompetency is made, however, the patient is almost automatically sent back to the hospital for the criminally insane. Until 1973, when a Supreme Court rule established limits on how long incompetent offenders could be detained in hospitals for the criminally insane, incompetent defendants who had never been convicted of a crime faced prolonged incarceration (McGarry et al., 1973).

Some psychiatrists and attorneys are concerned that the incompetency plea threatens the defendant's right to a speedy trial and removes the opportunity for plea bargaining and bail (Halpern, 1975). Others fear that the incompetency plea allows defendants who are not really sick to "beat the rap" (Burt and Morris, 1972). The few studies that have been done suggest that defendants who are found incompetent spend about the same amount of time under detention as those who are tried (Steadman, 1979).

In 1960 the Supreme Court ruled unanimously that the test for competency should be "whether the defendant possesses sufficient present ability to consult with his lawyer with a reasonable degree of rational understanding and whether he has an actual as well as a factual understanding of the proceedings against him" (*Dusky* v. *United States,* 1960). The majority of states have created statutes which, although they vary slightly in wording, have criteria that are basically equivalent to those created by the Supreme Court. The criteria for incompetency, while clearly related to the mental capacities of the defendant, do not necessarily require that a defendant be mentally ill. A person may lack the ability to consult with an attorney because of any physical or situational handicap which impairs communication. Whether the defendant understands the nature of the charges and is able to assist counsel in preparing a defense is as much a legal as a psychological determination. Only the attorney can determine how much assistance the defendant will need to give on such issues as direct examination of friendly witnesses or cross-examination of adverse witnesses.

Psychiatrists become involved in competency examinations either as part of their work in hospitals where such examinations are routinely done or when they are hired by the defense or prosecution. The psychiatrist who works for an institution for the criminally insane or who is court appointed must be aware that although he seems to be in a neutral position, his testimony may have consequences that the defendant will not welcome. It is always imperative that the psychiatrist explain the purpose of his examination to the defendant.

In preparing for testimony, the psychiatrist should try to determine how present emotional abnormalities may compromise the defendant's capacity to be aware of legal defenses, to relate in a cooperative manner with attorneys so that legal strategies can be planned, and to understand court procedures, the charges against him or her, and the roles of all the participants in the adversarial process. In addition, the psychiatrist should make predictions as to the possibility of unmanageable behavior during the trial and the defendant's capacity to seek self-interested rather than self-destructive outcomes in the process of litigation. (A depressed person who is undeserving of punishment, for example, may act in such a way as to increase the probability of being punished.) The psychiatrist may also help the court by relating any extant mental disability to impairments in the defendant's cooperation or understanding.

The ultimate determination of competency to stand trial is a legal matter which the court decides. (One critical example of this fact is that the court may not view amnesia as a criterion of incompetence even where such loss of memory is likely to be genuine.) Like any expert witness, the psychiatrist should not be committed to any particular outcome of the competency hearing, but should assume the posture of a servant of the court with an opinion that may be accepted or rejected.

As well as having a sense of the limitations of their contributions, psychiatrists must bear in mind the need to protect the defendant's legal interests. The psychiatrist who examines the defendant at the request of the court should make certain that the defense attorney consents to the examination. Patients should be examined as soon as possible and reports promptly sent to the referring court. The psychiatrist should inform the defendant's attorney if it appears that the defendant is unlikely to regain competency, in order to allow the attorney to find the most appropriate disposition.

Although heated arguments rage on as to whether the plea should be abolished, psychiatrists will continue to be asked to play roles in incompetency proceedings. This will, for some time, be an important role in forensic psychiatry.

THE INSANITY DEFENSE

Throughout most of the history of psychiatry's involvement with the criminal justice system, our most passionate and certainly our most popularized involvement has been with the issue of how the criminal's responsibility and punishability might be mitigated by insanity. The insanity defense has drawn the attention and energy of some of our best scholars in psychiatry, psychology, and law. While the insanity defense has fascinating philosophical and social implications, it does not directly affect the lives of many defendants. It is rarely used, and it is even more rarely successful.

Only a few psychiatrists will particiapte in an insanity trial during their careers. Nonetheless, all psychiatrists should know something about the issues involved, because they influence how we conceptualize the problems of mental illness and criminality.

Our legal system assumes that most individuals who violate the criminal law choose to do so. Ordinary offenders are assumed to possess free will. Because they have chosen to do wrong, they are deemed appropriate subjects for punishment. For centuries, however, Anglo-American law has also provided a means for excusing from punishment offenders who are believed to be so mentally disordered as to be unable to make law-abiding choices. Since such offenders are viewed as lacking free will, they are not held responsible for their criminal actions. In practice, their exculpation is accomplished through the use of the insanity defense, which requires that they be adjudicated so deranged as to lack free will. The successful insanity defense completely relieves the defendant of all responsibility for the crime. It does not usually, however, allow the person to go free. Other legal mechanisms outside the scope of the doctrine of culpability are generally invoked to incapacitate the individual who is found insane.

The insanity defense operates in an all-or-nothing manner. The defendant who pleads successfully is not guilty and has not in theory committed a crime. The unsuccessful defendant is likely to be punished, and even if there is powerful evidence as to the severity of mental illness, it may have little mitigating influence. The insanity defense draws a sharp line between different classes of offenders. It distinguishes the few extremely disturbed defenders who allegedly lack free will from the vast mass of offenders whose crimes are believed to be the product of choice.

Other legal mechanisms through which mentally disturbed offenders receive partial relief from criminal punishment most often result in a reduced sentence. These mechanisms are governed by the legal concept of partial responsibility. When this concept is invoked, the defendant is not found to be so disordered as to be totally absolved of responsibility, but is viewed as sufficiently disturbed to be less responsible than the "normal" offender.

Two doctrines of partial responsibility have been developed. *Diminished capacity* allows a defendant who is so mentally impaired as to be incapable of entertaining a *mental element** required for a particular crime to be found guilty of a similar but lesser crime and thereby to receive less punishment. *Diminished responsibility* allows the judge or jury to lessen the severity of punishment where the criminal act seems related to severe mental impairment. In some states the court is required by statute to consider a lesser sentence when certain crimes are committed by emotionally disturbed offenders. In most states the judge has the prerogative of using information regarding the offender's mental status at the time of the crime to reduce the severity of punishment. Recent Supreme Court decisions have directed trial courts to consider the defendant's mental abnormality and other psychological data as mitigating or aggravating factors in capital murder cases. The avoidance of the death penalty on the basis of psychiatric mitigating factors is an extreme example of the use of the doctrine of diminished responsibility.

The same rationale underlies both the insanity defense and the two partial responsibility doctrines: to the extent that the defendant is mentally ill and incapable of choice, the moral and utilitarian purposes of the law are not served by punishing him or her. There is no moral justification for punishing those who are incapable of obeying the law. It can also be argued that the punishment of an insane person who cannot choose does not serve the goals of either specific or general deterrence. Punishing a nonresponsible defendant who cannot make choices will not deter private vengeance. Nor will the punishment of a nonresponsible defendant provide a moral lesson for the public. The other goals of the criminal justice system, incapacitation and rehabilitation, can be served by invoking doctrines other than culpability and punishment.

The offender found not guilty by reason of insanity is technically not guilty of having committed a crime. In most jurisdictions, however, automatic commitment procedures are invoked at the point that the finding is made. Even if the person does not meet the usual requirements for civil commitment, he or she may still be sent to a hospital for the criminally insane. Where the mentally disordered offender is felt to be dangerous to others, the successful plea does not guarantee his or her freedom. Recent litigation would allow the person found guilty by reason of insanity to be freed when not committable under the ordinary civil statutes of the state (see, for example, *State* v. *Krol,* 1975). Such efforts lead to more efforts to argue the insanity defense as well as to new legislation requiring commitment for the person on grounds of insanity.

Insanity is a legal, not a medical, term. It describes a legal excusing condition which has two elements, some form of mental illness and some form of incapacity related to that illness. In most insanity tests it is incapacity rather than mental illness which is the more critical excusing condition. Insanity should never be equated with *mental illness* or *psychosis.* Many severely disturbed patients will not be found insane because they do not have the specific incapacities the court views as excusing conditions. One reason insanity is not equated with mental illness and is not defined in medical terms is to allow the judge and jury

*Preceptor's note: The classic legal conception of a crime involves two basic elements, the act (*actus reus*) and the mental element (*mens rea*). Both elements are necessary to establish a crime.

to consider moral issues in ascribing responsibility and guilt. The ultimate question, whether the offender is sane or insane, is always left to the judge or jury.

The Psychiatrist's Role

Psychiatric testimony in insanity cases serves three purposes: first, it supplies the court with facts concerning the offender's illness; second, it presents informed opinion concerning the nature of that illness; and third, it furnishes a basis for deciding whether the illness made the patient legally insane at the time of the crime under that jurisdiction's standards of insanity. The first two functions are relatively straightforward. The third is much more difficult.

For practical purposes, there are only two standards currently used in this country, the McNaughten Rule and the American Law Institute (ALI) Rule. The McNaughten Rule is essentially a cognitive test. The accused person's defense is simply, "I did not know what I was doing," or, "I did not know that what I did was wrong." The ALI test incorporates an emotional as well as a cognitive element. "I didn't know what I was doing or that it was wrong," *and* "I couldn't help it" (Brooks, 1973). The American Law Institute test allows a broader range of excusing conditions. Most psychiatrists also find it somewhat easier to relate their psychiatric knowledge to the ALI standard. The psychiatrist who testifies in an insanity case must know which test is being employed. He or she must try to provide testimony which will enable the judge or jury to determine whether insanity, as defined by the criteria of that test, is present or absent.

The psychiatrist may become involved in the insanity case as a defense witness, as a prosecution witness, or as an impartial witness appointed by the court. There are some special technical problems the psychiatrist encounters in preparing an insanity examination. The psychiatrist examines the defendant only after the crime has occurred, and thus has no firsthand knowledge of the patient's mental status at the time of the crime. By the time the psychiatrist conducts the examination, the defendant may already have been found competent to stand trial, and the acute condition alleged to have been presented at the time of the crime may have long since disappeared. Determining what a person's mental status was months or years ago is even more difficult when the patient's recollection of events is not good, or when the patient is motivated to distort facts. Often the psychiatrist must rely heavily on information obtained from others. It is helpful to examine the police report of the crime and to interview or read the statements of people who were in close contact with the patient preceding, during, or following the crime. Relatives can provide useful objective information concerning the patient's past history.

Participation in the insanity defense requires that the psychiatrist be extremely well prepared. To be a good witness, the psychiatrist must review every report available about the defendant and must interview all significant individuals who are available. He or she must spend many hours with the defendant reconstructing the details of the illness and the criminal event and how the illness and crime might be related.

The insanity defense engenders much controversy. Many attorneys, psychiatrists, and legislators feel that it should be modified or abolished. Four major positions are taken within the psychiatric profession.

(1) Some psychiatrists believe that the insanity defense should be abolished.

(2) Some believe that the standards to which testimony is directed should be modified so as to be more encompassing of psychiatric concepts. The goal of this group is to bring definitions of insanity closer to definitions of severe mental illness.

(3) Some psychiatrists believe that the insanity defense is currently used quite reasonably in this country, but they assert that psychiatrists have an undue burden when expected to testify conclusively as to the McNaughten or ALI standards. These psychiatrists believe that the expert witness should merely provide information to the court and not respond as an expert to the legal standards which determine insanity.

(4) Some psychiatrists, a distinct minority who define themselves as forensic psychiatrists, believe that current uses of the insanity defense are rational, that psychiatrists are quite capable of testifying under current standards, and that they should be willing to do so (Halleck, 1980).

Under the doctrine of diminished capacity, referred to earlier, the jury is asked to consider whether a sane defendant's mental abnormality at the time of a crime prevented him or her from entertaining the specific mental state (the necessary mental element) required by statute for conviction of that crime. In theory, at least, it should be possible to negate the presence of any type of intent because of mental abnormality. Carrying this kind of practice to its logical outcome, however, might result in total acquittal of some mentally abnormal offenders. But unlike the situation which exists when the defendant is adjudicated insane, there is no legal mechanism available to restrain or incapacitate people acquitted on such a basis. If acquitted, they would go free. Our courts and legislators have viewed this as an undesirable outcome.

Currently the diminished capacity defense is used primarily in homicide cases where offenses can be graded according to the mental element involved; the charge can be downgraded only to an extent that still allows the court to impose some form of punishment. In some states, particularly in California, psychiatrists testify as to the presence or absence of premeditation, malice, or intent, the elements which different grades of homicide require. Standards have been developed which define these emotional states in quasi-legal terms, and the psychiatrist testifies as to whether the defendant meets these standards. Here, as in the insanity defense, the psychiatrist faces the difficult task of speculating on the defendant's emotional state at the time of the crime.

THE ROLE OF PSYCHIATRY IN THE SENTENCING PROCESS

Even though a defendant has been found sane, the judge or jury may still want to consider the person's mental status in setting his or her punishment. Judges have considerable discretion in the sentencing process. They may consider the presence of emotional illness at the time of the crime as a mitigating circumstance justifying a lesser punishment. The court also considers the emotional needs of the defendant in choosing a correctional setting. A defendant who needs psychiatric treatment, for example, might best be placed in an institution where such treatment is available, even if it is not the institution to which the court ordinarily sends those who commit the crime of which he or she was convicted. Finally, the court is interested in speculations as to the offender's future conduct both in and out of prison. The courts are especially concerned with the offender's future *dangerousness.* Although the term is rarely defined, the courts usually use it to mean the risk that the offender will commit another serious crime.

Psychiatrists, just like parole and probation officers, are often requested to submit presentence reports to the judge. The issues which these reports are to address are never clearly stated. Generally, they will address issues of mitigation, the need for treatment, and the likelihood of future criminal behavior. Some jurisdictions have court clinics that give psychiatric advice on the sentencing decision. In others, psychiatrists give advice when the prosecution, the defense, or probation officers seek an evaluation of the defendant. Psychiatric consultation before sentencing is often quite informal. Most courts accept a written report, which may be incorporated into a probation report. The written report may later be supplemented by informal contact between the psychiatrist and the sentencing judge.

The psychiatric report can have a powerful impact upon the judge's decision, and no one monitors the extent of that impact. The material reported is not exposed to an adversarial process, and the defendant can neither know what the psychiatrist has said nor contest the accuracy of the psychiatrist's opinion. The possibilities for abuse of this psychiatric role are legion. In the absence of any clear criteria as to what the presentencing reports should and should not contain, they are open to many kinds of uncontested statements which reflect poorly on the defendant.

Ethically and scientifically, the most questionable statements are predictions of future conduct. Our capacity to predict violent behavior is notoriously unsatisfactory (Monahan, 1981). Yet if such predictions appear in a presentence report, they may well be taken seriously by a judge who overestimates psychiatric skills. The judge may "play it safe" by using the psychiatric report to justify a longer sentence.

This is one of many instances of psychiatric involvement in the criminal justice system where the psychiatrist is placed in a double-agent role. The psychiatrist will have allegiances both to the patient and to the court or other institutional agencies. Often allegiance to the agency will take precedence over the determination to serve the offender's best interests. Before interviewing the offender for a presentence report, the psychiatrist should fully inform the offender of his or her role and about the potential uses of the report. The offender has an absolute right to be informed of the risk that psychiatric reporting can result in a longer sentence. More difficult for the psychiatrist than informing the offender is assuring that he or she does not abuse empathy or authority to extract information which will be used to hurt the offender. In this most excruciating ethical dilemma, a psychiatrist must, on the one hand, make full use of professional skills to develop rapport and obtain maximum information, and, on the other hand, must observe some restraint in exercising these skills.

The Supreme Court has ruled that under the Eighth Amendment the sentence of death can be imposed only after a sentencing hearing in which the prosecution and the defense are permitted to introduce evidence on a wide variety of potentially aggravating and mitigating considerations. Some states have adopted statutes which permit psychiatric testimony relevant to such considerations. Furthermore, the Supreme Court has ruled that any examination to provide such testimony in a death sentence hearing must be consented to by defense counsel (*Estelle* v. *Smith*, 1981). Thus, the informal psychiatric involvement in sentencing which typifies noncapital cases is to some extent constitutionally prohibited in capital sentencing. We are developing an adversarial process in which psychiatrists are being called upon to assist both sides in exploring the existence of considerations for and against the imposition of the ultimate penalty.

Though standards vary from state to state, courts seek psychiatric testimony primarily to discover the presence of emotional abnormalities at the time of the crime or the likelihood of future dangerous conduct (Dix, 1980). When testifying on the first issue, the psychiatrist is involved in what might be called a mini-insanity defense, in which the impairments at issue are partially rather than totally excusing. When testifying as to dangerousness, the psychiatrist enters an exceptionally murky area. Our capacities to predict future violence are poor. Yet courts are likely to give much weight to a psychiatric prediction of future violence.

In death penalty hearings, complicated ethical problems confront the testifying psychiatrist. He or she must be fully aware of the limitations of predictive abilities, be willing to expose the testimony to adversarial scrutiny, and should always explain the difficulties of prediction. The psychiatrist must avoid giving conclusory opinions and should never declare an individual dangerous or not dangerous without providing the data upon which an opinion is based. In general, it is wisest simply to describe how a wide variety of biological, psychological, and social variables may have interacted to lead the defendant to commit the crime. Presenting such facts and opinions to the jury, without unnecessary or speculative conclusions, should allow jurors and the judge to separate mitigating and aggravating circumstances and to make their own decisions on conclusory issues.

Some further ethical issues involved in sentencing evaluations are also important to consider. These have come to light as a result of psychiatric involvement in death penalty hearings. First, a defendant may not have to submit to the examination by a psychiatrist employed by the prosecution unless the defendant has shown an intent to use psychiatric testimony on his or her own behalf. In some instances, psychiatric testimony procured by the prosecution has been based on records and interviews with the defendant's acquaintances, and the doctor has never examined the defendant. This practice is, in this author's view, ethically unacceptable.*

Second, in some jurisdictions there is ambiguity concerning the prosecution's ability to use information the defense develops during its preparation for trial or sentencing. The defendant must be made aware that the results obtained in an interview with a psychiatrist hired by the defense might ultimately be used by the prosecution. If the interview is to continue, the defendant must communicate an understanding of the risk and express a willingness to participate in spite of it.

A third ethical issue involves the use of material developed for some

*Preceptor's note: Although the ethical issues are quite different, psychiatrists and other physicans routinely testify in contested wills (testamentary capacity) without having examined the decedent.

other purpose, such as for a determination of competency to stand trial. At the sentencing hearing the psychiatrist should not base the opinion offered on an interview primarily conducted for other purposes. The Supreme Court has ruled that if defendant and defense counsel have not been informed that the interview was to be used for such purposes, it is inadmissable.

In general, the exposure of psychiatric sentencing testimony to the adversarial process has heightened attorneys' and psychiatrists' awareness of the many ethical dilemmas involved in any sentencing procedure. The American Psychiatric Association has appointed a task force to draw up ethical guidelines for psychiatric participation in sentencing. Until these guidelines are agreed to, psychiatrists must scrupulously adhere to conventional guidelines of informed consent and must be extremely modest about predictive abilities.

THE PSYCHIATRIST IN THE FORENSIC HOSPITAL

As a rule, defendants who are found incompetent to stand trial or found not guilty by reason of insanity are sent to specialized units. Certain sex offenders and some prison inmates who become psychotic while incarcerated are also sent to such units. Located either in a separate hospital, within a prison hospital, or within an ordinary mental hospital, these units are here grouped under the rubric of the forensic hospital.

At the forensic hospital, the psychiatrist has treatment, educative, and administrative functions. The treatment functions are rather straightforward, but they are more difficult to carry out than in the ordinary hospital setting. Treatment is difficult when individuals are under indeterminate restraint and have little or no capacity to influence those who will release them. In an ordinary mental hospital, the patient is rewarded for getting better with greater freedom. This reward is far from certain in the forensic hospital, making for bitterness on the part of patients who are less than enthusiastic about participating in the therapeutic process.

While educative functions in the forensic hospital are rather straightforward and usually appreciated, the administrative functions of psychiatrists in forensic hospitals are complicated. Psychiatrists have little or no influence in determining who will be sent to these hospitals. This is almost always a function of a court or correctional agency. At the same time, the psychiatrist has considerable power to make recommendations which will keep an individual under confinement. Any psychiatric statement that an individual is still incompetent, still mentally ill, or still dangerous will usually be accepted by courts and used as a justification for continued confinement. The situation is less certain, however, when the psychiatrist recommends release. Sometimes psychiatrists acting as administrators are given the power to act upon these recommendations. In other instances any psychiatric recommendation must be approved by judicial agencies. As a result of a number of recent lawsuits against psychiatrists who released patients who later committed violent crimes, the conventional wisdom today is that the court should take responsibility for approving the release of any individual hospitalized because of alleged dangerous tendencies.

THE PSYCHIATRIST IN THE CORRECTIONAL SETTING

As in the forensic setting, the psychiatrist in the correctional setting has treatment, educative, and administrative responsibilities. Even if rehabilitation is an elusive goal, the psychiatrist can provide helpful treatment. Some inmates are mentally ill and simply need conventional treatment to achieve palliation. Most inmates are depressed and often seek the assistance of a psychiatrist in order to survive the ordeal of punishment. In general, as long as the psychiatrist's treatment goals are modest and are not used as a justification for extending the length of the offender's sentence, they are highly useful and uncontroversial. Likewise, the correctional staff welcomes the psychiatrist as a teacher who will help them learn as much as they can about mental illness and human behavior.

The administrative functions of the psychiatrist in the correctional setting raise many of the double-agent problems that occur in other contexts. When the offender reaches prison, administrators must decide what type of security to impose and what educational, occupational, recreational and therapeutic program will be made available. The psychiatrist may be asked to help the prison classification committee in making these decisions. This is a useful service for the institution and can also be useful for the offender, but as is true in any double-agent role, the offender is entitled to full informed consent when the psychiatrist does an examination.

Even more often the psychiatrist is asked to evaluate offenders who have committed serious crimes or who have a history of emotional illness before they appear before a parole board. Here, the psychiatrist is asked to make predictions as to the offender's potentiality for recidivism and particularly for recidivism through violent behavior. Again, the inmate must be fully informed as to the purpose of the examination. Parole boards are becoming more aware of the difficulty of predicting recidivism or dangerousness and are not so likely to be powerfully influenced by the psychiatrist's recommendations.

Some offenders develop overt psychotic illnesses which cannot be treated in the prison milieu, and transfer to a forensic hospital becomes necessary. The psychiatrist plays a direct and not uncomplicated role in this kind of disposition. Some offenders vehemently resist the psychiatric labeling involved in transfer to a forensic unit. Others exaggerate the extent of their incapacity in order to get out of an uncomfortable situation in the prison. Often the psychiatrist must invoke humanistic and political as well as medical criteria in deciding whether or not to transfer a given offender. Overall, however, this role is relatively humane and useful.

Bibliographies to Part IV

Bibliography for the Introduction

Davis v. *Watkins,* 384 F. Supp. 1196 (N.D. Ohio 1974).

Donaldson v. *O'Connor,* 422 U.S. 563 (1975).

Eisenberg, T., and Yeazell, S.C. "The Ordinary and the Extraordinary in Institutional Litigation." *Harvard Law Review* 93 (1980): 465–517.

"Developments in the Law—Civil Commitment." *Harvard Law Review* 87 (1974): 1190–1406.

J.L. v. *Parham,* 412 F. Supp. 112 (M.D. Ga. 1976).

Jackson v. *Indiana,* 406 U.S. 715 (1972).

Lessard v. *Schmidt,* 349 F. Supp. 1078 (E.D. Wis. 1972).

New York State Association for Retarded Children, Inc. v. *Rockefeller,* 357 F. Supp. 752 (E.D. N.Y. 1973).

Parham v. *J.R.,* 99 S. Ct. 2493 (1979).

Paris, J.J. "The New York Court of Appeals on Rules on the Rights of Incompetent Dying Patients." *New England Journal of Medicine* 304 (1981): 1424–1425.

Pennhurst State School and Hospital v. *Halderman,* 101 S. Ct. 1531 (1981).

Rennie v. *Klein,* 462 F. Supp. 1131 (D. N.J. 1979).

Stone, A.A. "The Myth of Advocacy." *Hospital and Community Psychiatry* 30 (1979): 819–822.

Stone, A.A. "Recent Developments in Law and Psychiatry." In *The American Handbook of Psychiatry: Advances and New Directions,* 2d ed., Vol. VII, edited by S.H. Arieti and H.K.H. Brodie. New York: Basic Books, 1981.

Stone, A.A. "The *Tarasoff* Decisions: Suing Psychotherapists to Safeguard Society." *Harvard Law Review* 90 (1976): 358.

Suzuki v. *Quisenberry,* 411 F. Supp. 1113 (D. Haw. 1976).

Virginia Academy of Clinical Psychologists v. *Blue Shield of Virginia,* 469 F. Supp. 552 (D. Va. 1979).

Wyatt v. *Stickney,* 325 F. Supp. 781 (M.D. Ala. 1971).

Bibliography for Chapter 21

Aden v. *Younger,* 57 Cal. App. 3d 662, 129 Cal. Rptr. 535 (1976).

Aldrich, R.F., and Turner, J.A. *Dilemma: A Report of the National Conference on the Health Records Dilemma.* Washington, D.C.: Commission on Confidentiality of Health Records, 1978.

Allred v. *State,* 554 P. 2d 411 (Alaska 1976).

"Physicians' Tort Liability, Apart from Defamation, for Unauthorized Disclosure of Confidential Information About Patients." *American Law Reports* 3d 20 (1968): 1109–1122.

American Medical Association. "Confidentiality of and Patient Access to Medical Records." *State Health Legislation Report* 9 (May 1981): 13–23.

American Psychiatric Association. *Confidentiality and Third Parties.* Washington, D.C.: American Psychiatric Association, 1975.

American Psychiatric Association. "Model Law on Confidentiality of Health and Social Service Records." *American Journal of Psychiatry* 136 (1979): 137–144.

American Psychiatric Association. *The Principles of Medical Ethics with Annotations Especially Applicable to Psychiatry.* Washington, D.C.: American Psychiatric Association, 1981.

Appelbaum, P.S. "*Tarasoff:* An Update on the Duty to Warn." *Hospital and Community Psychiatry* 32 (1981): 14–15.

Appelbaum, P.S., and Roth, L.H. "In the Matter of PAAR: Rape Counseling and Problems of Confidentiality." *Hospital and Community Psychiatry* 32 (1981): 461–462.

Beigler, J.S. "The 1971 Amendment of the Illinois Statute on Confidentiality: A New Development in Privilege Law." *American Journal of Psychiatry* 129 (1972): 311–315.

Bellah v. *Greenson,* 141 Cal. Rptr. 92 (1977).

Caesar v. *Mountanos,* 542 F. 2d 1064 (9th Cir. 1976).

Code of Federal Regulations, 42, part 2 (1976).

Cooper, A.E. "The Physician's Dilemma: Protection of the Patient's Right to Privacy." *St. Louis University Law Review* 22 (1978): 397–432.

Curran, W.J. "Failure to Diagnose Battered-Child Syndrome." *New England Journal of Medicine* 296 (1977): 795–796.

Doe v. *Roe,* 400 N.Y.S. 668 (1977).

Eger, C.L. "Psychotherapists' Liability for Extrajudicial Breaches of Confidentiality." *Arizona Law Review* 18 (1976): 1061–1094.

Griswold v. *Connecticut,* 381 U.S. 479 (1965).

Grossman, M. "Insurance Reports as a Threat to Confidentiality." *American Journal of Psychiatry* 128 (1971): 64–68.

Gurevitz, H. "*Tarasoff:* Protective Privilege Versus Public Peril." *American Journal of Psychiatry* 134 (1977): 289–292.

Gutheil, T.G., and Appelbaum, P.S. *Clinical Handbook of Psychiatry and Law.* New York: McGraw-Hill Book Co. (1982), chapter 1.

H. v. *A.,* No. GD 78-28756, Civil Division, Court of Common Pleas of Allegheny County, Pa., June 1, 1981.

Hawaii Psychiatric Society v. *Ariyoshi.*

Horne v. *Patton,* 291 Ala. 701, 287 So. 2d 824 (Ala. 1973).

"Mental Health and Mental Disabilities Confidentiality Act." *Illinois Laws,* 1979, P.A. 80-1508.

In re B., appeal of Dr. Loren Roth, 482 Pa. 471, 394 A. 2d 419 (1978).

In re Lifshutz, 2 Cal. 3d 415, 85 Cal. Rptr. 829, 467 P. 2d 557, 44 A.L.R. 3d 1 (1970).

In re Pittsburgh Action Against Rape, No. 211 W.D. Misc. Dkt. 1980 (Pa. Sup. Ct., January 23, 1981).

Lipari v. *Sears, Roebuck and Co.,* 497 F. Supp. 185 (D. Neb. 1980).

Massachusetts Acts of 1979, chapter 214.

McIntosh v. *Milano,* 168 N.J. Super. 466, 403 A. 2d 500 (1979).

"Court Strikes Down California Statute Regulating ECT, Psychosurgery." *Mental Disability Law Reporter* 1 (1977): 119–120.

National Commission on Confidentiality of Health Records. *Rx (Confidentiality)* 2 (Summer 1978): 7.

Noll, J.O. "The Psychotherapist and Informed Consent." *American Journal of Psychiatry* 133 (1976): 1451–1453.

Pennsylvania Code, 55, section 7100 (1979).

Pennsylvania Statutes Annotated, 50, section 6014 (1978).

Privacy Protection Study Commission. *Personal Privacy in an Information Society.* Washington, D.C.: U.S. Government Printing Office, 1977.

"The Hippocratic Oath." In *Ethics in Medicine: Historical Perspectives and Contemporary Concerns*, edited by S.J. Reiser, A.J. Dyck, and W.J. Curran. Cambridge, Mass.: MIT Press, 1977.

Roe v. *Wade*, 410 U.S. 113 (1973).

Roth, L.H., and Meisel, A. "Dangerousness, Confidentiality, and the Duty to Warn." *American Journal of Psychiatry* 134 (1977): 508–511.

Sharfstein, S.S., Towery, O.B., Milowe, I.D. "Accuracy of Diagnostic Information Submitted to an Insurance Company." *American Journal of Psychiatry* 137 (1980): 70–73.

Shaw v. *Glickman*, 415 A. 2d 625 (Md. Ct. Spec. App. 1980).

Shwed, H.J., Kuvin, S.F., and Baliga, R.K. "Medicaid Audit: Crisis in Confidentiality and the Patient-Psychiatrist Relationship." *American Journal of Psychiatry* 136 (1979): 447–450.

Slovenko, R. "On Testimonial Privilege." *Contemporary Psychoanalysis* 11 (1975): 188–205.

Spingarn, N.D. *Confidentiality: A Report of the 1974 Conference on Confidentiality of Health Records.* Washington, D.C.: American Psychiatric Association, 1975.

Stone, A.A. "The *Tarasoff* Decisions: Suing Psychotherapists to Safeguard Society." *Harvard Law Review* 90 (1976): 358–378.

Sullivan, F.W. "Peer Review and Professional Ethics." *American Journal of Psychiatry* 134 (1977): 186–188.

Tarasoff v. *Regents of the University of California*, 17 Cal. 3d 425, 551 P. 2d 334, 131 Cal. Rptr. 14 (1976).

Taylor, L., and Newberger, E.H. "Child Abuse in the International Year of the Child." *New England Journal of Medicine* 301 (1979): 1205–1212.

Warren, S.D., and Brandeis, L.D. "The Right to Privacy." *Harvard Law Review* 4 (1890): 193–220.

Wigmore, J.H. *A Treatise on the Anglo-American System of Evidence in Trials at Common Law, 3d ed., McNaughton revision.* Boston: Little, Brown and Co., 1961, pp. 828–832.

Wise, T.P. "Where the Public Peril Begins: A Survey of Psychotherapists to Determine the Effects of *Tarasoff.*" *Stanford Law Review* 135 (1978): 165–190.

Woodman, D. "State by State: Protection of 'Privileged Communications' in Civil Cases." *National Law Journal* 1 (August 20, 1979): 22.

Bibliography for Chapter 22

Addington v. *Texas*, 441 U.S. 418 (1979).

Alabama, Code Tit., 22, § 52-01 (1980).

Alaska Stat., § 47.30.340.ii (1978).

American Psychiatric Association. *Diagnostic and Statistical Manual of Mental Disorders, 3d ed.* Washington, D.C.: American Psychiatric Association, 1980.

American Psychiatric Association. *Task Force Report 8: Clinical Aspects of the Violent Individual.* Washington, D.C.: American Psychiatric Association, July, 1975.

Application of Noel, 601 P. 2d 1252 (Kan. 1979).

Arizona Rev. Stat. Ann., § 36-501 (1980).

Arkansas Stat. Ann., § 59-1401 (1980).

Bell v. *Wayne County General Hospital at Eloise*, 384 F. Supp. 1085 (E.D. Mich. 1974).

Benham v. *Edwards*, 501 F. Supp. 1050 (N.D. Ga. 1980).

Bension v. *Meredith*, 455 F. Supp. 662 (D. D.C. 1978).

Bethany v. *Stubbs*, 393 So. 2d 1351 (Miss. 1981).

Braverman v. *United States*, 317 U.S. 99 (1942).

Buzzell v. *Commissioner*, 423 A. 2d 246 (Me. 1980).

California Welf. & Inst. Code, § 5008(h)(1), 5250, 5260, 5300 (1980).

Chell, B. "After a Decade of LPS—Uncertain Times in Mental Health." (1981) (unpublished manuscript).

Colorado v. *Taylor*, 618 P. 2d 1127 (Colo. 1980).

Colorado Rev. Stat., § 27-10-102, 27-10-107, 27-9402 (1980).

Colyar v. *Third Judicial District Court*, 469 F. Supp. 424, 434 (D. Utah 1979).

Commonwealth ex. rel. Finken v. *Roop*, 339 A. 2d 764 (Pa. 1975).

Connecticut Gen. Stat., § 17-176 (1979).

County Attorney Pima County v. *Kaplan*, 605 P. 2d 912, 914 (Ariz. Ct. Ann. 1980).

Davis v. *Watkins*, 384 F. Supp. 1196 (N.D. Ohio 1974).

Doe v. *Gallinot*, 486 F. Supp. 983, 991 (C.D. Cal. 1979).

Doremus v. *Farrell*, 407 F. Supp. 509, 515 (D. Neb. 1975).

Eckerhart v. *Hensley*, 475 F. Supp. 908 (W.D. Mo. 1979).

Ennis, B. "First Day's Address." In *Legal Aspects of Admission and Treatment: Proceedings of a Conference, April 23-25, 1975, Kansas City, 1978.*

Ennis, B.J., and Litwack, T.R. "Psychiatry and the Presumption of Expertise: Flipping Coins in the Courtroom." *California Law Review* 62 (1974): 693–751.

Estate of Chambers, 131 Cal. Rptr. 357 (Cal. 1977).

Estate of Roulet, 590 P. 2d 1 (Cal. 1979).

Eubanks v. *Clarke*, 434 F. Supp. 1022, 1028 (E.D. Pa. 1977).

Ex parte Ullmann, 616 S.W. 2d 278 (Tex. Civ. App. 1981).

Georgia Code Ann., § 88-501(b), (c) (1980).

Goedecke v. *State Department of Institutions,* 603 P. 2d 123 (Colo. 1979).

Goldy v. *Beal,* 429 F. Supp. 640 (M.D. Pa. 1976).

Gross v. *Pomerleau,* 465 F. Supp. 1167 (D. Md. 1979).

Haber v. *People,* 398 N.E. 2d 121 (Ill. App. Ct. 1979).

"Developments in the Law: Civil Commitment of the Mentally Ill." *Harvard Law Review* 87 (1974): 1190, 1212.

Hatcher v. *Wachtel,* 269 S.E. 2d 849 (W. Va. 1980).

Hawaii Rev. Stat., § 334-1, 334-53 (1980).

Heap v. *Roulet,* 590 P. 2d 1 (Cal. 1979).

Hill v. *County Board of Mental Health,* 279 N.W. 2d 838 (Neb. 1979).

Hoffman, P.B., and Foust, L.L. "Least Restrictive Treatment of Mental Illness: A Doctrine in Search of Its Senses." *San Diego Law Review* 14 (1977): 1110.

Holiday v. *Florida,* 386 So. 2d 316 (Fla. Ct. App. 1980).

Humphrey v. *Cady,* 405 U.S. 504 (1972).

Idaho Code, § 66-317 (1980).

Illinois Stat. Ann. Art., 91 1/2, § 119 (1980).

Illinois v. *Hill,* 391 N.E. 2d 51 (Ill. App. Ct. 1979).

Indiana Code Ann., § 16-14-9.1-1 (1980).

In re Ballay, 482 F. 2d 648, 659 (D.C. Cir. 1973).

In re Beverly, 342 So. 2d 481 (Fla. 1977).

In re D.W.H., 411 N.W. 2d 721 (Ind. Ct. App. 1980).

In re Farrow, 255 S.E. 2d 777 (N.C. Ct. App. 1979).

In re Field, 412 A. 2d 1032 (N.H. 1980).

In re Frick, 271 S.E. 2d 84 (N.C. Ct. App. 1980).

In re Hatley, 231 S.E. 2d 633 (N.C. 1977).

In re Henderson, 610 P. 2d 1350 (Colo. Ct. App. 1980).

In re Hogan, 232 S.E. 2d 492 (N.C. 1977).

In re Hop, 623 P. 2d 282 (Cal. 1981).

In re Hutchinson, 421 A. 2d 261 (Pa. Super. Ct. 1980).

In re Janovitz, 403 N.E. 2d 583 (Ill. App. Ct. 1980).

In re Ottolini, 392 N.E. 2d 736 (Ill. App. Ct. 1979).

In re Patterson, 579 P. 2d 1335 (Wash. 1978).

In re Sonsteng, 573 P. 2d 1149 (Mont. 1977).

In re Watson, 154 Cal. Rptr. 151 (Cal. Ct. App. 1979).

Interest of Henderson, 610 P. 2d 1350 (Colo. Ct. App. 1980).

Interest of Paiz, 603 P. 2d 976 (Colo. Ct. App. 1979).

In the Matter of Arnston, 614 P. 2d 1214 (Ore. Ct. App. 1980).

In the Matter of Barker, 600 P. 2d 958 (Ore. Ct. App. 1979).

In the Matter of Byrd, 386 N.E. 2d 385 (Ill. App. Ct. 1979).

In the Matter of Chapman, 385 N.E. 2d 56 (Ill. App. Ct. 1978).

In the Matter of Christofferson, 615 P. 2d 1152 (Ore. Ct. App. 1980).

In the Matter of Collins, 271 S.E. 2d 72 (N.C. Ct. App. 1980).

In the Matter of Conrad, 578 P. 2d 1 (Ore. Ct. App. 1978).

In the Matter of Dean, 607 P. 2d 132 (N. Mex. Ct. App. 1980).

In the Matter of Evans, 408 N.E. 2d 33 (Ill. App. Ct. 1980).

In the Matter of F.B., 615 P. 2d 867 (Mont. 1980).

In the Matter of Farrow, 255 S.E. 2d 777 (N.C. Ct. App. 1979).

In the Matter of Fields, 377 N.E. 2d 301 (Ill. App. Ct. 1978).

In the Matter of Gatson, 593 P. 2d 423, 426 (Kan. 1979).

In the Matter of Goedert, 591 P. 2d 272 (Mont. 1979).

In the Matter of Gregorovich, 411 N.E. 2d 981 (Ill. App. Ct. 1980).

In the Matter of Hernandez, 264 S.E. 2d 780 (N.C. Ct. App. 1980).

In the Matter of Hiatt, 262 S.E. 2d 685 (N.C. Ct. App. 1980).

In the Matter of Linderman, 417 N.E. 2d 1140 (Ind. 1981).

In the Matter of Mathews, 613 P. 2d 80 (Ore. 1980).

In the Matter of Nelson, 580 P. 2d 590 (Ore. Ct. App. 1978).

In the Matter of Newsome, 424 A. 2d 222, 225 (N.J. Super. Ct. 1980).

In the Matter of O'Brien, 600 S.W. 2d 695 (Mo. Ct. App. 1980).

In the Matter of Olson, 596 P. 2d 620 (Ore. Ct. App. 1979).

In the Matter of Oseing, 296 N.W. 2d 797 (Iowa 1980).

In the Matter of Powell, 407 N.E. 2d 658 (Ill. App. Ct. 1980).

In the Matter of Salem, 228 S.E. 2d 649 (N.C. Ct. App. 1976).

In the Matter of Snowden, 423 A. 2d 188 (D.C. App. 1980).

In the Matter of Torsney, 394 N.E. 2d 262 (N.Y. 1979).

In the Matter of Wagstaff, 287 N.W. 2d 339 (Mich. Ct. App. 1979).

Iowa Code, § 229.1(2)(1980).

Jackson v. *Indiana,* 406 U.S. 715 (1972).

Johnson v. *Solomon,* 484 F. Supp. 278 (D. Md. 1979).

Jones v. *Texas,* 610 S.W. 2d 535 (Tex. Civ. App. 1980).

Kansas Stat. Ann., § 59-2902 (1980).

Kinner v. *State,* 382 So. 2d 756 (Fla. Dist. App. 1980).

Lefave, W.R., and Scott, A.W., Jr. *Criminal Law.* St. Paul: West Publishing Co., 1972, pp. 447–478.

Lessard v. *Schmidt,* 349 F. Supp. 1078 (E.D. Wis. 1972); *vacated and remanded on other grounds,* 414 U.S. 472 (1974); *judgment reinstated,* 413 F. Supp. 1318 (E.D. Wis. 1976).

Lodge v. *State,* 597 S.W. 2d 773 (Tex. Ct. App. 1980).

Lux v. *Mental Health Board of Polk County,* 274 N.W. 2d 141 (Neb. 1979).

Lynch v. Baxley, 386 F. Supp. 378, 391 (M.D. Ala. 1974).

Markey v. Wachtel, 264 S.E. 2d 437 (W.Va. 1979).

Maryland Code Ann., Art. 59, § 12(a)(iii); 22(a)(4)(1980).

"General Comments Concerning the Mental Health Law Project's Model Civil Commitment Statute." Mental Disability Law Reporter 2(1978): 519, 527.

Montana Rev. Code Ann., § 53-21-102(14)(1980).

Moore v. Duckworth, 443 U.S. 713 (1979).

Nebraska Rev. Stat., § 83-1009 (1980).

New Mexico Code, § 43-1.11, 43.1.3 (1980).

North Carolina Gen. Stat., § 122-58.2 (1980) (1979 Sess. Laws, Ch. 915).

North Dakota Cent. Code, § 25-03.1-02 (1979).

Northern v. State Department of Human Services, 575 S.W.D. 2d 946 (Tenn. 1978).

Ohio Rev. Code Ann., § 5122.01 (1980).

Oregon Rev. Stat., § 27-10-107, 426.130 (1980).

O'Connor v. Donaldson, 422 U.S. 563, 575 (1975).

Parham v. J.R., 442 U.S. 584 (1978).

Pennsylvania ex. rel. Platt v. Platt, 404 A. 2d 410 (Pa. Super. Ct. 1979).

Pennsylvania Stat. Ann. Tit., 50, § 7301 (1980).

People v. Howell, 586 P. 2d 27 (Colo. 1978).

People v. Sansone, 309 N.E. 2d 733 (Ill. App. Ct. 1974).

Rennie v. Klein, 462 F. Supp. 1131 (D. N.J. 1978).

Reynolds v. Sheldon, 404 F. Supp. 1004 (N.D. Tex. 1975).

Rogers v. Okin, 478 F. Supp. 1342 (D. Mass. 1979).

Scopes v. Shah, 398 N.Y.S. 2d 911 (1977).

Sheffel v. Sulikowski, 403 N.E. 2d 993 (1980).

Sisneros v. District Court, 606 P. 2d 55, 57 (Colo. 1980).

Stamus v. Leonhardt, 414 F. Supp. 439 (S.D. Iowa 1976).

State ex. rel. Doe v. Madonna, 295 N.W. 2d 356 (Minn. 1980).

State ex. rel. Pifer v. Pifer, 273 S.E. 2d 69 (W. Va. 1980).

State of New Mexico Department of Hospitals and Institutions. "Guidelines for Clinical Determination of 'Dangerousness' Related to Mental Disorders" (1977).

State v. Hudson, 409 A. 2d 1349, 1351 (N.H. 1979).

State v. Krol, 344 A. 2d 289, 302, 305 (N.J. Sup. Ct. 1975).

Stone, A.A. (with Stromberg, C.) Mental Health and Law: A System in Transition. Rockville, Md.: National Institute of Mental Health (1975), pp. 25–27.

Suzuki v. Alba, 438 F. Supp. 1106, 1110 (D. Hawaii 1977).

Suzuki v. Yuen, 617 F. 2d 173 (9th Cir. 1980).

Szasz, T. The Myth of Mental Illness. New York: Harper & Row, 1974.

U.S. ex. rel. Matthews v. Nelson, 461 F. Supp. 707 (N.D. Ill. 1978).

Utah Code Ann., § 64-7-28 (1) (1979).

Vitek v. Jones, 445 U.S. 480 (1980).

Von Luce v. Rankin, 558 S.W. 2d 445 (Ark. 1979).

Walker v. Dancer, 386 So. 2d 475 (Ala. Civ. App. 1980).

Warren v. Harvey, 632 F. 2d 925 (2d Cir. 1980).

Washington Rev. Code Ann., § 71.05.020(B) (1979).

Wege v. Texas, 593 S.W. 2d 145 (Tex. Civ. App. 1980).

Welsch v. Likins, 373 F. Supp. 487 (D. Minn. 1974).

Welsch v. Likins, 550 F. 2d 1122 (8th Cir. 1977).

Wisconsin Stat. Ann., § 51.20 (1980).

Wyatt v. Aderholt, 503 F. 2d 1305 (5th Cir. 1974).

Wyoming Stat., § 25-3-101(ix) (1980).

Bibliography for Chapter 23

Alexander, G.J., and Szasz, T.S. "From Contract to Status Via Psychiatry." Santa Clara Lawyer 13 (1973): 537–559.

Amendments to the California Welfare and Institutions Code, Section 5326.75 (1976).

Appelbaum, P.S., Mirkin, S.A., and Bateman A.L. "Empirical Assessment of Competency to Consent to Psychiatric Hospitalization." American Journal of Psychiatry 138 (1981): 1170–1176.

Appelbaum, P.S., and Roth, L.H. "Clinical Issues in the Assessment of Competency." American Journal of Psychiatry 138 (1981): 1462–1467.

Appelbaum, P.S., and Roth, L.H. "Competency to Consent to Research: A Psychiatric Overview." Archives of General Psychiatry (in press).

Ashley, M., Sestak, R.M., and Roth, L.H. "Legislating Human Rights: Informed Consent and the Pennsylvania Mental Health Procedures Act." Bulletin of the American Academy of Psychiatry and the Law 8 (1980): 133–151.

"Young People, Sex, and the Law, Part Two: Teenagers' Access to Contraceptives." Children's Rights Report 2 (1978): 3–11.

Culver, C.M., Ferrell, R.B., and Green, R.M. "ECT and Special Problems of Informed Consent." American Journal of Psychiatry 137 (1980): 586–591.

Freedman, B. "Competence, Marginal and Otherwise: Concepts and Ethics." International Journal of Law and Psychiatry, in press.

Friedman, P.R. "Legal Regulation of Applied Behavior Analysis in Mental Institutions and Prisons." Arizona Law Review 17 (1975): 39–104.

Goldstein, J. "On the Right of the 'Institutionalized Mentally Infirm' to Consent to or Refuse to Participate as Subjects in Biomedical and Behavioral Research." In Appendix, Research Involving Those Institutionalized as Mentally Infirm. Bethesda, Md.: The National Commission for the Protection of Human Subjects of Biomedical and Behavioral Research, 1978, pp. 2-1–2-39.

Grisso, T., and Vierling, L. "Minors' Consent to Treatment: A Developmental Perspective." Professional Psychology 9 (1978): 412–427.

Grossman, L., and Summers, F. "A Study of the Capacity of Schizophrenic Patients to Give Informed Consent." Hospital and Community Psychiatry 31 (1980): 205–206.

Gutheil, T.G., and Appelbaum, P.S. Clinical Handbook of Psychiatry and Law. New York: McGraw-Hill Book Co., 1982.

In re Boyd, 403 A. 2d 744 (D.C. Ct. App. 1979).

In re Yetter, 62 D. & C. 2d 619 (1973).

In the Matter of the Guardianship of Richard Roe III, No. 2257 (Mass. Sup. Jud. Ct., 1981).

In the Matter of Quackenbush, 383 A. 2d 785 (Morris County, N.J., Probate Ct. 1978).

Kaufmann, C.L., and Roth, L.H. "Psychiatric Evaluation of Patient Decision-Making: Informed Consent to ECT." *Social Psychiatry* 16 (1981): 11–19.

Kaufmann, C.L., Roth, L.H., Lidz, C.W., and Meisel, A. "Informed Consent and Patient Decision Making: The Reasoning of Law and Psychiatry." Unpublished, 1982.

Lane v. *Candura,* 376 N.E. 2d 1232 (Mass. Appellate Ct., 1978).

McGarry, A.L., Schwitzgebel, R.K., Lipsitt, P.D., and Lelos, D. *Civil Commitment and Social Policy: An Evaluation of the Massachusetts Mental Health Reform Act of 1970. Crime and Delinquency Report: A Monograph Series.* Rockville, Md.: National Institute of Mental Health, Center for Studies of Crime and Delinquency, 1981.

"Back to the Middle Ages." *Medical World News,* May 14, 1971, p. 51.

Meisel, A. "The Expansion of Liability for Medical Accidents: From Negligence to Strict Liability by Way of Informed Consent." *Nebraska Law Review* 56 (1977): 51–152.

Meisel, A. "The 'Exceptions' to the Informed Consent Doctrine: Striking a Balance Between Competing Values in Medical Decision Making." *Wisconsin Law Review* (1979): 413–488.

Meisel, A., Roth, L.H., and Lidz, C.W. "Toward a Model of the Legal Doctrine of Informed Consent." *American Journal of Psychiatry* 134 (1977): 285–289.

Meisel, A., and Roth, L.H. "What We Do and Do Not Know About Informed Consent: An Overview of the Empirical Studies." *JAMA,* in press.

Michels, R. "Competence to Refuse Treatment." In *Refusing Treatment in Mental Institutions: Values in Conflict,* edited by A. E. Doudera and J.T. Swazey. Ann Arbor, Mich.: AUPHA Press, University of Michigan, in press.

Mills, M.J., Mills, L.C., and Berger, P.A. "Informed Consent: Psychotic Patients and Research." *Bulletin of the American Academy of Psychiatry and the Law* 8 (1980): 119–132.

Munetz, M.R., Roth, L.H., and Cornes, C.L. "Tardive Dyskinesia and Informed Consent: Myths and Realities." Paper presented at a meeting of the *American Academy of Psychiatry and the Law,* San Diego, Calif., 1981.

Report and Recommendations, Research Involving Those Institutionalized as Mentally Infirm. Bethesda, Md.: The National Commission for the Protection of Human Subjects of Biomedical and Behavioral Research, 1978.

Olin, G.B., and Olin, H.S., "Informed Consent in Voluntary Mental Hospital Admissions." *American Journal of Psychiatry* 132 (1975): 938–941.

Palmer, A.B., and Wohl, J. "Voluntary-Admission Forms: Does the Patient Know What He's Signing?" *Hospital and Community Psychiatry* 23 (1972): 250–252.

Pennsylvania Mental Health Procedures Act, 50 *Purdons,* Section 7101 (1976).

Pryce, I.G. "Clinical Research Upon Mentally Ill Subjects Who Cannot Give Informed Consent." *British Journal of Psychiatry* 133 (1978): 366–369.

Rennie v. *Klein,* 476 F. Supp. 1294 (D. N.J. 1979).

Rogers v. *Okin,* 478 F. Supp. 1342 (1979).

Rogers v. *Okin,* 634 F. 2d 650 (1st Cir. 1980) *cert.* granted 49 U.S.L.W. 3788 (No. 80-1417, 1981).

Roth, L.H., Meisel, A., and Lidz, C.W. "Tests of Competency to Consent to Treatment." *American Journal of Psychiatry* 134 (1977): 279–284.

Roth, L.R., Lidz, C.W., Soloff, P., and Kaufmann, K. "Competency to Consent to and Refuse Electroconvulsive Treatment: Some Empirical Data." Paper presented at a meeting of the *American Psychiatric Association,* San Francisco, Calif., 1980.

Roth, L.R., Appelbaum, P.S., Sallee, R., Reynolds, C.F. III, and Huber, G. "The Dilemma of Denial in the Assessment of Competency to Refuse Treatment." *American Journal of Psychiatry,* in press.

Schloendorff v. *Society of New York Hospitals,* 105 N.E. 92 (1914).

Soskis, D.A. "Schizophrenic and Medical Inpatients as Informed Drug Consumers." *Archives of General Psychiatry* 35 (1978): 645–647.

Sovner, R., Dimascio, A., Berkowitz, D., and Randolph, P. "Tardive Dyskinesia and Informed Consent." *Psychosomatics* 19 (1978): 172–177.

Stanley, B., Stanley, M., Lastin, S., Kane, J., and Schwartz, N. "Preliminary Findings on Psychiatric Patients as Research Participants: A Population at Risk?" *American Journal of Psychiatry* 138 (1981): 669–671.

Stone, A.A. "The Right to Refuse Treatment." *Archives of General Psychiatry* 38 (1981): 358–362.

Toulmin, S. "Agent and Patient in Psychiatry." *International Journal of Law and Psychiatry* 3 (1980): 267–278.

Bibliography for Chapter 24

Abraham v. *Winters,* C.A. No. J79-388R (D. Miss. 1981).

American Psychiatric Association: Position Statement on the Right to Adequate Care and Treatment for the Mentally Ill and Mentally Retarded. *American Journal of Psychiatry* 134 (1977): 354–355.

Appelbaum, P.S., and Gutheil, T.G. "Rotting with Their Rights on: Constitutional Theory and Clinical Reality in Drug Refusal by Psychiatric Patients." *Bulletin of the American Academy of Psychiatry and the Law* 7 (1979): 308–317.

Bassiouni, M.C. "Right of the Mentally Ill to Cure and Treatment: Medical Due Process." *DePaul Law Review* 15 (1966): 291–312.

Bazelon, D.L. "Foreword: A Symposium, A Right to Treatment." *Georgetown Law Journal* 57 (1969): 676–679.

Bell v. *Wolfish,* 441 U.S. 520 (1979).

Birnbaum, M. "Some Comments on the 'Right to Treatment.'" *Archives of General Psychiatry* 13 (1965): 34–45.

Bonneau, J.V. "Involuntary Civil Commitment and the Right to Treatment in Pennsylvania." *Villanova Law Review* 15 (1970): 951–971.

Boston University Center for Law and Health Sciences. *Developmental Disabilities/Mental Retardation: Case Law Manual.* Boston: Boston University Law School, 1981.

Bowring v. *Godwin,* 551 F. 2d 44 (4th Cir. 1977).

Brewster v. *Dukakis,* C.A. No. 76–4423-F (E.D. Mass., Dec. 6, 1978).

Burnham v. *Department of Public Health,* 349 F. Supp. 1335 (N.D. Ga. 1972).

Cocozza, J., and Melick, M.E. "The Right to Refuse Treatment: A Broad View." *Bulletin of the American Academy of Psychiatry and the Law* 5 (1977): 1–7.

Colorado Association for Retarded Citizens v. *Colorado,* C.A. No. 78-F-1182 (D.C. Colo., Nov. 9, 1978).

"Comment, Constitutional Right to Treatment for Patients Committed Under the Police Power." *Mental Disability Law Reporter* 3 (1979): 388–389.

"Comment, *O'Connor* v. *Donaldson:* The Death of the Quid Pro Quo Argument for a Right to Treatment?" *Cleveland State Law Review* 24 (1975): 557–571.

Community Psychiatric Centers of Oregon, Inc. v. *Grant,* C.A. No. 79–782 (D. Ore., May 22, 1980).

Creek v. *Stone,* 379 F. 2d 106 (D.C. Cir. 1967).

Cruz v. *Beto,* 405 U.S. 319 (1972).

Davis v. *Balson,* 461 F. Supp. 842 (N.D. Ohio 1978).

Davis v. *Baylor,* C.A. No. C-73-205 (N.D. Ohio, April 30, 1976, and Jan. 21, 1977).

Davis v. *Watkins,* 384 F. Supp. 1196 (N.D. Ohio 1974).

Davy v. *Sullivan,* 354 F. Supp. 1320 (M.D. Ala. 1973).

Director of Patuxent Institute v. *Daniels,* 243 Md. 16, 221 A. 2d 397 (1966).

Dixon v. *Harris,* C.A. No. 74-285 (D. D.C., Feb. 1980).

Dixon v. *Weinberger,* 405 F. Supp. 974 (D. D.C. 1975).

Doe v. *Klein,* M.C.D. No. L-12088-74 P.W. (N.J. Super., June 29, 1977).

Donaldson v. *O'Connor,* 493 F. 2d 507 (5th Cir. 1974).

Donaldson v. *O'Connor,* 519 F. 2d 59 (5th Cir. 1975).

Drake, J. "Enforcing the Right to Treatment: *Wyatt* v. *Stickney.*" *American Criminal Law Review* 10 (1972): 587–609.

Eckerhart v. *Hensley,* 475 F. Supp. 908 (W.D. Mo. 1979).

Evans v. *Washington,* C.A. No. 76-0293 (D.C. D.C., June 14, 1978).

French v. *Blackburn,* 428 F. Supp. 1351 (M.D. N.C. 1977), *affirmed summarily,* 443 U.S. 901 (1979).

Friedman, P., and Halpern, C.R. "The Right to Treatment." *Legal Rights of the Mentally Handicapped* 1 (1974): 286–297.

Garrity v. *Thomson,* C.A. No. 78-116 (D. N.H., Nov. 29, 1978).

Gauthier v. *Benson,* C.A. No. 75-3910-T (Mass. 1975).

Grant, G.M. "Donaldson, Dangerousness and the

Right to Treatment." *Hastings Constitutional Law Quarterly* 3 (1976): 599–627.

Halderman v. *Pennhurst State School and Hospital,* C.A. No. 74-1345 (E.D. Pa., March 17, 1978).

Halleck, S.L. *Law in the Practice of Psychiatry: A Handbook for Clinicians.* New York: Plenum Medical Book Co., 1980.

Halpern, C.R. "A Practicing Lawyer Views the Right to Treatment." *Georgetown Law Journal* 57 (1969): 782–817.

Harper v. *Cserr,* 544 F. 2d 1121 (1st Cir. 1976).

Harvard Law Review. "Mental Health Litigation: Implementing Institutional Reform." *Mental Disability Law Reporter* 2 (1977): 221–223.

Hoffman, B. "The Right to Refuse Psychiatric Treatment: A Clinical Perspective." *Bulletin of the American Academy of Psychiatry and the Law* 4 (1976): 267–274.

Holt v. *Sarver,* 442 F. 2d 304 (8th Cir. 1971).

Horacek v. *Exon,* C.A. No. 72-6-299 (D. Neb., Oct. 31, 1975).

In re Lee, C.A. No. 86 (JD) 1362 (Cook Cty. Cir. Ct., Juv. Div., Ill., Aug. 24, 1972).

In re Shepard, 1, 2-79 Wnab (Vermont, Wash. Cty. D. Ct., Aug. 31, 1979).

In re Wilson, 438 Pa. 425, 264 A. 2d 614 (1970).

In the Matter of Spring, 399 N.E. 2d 493 (Mass. App. 1979).

Inmates of Boys' Training School v. *Affleck,* 346 F. Supp. 1354 (D. R.I. 1972).

Katz, J. "The Right to Treatment: An Enchanting Legal Fiction?" *University of Chicago Law Review* 36 (1969): 755–783.

Kaufman, E. "The Right to Treatment Suit as an Agent of Change." *American Journal of Psychiatry* 136 (1979): 1428–1432.

Kittrie, N. "Can the Right to Treatment Remedy the Ills of the Juvenile Process?" *Georgetown Law Review* 57 (1969): 848–885.

Levine, R.S. "Disaffirmance of the Right to Treatment Doctrine: A New Juncture in Juvenile Justice." *University of Pittsburgh Law Review* 41 (1980): 159–204.

Lora v. *Board of Education,* 456 F. Supp. 1211 (E.D. N.Y. 1978).

Lottman, M.S. "Enforcement of Judicial Decrees: Now Comes the Hard Part." *Mental Disability Law Reporter* 1 (1976a): 69–76.

Lottman, M.S. "Paper Victories and Hard Realities." In *Paper Victories and Hard Realities: The Implementation of Legal and Constitutional Rights of the Mentally Disabled,* edited by V. Bradley and G. Clark. Washington, D.C.: The Health Policy Center of Georgetown University, 1976b.

Lottman, M.S. "Whatever happened to Kenneth Donaldson?" *Mental Disability Law Reporter* 1 (1977): 288–293.

Lynch v. *Baxley,* 386 F. Supp. 378 (M.D. Ala. 1974).

Martarella v. *Kelley,* 349 F. Supp. 575 (S.D. N.Y. 1972).

Massachusetts Association for Retarded Citizens v. *Dukakis,* C.A. Nos. 75-5023-T, 75-5210-T (Mass. 1975).

McEvoy v. *Mahoney,* C.A. No. 74-2768-T (Mass. 1974).

McGarry, A.L., and Kaplan, H.A. "Overview: Current Trends in Mental Health Law." *American Journal of Psychiatry* 130 (1973): 621–630.

"Memorandum, Glenn LL." Mass. Department of Mental Health, June 30, 1981.

"Memorandum." Mass. Department of Mental Health, Sept. 13, 1979.

Mills v. Board of Education of the District of Columbia, C.A. No. 1939-71 (D. D.C., June 9, 1975, and July 24, 1975).

Mills, M.J. "The Rights of Involuntary Patients to Refuse Pharmacotherapy: What Is Reasonable?" *Bulletin of the American Academy of Psychiatry and the Law* 8 (1980): 233–254.

Mills, M.J. "The Continuing Clinicolegal Conundrum of the Boston State Hospital Case." *Medicolegal News* 9 (1981): 9–18.

Morales v. Turman, 430 U.S. 322 (1977a).

Morales v. Turman, 562 F. 2d 993 (5th Cir. 1977b).

Morales v. Turman, 565 F. 2d 1215 (5th Cir. 1977c).

Morris, G.H. " 'Criminality' and the Right to Refuse Treatment." *University of Chicago Law Review* 36 (1969): 784–801.

Morris, G.H. "Legal Problems Involved in Implementing the Right to Treatment." Paper presented at a meeting of the *American Academy of Psychiatry and Law,* Ann Arbor, Mich., Oct. 19, 1972.

Nason v. Superintendent of Bridgewater State Hospital, 353 Mass. 604, 233 N.E. 2d 908 (1968).

Naughton v. Bevilacqua, 458 F. Supp. 610 (D. R.I. 1978).

Nelson v. Heyne, 491 F. 2d 352 (7th Cir. 1974).

Newman v. State of Alabama, C.A. No. 3501-N (M.D. Ala. 1972).

New York State Association for Retarded Citizens and Parisi v. Carey, C.A. No. 72-C-356/357 (E.D. N.Y. April 30, 1975).

"Note, Developments in the Law: Civil Commitment of the Mentally Ill." *Harvard Law Review* 87 (1974): 1190–1406.

"Notes, Implemental Problems in Institutional Reform Litigation." *Harvard Law Review* 91 (1977): 428–463.

"Note, The Nascent Right to Treatment." *Virginia Law Review* 53 (1967): 1134–1160.

"Note, The *Wyatt* Case: Implementation of a Judicial Decree Ordering Institutional Change." *Yale Law Journal* 84 (1975): 1338–1379.

"Note, *Wyatt v. Stickney:* A Constitutional Right for the Mentally Ill." *University of Pittsburgh Law Review* 34 (1972): 79–90.

O'Connor v. Donaldson, 422 U.S. 563 (1975) (Burger, C.J., concurring).

Parisi v. Rockefeller, 357 F. Supp. 752 (E.D. N.Y. 1973).

Pennhurst State School and Hospital v. Halderman, 49 U.S.L.W. 4363 (April 20, 1981).

Pennsylvania Association for Retarded Children v. Pennsylvania, 343 F. Supp. 279 (E.D. Pa. 1972) (consent decree).

Powell, W.J. "The Right to Treatment—A 'Fabled' Right Receives Judicial Recognition in Missouri." *Missouri Law Review* 45 (1980): 357–369.

Pugh v. Locke, 406 F. Supp. 318 (M.D. Ala. 1976).

Pyfer, E.L. "The Juvenile's Right to Receive Treatment." *Family Law Quarterly* 6 (1972): 279–320.

Ragsdale v. Overholser, 281 F. 2d 943 (D.C. Cir. 1950).

Ricci v. Greenblatt, C.A. No. 72-469-T (Mass. 1972).

Roberts, J.C. "Civil Restraint, Mental Illness and the Right to Treatment." *Yale Law Journal* 77 (1967): 87–116.

Rogers v. Okin, 478 F. Supp. 1342 (D. Mass. 1979).

Romeo v. Youngberg, C.A. No. 78–1982 (3d Cir. Nov. 24, 1980), No. 76-3429 (E.D. Pa., Jan. 9, 1979).

Romeo v. Youngberg, 644 F. 2d 147 (3d Cir. 1980). cert granted, 49 U.S.L.W. 3851 (May 18, 1981).

Roth, L.H. "Involuntary Civil Commitment: The Right to Treatment and the Right to Refuse Treatment." In *Psychiatrists and the Legal Process: Diagnosis and Debate,* edited by R.J. Bonnie. New York: Psychiatric Annals, Insight Communications, 1977, pp. 332–345.

Rouse v. Cameron, 373 F. 2d 451 (D.C. Cir. 1966). *reheard on other grounds,* 387 F. 2d 241 (D.C. Cir. 1967) (en banc).

Sas v. Maryland, 334 F. 2d 506 (4th Cir. 1964).

Saville v. Treadway, 404 F. Supp. 430 (M.D. Tenn. 1974).

Schever v. Rhodes, 416 U.S. 232 (1974).

Scott v. Plante, 532 F. 2d 939 (3rd Cir. 1976).

Shepherd, L.R. "Challenging the Rehabilitative Justification for Indeterminate Sentencing in the Juvenile Justice System: The Right to Punishment." *St. Louis University Law Journal* (1977): 21–55.

Sidles v. Delaney, C.A. No. C75-300A (N.D. Ohio, April 26, 1976).

Solesbee v. Balkcom, 339 U.S. 9 (1950) (dissenting opinion).

Stachulak v. Coughlin, 364 F. Supp. 686 (N.D. Ill. 1973).

Stamus v. Leonhardt, 414 F. Supp. 493 (S.D. Iowa 1976).

States v. Collier, C.A. No. GC71-6-K (N.D. Miss., Aug. 22, 1973).

Stone, A.A. *Mental Health and Law: A System in Transition.* U.S. Department of Health, Education, and Welfare Publication. Rockville, Md.: National Institute of Mental Health, 1975a, pp. 75–176.

Stone, A.A. "Overview: The Right to Treatment—Comments on the Law and Its Impact." *American Journal of Psychiatry* 132 (1975b): 1125–1134.

Stone, A.A. "Recent Mental Health Litigation: A Critical Perspective." *American Journal of Psychiatry* 134 (1977): 273–279.

Stone, A.A. "The Right to Refuse Treatment: Why Psychiatrists Should and Can Make It Work." *Archives of General Psychiatry* 38 (1981): 358–362.

Suzuki v. Quisenberry, 411 F. Supp. 1113 (D. Hawaii 1976).

Swann v. Charlotte-Mecklenburg Board of Education, 311 F. Supp. 265 (W.D. N.C. 1970), affirmed 402 U.S. 1 (1971).

Tippet v. Maryland, 436 F. 2d 1153 (4th Cir. 1971).

Twerski, A. "Treating the Untreatable—A Critique

of the Proposed Pennsylvania Right to Treatment Law." *Duquesne Law Review* 9 (1970): 220–228.

U.S. Constitution, Article III, Section 2.

U.S. v. *Pardue,* 354 F. Supp. 1377 (D. Conn. 1973).

Vitek v. *Jones,* 445 U.S. 480 (1980).

Welsch v. *Likins, C.A. No. 4-72-Civ. 451 (D. Minn., Oct. 1, 1974), 550 F. 2d 1122 (8th Cir. 1977).*

Wood *v.* Strickland, *420 U.S. 308 (1975).*

Woodward, B., and Armstrong, S. *The Brethren: Inside the Supreme Court.* New York: Simon and Schuster, 1979.

Wuori v. *Zitnay,* C.A. No. 75-80 (S.D. Maine, July 14, 1978).

Wyatt v. *Aderholt,* C.A. No. 72-2634 (5th Cir., Aug. 15, 1972).

Wyatt v. *Aderholt,* 503 F. 2d 1305 (5th Cir. 1974).

Wyatt v. *Hardin,* C.A. No. 3195-N (M.D. Ala., Feb. 7, 1975).

Wyatt v. *Ireland,* C.A. No. 3195-N (M.D. Ala., Oct. 25, 1979).

Wyatt v. *Stickney,* 325 F. Supp. 781 (M.D. Ala. 1971a).

Wyatt v. *Stickney,* 334 F. Supp. 1341 (M.D. Ala. 1971b).

Wyatt v. *Stickney,* 344 F. Supp. 373 (M.D. Ala. 1972a).

Wyatt v. *Stickney,* 344 F. Supp. 387 (M.D. Ala. 1972b).

Bibliography for Chapter 25

Anderson v. *Dunn,* 19 U.S. 204 (1821).

Bachrach, L. "Is the Least Restrictive Environment Always the Best? Sociological and Semantic Implications." *Hospital and Community Psychiatry* 31 (1980): 97–103.

Butler v. *Michigan,* 35 U.S. 380 (1957).

Community Mental Health Centers Act, P.L. 88–164, 77 *Stat.* 282.

Covington v. *Harris,* 419 F. 2d 617 (1969).

The Developmentally Disabled Assistance Act, 42 *U.S. Code* § 1060.

Dixon v. *Weinberger,* 405 F. Supp. 974 (D. D.C. 1975).

Halderman v. *Pennhurst State School and Hospital,* 446 F. Supp. 1295 (E.D. Pa. 1977).

Halderman v. *Pennhurst State School and Hospital,* 612 F. 2d 84 (1979).

Hospitalization of the Mentally Ill Act, 21 *D.C. Code* § 501 *et. seq.*

Lake v. *Cameron,* 364 F. 2d 657 (1966).

O'Connor v. *Donaldson,* 422 U.S. 563 (1975).

Okin v. *Rogers, cert. granted,* 101 S. Ct. 1972 (1981).

Pennhurst State School and Hospital v. *Halderman,* 101 S. Ct. 1531 (1981).

Romeo v. *Youngberg,* 644 F. 2d 147 (1980).

Shelton v. *Tucker,* 364 U.S. 479 (1960).

Wyatt v. *Stickney,* 325 F. Supp. 781 (1971).

Youngberg v. *Romeo, cert. granted,* 101 S. Ct. 2313 (1981).

Bibliography for Chapter 26

A.E. and R.R. v. *Mitchell* No. 78-466 (D. Utah, 1980).

Appelbaum, P.S., and Gutheil, T.G. "Drugging a Defendant: Armchair Ethics?" *Hastings Center Report* 9 (1979a): 4.

Appelbaum, P.S., and Gutheil, T.G. "Rotting with their Rights on: Constitutional Theory and Clinical Reality in Drug Refusal by Psychiatric Patients." *Bulletin of the American Academy of Psychiatry and the Law* 7 (1979b): 308–317.

Appelbaum, P.S., and Gutheil, T.G. "Drug Refusal: A Study of Psychiatric Inpatients." *American Journal of Psychiatry* 137 (1980a): 340–346.

Appelbaum, P.S., and Gutheil, T.G. "The Boston State Hospital Case: 'Involuntary Mind Control,' the Constitution and the 'Right to Rot.'" *American Journal of Psychiatry* 137 (1980b): 720–723.

Appelbaum, P.S., and Gutheil, T.G. "The Right to Refuse Treatment: The Real Issue is Quality of Care." *Bulletin of the American Academy of Psychiatry and the Law,* in press.

"Developments in the Law—Civil Commitment of the Mentally Ill." *Harvard Law Review* 87 (1974): 1190–1344.

Doe v. *Bolton* 410 U.S. 179 (1973).

Doe v. *Doe* 345NE2d995-1001 (Mass., 1979).

Ford, M.D. "The Psychiatrist's Double Bind: The Right to Refuse Medication." *American Journal of Psychiatry* 137 (1980): 332–339.

Griswold v. *Connecticut* 381 U.S. 479 (1965).

Gutheil, T.G. "Restraint v. Treatment: Seclusion as Discussed in the Boston State Hospital Case." *American Journal of Psychiatry* 137 (1980): 718–719.

Gutheil, T.G., and Appelbaum, P.S. "Substituted Judgment and the Physician's Ethical Dilemma: With Special Reference to the Problem of the Psychiatric Patient." *Journal of Clinical Psychiatry* 41 (1980): 303–305.

Gutheil, T.G., and Appelbaum, P.S. "The Patient Always Pays: Reflections on the Boston State Case and the Right to Rot." *Man and Medicine* 5 (1980): 3–11.

Gutheil, T.G., and Appelbaum, P.S. *Clinical Handbook of Psychiatry and Law.* New York: McGraw-Hill, 1982.

Hymowitz, P. and Spohn, H. "The Effects of Antipsychotic Medication on the Linguistic Ability of Schizophrenics." *Journal of Nervous and Mental Disease* 168 (1980): 287–296.

In the Matter of Guardianship of Richard Roe III, SJC-2257 (Mass., April 23, 1981).

In the Matter of Spring Mass. Adv. Sh. (1980) 1209.

Mackey v. *Procunier* 477F2d877 (9th CIR, 1973).

Meadow, A., Donlon, P.T., and Blacker, K.H. "Effects of Phenothiazines on Anxiety and Cognition in Schizophrenia." *Diseases of the Nervous System* 36 (1975): 203–208.

Mills, M.J. "The Rights of Involuntary Patients to Refuse Pharmacotherapy: What is Reasonable?" *Bulletin of the American Academy of Psychiatry and the Law* 8 (1980): 233–254.

Mills, M.J. "The Continuing Clinicolegal Conundrum of the Boston State Hospital Case." *Medicolegal News* 9 (1981): 9–18.

Plotkin, R. "Limiting the Therapeutic Orgy: Mental Patients' Right to Refuse Treatment." *Northwestern University Law Review* 72 (1977): 461–525.

Rachlin, S. "With Liberty and Psychosis For All." *Psychiatric Quarterly* 48 (1974): 410–420.

Rachlin, S. "One Right Too Many." *Bulletin of the American Academy of Psychiatry and the Law* 3 (1975): 99–102.

Rennie v. *Klein* 462 F. Supp. 1131 (D. N.J., 1979).

Rogers v. *Okin* 478 F. Supp., 1342–1389 (D. Mass 1979).

Rogers v. *Okin* No. 79-1648, 79-1649 (1st Cir., 1980).

Spohn, H.E., Lacoursiere, R.B., Thompson, K., and Coyne, L. "Phenothiazine Effects on the Psychological and Psychophysiological Dysfunction in Chronic Schizophrenics." *Archives of General Psychiatry* 34 (1977): 633–644.

Stone, A.A. *Mental Health and Law: A System in Transition.* New York: Jason Aronson, Inc., 1976.

Stone, A.A. "The Myth of Advocacy." *Hospital and Community Psychiatry* 30 (1979): 819–823.

Stone, A.A. "The Right to Refuse Treatment: Why Psychiatrists Should and Can Make It Work." *Archives of General Psychiatry* 38 (1981): 358–362.

Superintendent of Belchertown State School v. *Saikewicz* 373 Mass. 728 (1977).

Whitree v. *State*, 29ONYS2d486,501 (SUP. CT. 1968).

Bibliography for Chapter 27

Brooks, A. *Law, Psychiatry and the Mental Health System.* Boston: Little Brown, 1973.

Burt, R., and Morris, N. "A Proposal for the Abolition of the Incompetency Plea." *University of Chicago Law Review*, 40, No. 60 (1972).

Dix, G.E. "Clinical Evaluation of the 'Dangerousness' of 'Normal' Criminal Defendants." *Virginia Law Review* 62 (1980): 523–581.

Drope v. *Missouri*, 420 U.S. 162 (1975).

Dusky v. *United States*, 362 U.S. 402 (1960).

Estelle v. *Smith*, 101 S. Ct. 1866 (1981).

Halleck, S. *Law in the Practice of Psychiatry.* New York: Plenum, 1980.

Halpern, A.L. "Use and Misuse of Psychiatry in Competency Examination of Criminal Defendants." *Psychiatric Annals* Vol. 5, No. 4 (April 1975).

McGarry, L. *Handbook, Competency to Stand Trial and Mental Illness.* Rockville, Md: National Institute of Mental Health, 1973.

Monahan, J. *The Clinical Prediction of Violent Behavior.* Rockville, MD: National Institute of Mental Health, 1981.

Pate v. *Robinson*, 383 U.S. 375 (1966).

State v. *Krol*, 68, New Jersey, 236, 344, A.2nd 289 (1975).

Steadman, N. *Beating a Rap.* Chicago: University of Chicago Press, 1979.

Symonds, M. "Policemen and Police Work—A Psychodynamic Understanding." *American Journal of Psychoanalysis.* 32:2 (1972): 163–169.

Teplin, L. "Police Involvement with the Psychiatric Emergency Patient." *Psychiatric Annals* 103 (1980): 46–54.

V

Borderline and Narcissistic Personality Disorders

Part V

Borderline and Narcissistic Personality Disorders

Authors

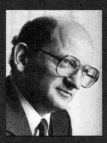

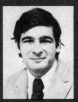

John G. Gund
Associate Professor
Harvard Medical Sc
at the McLean H

Otto F. Kernberg, M.D.,
Preceptor

Medical Director
The New York Hospital-
    Cornell Medical Center
Westchester Division
Professor of Psychiatry
Cornell University Medical
    College
Training and Supervising
    Analyst
Columbia University Center
    for Psychoanalytic Training
    and Research

Pearson Sund
Chief Psychopharma
McLean Hospital

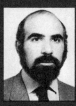

Larry J. Siever, M.D.
Staff Psychiatrist
Clinical Neuropharmacology Branch
National Institute of Mental Health

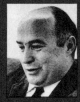

Jonathan O. Cole, M.D.
Chief, Psychopharmacology Program
McLean Hospital

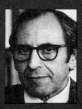

Arnold M. Cooper, M.D.
Director of Training and Professor
    of Psychiatry
The New York Hospital-Cornell
    Medical Center
Department of Psychiatry

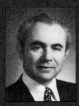

Paul H. Ornstein, M.D.
Professor of Psychiatry
University of Cincinnati
College of Medicine

Borderline and Narcissistic Personality Disorders

Introduction to Part Five
by Otto F. Kernberg, M.D.

The following chapters review and update our current understanding of borderline and narcissistic personality disorders, their clinical characteristics, differential diagnosis, and treatment. As far as current knowledge permits, the chapters also review the etiology and psychopathology of these disorders. Together, the chapters in this Part are intended to present a balanced view of a field that is rapidly changing and expanding. Because both borderline and narcissistic personality disorders have been subject to so much controversy over the past decade or so, the Part does not cover the field completely. Rather, important issues such as family treatment considerations and the entire area of hospital treatment are omitted in order to give adequate coverage to the most important controversial areas.

The diagnostic frame of the two categories considered in this Part is still a matter of controversy, as will be manifest in the chapters that follow. The serious problems remaining with regard to classifying personality disorders in general may underlie the fact that this group of disorders is probably the least well addressed of the DSM-III classifications. Dr. John Gunderson raises the problem of varying diagnostic preferences regarding the borderline personality disorder. His own preference, and the preference of most empirical researchers, is for the narrow or restrictive definition in DSM-III. Most psychotherapists working with borderline conditions, on the other hand, prefer a very broad definition, one that stresses psychodynamic, developmental, and characterological features. Between these two extremes lies the psychostructural approach of Michael Stone (1980) and the Preceptor (Kernberg, 1977; 1981). Gunderson's chapter explores these differences in the light of empirical research carried out in the last fifteen years.

Dr. Larry Siever's chapter on genetic factors complements Gunderson's critical review with a comprehensive review of the evidence currently available relating borderline personality disorders to the genetic predisposition for schizophrenic illness, affective disorders, and minimal brain dysfunction. Siever points to underlying genetic, organic, psychostructural, and psychosocial predispositions that transcend restrictive diagnostic categories and that may, in different proportions, codetermine clinical phenomenology.

In their review of the psychopharmacological treatment of borderline patients, Drs. Jonathan Cole and Pearson Sunderland stress the relation between the clinical characteristics of subgroups of these patients and their pharmacological response, again pointing to the still open issue of delimiting the borderline syndrome. They emphasize the tentative nature of the findings thus far and call particular attention to the studies made by Donald Klein, who defines subgroups of borderline patients in terms of their pharmacological response. Since this review provides practical guidelines for the psychopharmacological management of borderline patients, it should be of particular interest to the clinician.

The Preceptor, in his review of the psychotherapeutic treatment of borderline personalities, spells out a modified psychoanalytic procedure or psychoanalytic psychotherapy as the treatment of choice. He also describes supportive psychotherapy to be used when an expressive or exploratory mode is contraindicated.

The last three chapters of this Part deal with the pathogenesis, diagnosis, and treatment of narcissistic personality disorder. In contrast to borderline personality disorder, the narcissistic personality disorder is a clinically more circumscribed type of character pathology, and fewer controversies and disagreements surround its descriptive-phenomenological features. Since the narcissistic personality disorder has so far not been the subject of specifically designed empirical studies, its descriptions stem rather from clinical and theoretical analyses of character pathology or personality disorders in the context of psychoanalytic exploration. Within the psychoanalytic literature, theoretical approaches may be roughly described as stemming from object relations, ego psychology, and self psychology. These theories differ widely as to the underlying psychopathology of the narcissistic personality and the optimal treatment techniques. Nonetheless, the clinical descriptions overlap and for practical purposes coincide with the DSM-III criteria for Narcissistic Personality Disorder.

Dr. Arnold Cooper introduces this section with an examination of the contrasting psychoanalytic theories and techniques and places them in the context of a broader historical view of the psychoanalytic theories of narcissism. He reviews critically the ambiguities related to the very term *narcissism,* the long-standing controversies regarding the relative importance of environmental and inborn (drive-derived) features, and the relation between an objective, technically neutral and an empathic stance.

Dr. Paul Ornstein's and the Preceptor's chapters complement each other. They offer contrasting psychoanalytic views of the narcissistic personality, with Ornstein representing Heinz Kohut's theory, and the Preceptor discussing his own theory.

The very title of Ornstein's chapter, "On the Psychoanalytic Psychotherapy of Primary Self Pathology," reflects the latest shift in Kohut's thinking before his untimely death. What was previously called "narcissistic personality disorders" is now called "primary self pathology," a diagnostic category Ornstein contrasts with nonnarcissistic or "neurotic" characters whose symptomatology he calls "secondary self pathology." Ornstein summarizes Kohut's theories and points out that they began as an effort to understand narcissistic personality disorders. He concludes the chapter with a clinical illustration of a patient who, in his view, presents a primary self disorder and is treated with a psychotherapeutic approach that employs self psychology principles and technique.

The Preceptor's chapter on the narcissistic personality disorder presents his object relations-ego psychology theory of narcissism and the corresponding psychoanalytic and psychotherapeutic techniques. He amplifies the description of supportive techniques spelled out for borderline patients in his earlier chapter with a description of supportive psychotherapy with narcissistic personalities.

This Part, then, presents an overview of the field of borderline and narcissistic personality disorders and aims to convey new developments in this field together with the many controversies on crucial issues of etiology, psychopathology, and treatment.

Chapter 28

Empirical Studies of the Borderline Diagnosis
by John G. Gunderson, M.D.

INTRODUCTION

The long-standing diagnostic confusion about borderline patients has many causes, including the problems of defining enduring personality traits as pathological in the absence of specific symptoms and the problem of overcoming strongly entrenched beliefs about whether a discontinuity exists between psychosis and neurosis.

Because of these problems and because of the significance of the borderline disorders, the empirical research in the area is of fundamental importance. Although no epidemiological work has been done on the borderline personality disorders, prevalence estimates range from ten percent to thirty percent among persons seeking psychiatric care and from three percent to 35 percent of the general population. The only study giving data on consecutive admissions suggested that the prevalence there is between 8.5 percent and 17.9 percent (Kroll et al., 1981b). Perhaps even more significant than the prevalence of the disorders are the particularly troublesome problems they pose in treatment. The amount of difficulty borderline patients have created for mental health professionals is far disproportionate to their numbers. These difficulties provide both the incentive and the justification for the burgeoning efforts to improve our capacity to identify such persons and to deepen our understanding of the origins of the disturbing and dangerous treatment complications with which they are associated.

The literature providing descriptive accounts of patients diagnosed as borderline has been reviewed more or less extensively by a number of authors in the past decade (Grinker et al., 1968; 1977; Gunderson and Singer, 1975; Mack, 1975; Kernberg, 1975; Perry and Klerman, 1978; Meissner, 1978; Liebowitz, 1979; Stone, 1980). These reviews have all suggested that the phenomenology of such patients varies over time and that the resulting controversies about their identification enjoin the psychiatric field to isolate empirically what, if any, are the defining characteristics of this patient group. Guze (1975) in particular stated that the diagnostic confusion about borderline patients would not be resolved in the absence of more systematic research.*

Since a number of excellent reviews of the descriptive literature already exist and because these reviews have been integrated into subsequent research efforts, they will not be reviewed here. Rather, this chapter will review the systematic research on borderline patients, discuss what has been learned from the studies, and explore the major remaining questions. The review is divided into four parts. The first part is a review of studies which characterize borderline samples and test their discriminability from comparison groups. Second is a review of the diagnostic criteria which these studies have generated. Third is a review of various diagnostic instruments, and fourth is a review of the

*Editor's note: The reader may wish to look ahead for an enumeration of the author and Kolb's and others' criteria, which appears in Table 2 of this chapter (p. 426), and for a listing of DSM-III criteria, which appears in Table 4 of Siever's chapter (p. 450).

studies which have compared the various diagnostic schemes. Much of this work is summarized in its approximate chronological order in Table 1. The reader will find it helpful to refer to this table as the review proceeds.

CHARACTERIZATION AND DISCRIMINATION OF BORDERLINE PATIENTS

Systematic study of borderline patients began with the seminal study of *Grinker, Werble, and Drye* (1968). In that study, 53 borderline patients were selected on the basis of the diagnostic impressions of one outpatient psychiatrist. Using cluster analyses, the researchers described four subgroups within their sample: a neurotic border group, an "as if" group, a psychotic border group, and a core borderline group. The research used neither a structured means of data collection nor comparison groups. In a recent update of this work, Grinker et al. (1977) added 14 new borderline patients and largely affirmed their earlier findings. In addition, Grinker (1979) has compared his sample of borderline patients with a sample diagnosed as schizophrenic. Doing so, he has given new emphasis to the brief, quickly reversible, and ego-dystonic nature of the psychotic episodes found in borderline patients. Grinker concluded from his studies that "the borderline syndrome represents an independent entity deriving from a developmental defect" (Grinker, 1979, 51).

In another early effort, the author and a National Institute of Mental Health (NIMH) group, *Gunderson, Carpenter, and Strauss* (1975) used an operational definition of borderline to sort out a sample and compared it to a matched sample of schizophrenics on prognostic variables, signs and symptoms, and outcome at two and five years. The sample of borderlines had been referred to NIMH as possibly schizophrenic but had not been found to fulfill the criteria for that diagnosis. Although this study used reliable methods and collected data systematically, it did not assess many areas considered important for the borderline diagnosis. Moreover, the clinical diagnostic method of selecting the sample makes it difficult to generalize to other borderlines. The borderline patients were found to have more anger and more dissociative experiences than the schizophrenic group, but could not be discriminated from the schizophrenic patients on a series of prognostic variables. Both the NIMH study (Gunderson et al., 1975; Carpenter et al., 1977) and the earlier study by Grinker et al. (1968; Werble, 1970) provided follow-up data which indicate that borderline patients generally remain unemployed, unmarried, symptomatic, and subject to rehospitalizations. Thus, while these follow-up studies have shown that borderlines are not schizophrenic, they have underscored the serious morbidity of borderline patients.

In a third early study, *Willett et al.* (unpublished) used an operational definition for their borderline sample which was similar to the method used by the NIMH group. The sample was a group of male, military hospital inpatients whose diagnosis changed from a psychotic diagnosis to a nonpsychotic one during hospitalization. They compared these patients with patients diagnosed both on admission and at discharge as either psychotic or nonpsychotic. Notable among their findings was that the borderline patients were significantly more likely to be married and to abuse drugs than the psychotic patients, but the borderline group reported significantly less drug abuse than the nonpsychotic group. Not surprisingly, both the borderline and psychotic samples showed significantly more signs of thought disorder than the non-psychotic group. The only variable that distinguished the borderline patients from both nonpsychotic and psychotic patients was their greater expression of overt anger. Although the procedure used to select the sample in this study makes it difficult to compare the findings with those of others, the borderline sample does appear to have been similar to that of the NIMH study and to Grinker's psychotic border subgroup. Like both these studies, Willett's study confirms the prevalence of angry and depressive affect in borderline patients. However, as in the NIMH study, it also indicates that the depression is non-discriminating. The findings have added interest because they were derived from an all-male sample, whereas other study samples contain a preponderance of female subjects.

In an effort to build upon and compensate for some of the limitations of these previous research efforts, the author, *Gunderson,* began a study at McLean Hospital (Gunderson, 1977; Gunderson and Kolb, 1978; Kolb and Gunderson, 1980; Austin, et al., unpublished; Gunderson et al., 1981). They selected a sample of clinically diagnosed, "certain" borderline patients, used a semistructured interview specifically targeting those areas of functioning considered most typical for borderlines, and employed both schizophrenic and depressed comparison groups. Based on a review of published clinical descriptions, this study identified five areas of functioning as characteristically problematic for borderline patients: social adaptation, impulse and action patterns, affects, psychotic symptoms, and interpersonal relationships. In order to assess psychopathology systematically in these five areas, a Diagnostic Interview for Borderlines (DIB) was developed (Gunderson et al., 1981). A sixth area which the literature review had indicated could provide important information was psychological testing (Gunderson and Singer, 1975), but this was not assessed.

To make an initial comparison of a sample of borderline patients with samples of depressed and schizophrenic patients, matched on demographic variables, the author used a one-way analysis of variance on the 29 statements from the DIB (Gunderson, 1977). That study showed that only eight of the 29 statements failed to reveal significant differences with at least one control group. Moreover, all five sections of the DIB could be utilized to discriminate borderlines from one or both comparison groups. Subsequently, the author and Kolb (1978) compared samples using discriminant function analyses. In each instance, a discrete list of characteristics from the DIB could easily discriminate the borderline group from the comparison group. Concluding that their borderline sample had represented a definable syndrome, the authors consequently joined Grinker in the belief that this syndrome is a discrete form of personality disorder.

In a replication study using the DIB on comparable samples of depressed and schizophrenic patients, *Soloff and Ulrich* (1981) found that only six of the 29 DIB statements failed to differentiate their borderline sample from at least one comparison group. In almost all ways, their results echo those found in the author's analysis-of-variance study. When these researchers did discriminant functions, they found even higher discriminability of the borderline group from their comparison groups. Both studies found that the information from the

Table 1. Empirical Studies of Borderline Patients

Investigator	Inpt. (I) Outpt. (O)	Borderline Selection Criteria	N	Comparison Group	Selection Criteria	N	Type of Analysis	Level of Discr.	% Sensitivity and Specificity	Notes
1. Grinker et al., 1968	O/I	Clin.[2]	53	NA	NA	NA	Fctr. Anal.			Assessment on Ego fctn inferred from beh. obsv'n by RN's
2. Willett et al., unpublished	I	Severe dysfct'n with questionable psychosis	30	Psych.[3] Nonpsych.	Clin.	111 168	T-tests for: i) 5 Sx var's ii) 3 Demogr. var's	p<.05 for 3 of 10 compar's 3 of 10 compar's		All male sample
3. Gunderson et al., 1975	I	Severe dysfct'n with questionable psychosis	24	Schiz.	Clin. IPSS[4] Matching on demogr.	29	T-tests on: i) Sx fctrs ii) 6 Px var's iii) 5 var's outcome	p<.05 for 5 0 0		
Carpenter et al., 1977				Schiz. MDI Psych. Neurotic	Clin. IPSS	29 66 112 71	ANOVA of psychopathology profiles	p<.05 p<.05 p<.05 NS		PSE-SX Measures constituted 27 factors which formed the profiles.
4. Gunderson, 1977	I	Clin.	31	Schiz. Depr.	IPSS Clin.[5]	22 11	ANOVA for 29 DIB statements	p<.05 on 21		

Study		Criterion	N	Comparison group	Comparison Dx	N	Discriminant Fcts.	Result		Ratio
Gunderson and Kolb, 1978			29	Schiz. / Depr. / Non-BL	IPSS / Clin.[5] / Clin.	NA	appl of Fct. (c)	a) 100% / b) 95.4% / c) 86.8%	81.0%	
			32	Schiz / Depressive / Non-BL (incl MDI, pers dis) / Clin.	IPSS / Clin.[5] / Clin.	22 / 11 / 42 ; 20 / 10 / 38	Use of DIB ≥7 to determine dx'c sep'n	76.9% / 78.6% / 77.0%		73/85 / 73/100 / 73/81
Gunderson et al., 1981		DIB≥7	12–16	Non-BL	DIB ≤6	12–16	Correl'n dx between raters	85.7%		
5. Spitzer, et al., 1979a	0 (10% I)	Clin. Dx of BPD, BPO or BL Schiz	808	Non-BL (Mixed 55% Neur; 40% Pers. Dis; No Psych.)	Clin.	808	17-item set	88.0%		88/87
		Clin. Dx of BPO	234				9 unstable item set	80.9%		77/82
6. Perry and Klerman, 1980	0	Clin.	25	Non-BL (mixed)	Clin.	102	T-test of 129 items	p<.05 for 81		

Table 1. Continued

Investigator	Impt. (I) Outpt. (O)	Borderline Selection Criteria	Comparison Group N	Comparison Group	Selection Criteria	N	Type of Analysis	Level of Discr.	% Sensitivity and Specificity	Notes
Perry, unpublished			39			234	Dx'ic scores[6] on criteria attrb't to: i) Knight ii) Kernberg iii) Grinker iv) Gunderson v) Spitzer vi) Perry (BPS-II)	49/73 64/84 59/80 77/86 79/86 74/87		Gunderson, Spitzer, Kernberg, and Perry highly overlapping. (correl'n ≥0.9)
7. Sheehy et al., 1980	0	Clin.		Schiz. Neur. Pers. Dis. Non-BL.	IPSS Clin. Clin. Clin.	30 30 30 90	Discr. fct of 16 Sx checklist items	? ? ? 100%	93/76	Results consistently similar to Gunderson and Kolb
8. Kroll et al., 1981b	I	DIB≥7 DSM-III	21 10	Non-BL. Non-BL.	DIB≤6 RDC[7]	96 107	Correl'n betw DIB DX & i) Spitzer et al. item list unstable schztpl ii) DSM-III (RDC)	X^2 = NS p<.01 NS X^2=p<.01		Only sztpl items which were signif greater in BL's were ideas of ref. and social isol'n.
Kroll et al., unpub.	I	DIB≥7 DSM-III	7 4	Non-BL.	DIB≤6 Clin.	40 43	Corr'n betw Dx and DSM-III	87% agr. 93% agr.		English sample

Study									
Kroll et al., 1981a	I	DIB≥7	6–9	Non-BL	DIB≤6	21–24	Corr'n of Dx betw raters	90.0%	Replication of Gunderson '77 and Gunderson and Kolb '78
9. Soloff and Ulrich, 1981	I	Clin.	23	Schiz. Unipolar Depression	RDC	22 20	T-test on 29 DIB statements	p<.05 on 23	
				Schiz. Uni-Depr. Schiz. and Depr.		22 20 42	Discr. fcts of DIB Sct'n Series	97.8% 97.7% 96.9%	
10. Kernberg et al., 1981	I	Structural Interview	17	Non-BL (Psych.)	Structural Interview	15	Corr'n betwn Strct'Int i) DIB Dx	78% p=.004	
			17			12	ii) Psych test Dx	69% p=.016	
			17			15	iii) WAIS vs. Rorschach	72% p=.013	
		DIB≥7	13		DIB≤6	16	Corr'n betwn. DIB DX & i) Psych test Dx	76% p=.008	86% with DIB Cutoff ≥8
			14				ii) WAIS vs Rorschach	69% p=.044	75% with DIB Cutoff ≥8

Table 1. Continued

Investigator	Inpt. (I) Outpt. (O)	Borderline Selection Criteria	N	Comparison Group	Selection Criteria	N	Type of Analysis	Level of Discr.	% Sensitivity and Specificity	Notes
Koenigsberg, in press	I/O		14	Bl. outpatient	DIB≥7	18	T-test of 29 DIB statements	p<.05 on 6		
11. Kobele et al., unpublished	I	NA		Schiz. MDI Anorx. Nvs. Normals	RDC	18 8 8 9	Use of DIB score≥7 to detr'm Dx'c sep	Correct 17 8 8 9	/94 /100 /100 /100	

1. Sample diagnosed on outpatients, but hospitalized as part of study protocol.
2. Clin. means diagnosis based on clinical judgment.
3. Psych means psychotic.
4. IPSS refers to diagnoses made on criteria from the International Pilot Study of Schizophrenia.
5. Most fulfilled Feighner criteria for Primary Affective Disorder (Feighner et al., 1972).
6. Figures cited are based on separations achieved by using the upper quartile of scores on each of the criteria lists. The author used other cutoffs as well.
7. RDC refers to Research Diagnostic Criteria (Spitzer et al., 1977)

impulse/action pattern section and from the interpersonal relations section of the DIB were most valuable for discriminating borderlines from members of both comparison groups. Soloff and Ulrich speculated that their higher levels of prediction could be due to the fact that they used more homogeneous controls diagnosed according to Research Diagnostic Criteria (RDC). Further, they noted, the psychiatrist who did the DIB ratings had participated in preinterview screening of patients' charts, and this may have introduced bias. While affirming the value of the DIB in discriminating borderline from nonborderline patients, the authors cautioned, "Evaluation of consecutive or random admissions by raters blind to diagnosis and naive to theory would provide a more rigorous test of the DIB" (Soloff and Ulrich, 1981, 692).

Another group of studies has attempted to differentiate the borderline syndrome from other disorders. Work by *Kroll et al.* (1981b) and by *Kobele et al.* (unpublished) has shown that good discrimination is possible when the DIB is used to diagnose borderlines as compared to manic depressives and patients with anorexia nervosa and other types of personality disorders. Both Kroll et al. (1981b) and Kolb and the author (1980) note, however, that the most difficult discrimination is for patients with other types of personality disorder. Kroll et al. found that impulsiveness, especially self-destructiveness, brief psychotic episodes, and disturbed interpersonal episodes, were the most important discriminators of borderlines. They suggest that the DIB measures of social adaptation and affect were primarily useful as means of excluding schizophrenic patients.

Perry and Klerman (1980) designed a study similar to that of the author, but they did not use the DIB. They compared their sample of 18 outpatient borderlines with 102 outpatients given a variety of other diagnoses on 129 items, which were presumed to represent those of Knight (1953), Kernberg (1967), Grinker et al., (1968) and the author and Singer (1975). Using a one-way analysis of variance, they found that the borderline sample's results on 81 items were significantly different from all patients' results. In most respects, the same variables that the author had found discriminated his borderline sample from schizophrenic and depressed groups discriminated the borderline sample from the diagnostically heterogeneous comparison group in the Perry and Klerman study. These researchers noted, however, that affective instability seemed more prominent and more discriminating in their sample than it had been in the author's study. In contrast to their oft-quoted 1978 review, Perry and Klerman (1980) concluded that their results supported the descriptive validity of a borderline personality disorder.

Sheehy, Goldsmith, and Charles (1980) have reported yet another study searching for the discriminating characteristics of borderline patients. They devised a 16-item symptom checklist on the basis of the literature and the combined clinical wisdom of approximately twenty senior staff members of the outpatient psychiatric service at the Bronx Municipal Hospital Center. Over a one-year period, their symptom checklist was a routine part of the evaluation done by PGY III residents on all new outpatient clinic patients. Of particular importance was their inclusion of a comparison group composed of nonborderline patients with other personality disorders. Using a discriminant function analysis, they compared the symptom checklist profile of borderline patients with the profiles of each of the three comparison groups and with the profile for all other groups combined. Both with respect to the individual comparison group, and with respect to the combined comparison group, their findings were consistent with those reported by the author and Kolb (Gunderson and Kolb, 1978). Like Soloff and Ulrich, they found that the borderlines in their samples were even more discriminable from the nonborderlines than had the author and Kolb. Impulsivity, intense affects, and interpersonal difficulties were the most powerful in distinguishing the borderline patients from the others.

Each of the foregoing studies had been done exclusively on either inpatient or outpatient samples, leaving questions as to the comparability of their samples and the generalizability of their results. To address the issue, *Koenigsberg* (in press) compared DIB-diagnosed borderline inpatients with an outpatient sample. He found general agreement on their characteristics but noted that the inpatients were more likely to be involved in self-mutilative behavior and to be more intolerant of aloneness. Although these differences may help to explain why some borderline patients are hospitalized, he observed, the outpatient sample clearly represents the same clinical entity. This result validates the impression of similarity between the results obtained in the earlier outpatient and inpatient samples.

DEVELOPING DIAGNOSTIC CRITERIA

Grinker et al. (1968) employed a factor analysis to isolate the four characteristics which best defined their sample of borderlines. To look for the best overall discriminating characteristics of their borderline samples, subsequent investigators have used discriminant function analyses and comparison groups as large and heterogeneous as they could generate. Table 2 summarizes the results of five studies.

The author, *Gunderson, and Kolb* (1978) added nine patients with various other diagnoses to those of their initial two comparison groups. Their discriminant function analysis yielded 14 DIB statements which they then condensed into the seven criteria seen in Table 2. These seven criteria were able to discriminate the borderlines in this sample from all others with 86.8 percent accuracy. When the criteria were applied to an independent new sample of 29 clinically diagnosed borderline patients, they correctly identified 81 percent, suggesting that a reasonably identifiable syndrome exists in the patients that clinicians diagnose as borderline personality disorder. Two unresolved questions were the degree to which the discriminating variables found in this study are generalizable to other settings in which diagnostic habits may differ and to what extent they would hold up with other comparison groups. Subsequent investigations have provided results which bear on these questions.

Sheehy et al. (1980), in an outpatient study, found overall discriminators quite similar to those obtained by the author and Kolb. Although it proved elusive as far as reliability was concerned, Sheehy also found that an unstable identity was a useful criterion. Of special interest because they have not been tested by other investigators were the discriminating variables of absence of hypochondriasis and absence of obsessive/compulsive complaints.

Spitzer, Endicott, and Gibbon (1979a) aimed to develop an item list which could accurately distinguish between patients which clinicians diagnosed as borderline and patients they considered nonborderline (see also Table 1). As a basis for 11 of their 17 items, they used components or the entirety of all seven of the Gunderson and Kolb criteria. Spitzer et al. further divided nine of their 17 items into those which were called unstable and which were more characteristic of the borderline personality concept as described by Kernberg (1967) and by the author and Singer (1975). Eight of these nine items were components of the Gunderson and Kolb discriminant function. The ninth item, identity diffusion, was supported by the research of both Grinker and Sheehy. They sent both the 17-item and the nine-item lists to 4,000 members of the American Psychiatric Association and asked them to judge the lists' discriminating ability. The 808 who responded indicated that the 17-item list would accurately discriminate borderline from nonborderline patients 88 percent of the time, whereas the nine-item set would do so 80.9 percent of the time. Although Spitzer et al. made a somewhat controversial interpretation of their data (Siever and Gunderson, 1979; Sheehy et al., 1980), their results did support the notion of an identifiable borderline syndrome. Especially in view of the overlapping items in the more restricted unstable item set, their work very much confirms the specific findings in the reports of both the author and Kolb and Sheehy et al. Their work goes further, moreover, by suggesting how the borderline diagnosis is used throughout the country and how it is applied in outpatient as well as inpatient settings.

Perry and Klerman (1980) found that their borderline sample scored significantly higher on all nine unstable items from the Spitzer et al. study than did their nonborderline controls. Perry has also found a list of best overall discriminating variables which closely overlap with the other sets of criteria (Christopher Perry, personal communication). The fact that so much overlap has emerged from different original items on different samples, and where researchers used different forms of assessment and had a variety of raters, is impressive.

Despite the general consensus on criteria, several areas of disagreement remain. The first concerns the criterion of low achievement. Spitzer et al. found that, while it was moderately characteristic of borderline patients, low achievement had little discriminating power when they compared borderlines with controls. However, in both Soloff and Ulrich's replication with inpatients (1981) and Perry and Klerman's outpatient study (1980), the level of school and work achievement of their borderline patients appeared quite low, as it did in the author and Kolb's study (1978). In all of these studies low achievement helped discriminate borderlines from comparison samples. However, the studies by Kroll et al. (1981b), and by Soloff and Ulrich (1981), as well as that of the author, have found that the more general area of social adaptation, of which low achievement was one part, proved to be of little use in providing diagnostic information. While it appears that low achievement is characteristic of borderlines, it may lose its discriminating power or be less apparent in samples of borderline outpatients who are seeing private psychotherapists. On balance, then, the criterion of low achievement requires further evaluation.

A second area of remaining controversy concerns the inclusion of mild psychotic experiences. As has been noted, virtually every study done to date has found that this area provided useful discriminating information. The author and Kolb (1978) grouped several of their most discriminating variables into the criteria called mild psychotic experi-

Table 2. Empirically Derived Criteria For Borderline Personality

	Grinker et al, 1968	Gunderson and Kolb, 1978	Spitzer et al, 1979a (Unstable)	Sheehy et al, 1980	Kernberg et al, 1981*
AFFECT	1. Anger 2. Depression, loneliness	1. Heightened affectivity • anger • depression (nondiscriminating) • chronic dysphoria	1. Anger 2. Unstable affect • depression • irritability • anxiety 3. Chronic feelings emptiness/boredom	1. Poor affect 2. Intense feelings and impulses	NA
IDENTITY	3. Poor Self-identity	NA	4. Identity disturbance	3. Unstable sense of self	1. Identity diffusion
INTERPERSONAL RELATIONSHIPS	4. Anaclitic reln's	2. Disturbed close reln's • deval'n • manipulation • dependency • masochism 3. High socializ'n • intolerant of aloneness	5. Unstable intense reln's • deval'n • manipulation • idealization • shifting attitudes 6. Intolerant of aloneness	4. Devaluation and idealization 5. Periodic social isol'n	• devaluation • idealization (These are considered defenses. See 3 below.)
IMPULSIVITY	NA	4. Impulsivity • drug/ETOH abuse • promiscuity	7. Impulsivity • drug/ETOH 8. Physically self-damaging acts	6. Impulsivity 7. Drug/ETOH abuse 8. Unstable sex (promiscuity)	NA

PSYCHOSIS	NA	5. Manipulative suicide • mutilation • overdoses	• mutilation • suicide gestures • fights, accidents	NA	2. Intact reality testing • vulnerable to brief psychotic experiences • altered sense of reality • projection (These are considered defenses. See 3 below.)
		6. Mild Psychotic Experiences • dissociation • paranoid ideas • regressions • absence of any severe or widespread psychotic symptoms	(Dissociative experiences, ideas of reference, and paranoid ideas became part of the schizotypal item list.)	9. Projection and poor sense of reality	
MISC		7. Low achievement		10. Absence of hypochondriasis 11. Absence of obsessions/compulsion 12. Bizarre sexual fantasies	3. Primitive defenses • splitting • denial (See also above.)

*Kernberg's criteria are in the process of being empirically tested for their discriminating value.

ences. Sheehy et al. (1980) found that the use of projection with episodic reality disorders was a major discriminating characteristic. Perry and Klerman (1980) found that the borderlines scored higher on mild psychotic experiences than controls, as indicated by such items as episodic depersonalization and derealization, transient psychotic episodes, psychotic episodes in psychotherapy, distorted perceptions and ideas of others, and even the presence of psychosis at the time of the interview. In contrast to the author, neither Perry and Klerman (1980) nor Soloff and Ulrich (1981) found brief paranoid experiences helpful in discriminating. In summary, all these studies offer strong support for the inclusion of psychotic-like experiences as a diagnostic criterion for Borderline Personality Disorder. Spitzer et al. (1979a), however, separated the components of this area, such as brief paranoid experiences, ideas of reference, illusions, and dissociative reactions. They made each of them separate variables in a list of features which, they hypothesized, defined a separate and new form of personality disorder—schizotypal personality disorder. Their own results suggest that most patients with either borderline or schizotypal personality disorder will fulfill criteria for the other. Many investigators and clinicians believe that this removal of psychotic experiences from the criteria for borderline personality, also reflected in DSM-III (American Psychiatric Association, 1980), has diminished the value of the borderline diagnosis. (Gunderson, 1980; Sheehy et al., 1980; Kernberg, 1979; John Frosch, personal communication). They believe that psychotic experiences are central, critical features for understanding the underlying personality and the treatment problems found with borderline patients.

DIAGNOSTIC ASSESSMENT INSTRUMENTS

The number of diagnostic instruments available to help define samples of borderline patients has proliferated rapidly in recent years. Some aspects of these instruments are summarized on Table 3.

DIAGNOSTIC INTERVIEW FOR BORDERLINES (DIB) The first and most widely utilized instrument has been the DIB, developed by the author (Gunderson et al., 1981). The DIB is a semistructured interview specifically designed for achieving a reliable assessment of information considered relevant for the borderline diagnosis. Unlike most other structured interviews, the DIB places major emphasis on historical information. Even the more symptom-oriented sections on affects and psychosis include inquiries about more enduring behavioral patterns which extend into the past history. The interview consists of making a number of specific inquiries into related areas, and then rating a statement based on a summary impression from responses to these inquiries. Each statement involves one of 29 putative characteristics of borderline patients. The scores on these 29 statements are then converted into a scale of 0 to 2.0 for each of five sections of the interview. Together, then, the five sections give a potential total interview score of ten points. A total score of ≥ 7.0 is sufficient to determine a diagnosis of Borderline Personality Disorder. The reliability of diagnoses based on this total score is 0.87 to 0.90 (Kolb and Gunderson, 1980; Kroll et al., 1981a). Other studies of the DIB have shown a good reliability on the component parts of the interview (Gunderson et al., 1981; Kroll et al., 1981a; Koenigsberg, in press) and generally support the interview's construct validity as recognized statistically (Gunderson et al., 1981) and by using independent measures concurrently. These independent measures have included psychological test battery diagnoses (Kernberg et al., 1981), a variety of scales measuring depression, hostility, and impulsiveness (Soloff, 1981), and the MMPI (Kroll et al., 1981b). Although the author has stated that the DIB requires a reasonably seasoned professional rater, Kroll et al. (1981a) found that a nonprofessional could be trained to use it reliably.

As noted earlier, the author and Kolb (1978) took the best discriminating variables from their original sample of borderline patients and applied these to a new sample to test their ability to define those patients as borderline or nonborderline. Their criterion diagnosis for this sample was based on independently determined, but purely clinical diagnostic assessments. Although they found 81 percent accuracy in separating borderlines from nonborderlines by this criterion, the study was flawed by the degree to which the diagnostic viewpoint of the investigators may have influenced the clinical judgments of the people in their hospital setting. Thus, the more important test of the validity of those criteria awaited their subsequent adoption in the Spitzer et al. study (1979a). In any event, the seven criteria which made up the Gunderson and Kolb discriminant function have not been separated from the DIB onto a new form and had their psychometric properties independently worked out.

GUND-R SCALE In response to the need for a form which could identify a sample of borderline patients similar to that identified with the DIB, but which could be used retrospectively on hospital records, the author developed the Gund-R scale (Gunderson, unpublished). Preliminary work has suggested a good level of agreement between diagnoses reached with the Gund-R scale based on case records and diagnoses reached on the basis of DIB interviews. A form of concurrent validation has been achieved by taking samples of patients diagnosed as borderline or nonborderline on the Gund-R scale and demonstrating that those fulfilling borderline criteria have a distinct MMPI profile which allows them to be discriminated from other patient groups (Leach, unpublished). This profile coincides nicely with the MMPI profile which has been noted in samples of borderline patients diagnosed by the DIB (Kroll et al., 1981b) or by DSM-III criteria (Snyder et al., unpublished).

SPITZER ET AL. ITEM LIST As noted earlier, Spitzer et al. (1979a) developed a 17-item list which included many of the items which had emerged as most discriminating from the DIB studies. They considered their item list to be inclusive of at least two forms of personality disorder, namely, what they subsequently called unstable and schizotypal. The eight unstable items which subsequently became the criteria for Borderline Personality Disorder in DSM-III do not have reliability evaluations, except for the general reliability figures given for all Axis II Personality Disorder categories (Spitzer et al., 1979a). As noted, the probable unreliability of the use of the DSM-III criteria makes it difficult to interpret studies which rely on them to define their borderline samples.

SCHEDULE FOR INTERVIEWING BORDERLINES (SIB) Baron et al. (1981) have recently developed an interview called the Schedule for

Table 3. Diagnostic Assessment Instruments

Instrument Name	Type	Theoretical Basis	Application		Reliability			Validity		
			I	O	Interrater Var's	Dx	Test-retest	Construct	Concurrent	Replic'n[1]
1. DIB[2] (Gunderson et al., 1981)	Semi-strct'd interview	Discrete Personality Disorder	X	X	0.77	0.87-0.90		X	X	X
2. Gunderson and Kolb, 1978	Item list	"	X		0.75	0.81				X
3. Gund-R scale[3] (Gunderson, unpublished)	Item list	"	X						X	
4. Spitzer et al. (1979a)	Item list	Heterogeneous PD	X	X						
5. SIB[4] (Baron et al., 1981)	Structured interview	"			0.75-0.97[4]	0.88[4]	0.60-0.90[4]			

6. DSM-III (American Psychiatric Association, 1980)	Item list	Empirical[6] Discrete PD	X	X	0.50[4]	0.61[5]	0.54[5]	X
7. Structural Interview (Kernberg, 1977; 1981)	Interview	BPO[7]-all PD	X	X				X
8. BPS II[8] (Perry, unpublished)	Item list	Empirical		X	"adequate"			

1. Refers to studies employing concurrent and established measures of the same phenomena
2. Diagnostic Interview for Borderlines
3. A scale designed for retrospective application to clinical records
4. Schedule for Interviewing Borderlines—reliability figures only available on the "schizotypal" items
5. Based on reliability study for DSM-III categories of Personality Disorder
6. Scale based on empirical work without reflecting theoretical bias
7. Borderline Personality Organization
8. Borderline Personality Scale II

Interviewing Borderlines (SIB). The SIB is a structured interview which assesses the presence or absence of all 17 Spitzer et al. items. It is directed towards the here-and-now content information elicited by an interviewer. As such, SIB departs from the DIB's emphasis on ongoing historical patterns or Kernberg's emphasis on the here-and-now interactional observations. Because of its shorter time frame, it is better suited for measuring change over time of borderline criteria than other existing instruments. Thus far, Baron has reported reliability only on the schizotypal subset, entitled the Schedule for Schizotypal Personalities (SSP). There is little reason to believe the borderline (unstable) items will be discrepant from these. The investigators noted that the item coverage for schizotypal features found in both the Schedule for Affective Disorders and Schizophrenia (SADS) and DSM-III allowed an unacceptable (i.e., $r < 0.50$) interrater reliability. Using the SSP to reduce information variance, the reliability rose to the impressive levels seen in Table 3. In summary, the SSP subsection of the SIB appears to be a promising instrument with high reliability. The instrument awaits further psychometric development, however, especially with regard to the unstable components which are generally expected to define borderline samples. It must be noted, too, that the validity of the schizotypal diagnosis based on the DSM-III items and adopted in the SIB requires much more evaluation before it can be judged.

STRUCTURAL INTERVIEW Kernberg's Structural Interview is designed to test whether borderline patients respond to confrontation, clarification, and interpretation in ways which are hypothesized to discriminate them from patients who are either psychotic or neurotic (Kernberg, 1977; 1981). This diagnostic interview is based on here-and-now interactional features rather than on the content of the interview and the patient's historical patterns of behavior. Where historical information is used, it is mainly concerned with interpersonal relationships. The Structural Interview assesses three areas (reality testing, primitive defenses, and identity diffusion) which are generally considered to require higher level inferences than the areas scored in other instruments. Although some work has been completed in assessing the interrater reliability on the reality-testing area ($r = 0.81$), the methods for assessing reliability in the areas of identity diffusion and primitive defenses are still under development. Psychometric questions about the Structural Interview continue to make it difficult for others to learn to use it, and also make it difficult to generalize from conclusions. The potential advantage of the instrument is that the diagnosis rests upon features which Kernberg believes help to predict psychotherapeutic responsibility.

BORDERLINE PERSONALITY SCALE II (BPS II) The latest instrument is Perry's Borderline Personality Scale II (BPS II). The BPS II consists of a list of those 54 items which emerged from Perry and Klerman's analysis of variance and subsequently survived a replication study (Perry, unpublished). It represents a refinement of the earlier BPS I composed of all 81 items which had been found to differentiate borderline patients. The BPS II has a heavy emphasis on interview behavior, history of interpersonal relationships, and impulsive self-destructivity. The reliability of the items is unclear, but they were tested "for adequacy" prior to being included in the larger item set from which the BPS II was drawn. Perry reports that internal consistency is high and that his scale has the advantage that it can be reliably used by experienced nonprofessionals during unstructured clinical evaluations.

In summary, most of these diagnostic tools have been developed from item sets based on the clinical literature and other clinical impressions. The assessment methods vary from structured interviews (SIB), to semistructured interviews (DIB), to even less structured interviews (the Structural Interview), to item lists to be scored from unstructured clinical interviews (DSM-III, Spitzer et al., BPS II). As Stone (1980) has noted, the instruments also vary in their content emphasis, from the more traditional emphasis that Spitzer et al. place on symptoms to Kernberg's emphasis upon defense mechanisms, with the author's DIB coming somewhere between these extremes.

COMPARING DIAGNOSTIC SCHEMES

KERNBERG ET AL. STUDY Kernberg and his associates (1981) have completed studies comparing different methods of defining borderline samples. His own concept of the borderline category, which he calls borderline personality organization, is of a broad midrange form of psychopathology to be differentiated from two other forms of intrapsychic personality organization, namely, psychotic personality organization, on the one hand, and neurotic personality organization on the other. This contrasts with the concept of borderline personality as a discrete form of personality disorder, a concept embodied in the empirical studies by Grinker and the author. Otto Kernberg (personal communication) believes that this latter concept, which is closely represented by DSM-III criteria, roughly corresponds to that subtype of his concept of borderline personality organization which he calls infantile personality (Kernberg, 1967).

Kernberg et al. (1981) used the Structural Interview to make borderline diagnoses on a sample of patients who were also diagnosed as borderline or not by three other independent methods: the DIB, clinical diagnoses from psychological tests, and an operational diagnosis of borderline based on whether patients performed better on the WAIS than on the Rorschach. This study showed considerable overlap among all of the methods. The 78 percent overlap between patients diagnosed borderline by the DIB and those given this diagnosis by the Structural Interview suggests, in view of the contrasting concepts of borderline upon which each is based, that either the Structural Interview defines a narrower group than its theory would suggest or that the DIB defines a larger sample of persons than its theoretical basis would predict. It seems likely, however, that the overlap would be greater for inpatient samples than for outpatient samples. Among outpatients, more are likely to have personality disorders but not be sufficiently dysfunctional to meet DIB criteria, while they could meet Kernberg's psychostructural criteria and not need hospitalization (Koenigsberg, in press; Stone, 1980). Kernberg et al. (1981) also found, as expected, that the Structural Interview was the most inclusive diagnostic method and that the agreement between the DIB and psychological tests rose to 86 percent when the DIB cutoff was raised from seven to eight.

KROLL ET AL. STUDY Kroll et al. (1981b; unpublished) have completed studies comparing samples of consecutively admitted patients diagnosed borderline and nonborderline under RDC criteria as well as the DIB. They also employed a checklist of the 17 items from the original Spitzer et al. study. In two separate studies, Kroll et al. (1981b; unpublished) found a high degree of correlation between patients diagnosed as borderline or nonborderline using the DIB and those who were placed in these categories using the DSM-III criteria. When they broke the Spitzer et al. item list into items called unstable and those called schizotypal, they found that the DIB diagnosis continued to correlate highly with the unstable characteristics but not with the schizotypal ones. Despite the generally high degree of overlap between the borderline samples diagnosed by these two methods, they preferred the DSM-III criteria to the DIB because DSM-III defined a smaller number of persons as borderline.

COMPARISONS TO DSM-III Several other studies have compared borderlines diagnosed by DSM-III criteria to those diagnosed by DIB criteria and have confirmed the finding of a high degree of overlap. In contrast to Kroll et al., these studies showed that the DSM-III criteria appeared somewhat more inclusive than DIB criteria (Bradley, 1980 study, unpublished; Gunderson et al., unpublished).

In this regard, Stone has written extensively about his expectation that the DSM-III criteria for borderline are considerably more inclusive than those offered by the author or any other investigator, including Kernberg (Stone, 1979; 1980). Until a reliable means of using DSM-III criteria can be compared to the use of DIB, it is probably best to assume that the differences are related to rater variance. What differences ultimately do emerge should be small and should be largely due to the DIB's inclusion of brief psychotic-like experiences.

PERRY STUDY By far the most ambitious effort to compare diagnostic criteria for borderline patients has been the work of Perry (1981 study, unpublished). In his study, Perry drew up lists of criteria attributable to four major contributors in this area (Knight, 1953; Kernberg, 1967; Gunderson and Singer, 1975; Austin et al., unpublished). He subsequently added criteria derived from the Spitzer et al. study (1979a) which, as noted, overlap heavily with those derived from results of the author and Kolb (1978). His final list (BPS II) of 54 variables included those found to be the best discriminators from among those offered by the four contributors. A large sample of patients were then given clinical interviews in an outpatient clinical setting and were rated for the presence or absence of the criteria. Persons diagnosed as borderline and nonborderline by each set of criteria were then compared.

Perry believes that his results show that the patients diagnosed as borderline by Knight's criteria (1953) represent a separate group from those diagnosed borderline by any of the other methods. In particular he noted that the Knight concept of borderline seemed to overlap more with schizophrenia than any of the others. Not surprisingly, in view of their common origins and in view of the results cited above, Perry found a high degree of overlap between samples diagnosed borderline by the author's DIB criteria and DSM-III criteria. On the other hand, it is surprising, yet consistent with Kernberg's results (Kernberg et al. 1981), that he found a high degree of overlap between DSM-III, DIB and Kernberg's criteria. His own BPS II item list also correlated highly with these latter three sets of criteria. Grinker's concept (Grinker et al.

1968) seemed somewhat larger than these others and to have less clear boundaries.

Perry cautions against making a diagnosis of borderline based solely on assessment of the primitive defenses that Kernberg believes are characteristic of borderline personality organization. He found that using that assessment alone would lead to diagnosing a larger number of persons as borderline than would the other, more descriptive criteria. Perry concludes that his results "offer strong convergent evidence for the descriptive validity of the Borderline Personality Disorder" (Perry, unpublished, Abstract). A major problem with this study must be noted, however. It is unclear to what extent the items attributed to the various contributors are valid reflections of their concepts.

DISCUSSION

Most of the studies reviewed used newly developed instruments to assess variables the investigators considered to be characteristic of borderline personality based on the literature and their clinical experience. Instruments have varied from the more extensive, specially designed DIB, which uses trained, professional raters, to checklists, which were employed by relatively inexperienced raters, to an item list given to a large number of practicing psychiatrists. In each instance, in both inpatient and outpatient settings, discriminant function analyses and analyses of variance showed that borderline patients could be discriminated from nonborderlines. Moreover, wherever results could be compared between investigators, they tended to coincide strongly on the variables which were discriminating. The repetitiousness of these findings and the degree of discrimination from the variety of comparison groups allows the conclusion that a reasonably well-defined syndrome exists among patients diagnosed as borderline.

Such concordance among the findings is surprising in view of the disparate concepts behind the use of the term *borderline* and the frequent allegation that the borderline category is a wastebasket diagnosis. This concordance provides descriptive validity to the conclusion that a borderline diagnostic category does exist, a conclusion which virtually all investigators, many of whom began with serious doubts, have made. It is worth noting in this regard that the empirical studies of borderline patients have given the Borderline Personality Disorder a more solid basis than virtually all other DSM-III Personality Disorders, with the possible exception of Antisocial Personality Disorder. By way of contrast, another stepchild of the psychoanalytic tradition, the Narcissistic Personality Disorder, has achieved diagnostic status in DSM-III, despite its having had no empirical studies and despite the considerable controversy as to whether or not it is a trait more or less present in everyone.*

Questions concerning the borderline category do persist, however. One question already touched upon concerns the particular criteria which define the borderline syndrome. Whether or not low work or school achievement is a useful discriminating criterion is a remaining issue. The desirability of including brief psychotic experiences or episodic lapses in reality testing, a second issue, seems to be heavily

*Preceptor's note: For alternate viewpoints and further discussion of the narcissistic personality disorder, see the chapters by Cooper, Ornstein, and the Preceptor at the end of this Part.

supported by existing empirical evidence and calls for a revision in the DSM-III definition.

The second and broader question concerns the boundaries with psychotic disorders. There has been a gradual and steady shift in attention away from the question of whether the borderline syndrome can be discriminated from schizophrenia—it clearly can—and towards the question of the descriptive overlap with the affective disorders. With respect to the empirical studies already done, it was clear from very early on that depression was a highly characteristic but not very discriminating aspect of the borderline patient's phenomenology. A series of recent reports have indicated that many borderline patients will fulfill the diagnostic criteria for Affective Disorders (Stone, 1977; Cole, 1980; Akiskal, 1981; Carroll et al., 1981). The identification of patients who fulfill the diagnostic criteria for both Borderline Personality Disorder and Affective Disorders is a challenging and interesting frontier. Already, there are those who believe that affective disregulation may be responsible for much of the borderline's character pathology (Klein, 1977; Akiskal, 1981) and others, including Carroll et al. (1981) and the author, who believe that the borderline character pathology is primary and that antidepressant therapy is unlikely to affect it much.

A parallel concern is the need to delineate further the borderline syndrome from other personality disorders. Although such discrimination has repeatedly been shown to be possible (Spitzer et al., 1979a; Perry and Klerman, 1980; Sheehy et al., 1980), there is also evidence of overlap of patients fulfilling criteria for Borderline Personality Disorder with some of those fulfilling criteria for other Personality Disorders. Schizotypal Personality Disorder is the most glaring example of this, but there are also suggestions of overlap with other categories as well, including Narcissistic Personality (Kernberg et al., 1981), Antisocial Personality (Akiskal, 1981; Kroll et al., 1981b), and Histrionic Personality Disorders (Kroll et al., 1981b).

These results point to a critical and still unresolved conceptual question. To what extent do the current definitions of a borderline personality syndrome define a discrete personality disorder discriminable from other personality disorders, and to what extent is the syndrome reflective of a midlevel personality organization which encompasses a variety of more specific personality character types? Kernberg (1975) has written extensively about the concept of a midlevel personality organization and favors it as a means of sorting out patients who require or benefit from the treatment paradigm which he advocates. In contrast, the author advocates the concept of the borderline as a discrete type of personality disorder on the basis that the more narrowly defined group of patients presents specific and unique treatment issues and problems that require specific and, to some extent, unique treatment interventions (Gunderson, 1980; Gunderson et al., 1981). Such treatment issues and interventions would not fit the broader range of personality disorders encompassed by Kernberg's concept of borderline personality organization. Given that both conceptualizations look for validation primarily in terms of treatment issues and responses, their relative merits may await studies of treatment outcome.

Many psychoanalysts have in the past criticized Kernberg's concept as being overly broad and inclusive (Dickes, 1974; Meissner, 1978;

Mack, 1975; Robbins, 1976). Recently, the issue of its boundaries has been most sharply joined by debates over whether severe narcissistic disturbances represent a discrete personality disorder with its own developmental line (à la Kohut), or whether they should be subsumed along with most other serious character disturbances within the larger rubric of borderline personality organization (à la Kernberg).

This review has not wrestled with several other issues related to the diagnosis of borderline patients. For example, both Kroll et al. (1981b) and Andrulonis et al. (1981) have suggested descriptive differences between males and females. Nor has this review attempted to struggle with the emerging possibility of a subgroup with serious organic impairments as suggested by Akiskal (1981), Andrulonis et al. (1981), and Paulina Kernberg (unpublished). The broader question of the descriptive subgroupings proposed by Grinker originally and re-shuffled more recently by Austin et al. (unpublished) and Andrulonis et al. (1981) has been only alluded to. Finally, this review has not covered the rapidly expanding literature on the psychological test performance of borderline patients.

Despite persisting questions with respect to the integrity of the borderline diagnosis, as presently defined, the major impressions derived from the foregoing review are that so much work has been done on the subject in the past decade and that considerable progress has resulted. In 1970, enormous variability in the use of the term prevailed, and only one empirical study on borderline cases had been done. By 1980, at least twenty empirical studies were in progress in the United States alone. It is no longer a question of whether a syndrome exists nor even a question of who is designated borderline. The questions now are what meaning the syndrome has, whether the existing syndrome should be further divided, and what is the basis upon which such a division should occur (e.g., psychodynamics, psychopharmacological response, or familial prevalence).

Reflecting the changes in the past decade, the borderline category has moved out of the exclusive province of psychoanalysis and into the mainstream of psychiatry. The proliferating clinical and research studies reflect most of the major controversies within the field of psychiatry itself. Thus, lingering around the edges of the sober presentation of these empirical studies are such major controversies as psychodynamic versus symptom orientations to diagnosis, the relative power of bio-genetic and psychosocial determinants of adult psychiatric syndromes, and the debates within psychoanalytic theory involving the recent developments in self psychology and object relations.

Chapter 29 # Genetic Factors In Borderline Personalities†
by Larry J. Siever, M.D.

INTRODUCTION

Borderline Personality Disorder has only recently been defined as a diagnostic entity, but because of its widespread clinical usage and

†The author acknowledges Ms. Beverly Mucciardi, Mrs. Gloria Goldsmith, Ms. Lindy Rosloff, and Dr. John Gunderson for their assistance and suggestions.

diagnostic contiguity to the major psychoses, researchers had begun some time ago to explore its possible genetic underpinnings. While genetic factors are increasingly implicated in the etiology of the major psychoses, developmental influences remain the focus of interest for the personality disorders. Nonetheless, speculation and research into the respective etiologic roles of genetic factors and environmental factors in the genesis of borderline personality have been stimulated by its position in between the psychoses and personality disorders.

Genetic research pertaining to the borderline diagnostic area originally was primarily oriented towards elucidating the genetic transmission of schizophrenia (Siever and Gunderson, 1979), but these studies generally focused on the prevalence of psychiatric illness in the relatives of schizophrenics. Only recently have investigators begun to identify borderline patients as index cases and then to determine the prevalence of other diagnoses among their relatives. Studies utilizing these different approaches are critically reviewed here with suggestions as to promising avenues for future investigation.

The investigation of genetically determined biologic markers for the major psychoses has proved useful both in diagnosis and as a way of unraveling the etiology of the major psychoses. The extension of this strategy into the borderline diagnostic regions may be helpful in understanding the genetic or constitutional aspects of the borderline disorders and their relationship to the major psychoses. Although this is a new area of investigation, several interesting leads from recent studies are discussed as well.

STUDIES BASED ON BORDERLINE PROBANDS

STONE STUDIES The most relevant studies bearing on the genetics of borderline personality begin with a set of probands and determine the prevalence of different psychiatric disorders in their relatives. Stone (1977; 1979; 1980; 1981) was one of the first to study the family history of an index sample of borderline patients. He used psychostructural criteria according to the scheme of Kernberg (1967) to make his diagnoses and compared the borderlines to patients with psychotic or neurotic structures. A number of investigators agree that the psychostructural criteria for borderlines define a larger group of patients than do the operationalized criteria of Gunderson and Kolb (1978) (Stone, 1977; 1980; Gunderson, 1979; Kernberg, 1979) and that they lead to including a large number of patients that would also be diagnosed as having either classical or spectrum affective disorders (Stone, 1980). The psychotic patients in Stone's sample were mostly schizophrenic or had schizoaffective disorders.

In a study of inpatients, Stone compared the family history of 23 borderline inpatients with that of 23 psychotic inpatients. When possible, relatives were diagnosed by third-year residents according to a Genetic Data Sheet developed from the work of Winokur et al. (1969) and Spitzer et al. (1971). The borderline patients had no schizophrenic and 18 affectively ill relatives, while the psychotic probands had five schizophrenic and ten affectively ill relatives (Stone, 1977; 1980), a significant difference. In a parallel study of outpatients, a group of 23 somewhat healthier outpatient borderlines from Stone's clinical practice were compared to 25 neurotic outpatients. The borderlines had a significantly greater tendency to have relatives with major psychotic disorders and alcoholism than did the neurotic controls. It is interesting to note that the proportion of schizophrenic relatives among the borderline outpatients was greater than that among the borderline inpatients. Thus, while there was a marked predominance of affective disorders over schizophrenia among the relatives of the borderline inpatients, this was not so clearly the case among the relatives of the borderline outpatients.

This study was important in staking out a new area for genetic investigation and suggesting that the borderline disorders, previously conceptualized in terms of their relationship to schizophrenia, may be genetically closely related to the affective disorders. However, the results must be interpreted with some cautions and need to be extended in larger samples with a more rigorous methodology. The study left open the possibility that the increased number of affectively ill relatives of the hospitalized borderline sample, compared to the lesser number of such relatives of the hospitalized psychotic sample, might be due to the contribution of a subgroup of the borderline proband families with a high concentration of affectively ill relatives. This seems probable in that, according to Stone's data (1980), ten of the 23 psychotic probands, compared to 11 of the 23 borderline probands, had at least one relative with manic-depressive psychosis or schizoaffective disorder, not a significant difference. However, among the borderline probands, four had at least two manic-depressive relatives, while none of the psychotic probands had more than one such relative.

The raters in Stone's study, although blind to the probands' psychostructural diagnoses, presumably were not blind to either the hypothesis or the identity of the probands when rating the relatives. Thus, the possibility of rater bias cannot be excluded. Furthermore, the Genetic Data Sheet criteria, which are used to evaluate the relatives, have not been operationalized or standardized. Two final problems were that since the outpatient sample was drawn from Stone's practice, it may not have been respresentative, and it apparently was not evaluated blindly.

GUNDERSON AND KOLB STUDY Gunderson later applied his and Kolb's criteria (1978) to borderlines from the Stone sample. In addition to identifying most of the psychostructurally diagnosed borderline inpatients, their criteria identified as borderline a number of the psychotic probands that had not been diagnosed as borderline by the psychostructural criteria (John Gunderson, personal communication). One might then expect inpatient borderlines, as diagnosed by the Gunderson and Kolb Diagnostic Interview for Borderlines (DIB) (1978), to be more likely to have schizophrenic relatives than those diagnosed by psychostructural criteria. But this does not seem to hold true for the borderline outpatients in Stone's study (1977; 1980) who had schizophrenic relatives. Very few of these would satisfy the Gunderson and Kolb criteria (1978). There may thus be a subgroup of these outpatients with a more isolated schizotypal picture, patients who do not behave in a way that requires the intervention of hospitalization, and these schizotypal individuals might be more likely to have a genetic relationship to schizophrenia. As Stone (1980) points out, the more dramatic symptomatology and self-destructive behavior seen in hospitalized patients may select for those with an affective predisposition.

It would appear that the borderlines diagnosed by Gunderson and Kolb's criteria (1978) may include a subgroup which is genetically related to schizophrenia and of which the members are generally the more severely ill inpatients who would be considered psychotic by the psychostructural criteria. Kernberg's psychostructural criteria for borderlines (1967), on the other hand, may be met by some of the healthier outpatients, who may be more schizotypal in symptomatology and who would not satisfy the Gunderson-Kolb criteria (1978), and this group may also be genetically related to schizophrenia.

Those core borderlines who satisfy both sets of criteria seem to have primarily affective-disordered rather than schizophrenic relatives. Those borderlines with schizophrenic relatives seem to fall either in the more severely ill psychotic regions or in the more mildly schizotypal regions of the borderline diagnostic area. They would therefore not be universally considered borderline by the various sets of criteria. These individuals may show either a more stable schizoid adaptation or decompensate to an overt psychosis, in comparison to those borderlines with affectively ill relatives. The latter group, on the other hand, may show a recurrent, dramatic, affective-related symptomatology in a more "stably unstable" pattern.

Stone notes that many of the borderlines diagnosed by psychostructural criteria also satisfied Research Diagnostic Criteria (RDC) (Spitzer et al., 1975) for affective-related disorders, while other borderlines satisfied some but not sufficient criteria for an affective diagnosis (Michael Stone, personal communication). It might be expected that the affectively ill borderlines have relatives with affective disorders, as the affective disorders have already been shown to have a genetic component (Gershon et al., 1977). Moreover, even borderlines who fall short of satisfying affective disorder criteria have a genetic relatedness to the affective disorders (Stone, personal communication). Further research would be helpful to clarify what proportion of those borderline disorders have coexisting affective disorders, and how many individuals who fail to satisfy current research criteria for affective disorders also have an increased prevalence of affective disorders among their relatives.

AKISKAL STUDY Akiskal and his co-workers (1981) recently reported that of one hundred patients diagnosed as borderline by Gunderson and Singer's criteria (1975) and by DSM-III (American Psychiatric Association, 1980), 45 also had coexisting affective disorders, mostly of an atypical variety. Seventeen had first-degree relatives with a bipolar affective disorder, and another 17 had first-degree relatives with a major depressive disorder. In contrast, only three probands had a family history of schizophrenia. This study did screen for other diagnoses systematically, and it is of interest to note that not only did many of the probands also fulfill criteria for affective diagnoses, but 18 subjects were diagnosed as having agoraphobia or obsessive compulsive disorders, and 21 had either sociopathy or somatization disorder. Only nine had a "pure" schizotypal disorder, although 16 satisfied DSM-III criteria for Schizotypal Personality Disorder. A majority of the patients had a history of substance abuse. On follow-up from six to 36 months later, 37 percent had developed an affective-related episode, while a schizophrenia-related episode on follow-up was observed in only seven probands.

This study supports Stone's hypothesis (1980) that the borderline disorders may overlap with and have genetic factors in common with the affective disorders. Specific diagnoses were applied systematically to a large patient population. However, although the probands were diagnosed borderline according to both DSM-III and Gunderson and Singer's criteria (1975), a standardized operationalized interview does not yet exist for the DSM-III criteria for Personality Disorders. Furthermore, Gunderson and Singer's 1975 criteria for borderlines are unoperationalized, unlike the more recent criteria of Gunderson and Kolb (1978). Other diagnoses for the probands and relatives were presumably made according to DSM-III guidelines, but this is not made explicit. Furthermore, because many (37 percent) of these patients received multiple diagnoses, the degree of overlap of different diagnoses is sometimes difficult to determine, although of potential interest, as in the cases of three individuals in whom dysthymic disorder (a subaffective disorder) and schizotypal disorder coexisted. Unfortunately, the study also lacked a control group from the same clinic with which to compare the borderline probands' and their relatives' diagnoses. If, for example, subaffective or affective disorders, according to Akiskal's diagnostic schema, were to occur in a large proportion of general clinic psychiatric patients, regardless of other diagnosis, no specific relationship between the borderline disorders and affective disorders could be inferred.

The low percentage of borderline outpatient probands with schizophrenic relatives in this study diverges from Stone's findings (1977; 1980) that almost half of the affected relatives of his outpatient borderline sample were schizophrenic. Since the number of borderline probands with schizophrenic relatives is not stated, an explicit comparison is not possible, but again the results suggest that the psychostructural criteria applied to outpatients will include a greater number of schizotypal individuals with a genetic relatedness to schizophrenia.

ANDRULONIS ET AL. STUDY   Another recent study reporting the familial prevalence of psychiatric diagnoses in the relatives of borderline probands was undertaken by Andrulonis et al. (1981). They found that 42 percent of female patients and 22 percent of male patients had a positive family history for the affective disorders, while a family history of schizophrenia was low for all of their patients. In addition, 47 percent of male patients and 34 percent of female patients had a strong family history of alcohol or drug abuse, diagnoses which may in some instances be related to the affective disorders. The overlap between those borderlines with a positive history of affective disorders and those with a positive history of alcohol or drug abuse is not stated. It is interesting to observe the positive family history for affective disorders for this particular group of borderlines, since they may represent a rather different population from those in the previous studies. This group consisted of 91 hospitalized borderline patients who satisfied the criteria for borderline personality according to DSM-III, Gunderson et al. (Gunderson and Singer, 1975; Gunderson and Kolb, 1978), and Spitzer et al. (1979). Since the diagnoses were derived from hospital records and not from structured interviews, the diagnoses must be considered uncertain. Most of the patients were young (average age from 18 to 24, depending on the subgroup) and had been resistant to previous psychiatric intervention. A large proportion of the sample, 53 percent of the males and 13.5 percent of the females, had a positive history for minimal brain dysfunction (MBD) or learning disability.

Eleven percent of the sample had a positive history of brain trauma, encephalitis, or epilepsy. This contrasts with Akiskal's sample (1981), in which the prevalence of all organically related diagnoses was eight percent with four percent having epileptic disorders and four percent having Residual Attention Deficit Disorders, a DSM-III diagnosis related to MBD. Andrulonis et al. (1981) conclude that organic brain dysfunction, related either to MBD or to episodic dyscontrol (suggested to be a limbic dysfunction related to a subclinical seizure disorder) may characterize a subgroup of borderline patients. However, the prevalence of these disorders in a more representative sample and their overlap with affective-related disorders cannot be clearly determined from this pilot study.

TULIS STUDY One of the most recent studies, still ongoing, is the one Tulis and her associates (Tulis, 1980) are conducting at the New York Hospital-Westchester Division. (Their study is independent from Stone's [1980], although he also derived his samples from this hospital population.) In this study, the researchers reviewed the charts of fifty female patients who fit six of the eight DSM-III criteria for Borderline Personality Disorder, more than the five required to make the diagnosis by DSM-III. They aimed to test the hypothesis that this diagnosis may be genetically linked to either bipolar affective disorder or schizophrenia or, alternatively, that it may be primarily a function of maternal or early developmental failures (Tulis, 1980). The rates of manic-depressive psychosis, schizophrenia, neuroses, personality disorders, alcoholism, and suicide in the relatives of the fifty female borderlines were compared to the rates for these disorders among the relatives of one hundred female manic-depressive patients, one hundred female schizophrenic patients, and larger samples including one hundred males from each of the manic-depressive and schizophrenic groups. Only first-degree relatives were clinically diagnosed, and the diagnosis was based on family history information in the chart and on speaking with these patients' therapists (Elaine Tulis, personal communication). The raters were not blind to the probands' identities. Among the borderline probands were two who had a definite affectively disordered parent (one unipolar and one bipolar) and a third from an uncertain bipolar parent. This finding is significantly different from the baseline population rate only if the uncertain bipolar relative is included in the analysis. No certain schizophrenics were found among the first-degree relatives of this sample. No differences appeared in psychotic diagnoses between the relatives of the borderline probands and relatives of both groups of schizophrenic probands. The prevalence of all affective disorders in the relatives of the manic-depressives was significantly greater than in those of the borderlines, if the uncertain diagnosis is not included. A highly significant finding was the greater likelihood of treated neuroses, personality disorders, and particularly alcoholism in the relatives of the borderlines than in the relatives of the control groups. Parental psychopathology and unfavorable childhood environmental circumstances characterized the borderline sample.

This study is consistent with other studies in failing to find a genetic link between borderlines and schizophrenics, but it finds only a questionable relatedness between the borderlines and affective disorders. This may be because only first-degree relatives were considered, in contrast to Stone's study, and because diagnosis was based only on chart information rather than on a direct interview with the proband or relatives as in the previous studies. The study shares with the other studies, except for Stone's, the advantages of having used a substantial sample size and of having employed DSM-III criteria, but it has the disadvantage of not having used blind ratings.

DISCUSSION   It is unfortunate that no studies to date have identified a personality disordered control group. Two studies (Akiskal, 1981; Andrulonis et al., 1981) had no comparison group, while the other two (Stone, 1977; 1980; Tulis, 1980) had psychotic (schizophrenic and manic-depressive) control groups. If strong genetic ties do exist between borderlines and affective disorders, they might be obscured in a comparison between borderlines and affectively disordered control groups, due to the likelihood of a large number of affectively disordered relatives in the controls' families. It would be useful to know if probands with affectively disordered relatives are more numerous in the borderline group than in the nonborderline group or if, in fact, some relatedness to the affective disorders is characteristic of the broader spectrum of personality disorders.

At this point, the studies are too few and the methodology is too lacking to establish with confidence the character of genetic factors that may be important in the genesis of the borderline disorders. Further studies should use clearly defined populations for which the demographic characteristics and sources of referrals are explicitly stated. Standardized criteria, such as those of DSM-III and Gunderson and Kolb (1978), should be applied and preferably operationalized in a standardized interview such as the DIB (Gunderson and Kolb, 1978). The DIB has now been shown reliable in discriminating borderline patients from other diagnostic groups (Gunderson and Kolb, 1978; Soloff and Ulrich, 1981). Useful studies might also aim to determine the overlap with other borderline diagnostic systems such as those of Winokur et al. (1968; 1977), Kernberg (1967), and Liebowitz and Klein (1981). Relatives should be rated blindly, preferably by personal interview, and, again, diagnosed according to accepted standardized diagnostic criteria. Appropriate controls, including probands with other personality disorders, need to be introduced.

Cumulatively, these studies do not support the contention that borderlines as currently diagnosed have a genetic relationship to schizophrenia. Several of them have, however, suggested a genetic relationship to the affective disorders (Stone, 1977; 1980; Akiskal, 1981; Andrulonis et al., 1981) and to other personality disorders (Akiskal, 1981; Tulis, 1980). A large group of borderlines, in the range of half the samples in several studies (Stone, 1977; 1980; Akiskal, 1981; Andrulonis et al., 1981), have coexisting affective disorders. In at least a subgroup of these affectively disordered borderlines, it seems likely that their symptomatology is based in part on genetic factors shared with the more classical affective disorders. In other instances, it is less clear whether the affective symptomatology is primary or secondary to a primary character pathology. Another large proportion of these samples seems to have no diagnosable coexisting affective disorder or positive family history for affective illness. The relative sizes of each of these subgroups and the relationship between the affective psychopathology and the interpersonal and impulse-related symptomatology in borderlines remain open questions. The research reviewed next bears indirectly on the genetic relatedness of borderlines to both the affective disorders and schizophrenia, but these studies sharpen rather than resolve the question.

OTHER GENETIC STUDIES IN RELATION TO THE AFFECTIVE DISORDERS

Other studies of Akiskal and his colleagues (1977; 1980), have suggested a substantial relationship between the diagnosis of borderline and the subaffective disorders such as cyclothymic personality. Almost one-third of their cyclothymic patients had been diagnosed as borderline prior to entry into their affective disorders program. Many of these patients responded to lithium and had an increased prevalence of manic-depressives among their relatives (Akiskal et al., 1980). However, it is not clear how many would satisfy operationalized criteria for borderline personality disorder. Since only seven percent of the borderline patients were diagnosed as having a cyclothymic disorder, these two diagnoses appear to be separable but partially overlapping disorders. How it is that some cyclothymic patients demonstrate borderline psychopathology while others do not is another question that deserves further exploration. Another study demonstrated an increased prevalence of cyclothymic and related personality disorders in the biological relatives of affectively ill probands (Gershon et al., 1977).

Perhaps because of the lack of standardized criteria available for diagnosing borderlines and prevailing conceptions that borderlines were more closely related to schizophrenia, no available studies of manic-depressives or other affectively ill probands have looked explicitly for the presence of borderline diagnoses in their relatives. Such studies might be valuable in determining how closely linked borderline disorders are to more classically diagnosed affective disorders, or whether they reflect a largely independent genetic substrate. In the latter case, the atypical affective features would then be manifest as part of a separate constellation of personality traits.

OTHER GENETIC STUDIES IN RELATION TO SCHIZOPHRENIA

Borderline disorders were at first widely believed to be genetically related to schizophrenia. Bleuler (1924) noted in the early part of this century that a number of relatives of schizophrenics presented with an aloofness and constriction of affect similar in kind, although not in degree, to those features observed in schizophrenics. Overt schizophrenia, although present in relatives of schizophrenics, may not then be the only schizophrenia-related psychopathology in these families. In the 1940's, 1950's, and 1960's, researchers were using terms such as *borderline schizophrenia* (Noble, 1951; Ekstein, 1955), *latent schizophrenia* (Federn, 1947), *pseudoneurotic schizophrenia* (Hoch and Polatin, 1949), *ambulatory schizophrenia* (Zilboorg, 1941), *psychotic character* (Frosch, 1964), *borderline state* (Knight, 1953), and *schizotype* (Rado, 1962a; 1962b). This terminology reflects the attempt to define individuals who might not have an overt schizophrenic psychosis but who did manifest the decreased relational capacity and primary-process thinking observed in schizophrenia. Thus, when investigators such as Kety, Rosenthal, and Wender decided to study the genetics of the schizophrenic disorders, they included in their diagnostic schema the category of borderline or latent schizophrenia. They reasoned that this would increase their sensitivity in picking up disorders that symptomatically fall short of classical schizophrenia but might be genetically related to schizophrenia.

Genetic studies of schizophrenia that shed light on this issue are based on studies of twins, one of whom is schizophrenic, and family studies of schizophrenics, particularly studies of schizophrenics or offspring of schizophrenics who have been adopted away.

KETY, ROSENTHAL, AND WENDER STUDIES The best controlled investigations were the adoptive studies of Kety et al. (1968; 1975), Rosenthal et al., (1968; 1971), and Wender et al. (1974). These researchers collaborated in a series of studies that attempted to separate as much as possible the role of genetic factors from the role of environmental factors in the etiology of schizophrenia and that took advantage of the comprehensiveness of Danish adoptive records. In the extended family study, Kety et al. (1968; 1975) identified a sample of schizophrenics who had been adopted soon after birth. They were able to locate most of the biologic and adoptive relatives of these index probands, to compare the prevalence of schizophrenia between the two groups of relatives, and to compare this rate to the prevalence among corresponding relatives of a matched group of control adoptees.

Of particular interest to the topic of this review was the manner in which the diagnoses of schizophrenia were made (see Table 1). Note-

Table 1. Diagnostic Classification System Used in Adoptive Studies[1]

A. Definitely not schizophrenia (specify diagnosis).

B1. Chronic schizophrenia (chronic undifferentiated schizophrenia, true schizophrenia, process schizophrenia).

Characteristics:

(1) Poor prepsychotic adjustment; introverted; schizoid; shut-in; few peer contacts; few heterosexual contacts; usually unmarried; poor occupational adjustment.

(2) Onset: gradual and without clear-cut psychological precipitant.

(3) Presenting picture: presence of primary Bleulerian characteristics; presence of clear rather than confused sensorium.

(4) Posthospital course: failure to reach previous level of adjustment.

(5) Tendency to chronicity.

B2. Acute schizophrenic reaction (acute undifferentiated schizophrenic reaction, schizoaffective psychosis, possible schizophreniform psychosis, [acute] paranoid reaction, homosexual panic).

Characteristics:

(1) Relatively good premorbid adjustment.

(2) Relatively rapid onset of illness with clear-cut psychological precipitant.

(3) Presenting picture: presence of secondary symptoms and comparatively lesser evidence of primary ones; presence of affect (manic-depressive symptoms, feelings of guilt); cloudy rather than clear sensorium.

(4) Posthospital course good.

(5) Tendency to relatively brief episode(s) responding to drugs, electroshock therapy, etc.

[1]Reprinted with permission from Kety, S., Rosenthal, D., Wender, P., and Schulsinger, F. "The Types and Prevalence of Mental Illness in the Biological and Adoptive Families of Adopted Schizophrenics." In *The Transmission of Schizophrenia*, edited by D. Rosenthal and S. Kety. Oxford: Pergamon Press Ltd., 1968, 345–362.

Table 1.   Continued

B3.   Borderline state (pseudoneurotic schizophrenia, borderline, ambulatory schizophrenia, questionable simple schizophrenia, "psychotic character," severe schizoid individual).

Characteristics:

(1)   Thinking: strange or atypical mentation; thought shows tendency to ignore reality, logic, and experience (to an excessive degree) resulting in poor adaptation to life experience (despite the presence of a normal IQ); fuzzy, murky, vague speech.

(2)   Experience: brief episodes of cognitive distortion (the patient can, and does snap back, but during the episode the idea has more the character of a delusion than an ego-alien obsessive thought); feelings of depersonalization, of strangeness, or of unfamiliarity with or toward the familiar; micropsychosis.

(3)   Affective: anhedonia—never experiences intense pleasure—never happy; no deep or intense involvement with anyone or anybody.

(4)   Interpersonal behavior: may appear poised, but lacking in depth ("as if" personality); sexual adjustment—chaotic fluctuation, mixture of heterosexuality and homosexuality.

(5)   Psychopathology: multiple neurotic manifestations that shift frequently (obsessive concerns, phobias, conversion, psychosomatic symptoms, etc.); severe widespread anxiety.

C.   Inadequate personality.

Characteristics:

A somewhat heterogenous group consisting of individuals who would be classified as either inadequate or schizoid by DSM-II. Persons so classified often had many of the characteristics of the B3 category, but to a considerably milder degree.

D1, 2, or 3.

Uncertain B1, 2, or 3 either because information is lacking or because even if enough information is available, the case does not fit clearly into an appropriate category.

worthy is that they included, in addition to chronic schizophrenia and acute schizophrenic reaction, the diagnosis of borderline state. As the Table shows (B3), this latter category had its forerunners in the diagnoses of pseudoneurotic schizophrenia or "psychotic character." These investigators found that when the schizophrenic spectrum disorders, including chronic schizophrenia and borderline state, were tabulated as a group, they were more prevalent among the biologic relatives of the schizophrenic adoptees than among their adoptive relatives or among either the adoptive or biologic relatives of the controls. This indicates that genetic factors contributed to the onset of schizophrenia in these adoptees. The results suggest that although chronic schizophrenia may be found among the biologic relatives of schizophrenics, it is even more common to find borderline or less clearly diagnosable schizophrenics among these relatives (see Table 2) (Siever and Gunderson, 1979). Thus, the borderline diagnosis, as used by these investigators, appears to have a genetic relatedness to schizophrenia.

However, when relatives of the nine borderline probands are considered separately, no chronic schizophrenics can be observed in their biologic relatives. This may be because the borderlines have less of a

Table 2. Schizophrenia Spectrum Diagnoses of Biologic Relatives of Schizophrenic or Borderline Adoptees in the Danish Adoption Studies*

Diagnoses of Relatives	INDIVIDUALS			FAMILIES		
	Index	Screened Controls	P	Index	Screened Controls	P
Interview study with borderline probands only						
Chronic schizophrenic and borderline relatives	5/38 (13.2%)	2/113 (1.8%)	.011	3/9 (33.3%)	1/23 (4.3%)	.057
Borderline relatives only	5/38 (13.2%)	1/113 (0.9%)	.004	3/9 (33.3%)	1/23 (4.3%)	.057
Interview study with chronic schizophrenic probands only						
Chronic schizophrenic and borderline relatives	19/104 (18.3%)	2/113 (1.8%)	<.001	10/17 (58.8%)	1/23 (4.3%)	<.001
Borderline relatives only	13/104 (12.5%)	1/113 (0.9%)	<.001	9/17 (52.9%)	1/23 (4.3%)	.001
Interview study with chronic schizophrenic and borderline probands						
Chronic schizophrenic and borderline relatives	24/142 (16.9%)	2/113 (1.8%)	.001	12/26 (46.2%)	1/23 (4.3%)	<.001
Borderline relatives only	18/142 (12.7%)	1/113 (0.9%)	<.001	12/26 (46.2%)	1/23 (4.3%)	.001

*Derived from data from Kety et al., 1975.

genetic loading for schizophrenia than do the chronic schizophrenics. But it also raises the possibility that these borderline index cases may have had a somewhat different clinical picture, with different genetic underpinnings, than did the relatives of the chronic schizophrenics. Furthermore, only a small subsample of the borderlines had other borderlines among their relatives, suggesting that only a subgroup may have strong genetic determinants. This is consistent with the possibility that there are different subgroups of borderlines with varying clinical characteristics, reflecting different genetic contributory factors (Siever and Gunderson, 1979).

The other genetic studies of this group of investigators (Rosenthal et al., 1968; 1971; Wender et al., 1974) tend to suggest the same conclusions. The schizophrenic spectrum disorders seem to cluster in individuals genetically related to a schizophrenic (Siever and Gunderson, 1979), but this relationship is less clear for borderline index cases. In the adopted-away study (Rosenthal et al., 1968; 1971), for example, most of the borderlines were among the adopted-away offspring of the chronic schizophrenics. Furthermore, a number of borderlines were diagnosed among the offspring of the manic-depressive parents (Rosenthal et al., 1968; 1971; Siever and Gunderson, 1979). Wender et al. (1974), as part of the same series of investigations, demonstrated that a significant proportion of the offspring of chronic schizophrenics may become borderlines, whether reared by their biologic or by their presumably healthier adoptive parents.

OTHER STUDIES USING THE KETY ET AL. DATA BASE Various other investigators have taken advantage of the rich data set provided by these very important studies in an attempt to refine further the characterization of the borderline relatives of schizophrenics. These studies aid in clarifying the characteristics associated with a genetic relatedness to chronic schizophrenia and thus the relationship these characteristics have to current clinical conceptions of borderline personality.

Among the studies applied to this population are those of Rieder (1979) and Khouri et al. (1980). Both investigators found that borderline schizophrenia, as diagnosed by DSM-III (Rieder, 1979), or by the Symptom Scale for Borderline Schizophrenia (Khouri et al., 1980), could reliably identify the borderline relatives of schizophrenics in these and other adoptive studies (Kety et al., 1975; Rosenthal et al., 1971; Rieder et al., 1975).

Spitzer and his colleagues (1979), in the preparation of DSM-III, also used the adoptive study data. They were interested in defining the characteristics of these relatives as the basis for a new diagnosis: Schizotypal Personality Disorder (see review by the author, Siever, 1981). They saw this new diagnosis as providing a way of separating that usage of the borderline category that was most closely associated with schizophrenia from the other clinical usage of the category. They considered that the latter usage defined a personality disorder characterized by instability, not specifically related to schizophrenia. They developed an eight-item set of criteria that emphasizes schizotypal cognitive eccentricities and that is based on a scrutiny of characteristics of the borderline relatives of the extended family study (see Table 3).

From the clinical literature on borderline personality, they also developed an item set similar to the criteria of Gunderson and Kolb

Table 3. DSM-III Diagnostic Criteria for Schizotypal Personality Disorder

The following are characteristic of the individual's current and long term functioning, are not limited to episodes of illness, and cause either significant impairment in social or occupational functioning or subjective distress.

A. At least four of the following:

(1) magical thinking, e.g., superstitiousness, clairvoyance, telepathy, "6th sense," "others can feel my feelings." (In children and adolescents, bizarre fantasies or preoccupations)

(2) ideas of reference, self-referential thinking

(3) social isolation, e.g., no close friends or confidants, social contacts limited to essential everyday tasks

(4) recurrent illusions, sensing the presence of a force or person not actually present (e.g., "I felt as if my dead mother were in the room with me"), depersonalization or derealization not associated with panic attacks

(5) odd speech (*not* loosening of associations or incoherence), e.g., speech that is digressive, vague, overelaborate, circumstantial, metaphorical

(6) inadequate rapport in face-to-face interaction due to constricted or inappropriate affect, e.g., aloof, cold

(7) suspiciousness or paranoid ideation

(8) undue social anxiety or hypersensitivity to real or imagined criticism

B. Does not meet the criteria for Schizophrenia.

Source: American Psychiatric Association, 1980.

(1978). Their item set, however, did not include the psychotic-like phenomena, an essential part of Gunderson and Kolb's criteria. These items provided the basis for the current DSM-III criteria for Borderline Personality Disorder (see Table 4). Schizotypal and borderline item sets were incorporated into a questionnaire which 4,000 members of the American Psychiatric Association applied to their clinically diagnosed borderline patients. Although the two sets were partially independent, a majority (58 percent) of these patients met DSM-III criteria for both disorders, suggesting the two diagnoses overlap more frequently than they do not. This may be because psychotic-like characteristics, including referential ideation and unusual perceptual experience, are incorporated into the schizotypal criteria but not into the borderline criteria. If the impulsive, affectively unstable borderlines have a sufficient number of psychotic-like phenomena as well, they would satisfy both sets of criteria. These results thus leave open the question of how much and in what ways schizotypal individuals genetically related to schizophrenics may be different from clinically diagnosed borderlines.

A lack of clarity persists regarding the precise criteria that might be best applied to the borderline relatives of schizophrenics and how closely related these characteristics may be to criteria for borderline personality disorder derived from recent empirical studies (Gunderson and Kolb, 1978; Grinker et al., 1968; 1977).

In an effort to answer some of these questions, the author and Gunderson (Gunderson, Siever, and Spaulding, unpublished data) have reexamined the case records from the extended family study of Kety et al. (1975). Independent blind clinical diagnoses and DSM-III criteria for Schizotypal Personality Disorder and Borderline Personality Disorder were applied to 53 subjects with borderline and other personality

Table 4. DSM-III Diagnostic Criteria for Borderline Personality Disorder

The following are characteristic of the individual's current and long-term functioning, are not limited to episodes of illness, and cause either significant impairment in social or occupational functioning or subjective distress.

A. At least five of the following are required:

(1) impulsivity or unpredictability in at least two areas that are potentially self-damaging, e.g., spending, sex, gambling, substance use, shoplifting, overeating, physically self-damaging acts

(2) a pattern of unstable and intense interpersonal relationships, e.g., marked shifts of attitude, ideation, devaluation, manipulation (consistently using others for one's own ends)

(3) inappropriate, intense anger or lack of control of anger, e.g., frequent displays of temper, constant anger

(4) identity disturbance manifested by uncertainty about several issues relating to identity, such as self-image, gender identity, long-term goals or career choice, friendship patterns, values, and loyalties, e.g., "Who am I", "I feel like I am my sister when I'm good"

(5) affective instability: marked shifts from normal moods to depression, irritability, or anxiety, usually lasting a few hours and only rarely more than a few days, with a return to normal mood

(6) intolerance of being alone, e.g., frantic efforts to avoid being alone, depressed when alone

(7) physically self-damaging acts, e.g., suicidal gestures, self-mutilation, recurrent accidents or physical fights

(8) chronic feelings of emptiness or boredom

B. If under 18, does not meet the criteria for Identity Disorder.

Source: American Psychiatric Association, 1980.

disorders. Each of these cases was scored for the presence of 45 characteristics derived from the literature on borderline and schizotypal disorders, including criteria developed by Spitzer et al. (1979), Rieder (1979), Khouri et al. (1980), Grinker et al. (1968; 1977), and Gunderson and Kolb (1978). In the development of this clinical rating scale, the authors attempted to include a broader range of characteristics—including psychosocial functioning and quality of affect and interpersonal rapport—than had been used in the previous investigations. Those had focused selectively on cognitive-perceptual distortions with a psychotic flavor. In the index group of borderlines all but one of the subjects were diagnosed as borderline by both the clinical ratings and the DSM-III criteria for Borderline Personality Disorder, but this diagnosis applied to only a small minority of the borderline relatives of schizophrenics. The index cases in the extended family study appear to have been chosen in greater accordance with current clinical conceptions of borderline personality than were the borderline relatives of schizophrenics, who were rated blindly by the investigators after these relatives were located. Furthermore, as noted earlier, the borderline index cases did not have chronic schizophrenics among their relatives, while the borderline biologic relatives were found largely among the relatives of chronic schizophrenics. The borderline relatives, who by and large had received no psychiatric treatment, did not appear to manifest the impulsive, unstable, or self-destructive behavior observed in many of the index borderline cases, behavior which had, in many cases, led to their hospitalization. The index cases may have represented a more severe variant of the same syndrome observed in the borderline relatives, but it seems quite likely that, in fact, they represent a somewhat different diagnostic entity than do the borderline relatives. Both, however, shared sufficient cognitive peculiarities for the investigators to have given them the diagnosis of borderline state.

DSM-III criteria for Schizotypal Personality Disorder did not identify the borderline relatives of schizophrenics as sensitively as might have been expected, although they did so far better than did the criteria for Borderline Personality Disorder. Relatives of schizophrenics designated borderline by Kety et al. had poorer social adjustment, more eccentric behavior, and more affective and interpersonal detachment, but less discrete affective symptoms, impulse-related instability, and psychotic-like symptoms than all other subjects. This finding was true for the borderline relatives of schizophrenics, whether compared to disordered relatives, borderline index cases, affective-disordered relatives, or the several schizophrenic relatives.

DISCUSSION From the studies considered cumulatively, it appears that individuals genetically related to schizophrenics are likely to exhibit a chronically marginal social adjustment with identifiable eccentricities, a relative social isolation, and a detached interpersonal stance. This picture contrasts with the more dramatic and often self-destructive symptomatology which reflects affective and impulsive instability and is observed in individuals who satisfy the current DSM-III criteria for Borderline Personality Disorder or the operationalized diagnostic criteria of Gunderson and Kolb (1978). A focus on specific psychotic-like characteristics in the manner defined by the DSM-III criteria for Schizotypal Personality Disorder or in the symptom schedule of Khouri et al. (1980) may not clearly distinguish between the two groups. Individuals with Borderline Personality Disorder may have such discrete psychotic-like characteristics, whereas individuals genetically related to schizophrenics may actually show less discrete symptoms in the cognitive sphere and more chronic defensive guardedness, suspiciousness, and isolation. These characteristics may, in some cases, function to preclude the emergence of more obvious breaks with reality testing. An emphasis on quality of affect and interpersonal relatedness, now covered in only two of the Schizotypal Personality Disorder criteria, might help to define this group better. Furthermore, these studies offer no evidence that individuals who have a history of impulsive or affective instability and who may satisfy criteria for Borderline Personality Disorder have an increased prevalence of schizophrenia among their relatives. This suggests that the Borderline Personality Disorder, as defined by DSM-III, may not be closely related to schizophrenia.

Twin studies also may provide a powerful tool for analyzing the role of genetic influences in the etiology of a psychiatric disorder. Such studies applied to schizophrenics are reviewed more comprehensively elsewhere (Siever and Gunderson, 1979) and suggest that borderline disorders appear in the co-twins of schizophrenics but that the picture may not be uniform or easily defined. Investigators such as Gottesman and Shields (1972), Kringlen (1967), Essen-Moller (1970), Inouye (1963), Fischer (1972), Tienari (1963; 1971), Pollin et al. (1966), and Pollin and Stabenau (1968) report findings which suggest that attributes often associated with borderline psychopathology may appear in the co-twins of schizophrenics. These characteristics generally include chronic anxiety, introversion, paranoid ideation, decreased capacity for interpersonal closeness, and, in some instances, discrete psychotic-like symptoms, such as referential ideation. However, since most of the investigations did not classify these individuals with a systematic diagnostic scheme, they cannot at this point add to a more specific understanding of the relationship between borderline personality and schizophrenia.

BIOLOGIC MARKERS IN THE BORDERLINE DISORDERS

Another approach to elucidating the role of genetic factors in the development of the borderline disorders is to identify biologic abnormalities which might indicate an underlying genetic predisposition to the disorders. In some cases, however, the biologic findings may reflect an early biologic environmental insult or may be secondary to the clinical state and thus can not be considered genetic in origin.

Monoamine oxidase (MAO), one of the enzymes which metabolizes central brain amines, may be a biologic marker of some borderline disorders. It has been reported to have decreased activity in bipolar depressed patients (Murphy and Weiss, 1972) and in schizophrenics (Murphy and Wyatt, 1972). In community volunteers studied at NIMH, decreased MAO is associated with sensation-seeking behavior, history of depression, and family history of suicide (Buchsbaum et al., 1976; Coursey et al., 1979). Baron et al. (1980), in a study of student volunteers, have reported that individuals with low platelet MAO, when compared to those with high platelet MAO, showed an increased incidence of borderline schizophrenia as diagnosed by the Schedule for Interviewing Borderlines (SIB) (Baron, 1979). This interview schedule was designed to determine the presence of schizotypal features. Davidson et al. (1980), using a different design, found significantly lower platelet MAO activity in a sample of individuals with a diagnosis of borderline personality or of unipolar depression, compared to patients with depression secondary to chronic anxiety. One might expect low platelet MAO activity to be most closely associated with borderline psychopathology related to the affective disorders, for it is in patients with these disorders that low platelet MAO activity is most consistently observed. Furthermore, the psychopathology observed in student volunteers with low platelet MAO activity in the NIMH studies (Buchsbaum et al., 1976; Coursey et al., 1979) was affective in character. Elevated platelet MAO activity, on the other hand, has been observed in schizophrenia-related depressions (Schildkraut et al., 1978), as well as in the depressives with chronic anxiety described earlier (Davidson et al., 1980).

An abnormal early escape of plasma cortisol concentrations (or initial failure of suppression of cortisol), in response to the dexamethasone suppression test (DST), has been demonstrated to be characteristic of slightly over half of patients with endogenous depression (Carroll et al., 1981). Carroll et al. recently studied 21 patients who met the borderline criteria of Gunderson and Singer (1975) and Spitzer et al. (1979) and in whom the borderline diagnosis was considered primary by their treating clinicians. They found no unequivocal evidence for a concurrent affective disorder, although 13 of 21 of these patients (62 percent) had an abnormal DST. Carroll et al. (1981)

suggest that a significant number of patients may have a melancholic or endogenous depressive episode superimposed on a chronic borderline character disorder. While this may result in a confusing clinical picture, according to Carroll et al., it should not obscure the recognition that such individuals' melancholic episodes may have biologic underpinnings similar to those observed in more classic affective presentations, as reflected in an abnormal response to the DST.

Shortened latency to the onset of REM sleep has also been shown to be a characteristic of affectively disordered patients (Kupfer, 1978). Akiskal and colleagues (1980) have determined that subaffective dysthymic patients, who appeared to have clinical features akin to the primary affective disorders, and who responded to antidepressant medication, also showed shortened REM latency. Many of these patients clinically demonstrated borderline symptomatology. Akiskal et al. (1981) also studied eight outpatient borderlines with the same methodology. They found that the means on REM latency for the borderlines were not significantly different from those of eight affectively ill controls but that the means were significantly different from those of 12 nonaffective personality disordered controls. Thus, the shortened REM latency is a third marker for affective-related symptomatology and has increased prevalence among borderline patients compared to controls.

The author and his colleagues have recently shown an association between another genetically determined biologic marker, disordered smooth-pursuit eye movement (SPEM) (Holzman et al., 1974; 1980; Iacono and Lykken, 1979), and schizotypal characteristics in a non-psychiatrically defined community volunteer sample (Siever, Coursey, Alterman, Buchsbaum, and Murphy, unpublished data). SPEM impairment has been demonstrated in schizophrenics (Holzman et al., 1974; Lipton et al., 1980) and may be present in manic-depressives as well (Lipton et al., 1980). Interestingly, the author has found that student volunteers with impaired SPEM had a significantly greater number of schizophrenia-related characteristics than a high-accuracy SPEM control group (Siever, unpublished data). Of further interest, the characteristics that correlated with low-accuracy tracking included decreased rapport, flattened affect, and social introversion, very similar to those observed in the borderline relatives of the schizophrenics in the Kety extended family study (Kety et al., 1968; 1975; Gunderson, Siever, and Spaulding, unpublished data). However, the characteristics of instability and impulsivity associated with Borderline Personality Disorder, as defined by Spitzer et al. (1979), were not different between the low-accuracy and high-accuracy SPEM groups. Hence, this study suggests that a schizotypal adaptation may be related to a biologic genetic factor observed in schizophrenia and that the schizotypal adaptation is more marked by interpersonal and affective detachment than by positive psychotic-like symptoms.

Another biologic marker that has been related to schizophrenia and the affective disorders and applied to a borderline sample is susceptibility to motion sickness. Extremes of this tendency are associated with affective disorders, while schizophrenics fall in the middle range (Mirabile and Glueck, 1980). Andrulonis and colleagues (1981) found nonorganic female borderlines to cluster in the middle regions of this spectrum, suggesting they may be related to schizophrenic disorders.

Finally, borderline patients may show abnormal EEG and soft neurologic signs, suggesting organic brain dysfunction, perhaps related to the epileptiform disorders or to minimal brain dysfunction (MBD). One group found an increased prevalence of abnormal EEG's in a sample of hospitalized borderline patients (Cowdry et al., 1980). Andrulonis et al. (1981) showed that over half (53 percent) of their male borderline patients and 13.5 percent of their female borderline patients had a positive history for MBD or learning disability. These patients had a greater tendency to engage in antisocial acting-out behavior and alcohol or drug abuse. Several of them responded well to anticonvulsant medication (Andrulonis et al., 1981). These authors suggest that the threshold for impulsive behavior or destructive actions is lowered in these patients, due to excessive irritability of the limbic system, with resultant implications for characterologic development. In most cases, this phenomenon might result from environmental trauma, although genetic factors could conceivably play a role.

CONCLUSIONS

These studies suggest that genetic factors are important in the genesis of at least a subgroup of borderline disorders. Since the different diagnostic schema vary, however, it is difficult to determine what clinical characteristics define those borderlines who have genetic relatedness to schizophrenia or manic-depressive psychosis. The psychostructural criteria of Kernberg (1967; 1975) may select for patients with affective symptomatology or even diagnosed affective disorders, and these patients may be more likely to have a family history of affective disorders (Stone, 1977). The high prevalence of affectively disordered relatives in Stone's study (1980) may be due, then, to the affectively ill patients selected by the psychostructural criteria.

Gunderson's criteria (Gunderson and Kolb, 1978), on the other hand, include more psychotic-like phenomena that may, in some instances, indicate a genetic relatedness to schizophrenia, although they also select for individuals with coexisting affective disorders (Akiskal et al., 1981). Kety, Wender, and Rosenthal's criteria (Kety et al., 1968; 1975; Rosenthal et al., 1968; 1971; Wender et al., 1974) differ from current clinical conceptualizations of borderline. Because they could identify individuals related to chronic schizophrenics, they have been modified as a basis for the new DSM-III diagnosis, Schizotypal Personality Disorder. The outpatient borderlines with schizophrenic relatives diagnosed by psychostructural criteria in Stone's study (1980) may be related to the Schizotypal Personality Disorder as defined by DSM-III.

At present, the strongest genetic links observed in the borderline disorder are to the affective disorders. However, it seems likely that genetic influences related to the major psychoses do not account for a large proportion of the borderline diagnoses, at least as diagnosed by DSM-III criteria. The exact character of the overlap between these different criteria for borderline disorders, as well as how they may interdigitate with subgroups of borderlines with genetic links to the major psychoses, has yet to be determined. It would be of particular interest to select a broadly screened sample of borderlines, to diagnose them according to several of these schemas, and then to compare the clinical characteristics of those who had affectively disordered relatives, those with schizophrenic relatives, those with a high density of personality disordered relatives, and those with a largely negative family history.

Individuals with a genetic relatedness to schizophrenia and the affective disorders and who are clinically diagnosed borderline do seem to exist, as do individuals who may have coexisting personality disorders related to the major psychoses, disorders such as Schizotypal Personality Disorder or Cyclothymic Disorder. If the borderline syndrome is defined as a chronically, unstable, marginal psychosocial adaptation that is not exclusive of other diagnoses, then its coexistence with other psychiatric disorders, such as those on the schizophrenic or subaffective spectrum, seems quite possible. However, if it is defined as an independent entity, to be excluded if either an affective disorder or schizophrenia-related disorder is also present, then one might find that family histories of the major psychoses are lower.

Beyond the factors associating the borderline disorders with major psychoses, biologic factors, whether genetic or environmentally induced, may also be implicated in the etiology of borderline personality. This is suggested by the prevalence of borderlines among the relatives of the borderline probands in the adoptive studies (Kety et al., 1968; 1975; Rosenthal et al., 1968; 1971; Wender et al., 1974) and by the prevalence of other personality disorders among the relatives of the borderline probands in the studies of Tulis (1980). Biologic factors may underlie the characteristics of impulsivity and acting out and thus suggest a relationship to the epileptiform disorders, as suggested by the prevalence of abnormal EEG's and response to anticonvulsants. These phenomena, of course, may have an environmental rather than a genetic basis in many cases (e.g., early neurologic illness or trauma). Another possibility is that less specific genetic factors operate together with unfavorable environmental circumstances to inhibit mature ego development.

A final possibility is that there may be borderlines in whom genetic factors may either play such a small role in the development of the disorder or may be so nonspecific that these factors do not provide a meaningful perspective from which to view the disorder. Making a clear separation between the relative contributions of genetic and environmental factors in any disorder that evolves from an interaction of these two variables is, however, impossible. Adverse environmental milieus that interfere with the accomplishment of normal developmental tasks may predispose an individual to borderline psychopathology even without the presence of specific genetic vulnerability factors. At present, the division of borderline disorders into genetic or nongenetic disorders would be premature and unwise. On the other hand, defining subgroups of borderlines according to slight differences in clinical presentation, their genetic relatedness to other known major psychiatric disorders, or even their psychotropic medication and other treatment response could advance etiologic understanding. Dimensions of such subgroups might be based in part on the likely existence of schizotypal borderlines with a genetic relatedness to schizophrenia, affective borderlines with genetic affinities to the major affective disorders, "dyscontrol syndrome" borderlines related to the epileptiform disorders by virtue of either genetic factors or environmental insult, and a core group of characterologic borderlines who may have less specific or as yet poorly understood contributory genetic factors. What is required are careful studies which attempt to delineate the character and borders of these possible subgroups and to clarify the role of possible genetic factors within them.

Chapter 30 The Drug Treatment of Borderline Patients
by Jonathan O. Cole, M.D. and
Pearson Sunderland, III, M.D.

INTRODUCTION

Concept

The concept of the borderline patient is gradually developing to the point of providing clinicians with usable definitional criteria. Both Gunderson's Diagnostic Interview for Borderlines (DIB) (Gunderson and Kolb, 1978; Kolb and Gunderson, 1980) and DSM-III (American Psychiatric Association, 1980) reflect this conceptual development. In DSM-III the Gunderson concept is split into Borderline Personality Disorder and Schizotypal Personality Disorder. Perry and Klerman (1978) offer a comparison of the criteria which were available before these recent contributions.*

Although it was generally less clearly defined than it is today, the borderline concept has been popular with clinicians for a decade or more. The term tends to be used clinically as a label for those difficult patients who do not respond well to conventional therapies. The authors' experience at McLean Hospital suggests that such patients include those who are neither obvious chronic schizophrenics nor obviously suffering from endogenous depressions. When they fail to respond to treatment for more than two months, the staff begins to call them "borderline." Although this personality diagnosis is often justifiable, one wonders whether anger, impulsive acting out, suicidal attempts, interpersonal manipulation, identity disturbance, and mild psychotic experiences may not be the result of being cursed with a treatment-resistant depression and being treated unproductively in a psychiatric hospital. Could borderline traits be the depressed or neurotic patient's version of the symptoms of chronic institutionalization seen in schizophrenics? Obviously some patients have shown borderline characteristics since adolescence, but others do seem to develop them after having normal-appearing pre-illness adjustment. The longer one struggles with a treatment-resistant patient, the better chance one has to know the patient in depth and to make the distinctions necessary for a diagnosis of some type of borderline state.

Drug Treatment

Despite these reservations about how clinicians use the term *borderline* to express their frustration about difficult patients, many patients do exist who meet the criteria for the borderline state, and they

*Preceptor's note: See the preceding chapter by Gunderson for a review of the early and recent work in this area.

need appropriate treatment. What then can drug therapy offer to those who are correctly diagnosed borderline?

The question is impossible to answer on the basis of the published literature. To the authors' knowledge, only two papers address this issue specifically. The two reported using modern diagnostic criteria for borderline states and reviewed the results of treatment in actual patients. But the number of patients presented in the two papers totals only seven! Moreover, no controlled studies using clear criteria for borderline diagnosis exist either. The review which follows, therefore, covers not only the vestigial literature on drug therapy with borderlines but also reviews reports of the effectiveness of drugs in other clinical conditions which fall in the same no-man's-land between schizophrenia, depression, and neurosis as does the borderline condition. The authors believe that at least some patients considered borderline by some clinicians may fit within other rubrics for which a specific drug therapy has been proposed (Liebowitz, 1979). No specific drug therapy has been developed and tested especially for borderlines. In fact, the only helpful advice grows out of the older and vaguer definition of borderline state. To the extent that such patients fall diagnostically on the border of the older diagnostic entities such as schizophrenia or depression, for which effective drug therapies have been documented, it seems sensible to treat the borderline patient psychopharmacologically as though he or she were on the other side of the border and really had the more clearly treatable diagnosis.

Criteria

Although DSM-III specifies criteria for both Borderline Personality and Schizotypal Personality, the authors believe that the single set of criteria developed by Gunderson and his collaborators approaches more closely what clinicians mean when they use the borderline diagnosis. Gunderson's criteria have, moreover, recently been shown by an independent group to be reliable in differentiating borderline patients from patients with depression and patients with schizophrenia (Gunderson and Kolb, 1978).

Their seven criteria are (1) low achievement, (2) impulsivity, (3) manipulative suicide, (4) heightened affectivity, (5) mild psychotic experiences, (6) high socialization, and (7) disturbed close relationships. With these criteria in mind, the authors reviewed the drug treatment-response literature and prepared a table outlining the better studies in this generally unsatisfactory area (see Table 1).

STUDIES OF DRUG RESPONSE BY DIAGNOSIS

The diagnostic entities or semientities considered are borderline state, pseudoneurotic schizophrenia, Adult Attentional Deficit Disorder, emotionally unstable character disorder, rejection-sensitive dysphoria, impulsive anger, panic agoraphobia, and nonendogenous depression. The results of drug studies in each condition are presented, along with a review of the overlap between these conditions and the Gunderson criteria for borderline states.

Borderline Patients

The most interesting recent report on drug treatment in borderline patients by Brinkley, Beitman, and Friedel (1979) itself contains a reasonable literature review and presents descriptions of drug re-

Table 1. Psychopharmacological Studies of Borderline Patients

Study	Diagnosis	Sample Size	Drug Trial	Study Design	Response	Comments
Pennes (1954)	Pseudoneurotic schizophrenia	20	Amobarbitol 0.25 g—0.50 g iv Methamphetamine 20-40 mg iv Mescaline 0.4-0.6 iv LSD-25 0.01-0.12 mg	Single dose, multiple drug, open trial without placebo control	75% "normalization" of symptoms with amobarbitol and 55% with methamphetamine. "Intensification" with mescaline and LSD	Uncontrolled single dose study with phenomenologic outcome criteria
Vilkin (1964)	Chronic borderline	45	Diazepam 5 mg qd Trifluoperazine 2 mg qd Meprobamate/benactyzine 400 mg/2 mg qd	2-21 day flexible dose, multiple crossover study	Diazepam more effective	No diagnostic or outcome criteria described
Klein (1967)	Pseudoneurotic schizophrenia	32	Imipramine 300 mg qd Chlorpromazine 1200 mg qd	6-week study with randomly assigned placebo-controlled and fixed-dose regimens	Significant drug/placebo difference in favor of imipramine but not for chlorpromazine	Retrospective diagnoses in half of patients
Klein and Greenberg (1967)	Severe psychiatric disorders	13	Diphenylhydantoin 100 mg tid	4-week open trial without placebo control	No generally beneficial effect	No blood levels. Mixed diagnostic group of character disorders and psychoses

Study	N	Medication	Design	Results	Comments
Hedberg et al. (1971)	28	Tranylcypromine 20-30 mg qd Trifluoperazine 8-32 mg qd	8-week double-blind crossover studies using single doses and combination	50% pseudo-neurotic patients responded to tranylcypromine alone	Diagnostic criteria not clearly defined
Paykel (1972)	21	Amitriptyline 100-200 mg qd	4-week, flexible dose open trial without placebo control	Slight, but nonsignificant improvement	No placebo control. Unique diagnostic criterion
Rifkin et al. (1972b)	21	Lithium carbonate	6-week placebo crossover trial double-blind	Lithium carbonate was statistically significantly superior to placebo	Improvement measured via global mood swings with little follow-up
Wood et al. (1976)	15	Methylphenidate up to 60 mg qd	4-week double-blind placebo crossover design	60% favorable response	No controls and no operational diagnostic criteria
Liebowitz and Klein (1979)	14	Phenelzine 15-60 mg qd	6-month placebo controlled crossover study	Symptomatic improvement and progressive mood stabilization	Patients also received intensive psychotherapy concurrently. Study not complete

Pseudoneurotic schizophrenia

Depression and Personality disorder

Emotionally unstable character disorder

Adult minimal brain dysfunction

Rejection-sensitive dysphoria

Table 1. Continued

Study	Diagnosis	Sample Size	Drug Trial	Study Design	Response	Comments
Brinkley et al. (1979)	Borderline	5	Low dose neuroleptics: Perphenazine 16 mg qd Thiothixene 10 mg qd Thioridazine 25 mg qd	Case history	Important supportive role	Retrospective diagnostic criteria. Patients also received other drugs.
Wender et al. (1981)	Adult minimal brain dysfunction	60	Pemoline 18.75 mg to 150 mg	6-week double-blind parallel trial with pemoline and placebo	No statistically significant difference	Unique diagnostic criteria. Future differentiation may be possible using Parent Rating Scale (PRS)

sponse in five borderline patients. All improved substantially on low doses of antipsychotic drugs, responding with improved mood, behavioral stability, and decreased thought disorder. Typical successful drug dosages ranged from 16 mg/day of perphenazine to 10 mg/day of thiothixene or 25 mg/day of thioridazine. Benzodiazepines had been tried without adequate improvement in two of the patients, and doxepin had been only partially helpful in one. In these cases, the benzodiazepines relieved anxiety only somewhat, and the antidepressant relieved depression without affecting the other symptoms. The antipsychotics, however, produced general improvement in affect, thinking processes, and behavior.

An even more recent paper by Lyskowski and Tsuang (1980) describes two patients only, as examples of a drug-responsive borderline patient and of a borderline patient who did not require drug therapy. Unfortunately the first patient, who improved on 15 mg of trifluoperazine, had blunted affect, bizarre behavior, social withdrawal, and chronically inadequate social adjustment. He might have been called a simple schizophrenic or an ambulatory or latent schizophrenic several decades ago. Though he met DSM-III criteria for Borderline Personality Disorder, most clinicians would have identified him as requiring antipsychotic medication. The other patient was mainly depressed, with labile affect, a history of alcoholism, and a disordered psychosexual history. She is *not* documented to have received more than a minimal trial on antidepressants (150 mg/day of doxepin for an unspecified period). She can be inferred to have improved on several psychotherapies in the hospital, but the authors report no follow-up on her posthospital course. The authors do make the point that the DSM-III criteria can encompass some very different kinds of patients, a point with which the authors concur, but the study would have been more useful had it been more extensive and detailed.

Otherwise, the literature on drug response in patients described, however nonspecifically, as borderline is rather barren. Kernberg (1975) notes that tranquilizing medication (unspecified) may be necessary when anxiety interferes with psychotherapy, and Schmideberg (1959) notes that sedation, hypnotics, and placebos can be useful. Last et al. (1973) state that borderline patients are unresponsive to drug therapy, and Ostow (1962) adds that drugs tend to make matters worse. Dyrud (1972) writes that borderline patients like "euphoriants," while phenothiazines may lengthen periods of unpleasant affect. Schick and Freedman (1974), as well as Dyrud, suggest that borderline patients may misuse drugs to attempt to anesthetize themselves against unpleasant affects or to replace empty anhedonia with drug-induced stimulation. The authors' experience at McLean is that borderline patients often have a history of episodic abuse of recreational drugs.

The only published controlled study of drugs in patients described specifically as borderline is contained in a very brief note by Vilkin (1964). Diazepam tablets (5 mg) were more effective than either trifluoperazine tablets (2 mg) or a meprobamate/benactyzine combination (400 mg/2 mg) in a flexible dose, multiple crossover study. All 45 patients received each drug for periods ranging from two to 21 days. Since the author describes neither diagnostic nor outcome criteria, the study results are hard to interpret.

Pseudoneurotic Schizophrenia

Another group of relevant controlled studies involves patients diagnosed as pseudoneurotic schizophrenics (Hoch and Polatin, 1949). Such patients are usually described as having massive anxiety, anhedonia, agitation, and multiple neurotic symptoms (obsessions, compulsions, phobias) and as appearing psychotic at times. Generally, these patients do not have the more typical schizophrenic symptoms, such as delusions or hallucinations, or major disorganization of speech or thought.

Klein (1967) found that such patients respond better to imipramine than to chlorpromazine (CPZ). In his study, CPZ was usually pushed to over 1,000 mg/day, hardly a low-dose regimen. In a double-blind crossover study, Hedberg et al. (1971) compared trifluoperazine (8 to 32 mg/day), tranylcypromine (20 to 30 mg/day), and the combination. Their sample included 96 hospitalized "schizophrenic" patients, 28 of whom were judged to be "pseudoneurotic." All were to receive all three drug regimens, each for an eight-week period. Half of their 28 so-called pseudoneurotic patients did best on tranylcypromine alone. A minor reanalysis of their data suggests that only 16 percent of the 68 nonpseudoneurotic schizophrenics did best on tranylcypromine alone. On the antipsychotic alone, only 22 percent of the pseudoneurotic patients, as against forty percent of the nonpseudoneurotic patients, did best. Both studies of drug therapy in pseudoneurotic patients support the superiority of antidepressants over neuroleptics.

Pennes (1954) reports on the responses of pseudoneurotic schizophrenics, overt nonchronic, nonpseudoneurotic schizophrenics, and chronic schizophrenics to intravenous amobarbital (250 to 500 mg) and to intravenous methamphetamine (20 mg). Of the twenty pseudoneurotic patients, 75 percent showed clear improvement in symptoms after amobarbital and 55 percent after methamphetamine. The overt nondeteriorated schizophrenics showed almost as good a response to amobarbital (64 percent improved), while twenty percent of the pseudoneurotics and 36 percent of the overt schizophrenics were worsened by both drugs. Although the data in this study are not clearly presented, they suggest that pseudoneurotic patients may be more like depressives and might be expected to respond better to a stimulant than would "true" schizophrenics.

Adult Attention Deficit Disorder

Wood et al. (1976) have described a group of adults who resemble children with what is now called, under DSM-III, Attention Deficit Disorder (ADD) and what has also been called the hyperkinetic syndrome. ADD has also been called minimal brain dysfunction (MBD), but this is inappropriate, since most children with this disorder actually have no diagnosable neurological dysfunction. Adult patients, recalling their behavior as children, report typical hyperkinetic behaviors, and as adults they are overactive, anxious, emotionally overreactive, moody, and short-tempered, with low self-esteem, irritability, concentration difficulty, impulsivity, and trouble sticking to things. In a placebo-controlled study, 11 such patients showed clear improvement on methylphenidate in doses up to 60 mg/day. In a recent extension of this work Wender et al. (1981) report the results of a double-blind study of pemoline and placebo in sixty patients meeting similar criteria.

Twenty-seven of them had documentable histories of ADD in childhood, as determined by parent ratings, and only this subgroup showed a clear drug-placebo difference. Useful dosages of pemoline ranged from 9 to 150 mg/day. A period of dosage adjustment and development of tolerance to side effects was often necessary before response occurred. In a number of the patients, improvement was more obvious and striking to the spouse than to the patient. Most patients had marked mood lability as part of their total picture, and those who had been previously treated with lithium found the new drug's effect unpleasant. In summary Wender et al. (1981) propose that stimulant-responsive patients with Adult ADD or ADD, Residual Type, under DSM-III or under their own more detailed criteria should also have met the DSM-III criteria for ADD in childhood.

One of the authors has elsewhere reviewed the larger area of adult MBD (Cole, 1978). Adult MBD is also the subject of a recent book edited by Bellak (1979). In the latter work, Huessey (1979) describes successful use of imipramine in lower dosages (5 to 150 mg/day) in patients who may range from the MBD patients described by Wood et al. (1976) to schizophrenics in partial remission. Some of these patients were already on antipsychotic drugs.

Emotionally Unstable Character Disorder

Rifkin et al. (1972a) have identified a group of often younger female patients who show clear nonreactive mood shifts lasting from an hour to a day or two. At one time, they may show states of unaccountable depression with anhedonia, withdrawal and, often, suicidal ideation. At other times, the patients will be hypomanic—silly, giddy, overtalkative, socially intrusive, overoptimistic, driven, and angry when frustrated. Patients may perceive these periods of nonreactive mood shifts as unpleasant. In between these apparently "endogenous" affective shifts, the patients may show chronic maladaptive behavioral patterns, including rebelliousness, overdependency, drug abuse, promiscuity, or malingering. The mood swings themselves are ameliorated by CPZ or by lithium carbonate. Rifkin et al. (1972b) documented the latter effect in a double-blind crossover study in which emotionally unstable character disorder patients spent six weeks each on lithium and placebo. Fourteen were judged clearly better on lithium. However, the analysis of the intensity of the frequent mood shifts was statistically complex, and only the daily range in global mood showed a statistically significant drug-placebo difference.

In another report, Klein et al. (1977) had described these same patients to show increased mood stabilization on antipsychotics. They have recently suggested (1980) that thioridazine in doses of around 300 mg/hs is most effective and acceptable in this patient group. Nonaliphatic phenothiazines, e.g., trifluoperazine and fluphenazine, often produce irritability, but are sometimes preferred when thioridazine is too sedative. Klein et al. (1980) note that while antidepressants may occasionally help these emotionally labile patients a great deal, they often induce angry irritability instead of improving mood stability.

Rejection-Sensitive Dysphoria

Klein (1972; 1973) has identified this group of patients on the basis of their uniquely favorable response to monoamine oxidase (MAO) inhibitors. The group has been called both "rejection-sensitive dysphoria" and "hysteroid dysphoria." The main characteristic of this predominantly female patient group is marked dependence on external sources of admiration and approval. Patients are elated when given such attention and are desperately unhappy when it is withdrawn. They deny problems when happy and overreact when depressed. Their depressive phases lack endogenous characteristics. Even when well, the patients tend to be dramatic, social, seductive, exhibitionistic, and manipulative. They can be tearful, abusive, and vindictive and can abuse alcohol when rejected and therefore depressed. MAO inhibitors tend to stabilize these patients, making them less vulnerable to rejection and less likely to fling themselves into unwise romantic involvements (Klein, 1973). Klein adds that such patients may be more relaxed, less labile, and less irritable on low doses of trifluoperazine. On tricyclic antidepressants, they often become depersonalized and have somatic side effects or hypomanic symptoms.

It should be noted that phenelzine in doses of 45 to 60 mg/day often works in these patients. Occasionally, an increase up to 90 mg/day is needed to get a response, and the dose is cut back if insomnia and overstimulation become problems (Liebowitz and Klein, 1979). Also, if the patient has frequent, short but intense depressive episodes brought on by rejection, the use of a MAO inhibitor may have to be assessed as a prophylactic regimen rather than as a short-term treatment for acute depression. Theoretically, the drug should be both prophylactic and therapeutic, but in labile patients, the drug's ability to protect the patient against catastrophic overreactions to rejection may be the real clinical end point.

Klein (1972) also describes a separate group of "histrionic" or "hysteroschizophrenic" patients who are labile, agitated, erratic, and manipulative, and who show occasional delusions or hallucinations but are positively and negatively socially active in a rapidly changing fashion. He believes that these patients abuse sedatives and benzodiazepines and either are unresponsive to antipsychotic or antidepressant drugs or rapidly develop florid somatic side effects which cause the therapist to stop the medications. He further believes the patients learn to mimic a wide range of psychopathologies for manipulative purposes. He has not found any drug therapy particularly helpful. (For further discussion of these issues, see Klein et al., 1980).

Impulsive Anger

Uncontrollable angry outbursts are occasionally part of the borderline picture. Sometimes these outbursts are excessive reactions to minor provocation, and sometimes they seem like unprovoked affective explosions. Three pharmacological approaches to treating angry outbursts and/or chronic anger and irritability are discussed.

Neuroleptic drugs certainly reduce anger and hostility in schizophrenic patients. Whether they are as effective in borderline or related conditions is less certain, but the case reports of Brinkley et al. (1979) suggest that they may be. The authors suspect that the neuroleptics are the drugs most commonly used to attempt to control nonpsychotic anger in psychiatric inpatients, but their efficacy for this purpose should be better evaluated. Acute doses of parenteral chlorpromazine or sodium amobarbital, of course, can temporarily stop uncontrolled prolonged anger by putting the patient to sleep.

An ongoing series of studies, mainly uncontrolled (Tupin et al., 1973), is examining the ability of lithium carbonate to reduce impulsive anger and violence. Sheard (1976) has done the only well-controlled and clearly positive study in institutionalized violent offenders. Both he and Shader et al. (1974) review the literature well and present useful case examples. The case Shader discusses does appear to represent an extreme instance of the Borderline Personality Disorder. When it works well, lithium appears to reduce the patient's irascibility and impulsive anger without the sedation or lethargy common to most neuroleptics.

A third approach grew out of the ground swell of interest in psychiatric uses of the anticonvulsant, diphenylhydantoin, about 15 years ago. Stephens and associates (1970) at Johns Hopkins treated a range of psychiatric outpatients with this drug and found the best responses in angry, irritable, anxious patients with good ego strength. In a double-blind, controlled study comparing diphenylhydantoin and placebo in a group of outpatients selected on this basis, these researchers confirmed their preliminary clinical hypothesis.

Monroe (1970) has studied a different, but probably related group of patients who show brief or prolonged episodes of unusual behavior, violent, bizarre, or epileptoid. This behavior sometimes resembles acting out and is usually separable from the patient's interepisode behavior and personality. Patients with these "episodic behavioral dyscontrol disorders" sometimes show EEG abnormalities either during conventional recording or after special drug activation. Monroe notes that the episodes are occasionally worsened by neuroleptics, which lower seizure threshold, and are helped either by anticonvulsants, such as diphenylhydantoin or primidone, or by benzodiazepines, or sometimes by a combination of these drugs. He tends to use anticonvulsants first in episodic behaviors which present more like seizure equivalents, and chlordiazepoxide in more prolonged and psychiatric-appearing abnormal behavioral episodes.

Panic Agoraphobia

Patients with sudden, severe, and frequent panic attacks of overwhelming anxiety, usually accompanied by a variety of somatic symptoms, often develop secondary phobias. They fear being left alone or going out into unprotected situations (agoraphobia), and they often go beyond this state to have chronic anxiety and somatic symptoms in between the panic attacks. They may become manipulative in social relations to avoid being left alone, are subject to intense affects, and can show secondary depression (Klein, 1964). In taking histories from such patients, the initial panic attacks may be lost in the potpourri of secondary symptoms. While this syndrome may not often be mistaken for Borderline Personality Disorder, its response to tricyclic antidepressants (Zitrin et al., 1978) and perhaps even better to MAO inhibitors (Sheehan et al., 1980) is only gradually being appreciated.

Depressive Disorders

Although most borderline patients do not resemble those with old-fashioned, endogenous retarded depressions, many do have significant degrees of depression and related symptoms. Under DSM-III patients can qualify for Major Affective Disorder and Dysthymic Disorder, as well as for Borderline Personality Disorder or Schizotypal Personality

Disorder. To date no study of drug treatments in depression has subdivided from its group of patients a group meeting either DSM-III or Gunderson criteria for borderline states.

Nevertheless, some evidence suggests that such patients can respond to antidepressants. Paykel (1972) relates depressive subtypes to patients' response to amitriptyline and describes a group of younger patients with milder depressions and personality disorder who responded well to that tricyclic, as demonstrated by a fifty percent reduction in global illness score. Quitkin et al. (1979), in their review of the efficacy of MAO inhibitors, note that seven of the eight controlled studies of phenelzine in the vaguely defined conditions of atypical or neurotic depression demonstrate the superiority of phenelzine to placebo. Stewart et al. (1981) report on the superiority of desipramine to placebo in mildly depressed patients who could not ordinarily have qualified for conventional outpatient studies of antidepressant drugs because of their low scores on the Hamilton Depression Scale.

Thus, there is growing evidence that atypical, neurotic, personality-disordered, or mild depression can respond well to tricyclics or MAO inhibitors. This suggests that borderline patients with depression may benefit from antidepressant drug therapies.

OTHER ISSUES

Three years ago, Gunderson's group screened a number of McLean Hospital admissions for Borderline Personality Disorder using Gunderson's DIB (Gunderson et al., 1981). Sixty-two patients qualified for the diagnosis. Two years later their charts were reviewed for evidence of response to drug therapy, and they are now being reviewed again for the possibility that other psychiatric diagnoses may have coexisted. While this work is not complete, at least 15 of the patients also met DSM-III criteria for Major Depression, and 16 others met DSM-III criteria for either Dysthymic Disorder or Atypical Depression. Few patients identified as borderline had systematic adequate trials on both tricyclic antidepressants and antipsychotics, and such drugs as lithium or MAO inhibitors were almost never used. Moreover, when tricyclics were given, doses were often rather low, and treatment lasted only three or four weeks. In the sample as a whole, all that can be said at this point is that antipsychotic medication was judged useful more often than were the tricyclics, although both occasionally led to improvement. Overall, however, patients treated without any systematic pharmacotherapy were doing as well on discharge as were drug-treated patients. Given that this was not a systematic, controlled study and that patients receiving drug therapies may well have been more disturbed than those treated without drugs, the retrospective chart review serves mainly to underline the fact that no single drug class is clearly effective in the large proportion of borderline patients. It does suggest that occasional patients are helped by either antipsychotics or tricyclics. Another point made by the review, also made by DSM-III, is that Borderline Personality Disorder can coexist with other clinical syndromes, such as Major Depression.

Problems in Pharmacotherapy

Patients who fit or approximately fit the criteria for Borderline Personality Disorder, even if they also qualify for other more conventional disorders, such as depression, hypomania, or panic agoraphobia, are often worrisome candidates for drug therapy. Their anger, impulsivity, and manipulativeness may make the psychiatrist worry about the likelihood that the patient will never agree to take the proposed drug at all. The psychiatrist may also be concerned that if the patient does take the drug, it may become the focus of acting out. Some clinicians even suspect that borderline patients are particularly likely to develop side effects or are inclined to magnify them. Thus, both drug manipulation and drug compliance are anticipated problems. Worse still, in patients with a history of impulsive suicide attempts, the real possibilities exist that the patient will overdose dramatically in a suicidal gesture or that he or she will take excessive and dangerous amounts of the drug to suppress transitory feelings of desperation.

Two solutions are possible. One is that a skillful psychotherapist can achieve enough of an alliance with the patient to the point that he or she will be able to handle most life problems realistically, including any problems associated with drug taking. The other possible solution is that the patient, given an adequate dose of an appropriate and effective drug, will be so improved that prior unstable, impulsive, and self-destructive behavior will cease.

CONCLUSIONS

Having scanned possible pharmacotherapies for a variety of psychiatric conditions which fall outside the more rigorous definitions of Major Affective Disorder or schizophrenia, one must still determine what pharmacotherapy, if any, to select for a given borderline patient. This determination should begin with the complex job of getting a detailed history and knowing the patient well. Then one can try to match the symptoms and behaviors elicited with the range of conditions that appear to overlap with the borderline syndrome. An important consideration is the patient's individual history of past responses to prescribed or recreational drugs.

Table 2 correlates the various diagnostic groups discussed in this chapter to Gunderson's criteria for borderline personality disorder (Gunderson and Kolb, 1978), and Table 3 presents a possible approach to pharmacologic decisions. The reader should bear in mind that the evidence about drug therapies suggested in Table 3 is relatively weak. Since the evidence at best stems from one or two controlled studies and at worst from the reported clinical experience of a single senior clinician, the table is an armchair effort. The authors have used some of the principles in inpatient and outpatient consultations on hard-to-diagnose patients. Over the past three years, the senior author has seen a handful of patients who qualify for adult ADD (MBD) and respond to stimulants, or who qualify for emotionally unstable character disorder and respond to lithium. He has yet to see a clear case of rejection-sensitive dysphoria. The episodic dyscontrol inpatients seen have had their angry outbursts reduced by low-dose antipsychotics. A few outpatients with primary anger and relatively good ego strength have responded to diphenylhydantoin. In general, patients with atypical depressions often respond to tricyclics but sometimes develop intolerable side effects and may, then, do better on a MAO inhibitor.

Unfortunately, this whole area is still in flux, and this mapping of a bumpy terrain is the best that can be done at present. The ideas and

Table 2. Characteristics of Borderline Personality Found in Related Conditions

Borderline Personality Disorder Criteria (Gunderson and Kolb, 1978)	Pseudoneurotic schizophrenic	Adult Attention Deficit Disorder	Emotionally unstable character disorder	Rejection-sensitive dysphoria	Panic agoraphobia	Episodic behavior dyscontrol
1. Low achievement	+	+	+	?	?	+
2. Impulsivity	?	+	+	+	?	+
3. Manipulative suicide	+	?	+	+	?	?
4. Heightened affectivity	+	+	+	+	+	+
5. Mild psychotic experiences	+	?	?	+	+	+
6. High socialization	?	+	+	+	+	?
7. Disturbed close relationships	+	+	?	+	+	?

Table 3. Drug Therapy in Borderline States

BORDERLINE STATES	SPECIFIC QUALITIES OF STATES	POSSIBLE PHARMACOTHERAPIES
DEPRESSION PROMINENT	(1) Persistent	Tricyclic or MAO inhibitor
	(2) Rapid brief mood swings, depressed and hypomanic	Lithium or thioridazine
	(3) Precipitated by rejection, relieved by attention, histrionic	Phenelzine
	(4) Mixed with distractibility, restlessness, poor attention span	Stimulants
IMPULSIVE ANGER PROMINENT	(1) Chronic-severe	Antipsychotic
	(2) Chronic-mild	Diphenylhydantoin
	(3) Brief, episodic	Lithium or anticonvulsant
	(4) Mixed with restlessness, short attention span	Stimulants
THOUGHT DISORDER, SCHIZOPHRENIC PSYCHOPATHOLOGY	(1) Chronic	Low dose antipsychotics
	(2) Episodic mixed with multiple neurotic symptoms	Tricyclic or MAO inhibitor
	(3) Episodic, brief, different from patient's usual state	Anticonvulsant

suggestions presented are intended to lead to better studies, as well as to suggest more varied and targeted pharmacotherapeutic trials in individual patients.

Bothersome hints of patient resistance to pharmacotherapy appear in several papers on such diverse but related conditions as adult ADD (MBD), emotionally unstable character disorder, and rejection-sensitive dysphoria. Some of these patients, after a good response to medication, will apparently stop taking it, perhaps to recapture the highs or excitement of the pretreatment state. Of course, depressives, manics, and schizophrenics not uncommonly do the same thing, and perhaps for the same reasons.

The authors nonetheless believe that a reasonable drug is worth trying if it offers at least some hope of substantially improving the patient's disruptive dysphoric state, and particularly if attempts at short-term psychotherapy have proved inadequate. In fact, one reason for hospitalizing a borderline patient may be the opportunity the hospital provides for stabilizing the patient on a new medication and for determining whether the response is good enough to allow the patient to be treated with that drug in the community.

The authors hope that somewhere double-blind, controlled studies of drug therapies are being done with patients who meet explicit criteria for borderline states. If such studies are not yet under way, they should be planned. The next review of this area or some review in the next five years would then not have to range as far and come up with as little as this review.

Chapter 31

The Psychotherapeutic Treatment of Borderline Personalities
by Otto F. Kernberg, M.D.

RECENT LITERATURE

Because major contributors to the study of the psychotherapeutic treatment of borderline conditions gravitate toward a broad definition of borderline personality, the patients they write about might be classified under different headings in DSM-III (American Psychiatric Association, 1980) and by researchers who gravitate to a narrower definition.

Rinsley (1980) and Masterson (1976; 1978; 1980), for instance, concern themselves primarily with patients who, in the author's view (Kernberg, 1975), correspond to the infantile personality. Their patients also seem to correspond with Gunderson's concept of borderline personality disorder* and with what DSM-III designates the Histrionic Personality Disorder and the Borderline Personality Disorder *per se.* Rosenfeld (1979a; 1979b) focuses mostly on borderline patients with predominantly narcissistic and paranoid features, comparable to what DSM-III describes in the criteria for Narcissistic Personality Disorder and Paranoid Personality Disorder. Fairbairn (1954) and Rey (1979)

*Preceptor's note: For a full discussion of Gunderson's concept, see his chapter on empirical studies of the borderline diagnosis.

focus mostly on the schizoid features of borderline conditions characteristic of the Schizoid Personality Disorder in DSM-III. In short, the literature on intensive psychotherapy of borderline conditions covers a spectrum of psychopathology related to the various types of character pathology or personality disorders. In the author's view (Kernberg, 1975; 1980b), they have in common the structural characteristics of borderline personality organization, and in all of these other authors' views, they share common genetic (in a psychoanalytic sense) and developmental features.

Mahler (1971; 1972; Mahler and Kaplan, 1977) has provided the clinical and theoretical framework for these genetic and developmental features. The clinical descriptions in the works of the psychotherapists mentioned and in the works of others who have carried out intensive psychotherapy with borderline patients have all included features common to patients with borderline pathology (Bion, 1967; Green, 1977; Khan, 1974; Little, 1981; Volkan, 1976; Winnicott, 1958; 1965). With the exception of Bion, these authorities all make a distinction between the way they treat borderline patients and the way they treat neurotic patients, patients with nonborderline character pathology, and psychotics. Elsewhere the author has attempted to synthesize the clinical characteristics of borderline patients, developing, in the process, an explanatory frame of reference that links their descriptive and structural characteristics with their transference developments and the psychotherapeutic process (Kernberg, 1975; 1976a; 1976b; 1978; 1980a). Not coincidentally, the psychoanalysts and psychotherapists mentioned have reached a similar conclusion to that of the author. Psychoanalytic object relations theory constitutes a valuable frame of reference and provides an explanatory formulation for both the clinical characteristics of these patients and for their psychotherapeutic process.

In the past, under the influence of Knight's pioneering work (1954a; 1954b), the treatment considered optimal for borderline patients was supportive psychotherapy. Gradually, however, a majority of clinicians who worked intensively with borderline patients shifted to a psychoanalytic (or expressive) psychotherapeutic approach for most of those patients. Unmodified psychoanalysis was still considered possible for some patients.

In addition to the gradual accumulation and published descriptions of clinical experience, one major research project may have contributed to the current preference for expressive psychotherapy. The Menninger Foundation's Psychotherapy Research Project (Kernberg et al., 1972) attempted to compare the effects of psychoanalysis, expressive psychotherapy, and supportive psychotherapy, representing the entire spectrum of psychoanalytically derived psychotherapies, for both patients with "good ego strength," mostly neurotic character pathology and symptomatic neuroses, and patients with "ego weakness," reflecting the borderline spectrum of character pathology. The project supported the conclusion that the best treatment for patients with ego weakness may be an expressive approach, with little structure provided during the treatment hours, combined with as much concomitant hospitalization (environmental structuring) as the patient needs. This approach contrasts with a purely supportive treatment, in which a good deal of structure is provided during the treatment hours and in which there is no hospital support.

It is hard to evaluate the extent to which the findings of this project contributed to the gradual shift from supportive to expressive psychotherapy as the treatment of choice, and further research on long-term psychotherapy of borderline conditions is badly needed. Nonetheless, it is probably safe to conclude that, with the exception of Zetzel (1971) and Grinker (1975), a practical consensus now exists that the psychotherapy of borderline patients should be carried out in an expressive, long-term modality.

A source of some confusion in the literature on the psychotherapy of borderline personality is that some writers tend not to differentiate expressive psychotherapy from psychoanalysis, while others make a sharp distinction in this regard. In the author's view, those who tend to blur the distinction, such as Giovacchini (1979a; 1979b), Little (1981), Searles (1979), and Winnicott (1958; 1965), actually modify their technique sufficiently so that what they do in practice is not standard psychoanalysis. The advantage, in the author's view, of clearly separating expressive psychotherapy from psychoanalysis is that it permits a sharper delimitation of a specific psychotherapeutic approach for borderline patients.

This review would be unbalanced, however, without mentioning that clinical practice often diverges from the clear predominance of recommendations for expressive treatment in the literature. A large number of borderline patients, perhaps the majority, are treated with a mixture of expressive and supportive techniques or in a treatment modality that employs infrequent sessions (one per week or less), signifying a shift from an intended expressive modality to a supportive modality. The clinical effectiveness of crisis intervention and brief hospitalization, along with clear and firm environmental structure, illustrates that a supportive approach is helpful, at least for short-term types of psychotherapy. Another everyday clinical observation is the outpatient maintenance of many borderline patients by means of a long-term supportive psychotherapeutic relationship.

CLINICAL CHARACTERISTICS OF BORDERLINE PATIENTS IN THE PSYCHOTHERAPEUTIC SITUATION

Perhaps the most striking clinical characteristic of patients with borderline personality organization is the *premature activation in the transference of very early conflict-laden object relations* in the context of ego states that are dissociated from each other. Each of these ego states seems to represent a full-fledged, highly developed, regressive transference reaction, within which a specific internalized object relation is activated. This contrasts with the more gradual unfolding of internalized object relationships as regression occurs in the typical neurotic patient.

The ordinary transference neurosis is characterized by the activation of the patient's infantile self: the patient reenacts the emotional conflicts of this infantile self with the parental objects experienced in infancy and childhood. In contrast, the self- and object representations of borderline patients are activated in the transference in ways that do not permit the reconstruction of infantile conflicts with the parental objects as perceived in reality. With these patients, the transference reflects a multitude of internal object relations of dissociated or split-off aspects of the self with dissociated or split-off object representations of a highly fantastic and distorted nature.

The basic cause of these developments in borderline patients is the patients' failure to integrate the libidinally determined and the aggressively determined self- and object representations (Kernberg, 1975; 1976a; 1980a). The problem is that the intensity of aggressively determined self- and object representations makes integration of these with libidinally determined self- and object representations impossible. Because of the implicit threat to the good object relations, bringing together extremely opposite loving and hateful images of the self and of significant others would trigger unbearable anxiety and guilt. Therefore, an active defensive separation of such contradictory self- and object images occurs. In other words, *primitive dissociation or splitting* becomes a major defensive operation.

In working through the transference developments with borderline patients, the overall strategic aim is to resolve these primitive dissociations and thus to transform the primitive transferences into the higher-level transference reactions characteristic of the neurotic patient. Obviously, this requires intensive, long-term treatment along the lines the author has suggested, usually not less than two or three sessions a week over years of treatment (Kernberg, 1975; 1976a; 1976b).

The conflicts that typically emerge in connection with the reactivation of these early internalized object relations may be characterized as a pathological condensation of pregenital and genital aims under the overriding influence of pregenital aggression. Excessive pregenital aggression, and especially oral aggression, tends to be projected and determines the paranoid distortion of the early parental images, particularly those of the mother. Through projection of predominantly oral-sadistic and also anal-sadistic impulses, the mother is seen as potentially dangerous, and hatred of the mother extends to a hatred of both parents, which the child later experiences as a "united group." A "contamination" of the father image by aggression primarily projected onto mother and a lack of differentiation between mother and father tend to produce a dangerous father-mother image and a later conceptualization of all sexual relationships as dangerous and infiltrated by aggression. Concurrently, in an effort to escape dangerous dependency from oral rage and fears, a "flight" into genital strivings occurs; this flight often miscarries because of the intensity of the pregenital aggression which contaminates the genital strivings (Heimann, 1955a).

The transference manifestations of patients with borderline personality organization may at first appear completely chaotic. Gradually, however, repetitive patterns emerge. Reflecting primitive self-representations and related object representations under the influence of the conflicts mentioned above, they appear in the treatment situation as predominantly negative transference. The defensive operations characteristic of borderline patients (splitting, projective identification, denial, primitive idealization, devaluation, and omnipotence) become the vehicle of the transference resistance. The fact that these defensive operations have in themselves ego-weakening effects is a crucial factor in the severe regression that soon complicates the transference developments.

Once a borderline patient embarks on treatment, the crucial decompensating force is the patient's increased effort to defend against the emergence of the threatening primitive, especially negative, transference reactions. The patient intensifies his or her use of the very defensive operations that have contributed to ego weakness in the first place. One main "culprit" in this regard is the mechanism of *projective identification,* described by Melanie Klein (1946) and others, namely, Heimann (1955b), Money-Kryle (1956), Rosenfeld (1963), and Segal (1964). Projective identification is a primitive form of projection, called upon mainly to externalize aggressively invested self- and object representations. Empathy is maintained with external objects onto whom the projection has been made and is linked with an effort to control the object, now feared because of the projection.

In the transference this is typically manifest as intense distrust and fear of the therapist, who is experienced as attacking the patient. The patient feels empathy with the projected intense aggression and tries to control the therapist in a sadistic, overpowering way. The patient may be partially aware of his or her own hostility, but generally feels it is simply a response to the therapist's aggression and that being angry and aggressive is justifiable. The patient behaves as if life depended on keeping the therapist under his or her control. The patient's aggressive behavior, at the same time, tends to provoke counteraggressive feelings and attitudes from the therapist. It is as if the patient were pushing the aggressive part of his or her self onto the therapist and as if the countertransference then represented the emergence of this part of the patient from within the therapist (Money-Kryle, 1956; Racker, 1957).

What the patient projects in a very inefficient and self-defeating way is not pure aggression, it must be stressed, but rather a self-representation or an object representation linked with that drive derivative. Primitive self- and primitive object representations are actually linked by a specific drive derivative or affect state, and these self-object-affect states constitute the basic units of primitive internalized object relations (Kernberg, 1976a). What characterizes borderline patients is that they oscillate rapidly between moments of projection of a self-representation while remaining identified with the corresponding object representation, and other moments of projecting the object representation while identifying with the corresponding self-representation. A patient may, for example, project a primitive, sadistic mother image onto the therapist while experiencing him- or herself as the frightened, attacked, and panic-stricken little child. Moments later, that patient may experience him- or herself as the stern, prohibitive, moralistic, and extremely sadistic primitive mother and see the therapist as the guilty, defensive, frightened, but rebellious little child (see Racker, 1957, on the subject of "complementary identification").

This can be dangerous. Influenced by the intense aggression that the patient expresses, the transference-countertransference relationship may actually come close to reconstituting the originally projected interaction between primitive internalized self- and object representations. Under these circumstances, vicious cycles may develop: the patient projects aggression onto the therapist and, under the influence of the projected aggressive drive derivatives, reintrojects a severely distorted image of the therapist, thus perpetuating the early pathological internalized object relationship.

The rapidly alternating projection of self-representations and object representations, reflecting early pathological internalized object relations, produces a confusion of what is inside and outside in the patient's experience of the interactions with the therapist. It is as if the patient maintained a sense of being different from the therapist at all times, while concurrently exchanging personalities with the therapist. This frightening experience reflects a breakdown of ego boundaries in the interaction and consequently leads to a loss of reality testing in the transference. This loss of reality testing in the transference interferes with the patient's capacity to distinquish fantasy from reality, past from present, and projected transference objects from the therapist as a real person. Such circumstances seriously threaten the possibility that a "mutative interpretation" (Strachey, 1934) will be effective. Clinically, this incapacity to distinguish fantasy from reality appears as the patient experiencing something such as "Yes, you are right in thinking that I see you as I saw my mother, and that is because she and you are really identical." At this point, what has been referred to as a "transference-psychosis" is reached.

The term *transference psychosis* should, the author believes, be reserved for the loss of reality testing and the appearance within the transference of delusional material that does not affect very noticeably the patient's functioning outside the treatment setting. Hospitalization may sometimes be necessary for such patients, and at times it is quite difficult to separate a transference-limited psychotic reaction from a broader one. Nevertheless, in many borderline patients this de-limitation is quite easy, and it is often possible to resolve the transference psychosis in the psychotherapeutic treatment (Holzman and Ekstein, 1959; Little, 1951; Reider, 1957; Romm, 1957; Wallerstein, 1967).

Control of *transference acting out* within the therapeutic relationship assumes central importance. As this acting out of transference becomes a principal resistance to further change, the therapist should introduce parameters of technique to control the acting out. These parameters may give rise to the danger of starting a vicious cycle of projection and reintrojection of the patient's sadistic self- and object representations, and the therapist may appear to the patient as prohibitive and sadistic. The therapist can counteract this danger by interpreting the transference situation, then introducing the structuring parameters as needed, and finally interpreting the transference situation, again without abandoning the parameters. Some aspects of this technique have been illustrated in a different context by Sharpe (1931), who demonstrates how to deal with acute episodes of anxiety.

Because the transference acting out appears to be such a meaningful reproduction of the patient's past conflicts, fantasies, defensive operations, and internalized object relations, the therapist may be tempted to interpret the repetitive acting out as evidence of a working through of these conflicts. The repetition compulsion expressed through this transference acting out cannot be considered working through, however, as long as the transference relationship provides the patient with instinctual gratification of pathological, especially aggressive, needs. Some patients, indeed, obtain much more gratification of their pathological instinctual needs in the transference than would ever be possible in their extratherapeutic interactions. At this regressed level, the patient's acting out overruns the therapist's effort to maintain a climate of abstinence.

The question of *insight* in borderline patients deserves discussion. In some borderline patients, one finds what at first looks like insight into deep layers of the mind and into unconscious dynamics. Unfortunately, this is actually an expression of the ready availability of primary-process functioning which is part of the general regression of their ego struc tures. Insight that comes without any effort, that is not accompanied by any change in the patient's intrapsychic equilibrium, and, above all, that is not accompanied by any concern on the patient's part for the pathological aspects of his or her behavior or experience is question able insight. Authentic insight is a combination of the intellectual and emotional understanding of the deeper sources of one's psychic ex periences, accompanied by concern for and an urge to change the pathological aspects of that experience.

EXPRESSIVE PSYCHOTHERAPY WITH BORDERLINE PERSONALITY ORGANIZATION

Using Gill's (1954) specifications, psychoanalysis may be defined by three technical essentials: first, the analyst's position of technical neu trality; second, the use of interpretation as a major psychotherapeutic tool; and third, the systematic analysis of the transference. In fact, a spectrum of psychoanalytic psychotherapies ranging from psycho analysis to supportive psychotherapies can be differentiated in terms of these three basic features. (Supportive psychotherapy as it applies to borderline patients is dealt with in the final section of this chapter.)

Expressive psychotherapy for borderline conditions may be de scribed in terms of these three technical essentials. Because primitive transferences are immediately available, predominate as resistances and in fact determine the severity of intrapsychic and interpersonal disturbances, they can be and need to be focused upon immediately starting with their interpretation in the "here and now." Genetic reconstruction should be attempted only at late stages of the treatment when primitive transferences determined by part-object relations have been transformed into higher-level transferences or total-object rela tions. At that point, the transferences approach the more realistic experiences of childhood that lend themselves to such recon structions. Interpretation of the transference requires maintaining a position of technical neutrality, for primitive transferences cannot be interpreted without a firm, consistent, and stable maintenance of reality boundaries in the therapeutic situation. The therapist must also sustain an active caution against being sucked into the reactivation of patho logical primitive object relations by the patient. Insofar as both transfer ence interpretation and a position of technical neutrality require the use of clarification and interpretation and contraindicate the use of suggestive and manipulative techniques, clarification and interpreta tion are maintained as principal techniques.

Transference analysis, however, in contrast to psychoanalysis proper, is not systematic. Transference analysis must focus both on the severity of acting out and on disturbances in the patient's external reality, which may threaten the continuity of the treatment as well as the patient's psychosocial survival. Because of this and also because the treatment, as part of acting out of primitive transferences, easily comes to replace life, transference interpretation must be codetermined by three sets of factors—(1) the conflicts predominating in immediate reality, (2) the overall specific goals of treatment, as well as the consistent differentiation of life goals from treatment goals (Ticho 1972), and (3) what is immediate prevailing in the transference.

In addition, technical neutrality is limited by the need to establish parameters of technique (Eissler, 1953). In certain cases such para meters include structuring the external life of patients who cannot function autonomously during long stretches of their psychotherapy. Technical neutrality is therefore a theoretical baseline from which deviations occur again and again, to be reduced by interpretation. The therapist's interpretation of the patient's understanding (or mis-understanding) of the therapist's comments is an important aspect of this effort to reduce the deviations from technical neutrality.

With these cautions and observations in mind, the three technical essentials and the specific effects of these techniques on borderline personality organization can be examined in greater detail.

INTERPRETATION Interpretation is a fundamental technical tool in psychoanalytic psychotherapy with borderline patients. In fact, in order to protect technical neutrality as much as possible, suggestion and manipulation are practically contraindicated here. An exception is made when the potential for severe acting out requires structuring the patient's external life and using a team approach, which implies setting limits and other interventions in the social field. Such social structuring and interventive efforts should be considered parameters of technique, to be interpreted as soon and as comprehensively as possible toward their gradual dissolution.

Some have questioned whether patients with severe psychological illness and ego weakness can in fact respond to interpretation. Do these patients accept the interpretations because of their actual meaning or because of their magical, transference meanings? Empirical evidence indicates that patients with severe psychological illness are indeed able to understand and integrate interpretive comments, particularly if the patient's distortions of the therapist's interpretations are examined and interpreted in turn (Frosch, 1970). In other words, the patient's difficulty in integrating verbal communications is in itself a product of primitive defensive operations, and this difficulty can be interpreted, particularly as the defensive operations are activated in the patient's reactions to the therapist's interpretations.

However, the very fact that the patient's interpretations of the therapist's interpretations must be explored so fully results in clari-fication taking precedence over interpretation. This technical demand creates quantitative differences between expressive psychotherapy and psychoanalysis.

MAINTENANCE OF TECHNICAL NEUTRALITY This is an essential technical tool, an indispensable prerequisite for interpretive work. Technical neutrality by no means excludes empathy. At times the patient's regressive aggression in the transference brings about coun-teraggressive reactions in the therapist. Under such circumstances, technical neutrality depends on the therapist's emotional capacity to maintain an empathic attitude or "holding" action (Winnicott, 1958) and his or her cognitive capacity to integrate or "contain" (Bion, 1967) the fragmentarily expressed transferences.

The patient's potential for severe acting out, however, and the development of life- or treatment-threatening situations or both may require structuring, not only of the patient's life but of the psycho-therapy sessions themselves. Technical neutrality is thereby constantly interfered with, threatened, or limited, and a good part of the therapist's efforts will have to concentrate on returning, again and again, to the

returning to

point of technical neutrality. Again, this reduction in technical neutrality represents a quantitative difference from psychoanalysis proper.

TRANSFERENCE ANALYSIS As mentioned earlier, transference interpretation is limited in these cases and is codetermined by a constant focus on the immediate reality of the patient's life and the ultimate treatment goals. Also, because the interpretation of primitive transference gradually leads to the integration of part-object relations into total-object relations, and, by the same token, to a transformation from primitive transference to an advanced or neurotic transference, relatively sudden shifts occur in the transference of borderline patients. More neurotic or advanced transferences, reflecting more realistic childhood developments, appear at first infrequently and then with increasing frequency throughout the treatment. The shifting of transference phases throughout the treatment gives an overall timelessness to genetic reconstructions and interferes with their historical placement. The transference must therefore be interpreted in an atemporal "as if" mode over extended periods of time, an additional reason for considering transference interpretation in these cases less than systematic, and therefore different from the standard psychoanalytic situation.

Nevertheless, while transference analysis is less than systematic under these conditions, the interpretation of defensive constellations is quite systematic. In contrast to exploratory psychotherapy with better-functioning patients, where certain defenses may be selectively interpreted and others are not touched, the systematic interpretation of defenses in severe psychopathology is crucial to improving ego functioning and to transforming and resolving primitive transferences. The interpretation of the constellation of primitive defensive operations centering around splitting, therefore, should be as consistent as possible, given their detection in the patient's transference and in his or her extratherapeutic relationships.

Guidelines for Managing the Transference

Given these introductory statements, a more comprehensive outline concerning the management of the transference in the expressive psychotherapy of borderline patients follows.

(1) *The predominantly negative transference of these patients should be systematically elaborated only in the here and now, without attempting to achieve full genetic reconstructions.* With borderline patients, the lack of integration of the self-concept and lack of differentiation and individualization of objects interfere with the ability to differentiate present and past object relationships. Patients confuse transference and reality and fail to differentiate the therapist from the transference object. Full genetic reconstructions, therefore, must await advanced stages of the treatment.

(2) *The typical defensive constellations should be interpreted as they enter the transference,* for their interpretation strengthens the patient's ego and brings about structural intrapsychic change, which contributes to resolving the borderline personality organization.

(3) *Limits should be set in order to block acting out of the transference, with as much structuring of the patient's life outside the hours as necessary to protect the neutrality of the therapist.* Although interventions in the patient's external life may sometimes be needed, the therapist's technical neutrality is essential for the treatment. Moreover, it is important to avoid allowing the therapeutic relationship, with its gratifying and sheltered nature, to replace ordinary life, lest primitive pathological needs be gratified in the acting out of the transference during and outside the hours.

(4) *The less primitively determined, modulated aspects of the positive transference should not be interpreted.* Respecting the milder, modulated aspects of the primitive transference fosters gradual development of the therapeutic alliance. With borderline patients the focus on interpretation should be on the primitive, grossly exaggerated idealizations that reflect the splitting of "all good" from "all bad" object relations. These must be interpreted systematically as part of the effort to work through the primitive defenses.

(5) *Interpretations should be formulated so that the patient's distortions of the therapist's interventions and of present reality, especially of the patient's perceptions in the hour, can be systematically clarified.* In other words, the patient's magical utilization of the therapist's interpretations needs to be interpreted.

The strategy of interpretation of the transference with borderline patients may be conceived of as requiring three consecutive steps. These three steps represent, in essence, the sequence involved in working through the primitive transferences and, as part of their working through and eventual resolution, their transformation into advanced or neurotic transferences.

The *first* step consists of the psychotherapist's efforts to reconstruct, on the basis of his or her gradual understanding, the nature of the primitive or "part-object" relation that has become activated in the transference. The therapist needs to evaluate what, at any point, from within the contradictory bits of verbal and behavioral communication of the patient's confused and confusing thoughts, feelings, and expressions, is of predominant emotional relevance in the patient's present relation with him or her. In other words, the therapist, by means of the interpretive efforts, transforms the prevalent meaninglessness or futility in the transference, what literally amounts to a dehumanization of the therapeutic relationship, into an emotionally significant, although highly distorted and fantastic, transference relationship.

As a *second* step, the therapist must evaluate this crystallizing predominant object relation in the transference in terms of the self-representation and object representation involved, and clarify the affect of the corresponding interaction of self and object. The therapist may represent one aspect of the patient's dissociated self- and/or primitive object representation, and patient and therapist may exchange their enactment of self- or object representation. These aspects of the self- and object representations need to be interpreted, and the respective internal object relation must be clarified in the transference.

As a *third* step, the particular part-object relation activated in the transference has to be integrated with other part-object relations, reflecting other related and contradictory, defensively dissociated part-object relations, until the patient's real self and his or her internal conception of objects can be integrated and consolidated.

Integration of self- and object representations, and thus of the entire world of internalized object relations, is a major strategic aim in the treatment of patients with borderline personality organization. Integration of affects with their related, fantasied or real, human relations involving the patient and significant objects is another aspect of this work. The patient's affect dispositions reflect the libidinal or aggressive investment of certain internalized object relations, and the integration of split-off, fragmented affect states is a corollary of the integration of split-off, fragmented internalized object relations. When such a reso lution of primitive transferences has occurred, the integrative affec dispositions that then emerge reflect more coherent and differentiated drive derivatives. The integrated object representations then reflect more realistic parental images as perceived in early childhood. At this point, the borderline patient may be helped to come to terms more realistically with the past, in the context of profound transformations in the relation with the therapist and significant others in his or her present life.

SUPPORTIVE PSYCHOTHERAPY: A REEVALUATION

Supportive psychotherapy, in contrast to psychoanalysis and expres sive psychotherapy, does not use interpretation, only partially uses clarification and confrontation, and, for the most part, uses suggestion and "environmental intervention." The author is now replacing the older concept of "manipulation" (Bibring, 1954) with that of environ mental intervention for a reason that will become clear in what follows. In supportive psychotherapy, the therapist must remain acutely aware of the transference, monitor its developments, and carefully consider transference resistances in relation to his or her technique in dealing with patients' character problems and their connection to life difficult ies. But transference is not interpreted here, and the use of suggestion and environmental intervention implicitly eliminates technical neutral ity altogether.

What follows are tentative conclusions based upon the findings of the Menninger Project, a critical review of the general literature on sup portive psychotherapy detailed elsewhere (Kernberg, in press), and personal clinical experiences with borderline patients in supportive psychotherapy carried out in various inpatient and outpatient settings. The specific literature on supportive psychotherapy of borderline conditions is very scanty. The "purely" supportive approaches earlier recommended by Knight (1954b) and Zetzel (1971), and still sup ported by Grinker (1975), have shifted to the recommendation that supportive techniques be used only for the initial stages of psycho analytic psychotherapy with borderline conditions (Masterson, 1978). Adler and Buie (1979), Modell (1976), and Volkan (1979) stress the supportive effects of the holding function of the therapist, but propose an essentially expressive technique for borderline patients from the beginning of the treatment.

On the basis of the findings of the Menninger Project, the author has proposed rejecting the traditional assumption of Knight (1954b) or Zetzel (1971), among others, that the more distorted or weak the patient's ego, the more supportive the treatment needs to be (Kern berg, 1975; in press). The author questions the long-standing tradition of mixing expressive and supportive techniques, particularly when working with borderline personality organization. The main reason for rejecting this combined technique is the consistent clinical obser vation that the use of supportive techniques eliminates technical neutrality and, by the same token, eliminates the possibility of inter pretation of the transference. Because the borderline patient induces in the therapist strong emotional currents which in turn tend to cause the therapist to abandon a position of technical neutrality, particularly in the most intense transference developments, interpretation of these central transference areas becomes impossible. At the same time, in an effort to maintain an essentially analytic attitude while mingling expressive and supportive techniques, the therapist tends to restrain him- or herself in the use of supportive measures, thus weakening both the expressive and the supportive features of the psychotherapy.

Indications and Contraindications

For all the foregoing reasons, the author believes that when psychotherapy is being considered, it is preferable first to evaluate indications and contraindications for expressive psychotherapy. Strictly speaking, it may in fact be preferable in some cases to raise the question whether psychoanalysis itself is indicated and whether the patient is analyzable. If psychoanalysis is not indicated, as is true for the majority of borderline patients, the next question is whether expressive psychotherapy is indicated or whether it is contraindicated in the particular case. Only if all expressive modalities are contraindicated should supportive psychotherapy be considered and a strictly defined supportive technique adopted. A patient's apparent lack of time, motivation, capacity for introspection, and psychological mindedness—all of which would, if excessive, contraindicate expressive psychotherapy—should be probingly evaluated before settling on supportive psychotherapy.

It is advantageous in all cases to carry out this initial evaluation of the patient using an expressive approach and to give oneself sufficient time before making the decision to undertake supportive psychotherapy. An expressive approach to the diagnostic study facilitates the evaluation of indications and contraindications for the entire spectrum of psychoanalytic modalities of treatment. This approach also leaves the road open for expressive psychotherapy or psychoanalysis: it is easy to shift from an expressive to a supportive modality of treatment, but it is extremely difficult to move in the opposite direction.

The patient's past history of psychotherapeutic engagements may be fundamental in evaluating his or her capacity for undergoing expressive therapy, and for participating in psychotherapy at all. Several other issues may tilt the balance toward a supportive rather than an expressive mode. If the patient's illness is providing a considerable degree of secondary gain, or if the patient presents severe antisocial features, the prognosis for expressive psychotherapy is not good. Other issues militating against expressive therapy include disorganization of external life circumstances severe enough to require major environmental interventions; a general sense of urgency for such environmental interventions because of potentially damaging developments in the patient's current life; a chronic absence of actual object relations (patients with severe social isolation); and the presence of severe nonspecific manifestations of ego weakness, such as lack of anxiety tolerance, impulse control, or sublimatory channeling.

The severity of some of these features, however, may also contraindicate supportive psychotherapy, for example, chronic lying, even without an antisocial personality structure; a history of negative therapeutic reactions, with violent aggressive behavior and destructive or self-destructive acts, during past psychotherapy with skilled therapists;

and relentless masochistic acting out. These findings may raise doubts as to whether any kind of psychotherapy could be initiated on an outpatient basis. A period of brief or even extended hospitalization may clarify these issues and significantly broaden the potential range for all psychotherapeutic interventions. Supportive psychotherapy is an ideal modality for crisis intervention, and to combine a supportive technique in the sessions with direct interventions in the patient's environment provides an effective time-limited treatment.

Treatment Goals

Early in the consultation or at the start of treatment, whether the modality is long-term supportive psychotherapy, expressive psychotherapy, or psychoanalysis, the general goals and specific objectives of the treatment should be specified. Also important are to define at least one area in which patient and therapist are in agreement regarding such goals, to separate treatment goals from life goals (Ticho, 1972), and to clarify with the patient that psychotherapy is work carried out jointly between patient and therapist. The therapist's function is to contribute knowledge that may help the patient to understand him- or herself and his or her conflicts better and to work accordingly on conflicts and problems in reality. These requirements pertain most importantly to supportive psychotherapy, precisely because opportunities for systematic analysis of the patient's primitive transferences and magical perception and expectations are less available there than in an expressive psychotherapy. Specifications of goals and expectations can create a rational basis for the supportive treatment and constitute a boundary of reality against which transference distortions may later be diagnosed and modified. The patient's continuing responsibilities for his or her own life should be spelled out, and, if the need for external support is anticipated, its structure and relation to the treatment should be defined.

One major advantage of supportive therapy is that the frequency of sessions can be adjusted from two to three per week, to one every other week, or even less. The less frequent the sessions, however, the more important it is to evaluate the work the patient carries out between the treatment hours, and the more important it is that the therapist actively connect the contents of one session with another. The therapist must fully explore the patient's life and the conflicts and patterns of interactions outside the treatment hours, and in the process must challenge vagueness, lack of information, and the distorting effects of primitive mechanisms of denial, fragmentation of emotional experience, devaluation, and so forth. Such an active exploration of the patient's life, in contrast to the therapist's passive submission to the patient's defensive suppression or vagueness, tends to highlight the patient's primitive defense mechanisms and their resistance functions, and the exploration thus constitutes a first step in a challenge to such defensive operations.

The goals and objectives of supportive psychotherapy may range from ambitious to modest. But even modest goals may exceed the patient's capacities. A modest goal for the patient who may not be able to function independently in the foreseeable future should be to permit him or her to function autonomously within his or her limitations, facilitated by ongoing psychotherapeutic support. In other cases, supportive psychotherapy may permit the patient gradually to seek out and make use of alternative supportive environmental structures, and the psychotherapy can end when the patient is able to replace it by these other supports (Robert Michels, personal communication).

It is generally preferable to set goals and objectives that aspire to an increase in the patient's level of functioning and autonomy, and to shift into a more "custodial" form of supportive psychotherapy only when it becomes clear that the patient's capacity for cooperation and intrapsychic and psychosocial resources are insufficient to the more ambitious goals. In all cases, one must be alert to the presence of secondary gain of treatment in the form of chronic social parasitism.

Techniques

The basic technique of supportive psychotherapy consists of the exploration in the here and now of the patient's primitive defenses. The objective of this exploration is to help the patient achieve control over the effects of defenses through nonanalytic means and to foster a better adaptation to reality as the patient becomes aware of their disorganizing effects. In the process, manifest and suppressed (as opposed to unconscious and repressed) negative transferences can be highlighted, reduced by means of consistent examination of the reality of the treatment situation, and utilized for clarification of related interpersonal problems in the patient's life.

Consider, for example, a patient with paranoid personality, who uses projective identification, who is hypersensitive to criticism, and who experiences him- or herself as being attacked by others, while unconsciously provoking them into such attacks, and as being sadistically controlled, while subtly exerting such control over others. Such a patient may be gradually helped by focusing in a tactful, persistently challenging, yet nonthreatening way on how the patterns of his or her interactions with others tend to repeat themselves. The analysis of these difficulties with others will naturally be helped by the fact that the therapist has already observed similar behaviors in the treatment relationship. Very often, however, the systematic analysis of the patient's behavior in relation to others may be the first stage of a later exploration of the same behavior in the treatment situation. In other cases, to the contrary, early exploration of the transference in the here and now should precede the exploration of these issues in extratherapeutic interactions. This is particularly necessary when negative transference developments predominate, when these developments may threaten the continuity of the treatment, and when they are a major challenge to the treatment alliance in supportive psychotherapy.

Or consider the patient whose splitting operations are reflected in shifts from primitive idealization to total devaluation of others. The therapist may show the patient how these predictable sequences tend to weaken the objectivity of the patient's judgment of others and tend to threaten his or her relationships with such others. The therapist can also show the patient how a critical reflection about any total and extreme judgment of others may help to discriminate his or her reality.

Still another example is the need to clarify the denial manifest in a patient's neglect of serious work responsibilities, together with magical assumptions that what is denied will not have any predictable effects.

There is an important difference between a therapist's giving a patient advice on how to handle his or her life and the therapist's helping the patient to understand how certain "automatic" ways of functioning are detrimental to his or her interests. The therapist should not give a patient advice about issues that the patient may be able to handle but is defensively avoiding. The therapist's function is to acquaint the patient with the behavioral manifestations of the primitive defenses and their effects upon his or her evaluation of reality and decision-making processes.

In this connection, supportive psychotherapy can in fact be very "permissive" in increasing the patient's internal freedom for decision making by confronting him or her with internal contradictions. On the other hand, what often looks like the therapist's tolerant, permissive attitude may actually reflect the therapist's unconscious collusion with the patient's self-defeating tendencies.

In contrast to the therapist's position of technical neutrality in psychoanalysis and his or her constant reference to technical neutrality in expressive psychotherapy, the therapist who is practicing supportive psychotherapy is deliberately partisan to the needs of external reality and mindful of the patient's emotional needs. In other words, the therapist is promoting both adaptation and impulse expression. Occasionally, when adaptation conflicts with impulse expression, the therapist should acknowledge the conflict and be available to explore it with the patient.

Another general principle of supportive psychotherapy is to refrain from the use of advisory, "supportive" statements and environmental "manipulation," if to do so would exploit unanalyzed primitive transference dispositions. Clarification, confrontation, and environmental intervention, as well as the therapist's direct opinion on matters in which the patient objectively needs advice should all operate through rational channels. They should convey that the therapist has confidence in the patient's own critical judgment and in the patient's capacity for understanding and for using that understanding constructively.

Here the author is rejecting the traditional concept of "manipulation" as one supportive technique, in spite of its benign use by psychoanalysts interested in supportive psychotherapy. Manipulation conveys a denigrating attitude both toward patients and toward supportive psychotherapy. We certainly cannot avoid the suggestive effects of rational interventions, or, at a deeper level, powerful yet undiagnosed transference reverberations related to all we say and do during the patient's treatment in supportive psychotherapy. Nevertheless, by providing information and carefully considered and limited advice, and by directly expressing support on the basis of rational considerations, supportive effects may be obtained while the boundaries of reality in the treatment situation may thus be reinforced. Only against these boundaries of reality can we detect primitive defenses and transference distortions in the treatment and the patient's acting out in external reality.

This also means that when we wish to introduce medication as part of supportive therapy, we should explain its rationale and what the patient can expect from it. Medication should be used in pharmacologically effective doses rather than for placebo effects. If placebo effects do develop, they should be diagnosed without necessarily interpreting them, but without attempting to exploit them either. The therapist must maintain the internal logic and consistency of his or her conceptual scheme and techniques and of the verbalized understandings that define the goals and responsibilities of patient and therapist in the treatment situation.

At the start, one must define the major issues in the patient's life and psychopathology that are to be explored and modified in the course of treatment. This is a precondition both for the definition of the treatment objectives and for defining the roles of patient and therapist in obtaining the objectives. The goals of treatment should be realistic, to be achieved by mechanisms that can be explained to the patient and discussed. One should not assume that, simply by getting together, the patient and therapist will magically and jointly bring about a solution of the patient's problems. It is important to raise the question early whether direct environmental intervention is warranted or necessary, how it will be carried out, and whether any limits to the patient's behavior need to be set as a precondition for treatment. Severely destructive or self-destructive tendencies in the patient's immediate life may require such realistic preconditions.

The therapist must stress the patient's responsibility for honest communication to the therapist and the expectation that the patient will carry out work between the sessions. In addition, the therapist should set up a way of monitoring and evaluating, from session to session, how the treatment is influencing the patient outside the hours. Ideally, the patient should be expected to keep the therapist well informed about developments in his or her life, and to communicate promptly and fully on areas of conflicts and problems. The patient's difficulties in this regard or failure to achieve such a level of cooperation requires careful exploration.

Indications and contraindications for psychopharmacological treatment or other special therapeutic techniques should be evaluated fully in the initial stages of treatment, rather than introduced haphazardly and later on in response to the patient's failure to improve. In other words, a strategic integration of various treatment techniques as part of an overall treatment plan is preferable to a disorganized throwing in of new modalities in response to transference—and countertransference—developments.

Noninterpretive Transference Interventions

One major problem in the practice of supportive psychotherapy may be the therapist's unwarranted imitation of psychoanalytic technique. If the therapist conveys the sense of "sitting back" and leaves entirely to the patient the initiative for structuring the content of the hours, subtle forms of transference acting out are fostered. The patient shifts into a passive-dependent attitude toward the treatment, and primitive defenses go underground in the transference.

What follows are some practical considerations regarding noninterpretive transference interventions in supportive psychotherapy. As a most general statement, moderately intense positive transferences may be utilized for psychotherapeutic work, but intense primitive idealization must be treated cautiously because of the concomitant devaluation processes that are usually active in some other area of the patient's life. Latent negative transferences must be detected for strategic planning. Manifest negative transferences must be actively explored, clarified, and reduced by a realistic and full examination of the relevant conscious and preconscious fantasies, feelings, and behaviors, and by reinforcing reality considerations.

The therapist must be mindful that, insofar as he or she tolerates the patient's expression of intense ambivalence, he or she is carrying out a "holding" function in Winnicott's (1958; 1965) sense. Such holding reassures the patient of the therapist's permanence. The patient discovers that the therapist does not crumble under the impact of the patient's aggression and that it is possible to maintain a good relation with the therapist even in the presence of frustration and anger. All of these understandings reduce the patient's fears over his or her own impulses and foster strengthening of integrative ego functions.

In all types of treatment, work with the transference starts with conscious and preconscious tranference manifestations. This work continues until the patient's here-and-now fantasies about the therapist are explored and clarified. In the case of supportive psychotherapy, however, in contrast to the other two modalities, this exploration is not connected interpretively with the patient's unconscious relation to the therapist or with his or her unconscious past. It is instead used for confronting the patient with the reality of the treatment situation and with parallel distortions in the patient's external life. The beginning of work with transference manifestations is the same in all three modalities of treatment. The end point is very different. If a patient in supportive psychotherapy presents the therapist with very primitive regressive fantasy material, the communication is not neglected, but it is traced back to reality issues. In expressive psychotherapy, the direction is reversed: the usual path is from reality to the exploration of the underlying fantasy.

PROGNOSTIC CONSIDERATIONS

There are few systematic studies of prognostic features in the long-term psychotherapy of borderline conditions. The psychotherapy research project of the Menninger Foundation indicated that those patients with low initial ego strength, and particularly low initial quality of interpersonal relationships, showed the least improvement (Kernberg et al., 1972). On the basis of a detailed clinical evaluation of the patient population of that project, the author suggested that prognostic features included the predominant type of character constellation; certain ego and superego distortions reflected in individual character traits; self-destructiveness as a character formation; the particular type and intensity of negative therapeutic reactions; the degree and quality of superego pathology; and the quality of the patient's object relationships (Kernberg, 1975).

In evaluating the distribution of personality types among borderline office patients with respect to treatment outcome, Stone (unpublished) had findings in agreement with the prognostic considerations the author had suggested. Borderline patients with personality types of a predominantly hysteric, obsessive, depressive, phobic, infantile, and passive type had a rather successful outcome. In contrast, the majority of borderline patients with personality types that were predominantly paranoid, narcissistic, schizoid, explosive, hypomanic, inadequate, and antisocial ended in treatment failure. Masterson (1980) stressed the prognostic importance of the degree of early-life stress, the level of early ego development, the degree of mastery of early developmental tasks, and the effectiveness of early social relationships (object relations).

While there are other prognostic references sprinkled throughout the literature on intensive psychotherapy of borderline conditions, the evidence regarding most postulated prognostic features does not yet seem to be conclusive. The author's present view, probably consonant with that of Masterson and of Stone, is that the two most important prognostic indicators are the presence of antisocial features—which definitely worsen the prognosis for psychotherapeutic treatment—and the quality of object relations—which is in direct relation to a favorable prognosis. In addition, the development of negative therapeutic reactions is an important process variable with significant prognostic implications. The importance of other personality and environmental variables and of the techniques, skill, and personality of the therapist, as well as his or her countertransference, all require further systematic research. The relationship between the process and outcome of long-term psychotherapy remains an area that is as underrepresented in the psychotherapy research literature as it is crucial in the daily clinical practice of the psychiatrist and psychoanalyst.

Chapter 32

Narcissistic Disorders Within Psychoanalytic Theory
by Arnold M. Cooper, M.D.

INTRODUCTION

In recent decades growing interest in the psychoanalytic theory of narcissism and the self, and an increasing concern with the description and treatment of narcissistic disorders, have been major sources of new ideas and new data in psychoanalysis. This interest in narcissism and its disorders stems from multiple sources. Freud's usage of the term and the concept of narcissism left many areas of unclarity and ambiguity which later workers have sought to remedy. At the same time, conceptualizations of narcissism and the self seemed increasingly central in attempting to understand psychic development, the genetics and dynamics of psychopathology, and aspects of the phenomenology of the psychoanalytic process. The data of researchers in early infancy and childhood, the growing criticism of propositions of classical metapsychology, and the influence of the British object relations theorists all helped to fuel the growing interest in narcissism. There has also been a growing conviction on the part of psychoanalysts and observers of culture that disorders of narcissism have become increasingly prevalent in our time, replacing the neurotic disorders that Freud described.

One might say, then, that the need to restore theoretical coherence to many psychoanalytic propositions, a dissatisfaction with aspects of current theory, and the need to enhance our understanding of and therapeutic effectiveness with narcissistic disorders have combined to refocus our attention on the concepts of narcissism and narcissistic disorders. Against this background, the work of Heinz Kohut, with its central emphasis on the self, generated enthusiasms and controversies which in turn stimulated the efforts of psychoanalysts to supply confirming or negating data. It is probably fair to say that narcissism has been the fulcrum of the major psychoanalytic researches of at least the past decade. These researches into narcissism and the self have penetrated almost every aspect of psychoanalytic theory with a most productive reexamination of basic psychoanalytic ideas.

HISTORY

In an excellent review, Pulver (1970) has pointed out the many differing meanings assigned to the term and concept of *narcissism*, initially in Freud's writings and subsequently throughout the analytic literature (consult Pulver for a full review of Freud's writings on narcissism). Clinically, Freud referred to narcissism as a sexual perversion, characterized by treating one's own body as a sexual object, or as a basis for homosexual object choice in seeking a body like one's own. Genetically, he used the term to refer to a developmental stage of libidinal investment in the self. In terms of object relationships, narcissism referred either to a form of object choice in which aspects of the self predominate over the actual aspects of the object, or to a state of relative absence of object relations. Freud also used narcissism to denote aspects of self-esteem, on the economic assumption that self-esteem rises as the self is narcissistically cathected. Further, he used narcissism to characterize a mode of infantile thinking characterized by magical, omnipotent thought. To complicate matters further, Freud blurred distinctions between the concepts of ego and self, using the word *ICH* for both meanings. Thus, it was often unclear whether Freud was referring to a structural entity or giving a more holistic description (Laplanche and Pontalis, 1973).

The concept of narcissism was essential to Freud as he expanded his psychoanalytic purview, partly in response to criticisms of Jung and Adler, to include consideration of the self, ego development, the capacity for idealization, and the range of behaviors not adequately described as derivatives of the sexual instincts. In effect, the work on narcissism was a starting point for the development of ego psychology as elaborated by other theorists. Furthermore, Wilhelm Reich used the concept of narcissism as the basis for his important work on character. "Character is essentially a narcissistic protection mechanism . . . against dangers . . . of the threatening outer world and the instinctual impulse" (Reich, 1949, 158). The many differing meanings contained within the term narcissism parallel the changing frames of reference of the analytic point of view—topographic, developmental, economic, genetic, dynamic, and structural.

In a general way, Freud attempted to maintain a distinction between the transference neuroses and the narcissistic neuroses. Whether Freud derived this division clinically or theoretically is not entirely clear. The transference neuroses, amenable to psychoanalytic treatment, comprised those psychological disorders in which, within the psychoanalytic situation, the individual would, predictably, form a definable, intense attachment to the therapist. The distortions and resistances represented in this attachment recapitulated earlier attachments and the specific drive-defense conflicts around these attachments. The vividness of the transference, especially in its fully developed form as a transference neurosis, provided an opportunity to explore the genetics and dynamics of the distortions which contributed to the maladaptive life behaviors. The narcissistic neuroses, in contrast, referred to those disorders in which, within the analytic situation, the patient seemed unable to form an intense and relatively stable attachment towards the therapist.

The theory of libido economics required that narcissistic individuals have invested excessive available libido onto their own selves, and show a consequent impoverishment of libidinal investment in objects, as manifested in the failure to form object attachments. Most analysts today would agree that narcissistic character disorders have transference manifestations characterized by an apparent shallowness or absence of attachment, but this phenomenon is not understood in terms of libido economics. On the other hand, the more severe borderline and schizophrenic disorders are liable to show the most intense, although the most distorted, transferences.

Another way to characterize the distinction between the classical neurotic disorders and the narcissistic disorders is in terms of the origin and nucleus of pathology as oedipal in the former and preoedipal in the latter. Patients with more severe characterologic pathology are fixated in dyadic preoedipal conflicts, leading to failure of adequate structure formation at oedipal levels and to particularly severe distortions of oedipal triangular relationships. The question of the nuclear role of the Oedipus complex was of concern to Freud. In 1931, in his paper "Female Sexuality," Freud described his discovery that preoedipal events accounted for the nuclear pathology of certain neurotic disorders in women (Freud, 1961a). Although he had in 1905 described the Oedipus complex as a "shibboleth" of psychoanalysis (Freud, 1961b), Freud stated in 1931 that he should now question or abandon that position. But he did suggest that the description of the Oedipus complex could be expanded to include preoedipal events. The issue of the core role of the Oedipus complex has remained an important debate in psychoanalytic literature and is one of the many current controversies encompassed within the study of narcissistic disorders.

Although a detailed further history of the concept of narcissism is beyond the scope of this chapter, a few additional points are noteworthy. Heinz Hartmann (1950) attempted a sharper distinction between self and ego in an effort to clarify some of the problems of the concept of narcissism. In essence, his work and the later elaborations by Jacobson separated the concepts of self as person, ego as structure, and self-representation as a subsystem within the structural schema. Narcissistic pathology represented a disorder of libidinal investment of the self rather than of the ego. Spruiell (1981), in agreement with Laplanche and Pontalis (1973), suggests that this attempt to remove the ambiguity of Freud's use of *ICH* as both self and ego has been a step backwards and has retarded understanding of problems in narcissism.

While psychoanalysts have not yet achieved agreement on the theory and dynamics of narcissism, several general tendencies can be discerned. First, there is a recognition that issues of *narcissism*, defined either as a "concentration of psychological interest upon the self" (Moore and Fine, 1968, 57) or as self-esteem regulation, are aspects of all psychopathology. All disorders of the psyche have effects upon the self-representation and the nature of self-esteem regulation and are in turn affected by these functions. Second, narcissism, in the sense of self-interest, is increasingly recognized as being an aspect of healthy, normal functioning, rather than as being only an archaic developmental phase. Residues of infantile grandiosity and idealization are contributors to the capacity for enthusiasm and creativity in healthy adult life. Third, narcissistic configurations can present as regressive defenses against higher-level oedipal pathology and may not in themselves be indicative of primary disorders of the self.

Despite the many attempts to clarify the concept of narcissism, a mixture of meanings continues to be given to the term in the psychoanalytic literature. It is probably not possible to separate the usage from its origins in libido energic theory, and this theoretical viewpoint is incompatible with the views of the many analysts today who are seeking terminology that is more experience-close.

While ego psychologists have struggled with the integration of concepts of narcissism into the structural scheme, other theorists have attempted other solutions to the problems of conceptualizing narcissism. With many differences between them, psychoanalysts as diverse as Sullivan (1953), Horney (1939), Rado (1956), Winnicott (1965), Erikson (1963), and Fairbairn (1954) have, in various ways, suggested that the construction of the self, or an equivalent thereof, was a central task of all psychic development, and that this self develops interactionally through transactions with the caretaking individual. Each of these theorists regarded the task of maintaining the wholeness of the self as the primary goal of psychic development. Failures are variously characterized as developments of a "bad me" or a "false self" or an "inflated self" or, in a somewhat different vein, "identity diffusion." Rather than discussing each of these concepts in the detail they perhaps deserve, the author later reviews Kohut's concept of the central role of the self. His work has pioneered the current interest in narcissism, although many of his ideas were, of course, expressed by the other workers.

DISORDERS OF NARCISSISM

The Narcissistic Personality Disorder is a category in DSM-III (American Psychiatric Association, 1980). It is generally agreed that individuals with this personality disorder display disordered behavior in their self-centered grandiosity, their inability to maintain loving relations with others, and the instability of their self-esteem. Their grandiosity may be conspicuous or subtle, may express itself openly in exhibitionistic claims for attention, or may be partially hidden in attitudes of self-depreciation and shyness. They tend to be self-centered and self-important. They see all life events in terms only of their impact on themselves and crave attention and love as if they constantly needed to confirm their own grandiose fantasies.

Narcissistic characters may initially present a surface picture of attractive charm, but they lack the capacity for sustained loving attitudes or empathic concerns for other persons. Indeed, their relationships are characterized by deep mistrust, angry and envious feelings of others' successes—often poorly hidden—and an inability to experience positive feelings deeply or to share these feelings with others. Relationships tend to be characterized by an oscillation from initial overidealization and unrealistically inflated expectations from the other person, to eventual cynicism and bitter disappointment as the feet of clay are "discovered." Underneath their apparent charm may lie exploitive demands and a basic coldness towards others, with a lack of intimate connection with the other person and a one-sided demand that the other gratify the needs of the narcissist and ask nothing in return. Kernberg (1975) considers that narcissistic persons do not experience genuine depression with real sadness when confronted with loss, but rather experience resentment and vengeful wishes. Angry envy tends to color their relationships to persons who are not being idealized. Their inability to experience or respond with appropriate empathy to the needs of another is conspicuous.

Self-esteem tends to oscillate according to the immediate level of success in winning outside approval. There is an apparent inability for satisfying self-reward. Often these persons are capable of genuine achievement, even brilliance, but their gratification does not come from their own satisfaction with their work; rather, they measure themselves in the radiance of others' admiration. Their own work often leaves them feeling bored, and they seem to lack genuine enthusiasm and joy. Their emotional lives lack depth, and perverse activities are frequently present. Depression is common, as is hypochondriasis, and they experience a heightened susceptibility to feelings of injury when their unwarranted feelings of entitlement are not gratified. Frequently, advancing age and loss of youthful beauty present a crisis with a sense of failure and hopelessness.

The diagnosis of a narcissistic personality disorder can often be made in initial interviews. Not infrequently, however, a trial period of psychoanalytic treatment is required in order to reveal the narcissistic transference manifestations of narcissistic pathology. Narcissistic personality disorders occur in a wide range of severity, at one pole merging with borderline disorders, and at the other merging with oedipal conflictual disorders. Many variations in presenting symptomatology are also noted, including varying degrees of sociopathy, compulsiveness, and perversion.

PSYCHOANALYTIC THEORIES OF NARCISSISTIC DISORDERS

The deepening investigations of the origin and nature of disorders of narcissism have led to sharp differences among psychoanalytic theories about the tasks and organization of early psychic development. This ongoing controversy can be typified by brief descriptions of the work of Heinz Kohut and Otto Kernberg.

The Work of Kohut

Heinz Kohut constructed a unified theory of human behavior and an increasingly abstract metapsychology. The central concept in his recent work (1977) is that of the bipolar self, a mental organization of the self composed on one end of tendencies towards ambition and exhibitionism, and on the other of ideals and goals. These two poles of the self are linked by a tension arc of talents and skills. In the case of satisfactory development, primitive grandiosity and primitive idealization are tempered into enthusiastic ambitions, fueling the development of talents which enable the joyful achievement of desired values and goals. In order for development to proceed along these lines, the infant requires an appropriate relationship with the mothering person who is capable of the empathic responsiveness which feeds the needs of the developing self. The infantile grandiosity requires empathic "mirroring," an approving responsiveness or "the gleam in the eye" which feeds the child's sense of effectiveness and initiative. The child's primitive idealizing tendencies require a parent or parents capable of tolerating the idealized capacities for power and omniscience with which the infant must endow the caretaker in order to borrow needed strengths. Under satisfactory circumstances of empathic mothering, a cohesive, vigorous self will develop as a relatively autonomous center of initiative and creative joy. In Kohut's view, failures of appropriate self development are a consequence of a failure of empathic responsiveness from a responsible parent.

Kohut has posited that the development of the self proceeds through the internalized bonding of self and other, with the other perceived as a *selfobject*. The term *selfobject* refers to the mode in which another individual is "used" and internalized to provide not yet developed or missing parts of one's own self. To the extent that the other is perceived as a selfobject, the person is not perceived for his or her own qualities but is perceived as a needed aspect of the incomplete self. Kohut originally used the concept of the relation to the selfobject to describe a developmental stage and later expanded it to describe an ever changing, but lifelong human need (Kohut, 1980). All individuals live in a sea of selfobjects, strengthening their selves by varying degrees of internalization and merger with aspects of others. In "healthy" adult life this use of a beloved as a selfobject does not prevent the simultaneous recognition of the other as separate and as an object of one's own empathic interest.

According to Kohut, the construction of the cohesive bipolar self is the primary organizing sequence of psychic development. Its organization precedes drive organization, and it is not inherently conflictual. In this view, drive manifestations and tripartite structure are second-order products that emerge as the self develops its own hierarchic complexity. In the event that progressive and appropriate self development fails to occur due to failures of empathy on the part of the caretaker, the individual experiences fears of annihilation or of self-fragmentation. It is under these conditions that pathological manifestations of sexual and aggressive drives will appear as "disintegration products."

Within Kohut's conceptual framework, narcissistic personality disorders would include those individuals who have basically achieved a coherent and stable self (they are neither schizophrenic nor borderline), but in whom the self lacks sufficient cohesiveness or robustness. Because of this lack, such individuals under stress experience a threat of fragmentation of the unified self organization.

This imputed priority of self organization carries several implications:

(1) Intrapsychic conflict appears only relatively late in development, i.e., at the oedipal stage if development proceeds appropriately. It may further be implied that even the oedipal phase need not be a time of major intrapsychic conflict if the self is sufficiently robust.

(2) There is basically only one disorder in psychic life, a disorder of self organization. Other manifestations of psychopathology with drive-defense conflictual configurations are secondary to failures of the self.

(3) Narcissistic pathology is not conflict pathology, since conflict is not a significant element in psychic development until the oedipal phase. Narcissistic disorders represent an *arrest* of self development. Pathology of the self is therefore a deficiency disorder due to the failure of aspects of the self to develop, secondary to defects in early empathic responsiveness.

(4) Treatment will be significantly altered if the task is one of creating *missing* self structure rather than resolving intrapsychic conflict. (Treatment will be discussed briefly in a succeeding section.)*

*Preceptor's note: See also the following chapters by Ornstein and by the Preceptor for alternate views of treatment, with Ornstein describing an approach derived from Kohut.

(5) The nature of man is perceived differently from traditional psychoanalysis. Kohut envisioned his man as Tragic Man struggling to achieve his creative potential in the universe, versus Freud's vision of Guilty Man struggling to escape from inner conflict. While Freud sought to help man escape from neurotic suffering into ordinary human misery, Kohut hoped to help man to achieve joy and creativity. The mark of healthy functioning for Kohut and his followers is the capacity for joyful, enthusiastic creative activity.

(6) Kohut placed very special emphasis on the empathic-introspective point of view in psychoanalysis, insisting that all of our data collection occurs through our empathic perceptions and that these must also guide our therapeutic interventions. In his view, positivistic attempts to separate the observer from the observed have been responsible for errors in the development of analytic theory and technique.

The Work of Kernberg

Otto Kernberg presents another point of view in attempting to deal with the theoretical and technical problems raised by the narcissistic personality disorders (Kernberg, 1975; unpublished[a]; unpublished[b]). Though much closer in many of his writings to more traditional ego psychological viewpoints, Kernberg has nonetheless also differed sharply, if more subtly, with some of the traditional metapsychological views. Kernberg has leaned heavily on the work of Mahler, Jacobson, and the British School of object relations theorists. He describes the self as a component of early ego development originating in an un-differentiated internalized fusion of self and object. Over time, with the experiences of satisfaction and frustration, in interaction with objects, a separation of self and object begins to occur.

This view, held by many analysts, differs from Freud's original view of earliest narcissism being entirely invested in the self and only later in the object. In Kernberg's view (unpublished[b]), the earliest unit of motivation is a conglomeration of affect activation, the memories and cognitions associated with the affects, and the object relations matrix in which they are aroused. These complex states are, over time, sorted into generally loving or hating, or libidinal or aggressive, tendencies towards both self and object. All early infantile experience contributes to the differentiation and integration of internalized self- and object representations. In the course of normal development, there is a structural tension of the superego (the internalization of idealized self- and object images) and the ego (the representation of actual self- and object images). In the case of narcissistic personality disorders, the differentiated internalized self- and object representations are fused again as a defense against anxieties arising in interaction with the caretakers. The narcissistic disorders represent pathological re-fusion of ideal self-images, ideal object images, and actual self-images, all for the purpose of attempting to destroy a hated and feared actual object.

Narcissism, therefore, regularly carries with it not only distortions of the self, but also of the superego. According to Kernberg, the narcissistic character is in effect saying, "I do not need to fear that I will be rejected for not living up to the idea of myself which alone makes it possible for me to be loved by the ideal person I imagine would love me. That ideal person and my ideal image of that person and my real self are all one, and better than the ideal person whom I wanted to love me, so that I do not need anybody else anymore" (Kernberg, 1975, 231). Some of the consequences of this internal rearrangement include a denigrated self-image, viewed as fearful, hating, empty, and weak, and an attempt to project it onto the object, who is then viewed as dangerous and depriving. Where Kohut describes the mother of the narcissist as unempathic, Kernberg describes the parental figure as cold and aggressive. Kernberg sees the narcissistic structure as one designed to maintain dangerously feeble self-admiration by depreciating others and avoiding acknowledgment of dependency. Kernberg's view of the narcissistic disorders differs in very significant ways from Kohut's:

(1)   He views the self as an aspect of ego development.

(2)   The danger situation arising out of the unresponsiveness of a cold mother leads to rage, with a consequent predominance of splitting mechanisms which prevent an integration of idealized and actual selves and idealized and actual objects.

(3)   The predominance of rage and the attempt to maintain perfection in isolation, rather than experience the danger of intimacy, are the presenting configurations in analysis.

(4)   The issue is one of conflicts and drive-defense constellations, rather than one of a failure to develop aspects of a structure.

(5)   The narcissistic self is not a self which has been arrested at a phase of development requiring a resumption of growth, as Kohut implies. Rather, the narcissistic self is a pathologically distorted adult self requiring a change in organization.

(6)   Kernberg attempts to blend object relations theory with structural theory and to maintain the concepts of instinctual drives by deriving drives from motivating affects, rather than, as Freud did, regarding drives as primary biological givens.

CRITIQUE

The many analysts who, with varying degrees of difference, are pursuing ideas derived from Kohut's work continue to present a rapidly changing psychoanalytic landscape, as did Kohut himself. Several things seem clear to this observer. Similar to Edmund Bergler (1949) before him, Kohut worked to derive a unitary theory of psychopathology based upon narcissistic injury, or defective development of the self, as the source of all other forms of pathology. In fact, all other pathological constellations may be viewed as attempts to repair the basic pathology of the self. Kohut never did, perhaps, entirely give up the idea of "complementarity" which he had put forth in his early work, suggesting that Freud's structural schema for intrapsychic conflicts applies at the level of oedipal pathology, while his own schema of self pathology applies to developmental vicissitudes prior to that time. His more recent work, however, did demonstrate an increasing, and probably necessary, tendency to view the oedipal stage as a further developmental vicissitude of self development. Unlike Bergler, who claimed a basic neurosis deriving out of injured narcissism and the masochistic defenses against it, Kohut claimed a basic self pathology, nonconflictual in nature, from which drives and conflict issues are derivatives.

Increasingly, without explicit attack for the most part, he abandoned traditional metapsychology. Although he attempted originally to describe empathically derived experience-near phenomena, the concept of the bipolar self is a high-level abstraction, as are the secondary concepts of selves which are fragmented or enfeebled. The de-emphasis of psychic conflict led some to declare that Kohut's work, although interesting, is not psychoanalytic (Stein, 1979), but this seems to beg the question of the proper place of his work. Kohut chose to redefine psychoanalysis as the study of complex mental states rather than as the study of intrapsychic conflict. This is an appropriate strategy if one can demonstrate that intrapsychic conflict does not include the entirety of interesting developmental, genetic, and dynamic propositions and the range of phenomena occurring in transference.

Kernberg, attempting to meld object relations theory and structural theory, has come to quite different conclusions about the underlying structures of narcissism. It is possible, the author believes, to argue that Kernberg, deriving initial motivational states from affects and their object relations dispositions, as did Rado (1956) and Kardiner et al. (1959) before him, has effectively eradicated drive theory as it has been traditionally known in the psychoanalytic literature. The fact that all affective tendencies can roughly be organized along lines of hating or loving does not resurrect instinct theory as we have known it. Kernberg agrees with Kohut, insisting upon the interaction of infant and object as the essential matrix out of which all internal structure derives. After that, it is clear that their agreement breaks down. Perhaps the most significant question pertains to the issue of deficit pathology and resumption of normal growth which has been arrested, versus conflict pathology and the correction of pathological growth which has occurred.

Clearly, clinical data are needed to resolve this issue, but obtaining the data is problematic. First, all case presentations are so sketchy that they are subject to several interpretations, including the case of Mr. Z. (Kohut, 1978; 1979). Second, Kohut's empathic treatment mode calls for an early, noninterpretive phase of analysis, which could go on for a very significant period, long enough to permit narcissistic regression in the transference to the point of arrested development of grandiose and idealizing tendencies. In Kohut's view, too early interpretation of the defensive aspects of the narcissistic rage, denigration, coldness, lack of curiosity, and so forth in the transference, would recreate the unempathic infantile situation which led to these configurations and force the patient towards a compliant but superficial change. Kohut believed that traditional interpretive technique would not permit full narcissistic regression within the transference. Further, the traditional technique would inhibit the opportunity for the growth-enhancing and transmuting internalizations that occur when the narcissistic transferences are worked through in terms of the failures of the analyst to meet the patient's demands for empathy.

Since individuals who are not already sympathetic to Kohut's ideas will not, in fact, could not, attempt to do analysis as he recommended, neutral replication of the data is not possible. Such issues as deficit vs. conflict, or narcissistic rage as primary pathology vs. manifestation, will continue to elicit data and debate. Kohut was accused of avoiding analysis of rage, of encouraging the positive transference and over-idealization, and of creating a corrective emotional experience. Although he answered these charges (Kohut, 1977), the fact that he did not engage in gross analytic errors does not demonstrate the correctness of his methods. Meanwhile, differences in view and differences in treatment method are sharp, and we must continue to collect data.

Kohut left his theoretical writings with a difficulty in the concept of the self. Deliberately undefined, the concept is anthropomorphized with numerous adjectives (e.g., vigorous, feeble, fragmented, cohesive, joyful, and so forth) which lack clear reference in terms of the intrapsychic structure. Is the self the sole psychic structure prior to the oedipal period? The proposed relationships of self, whole person, self-selfobject matrix, ego, and self-representation are confusing. When the self is "enfeebled," for instance, is it the self that registers and responds to this enfeeblement of itself, or are there other parts of the psyche which are involved in the process? If there is only one structure of the mind, the self, we clearly have no way of discussing complex mental states, and Kohut did not describe clearly how the structures of the self are hierarchically organized through transmuting internalizations.

The author has focused on the work of Kohut in this section not necessarily because the work of other contributors to our concepts of narcissism are not equally subject to question, but because Kohut's propositions arose most clearly out of the clinical study of the narcissistic character disorders. Moreover, the vigor and freshness of his work continues to spur much of our current discussion.

EMPATHY

One of the more valuable by-products of recent work on narcissistic disorders has been a resurgence of interest in the nature of empathy and a reexamination of its role in psychoanalysis (Buie, 1981). Kohut insisted that the infant thrives precisely to the degree that the parent is capable of empathic responsiveness, and that empathy is a limiting dimension for the entire psychoanalytic enterprise, both as to scientific collection of data on complex mental states and as to therapy. The field itself therefore cannot advance beyond its capacity for psychoanalytic empathy. Furthermore, in Kohut's view, the narcissistic disorders, being preconflictual, are analyzable only through a finely tuned empathic responsiveness on the part of the analyst.

Kohut defined psychoanalysis as a "psychology of complex mental states which with the aid of the persevering empathic-introspective immersion of the observer into the inner life of man, gathers its data in order to explain them" (1977, 302). Implied in this is the view that any efforts, during data gathering, to adopt a positivist stance that would separate the observer from the observed will lack psychoanalytic scientific validity and will yield false data.

Kohut was careful both to discern that the empathic stance does not include verification of its findings and to distinguish empathy from sympathy or sentimentality (one can, for example, use empathic understanding of another person to exploit his or her vulnerability). This empathic use of the self for understanding the inner life of another distinguishes psychoanalysis from all other data-collecting fields. With respect to verification, Kohut emphasized that introspection is only a mode of data collection, not a method of data analysis. Once the data have been retrieved through the use of the empathic-introspective point of view, they must be further understood through processes of verification and systematization. The usual theoretical and scientific cognitive processes would then pertain.

Kohut, as have others, also insisted that the events within the transference are interactional and that the patient does not produce transference distortions in a vacuum. The patient who responds with rage to the analyst's analytical silence cannot be presumed to be responding defensively. Rather, the analyst's task is to place him- or herself in the patient's shoes in order to understand the patient's experience of the analyst's silence, in the light of the patient's own history. The patient's reaction may well represent an experience of self-fragmentation or a failure of self-regulation because of his or her sense of the analyst's lack of interest, rather than, for example, a defensive anger to force the analyst to provide oral supplies. Schwaber (1980) has given sensitive examples of how the patient's responses in an analytic hour always involve cues from the analyst. The analyst is never simply a neutral figure and must understand these cues from the patient's point of view, and not try to give the "correct" response that fits some preconceived observer idea.

There has been and continues to be much discussion about the extent to which Kohut and his followers have been collecting data empathically or distorting data. Nonetheless, it seems to this observer that Kohut and his followers have raised the consciousness of the analytic community to the importance of examining both the empathic stance of the analyst and the analyst's role in the here-and-now transference responses of the patient. A new interest has arisen in the modes of warmth, concern, and responsiveness to the patient's experiences without, in the process, having to gratify the patient's demands. None of these issues are new (Stone, 1961), but work with narcissistic disorders has refocused our attention upon them. Similarly, while our understanding of the developmental, genetic dynamics and structural aspects of empathy have been enhanced, we are still far from achieving the goal outlined by Schafer in 1959: "Further development of the theory of the self in relation to id, ego, superego and reality may make possible a systematic formulation of empathy in terms of selves in relation to each other" (Schafer, 1959, 347).

SUMMARY

The chain of events beginning with Freud's 1914 paper, "On Narcissism: An Introduction" (Freud, 1957), has in recent decades led to a concentration of psychoanalytic interest in the problems of the narcissistic disorders, the nature of narcissism, the role of the self in all human activity, and an intensive scrutiny of both the theory and the technique of psychoanalysis. These researches have greatly enhanced our understanding of the nature, origin, and therapy of the narcissistic disorders and have led us to a new appreciation of the role of narcissism in health. Perhaps most importantly, the works have fostered a controversy within mainstream psychoanalysis concerning the nature of our metapsychology and the essence of the psychoanalytic situation.

Heinz Kohut began with observations on the narcissistic disorders, which he attempted to explain in terms compatible with traditional metapsychology, and ultimately moved to a new explanatory system of the mind based on the development of the self, which is far removed from usual concepts of intrapsychic conflict. The dispute between Kohut and Kernberg has served to highlight aspects of this development. Some authors have expressed the view that the newer theories of Kohut, based on a deficit psychology of the self, are compatible with more traditional oedipal conflictual theories of mental function (Wallerstein, 1981) or that the theories each pertain to specific phases of development.

It is not clear that this is so. As self psychology develops, it seems increasingly to represent a culmination of tendencies in psychoanalysis toward a theory that is less reductionistic, more existential, more environmental, less mechanistic, less conflictual, and perhaps less deterministic. Together these tendencies would very significantly alter the terms of traditional psychoanalysis, and they may represent a new metapsychology which is not compatible with the older one. Only continued testing will demonstrate which theories serve us best. Meanwhile, we enjoy new therapeutic optimism with regard to the treatment of self disorders, new insights into early development, and renewed research vigor. At this point in the development of our knowledge, cross-cultural developmental studies could help to shed considerable light on the correctness of the contending theories concerning the development of the self and the self disorders.

Chapter 33 On the Psychoanalytic Psychotherapy of Primary Self Pathology
by Paul H. Ornstein, M.D.

INTRODUCTION:
ON THE PSYCHOANALYTIC PSYCHOTHERAPIES

In the short span of a decade and a half, Kohut's self psychology expanded and transformed the domain of psychoanalysis. This expansion and transformation also had, and continues to have, a considerable impact upon the conduct and process of psychoanalytic psychotherapy. Although the main focus of the chapter is upon psychoanalytic psychotherapy *per se*, the exposition moves freely back and forth between psychoanalysis and psychotherapy. From the outset, the author emphasizes the similarities rather than the differences between psychoanalysis and psychoanalytic psychotherapy (Ornstein and Ornstein, 1976). Such an approach is based upon the author's view that psychoanalysis, intensive psychoanalytic psychotherapy, and brief focal psychotherapy lie on a continuum.

The continuum idea is buttressed by the fact that the same personality theory, the same theory of psychopathology, the same basic theory of cure, and the same basic therapeutic approach guide our interventions in each of these treatment processes. The differences should certainly not be obscured and may be of considerable magnitude. Differences in the setting (e.g., the frequency of sessions, the use or nonuse of the couch, the open-endedness or definite limitations to the number of sessions, and so forth) and differences in the goals of the treatment will determine, to a large extent, the nature of the process that will be set into motion within each analyst- or therapist-patient relationship. While the setting and the goals do generally codetermine the nature of the evolving treatment process, the process is infinitely more profoundly determined by the patient's capacities to remobilize infantile and childhood needs, wishes, and fantasies, and by the particular analyst's or therapist's understanding and interpretations of them. What actually determines the nature of the therapeutic process, therefore, is the proper climate of safety and responsiveness offered by the therapist, the climate within which that patient can remobilize the thwarted need to grow, along with the internally elaborated obstacles to this growth. The setting and the goals will determine *how much* of this thwarted need to grow and the internalized obstacles can unfold, be worked through, and be resolved in each treatment modality.

Thus, while the quantitative and qualitative differences in the three treatment approaches are well known, focusing on the similarities has heuristic value. To summarize in familiar language, transferences are mobilized—to a greater or lesser extent—in each treatment modality. These transferences revive the patient's core problems along with their infantile and childhood maladaptive solutions, as well as the patient's efforts at new solutions. If the therapist responds to these from within fundamentally the same clinical-theoretical vantage point, guided by the emerging process and regardless of the setting, we may then speak of the psychoanalytic psychotherapies on a continuum. The differing goals and settings in the psychoanalytic psychotherapies do not *fundamentally* alter the nature of the therapeutic interventions—understanding and interpretations.

THE EVOLUTION OF PSYCHOANALYTIC SELF PSYCHOLOGY

The following brief overview of the evolution of Kohut's self psychology aims to expand our appreciation of his more recent formulations and to point towards the direction of further developments, as these now affect the analysis of both primary and secondary self pathology, i.e., the narcissistic disorders and the neuroses.

It is common knowledge that Kohut's work began as a response to his perception (shared by many of his contemporaries) that a widening gap existed between the clinical practice and theory of psychoanalysis. This gap was perhaps nowhere wider than in the attempts to treat narcissistic disorders, which were then generally considered unanalyzable within the mainstream of psychoanalysis. A large number of significant contributors made numerous efforts to narrow this gap and to extend psychoanalysis—more or less successfully and with a variety of modifications—to encompass some of the narcissistic disorders.[1]

What distinguishes Kohut's contributions from other approaches to the same group of patients has to do with his discovery of the two forms of specific selfobject transferences, the mirror transference and the idealizing transference. The mobilization of one of these transferences (or both of them, in a particular sequence) makes possible the psychoanalysis of primary self pathology without parameters and enables us to gain the necessary therapeutic leverage for intensive psychoanalytic psychotherapy or focal psychotherapy.

[1]These efforts are represented in the works of the many psychoanalysts whose divergent points of view have recently been summarized by Moore (1975). The most important contributions are represented in the works of Lampl-de-Groot (1962; 1963), Lichtenstein (1964; 1977), Rosenfeld (1964), and Kernberg (1975; 1976; 1980).

Development of the Theory

In *The Analysis of the Self* (1971) Kohut discussed a group of patients who were suffering from hitherto unanalyzable narcissistic personality or behavior disorders. The patients developed those archaic selfobject transferences which made their analysis possible and thereby furnished the observational data for Kohut's initial clinical and theoretical contributions. At that early stage of his work, Kohut defined the self as the content of the mental agencies, id, ego and superego—self psychology in the narrower sense. Kohut thus embedded his innovations in ego psychology, and expressed them in the language of classical metapsychology. Self psychology in the narrower sense was therefore at first viewed by many as applicable only to a group of patients whose psychopathology was rooted primarily in "deficit" and not in "conflict."

Furthermore, many considered this psychology of the self in the narrower sense (deficit psychology) to be an addition to and thus an expansion of classical ego psychology (conflict psychology). By juxtaposing these two psychologies and not attempting a forced or premature integration, Kohut deliberately left the door open for further developments within self psychology.[2] At the time, the former was held relevant for the understanding and treatment of the whole spectrum of narcissistic disorders, and the latter was held relevant for the understanding and treatment of the whole spectrum of neurotic disorders. The simple juxtaposition of these two psychologies thus resulted from the fact that self psychology initially did not claim new insights or new treatment approaches for the neuroses and neurotic personality disorders, the classical domain of psychoanalysis. This fact might account in part for the relative ease and speed with which many aspects of *The Analysis of the Self,* certainly its clinical insights and treatment principles, were viewed as significant expansions of psychoanalysis.

Objections to the complementarity of the two psychologies arose from many quarters. The recurrent claim was that conflicts, rather than deficits, were ubiquitously at the root of psychopathology, throughout the whole spectrum of nosologic entities. Hence, the critics claimed that the valid insights and treatment principles of self psychology in the narrower sense could be readily absorbed by contemporary psychoanalysis. But these claims were primarily theory based and did not seem to take into consideration the compelling clinical data observable in stalemated or second analyses, which could easily refute such claims (see, for instance, "The Two Analyses of Mr. Z.," Kohut, 1979).

---

[2]The sharp demarcation suggested by Kohut's formulations between the two psychologies had long been criticized on the basis of observations that in the clinical situation we have always encountered and dealt with a mixture of oedipal and preoedipal (structural and prestructural) constellations. The clinical and theoretical issues involved in the idea of a "mixture" of transferences cannot be adequately discussed here. It should only be mentioned that the argument *for* the sharp demarcation was empirically buttressed. The spontaneous clustering of analytic data around predominant themes usually led to the emergence of cohesive transferences. When there was no premature interference with this spontaneous emergence and clustering of themes, a more or less clearly delineated mirror transference, or an idealizing transference, or an oedipal transference neurosis established itself. The accent, methodologically, is on "no premature interference." Those who claim not to observe such spontaneous clustering will have to examine their approaches for the possibility of premature interference with such more or less clear-cut transferences. For a different resolution of the problem of two psychologies, see what follows in the chapter.

Further developments of self psychology, not hampered by efforts at integration, proceeded along different lines. Further study of the earlier reported appearance of oedipal themes provided the additional empirical data for the recognition of the *oedipal selfobject transferences.* These oedipal themes arose *de novo*, rather than being remobilized from infancy, and appeared at the end of successful analyses of patients with primary self pathology. Adding weight to the data was the subsequent inclusion in the self psychology research of the neuroses and neurotic personality disorders. The working through of these oedipal selfobject transferences permitted a reevaluation of the structure, form, content, position, and significance of a *normal oedipal stage* in development. This, in turn, brought new insights regarding the etiology of the ubiquitous, transient, and potentially pathogenic *oedipal conflicts* and of the pathological Oedipus complex which is at the root of the neurotic disorders.

By encompassing the neurotic spectrum of disorders, this broadening of the clinical base of self psychology brought with it considerable further expansion of theoretical insights. The expansion culminated in Kohut's articulation of self psychology in the broader sense in "The Restoration of the Self" (Kohut, 1977).

The Concept of the Selfobject

At the center of this advance was again the concept of the selfobject. The first delineation and working through of the mirror transference and the idealizing transference gave rise to the reconstruction of the role and functions of the *archaic* (mirroring and idealizing) *selfobjects* in structure building in infancy and childhood (Kohut, 1968; 1971). Here, too, the delineation and working through of the oedipal selfobject transference gave rise to the reconstruction of the role and functions of the *oedipal* (mirroring and idealizing) *selfobjects* in bringing about further structuralization and consolidation, including the feminine or masculine aspects of the self. The rudimentary self and its archaic, empathic selfobjects form that experiential unit in which the self emerges, develops, attains its cohesiveness, vigor, and vitality, and acquires those nuclear structures and functions—ambitions, skills and talents, and ideals—which constitute the bipolar self.

The drives are considered here as building blocks or constituents of the self. This is a decisive departure from earlier developmental concepts in psychoanalysis, in which the drives were seen as primary configurations. In the earlier concepts, the drives' inevitable clash with the external world, the socializing efforts of the parental imagos, led to the differentiation and development of ego and superego functions. Hence, although the need for a concept of an ego not born out of conflict was later recognized, this latter view assumed the primacy and ubiquity of drive-related conflicts and did not clearly differentiate between normal and potentially pathogenic or pathological conflict.

In contrast, self psychology assumed an *a priori* fit between the rudimentary self and its selfobjects. Conflicts arise secondarily, from inevitable traumatic disturbances in the selfobjects' empathic "intuneness," in their ability to perform their manifold and complex phase-appropriate functions. Self development, then, is not a matter of taming the drives, but of whether or not the selfobjects respond optimally and phase-specifically to the unfolding, innate potentials. Only in such a climate of optimum responsiveness will selfobject functions be progressively transformed, through transmuting internalizations, into permanent psychic structures.

As should be evident, the concept of the selfobject is pivotal. It is at once an empirically derived clinical concept, a relatively experience-near theoretical concept, and a reconstructively derived developmental concept, which also serves as a more firmly anchored bridge between the intrapsychic realm and social reality. As an empirically derived clinical concept, the idea of the selfobject captures the various, empathically observable, subjective experiences in the mirror transference and the idealizing transference. As a relatively experience-near theoretical concept, it guides us in formulating psychoanalytic propositions more in keeping with what usefully orders our patients' idiosyncratic self experiences. These propositions can also allow us to arrive at useful generalizations that are anchored in and can be related back to patients' subjective experiences.

As a reconstructively derived developmental concept, the selfobject concept further underlines the fact that psychoanalysis is a developmental psychology par excellence. It guides us to recognize the developmental analogues in the transference and to pinpoint the arrests, derailments, and deficits in the bipolar self, as well as its successfully operating compensatory structures and its unsuccessfully operating defensive structures. Significantly, as a developmental construct, it also permits a renewed longitudinal study of infant-mother pairs and of the process of parenting, and it enables the validation or modification of clinical, theoretical, or developmental formulations on the basis of data derived from outside the treatment situation. Here and in the transposition of the psychoanalytic investigative method into the broader sociocultural and political-historical realms, the selfobject serves as a new bridging concept.

Additional observations and growing insights into the nature of selfobjects suggest that, beyond their earliest structure-building and later structure-consolidating functions, they also have lifelong sustaining functions (Kohut 1977; 1978; Basch, 1979; Ornstein, A., unpublished). Selfobjects constitute the emotional nutriment of the human environment. Kohut expressed this recently by stating that: "In the view of self-psychology man lives in a matrix of selfobjects from birth to death. He needs selfobjects for his psychological survival, just as he needs oxygen in his environment throughout his life for physiological survival" (Kohut, 1978, 478). Self psychology thus sees a continuous development from archaic to mature selfobjects, in contrast to a developmental line from symbiosis to autonomy as an end point. Thereby it opens the way for a study of the role and function of selfobjects throughout the life cycle.

Self Psychology Compared with Classical Psychologies

With the combined study of both primary and secondary self pathology (i.e., the narcissistic disorders and the neuroses), and the resulting concept of the bipolar self, the psychology of the self in the narrower sense was transformed into self psychology in the broader sense. In this revision and expansion the self is no longer viewed merely as the content of id, ego, and superego. It is a supraordinate constellation, which encompasses the development of the personality and its functioning in health and illness independently of the constructs of ego psychology.

What, then, had become of the complementarity between self psychology (with its focus on the primacy of deficit) and ego psychology (with its focus on the primacy of conflict)? As noted, the complementary juxtaposition of these two psychologies was an inevitable pragmatic or tactical solution. At the time, self psychology had developed a comprehensive theory and treatment for primary self pathology but was only beginning to encompass the neurotic disorders. During this transitional phase, while the classical formulations were enriched by the psychology of the self in the narrower sense, their original tenets prevailed as the means for understanding and treating the neurotic disturbances.

Maintaining this creative tension between two psychologies did, as noted, lead to further progress (Basch, 1979; Kohut, 1977; 1978; 1980; Ornstein, A., unpublished). This progress came on the basis of a clinical experience, with the emergence of oedipal themes (*de novo*) at the end of successful analyses of primary self disorders, and with the working through of oedipal selfobject transferences. These developments then led to the recognition that the normal oedipal stage is a less violent, a much quieter, and a more joyful achievement than previously conceived. Provided the oedipal selfobjects are capable of taking pride and pleasure in, and of mirroring, the oedipal strivings and achievements of the child, the conflicts of this period will be mild and transient. Unempathic responses or traumata from the side of the selfobjects will intensify these conflicts, and this in turn will lead to a pathological Oedipus complex, to be revived in the oedipal selfobject transference in the analysis. Pathogenic oedipal conflicts and the pathological Oedipus complex represent "breakdown products" of an enfeebled self, and they result in intense castration anxiety, with its complex defenses as one manifestation.

Ultimately, then, throughout the entire spectrum of psychopathology, the crucial determinants are the nature of the self-selfobject relations and the phase-appropriate selfobject responses, i.e., the supplying of the phase-specific functions. These factors will determine favorable developments versus arrest, derailment, and the ensuing deficit in the bipolar self.

We have now come full circle in psychoanalysis. Ego psychology and its extensions in object relations theory attempted to encompass the whole spectrum of psychopathology, but these conceptualizations aided the analysis of only a relatively small segment of this spectrum (Ornstein, P., 1974). The further away we have moved from the neuroses toward the psychoses in this spectrum, the more difficulty with these conceptualizations we have encountered, both in the understanding of the conditions and in the treatment process. But despite the widely acknowledged therapeutic failures, drive- and object-related conflicts and defenses have retained their enormous appeal and served as a unified way of viewing all of psychopathology. (For examples of recent significant modifications in the definition of conflict, in order to retain this unified view, see Sandler, 1974; 1976; and Wallerstein 1979; unpublished.)

Self psychology in the broader sense, with the supraordinate bipolar self as its core construct, can now encompass the entire spectrum of psychopathology. Psychoanalytically, it encompasses those with a capacity to mobilize a sustained and cohesive archaic or oedipal self-object transference. Psychotherapeutically, it encompasses those who do not have the capacity for such a sustained and cohesive transference but who do have transference reactions, nevertheless, of the same quality and content. Conceptually, self psychology offers an alternative unified view of all psychopathology which is open to further empirical study.

ON THE NATURE OF SELF PATHOLOGY IN THE BIPOLAR SELF

The following overview of the structural components and functions of the bipolar self indicates briefly and schematically the nature of primary and secondary self pathology. The concept of the bipolar self was implicit in self psychology from the very outset (Kohut, 1966; 1968; 1971). The two major groups of transferences reflected the separate origins of the two aspects of the developing self.

(1) *The grandiose-exhibitionistic self* develops from within the matrix of its *mirroring selfobject,* to constitute the pole of *self-assertive ambitions.* This line of development leads to the acquisition of the capacity for relatively independent self-esteem regulation, to the capacity for the enjoyment of physical and mental activities, and to the capacity for the free pursuit of ambitions and purposes, the striving for power and success.

(2) *The idealized parental imago* develops within the matrix of its *idealized selfobject,* to constitute the pole of internalized *values, goals, and ideals.* This line of development leads to the capacity for self-soothing and self-calming and to the idealization of internalized goals and values, which are thereby accorded a strength-giving role within this pole of the self.

The developmental transformations of the grandiose-exhibitionistic self and of the idealized parental imago will also contribute to the attainment of such higher mental functions as empathy, humor, creativeness and wisdom, and these will be at the disposal of the cohesive, fully structuralized bipolar self. The inevitable tension between ambitions and ideals will activate innate talents and skills, the intermediate structures between the two poles, in the service of fulfilling the inner design or the life program laid down in the nuclear self. Kohut and Wolf summarize these important relationships:

> Once the self has crystallized in the interplay of inherited and environmental factors, it aims toward the realization of its own specific program of action—a program that is determined by the specific intrinsic pattern of its constituent ambitions, goals, skills and talents, and by the tensions that arise between these constituents. The patterns of ambitions, skills, and goals; the tensions between them; the program of action that they create; and the activities that strive toward the realization of this program are all experienced as continuous in space and time—they are the self, an independent center of initiative, an independent recipient of impressions (Kohut and Wolf, 1978, 414).

Obviously, if any one of the functions described above, or a combination of them, is available to the self in only a rudimentary form, a circumscribed and mild or a broadly based and severe deficit may arise. A variety of *defensive structures* develop, covering the void and representing the surface manifestations of the deeper structural defects. At times the structural defect is more prominent in one or another of the two poles, but severe primary self pathology is generally the result of deficits in both.

Should the bipolar nuclear self attain its cohesiveness, vigor, and vitality in relation to both the mirroring and idealized selfobjects, *primary structures* develop in the self. Should such felicitous development be thwarted in one or the other line of development or both, a variety of *defensive structures* will cover the underlying deficits. Should it be possible, however, for the infant or child whose needs have not been met in the original mirroring selfobject matrix to turn to the idealized selfobject, this offers another chance at acquiring *compensatory structures* in at least one pole of the self. Another possibility when earlier mirroring needs have not been met is that later ones, if adequately responded to, will lead to acquiring compensatory structures within the same pole of the self. The same applies to early and later idealizations. Inevitably, each cohesive self has a certain combination of primary, compensatory, and even some defensive structures. The less defensive structures are present, the more effectively can the cohesiveness of the primary and compensatory structures be maintained, thus safeguarding the functional integrity of the self.

Even when the oedipal stage of development is reached with a predominant mixture of primary and compensatory structures (a reasonably cohesive bipolar self), inadequate or faulty response or other, more actively inflicted traumata may yet undermine further structuralization in the self. A self that is thwarted in its oedipal strivings by a lack of adequate mirroring and acceptance, or by the unavailability of idealized oedipal selfobjects, may then become secondarily entangled in the conflicts that are thus engendered. These oedipal conflicts will then, as is well known, inhibit or otherwise interfere with self-assertive aggression, block the proper use of one's talents and skills, and interfere with the necessary consolidation of values and ideals, leaving the self bereft of inner strength in one or both of its poles.

Kohut and Wolf (1978) recently summed up the essential characteristics and the etiology and pathogenesis of primary and secondary disturbances in the self and offered some concise, relevant clinical illustrations. Among the many noteworthy contributions in their essay were the clinical descriptions of various configurations of self disorders, such as the "understimulated self," the "fragmenting self," the "overstimulated self," and the "overburdened self." In addition, they made significant forward steps regarding a psychoanalytic characterology when they described the "mirror-hungry," "ideal-hungry" and "alter-ego-hungry," "merger-hungry," and "contact-shunning" personalities. All of these were based on specific selfobject transference configurations. Aside from the poignancy of the descriptions themselves, the clear-cut transference-rootedness of these character types encountered in psychoanalysis enhances the therapeutic leverage available for their treatment, a feature generally missing in psychoanalytic characterology.

ON THE CONDUCT AND PROCESS OF TREATMENT: CLINICAL ILLUSTRATION

Instead of elaborating on the technical principles of treatment of narcissistic behavior and personality disorders, which were so succinctly described by Kohut and Wolf (1978), the author offers a clinical vignette from a long-term psychotherapy experience for illustration. No one clinical sample, especially in a highly condensed form, can illustrate all possible configurations of pathology or treatment process. Here, the very circumscribed aim is to highlight the fundamental shift in our mode of listening and observation and thus to demonstrate what has allowed us to gain new empirical data, as well as to reinterpret previously established ones. More specifically, the clinical data show certain aspects of a selfobject transference configuration in which previously thwarted developmental needs were freed up for some belated growth and maturation.

> **CASE EXAMPLE** Mrs. B. was a 28-year-old married woman when she entered treatment because she feared that she might seriously injure her two young children. She would severely beat them whenever she became uncontrollably enraged. Relatively innocuous events could precipitate her temper outbursts. This particular symptom became much attenuated over a three-year period of her treatment. However, there remained in her a profound sense of "badness," a feeling she had had about herself all her life.
>
> Mrs. B. had a history of severe "masochistic" acting out. She had actively sought out situations where she would be assured physical suffering, such as sleeping with widely opened windows in the winter so she would freeze, and other, rather bizarre forms of what may seem to the external observer as self-punishment. She had a history of severe depressions and hospitalizations following suicide attempts. None of this, however, had occurred during the present treatment until the third year, when her therapist, a woman, took a month off from work in order to have surgery. The patient had known of this ahead of time.
>
> Following the suicide attempt, the patient said that she had tried to kill herself because she feared that in the future, instead of her being able to depend on her therapist, the therapist would have to depend on her. This seemed to happen to all her friends, she said. She always ended up having to look after them.
>
> It stood out in her background history, the therapist believed, that the patient's mother may have been psychotic. She was certainly not able to tolerate strong affects either in herself or in her child. When upset, she would withdraw and lock herself into a closet, a circumstance which apparently occurred with some frequency. Mrs. B. remembered herself as a withdrawn and unhappy child. An early memory depicted her going into her bedroom, at age four or five, and banging her head on the floor.

The therapist reported this clinical vignette with some frustration. The problem was obviously complex: masochism, depression, suicide. The therapist was particularly distressed that the patient's depression and suicidal ideation continued even after her return from surgery and that she could not help the patient make contact with her repressed rage in the transference. The therapist considered this to be essential for the prevention of further suicide attempts. The patient insisted at first that she did not feel any rage, but rather a sense of helplessness, which she connected with her fear that her therapist would no longer be available to her and that instead the therapist would need the patient to care for *her*.

The therapist's position that it was important for Mrs. B. to face her rage was a crucial one in determining the therapeutic atmosphere and further progress of the treatment. Putting the interpretive emphasis on the patient's rage was in keeping with the therapist's assumption that repressed rage was responsible for the patient's severe masochism, for her temper outbursts, and now for her suicide attempt. The therapist was determined to make this unconscious affect conscious, since as long as it remained unconscious, she feared that it might still be turned against the self and acted out in the form of suicide. When the patient did not respond favorably to the interpretations guided by these assumptions, the therapist saw this as an irreparable break in the therapeutic alliance. The therapist was further distressed and puzzled about the fact that when the patient later on in the treatment did feel and was able to express her rage and haughtily withdrew from her, Mrs. B.'s depression, helplessness, and suicidal ideas did not cease.

The supervisor, who was first consulted at this point, understood the situation differently. The patient's rage and emotional withdrawal from the therapist were not an expression of a break in the therapeutic alliance, but a disruption of what was until then a well established, reasonably safe, protective, and strength-giving relationship with a powerful, Rock-of-Gibraltar-like, and reliably available therapist. We might now call this a "silent merger with an idealized selfobject," a merger that went unrecognized and that was therefore not systematically interpreted. The ordinary fluctuations and relatively minor disruptions of the transference prior to the therapist's surgery had not interfered with this patient's ability to experience her therapist's ongoing emotional availability. The therapist's illness, however, and her one-month absence, proved to be a major disruption. The patient reacted at first with helplessness and then with disappointment and rage at the traumatic loss of the therapist's "strength and perfection." The therapist became the "sick mother," on whom the patient could not depend. Rather, she anticipated that from then on she would have to be responsive to the therapist's needs.

Although the therapist's surgery and absence was a repetition of the childhood trauma, it must be noted, the patient's reaction to the therapist was *not* a repetition of her childhood behavior. As a child, she protected her mother from her rage reactions and tried to make herself innocuous to the mother by withdrawing into isolation and loneliness. But this led the five-year-old child to engage in solitary head banging for self-stimulation and for alleviating her feeling of being cut off from her mother. She was eventually able to express her rage openly at the therapist, which indicated the undoing of the childhood solution. The patient was able to express the rage because of her increased sense of safety established in the three years of treatment and then reestablished a few months after the therapist's return.

The therapeutic task then was to offer the kinds of reconstructive interpretations that would put the patient's rage, helplessness, and despair into the current transference context, as well as into its original genetic context. The differentiation between the transference and the genetic context is emphasized here to indicate that the transference is not a simple repetition of the past. While the therapist's absence reactivated the childhood affects associated with the mother's vulnerability and emotional unavailability, the patient's reaction went *beyond* the childhood solution. She now felt free to express her rage and disappointment with the therapist. With this expression, she indicated that she desperately needed to remain in contact with the "absolute perfection" of the therapist in order to regain and safeguard the vitality and vigor of her own psychic functioning.

The interpretation of the disrupted merger transference, and the patient's responses to this, included reconstructing the original circumstances in which the patient, as a child, could not express rage without fear or further isolation from the mother. Such an emphasis on the phase-appropriateness and legitimacy of the rage and fear in the transference usually helps the patient to accept the legitimacy of a childhood demand for an accepting and responsive emotional environment. The patient, then, instead of feeling contemptuous toward the enraged (bad) childhood self, can accept the frustrated child's demand for unconditional acceptance within the therapist-patient relationship. With the aid of empathic reconstructive interpretations, the patient can also be helped to accept the limitations of the therapist's "perfection," and eventually this helps the patient to accept the limitations of the original environment. Asking patients prematurely to accept the limitations of their original environments, by calling attention to the anachronistic nature of their reactions, deprives them of experiencing the legitimacy of their childhood wishes within the therapist-patient relationship. The therapist's empathy toward the angry and fearful child within the adult patient, conveyed through reconstructive interpretations, leads to insight which the patient then utilizes in developing his or her own empathy toward the original environment and the childhood self.

An Assessment of the Approach

This approach must be sharply differentiated from relying on the so-called therapeutic alliance to maintain and complete the working through of the transference. The concept of the therapeutic alliance seems to require that the patient summon adult ego capacities, distinguish between past and present, and then undo the transference distortions that inevitably enter every treatment process. From this vantage point, therapists usually try to repair the strain or break in the therapeutic alliance by fostering the "real relationship." They alter their own behavior or introduce a current contextual reality, external to the patient's self experience, or both. A preferable alternative, open to empirical study and verification, is to offer reconstructive interpretations of the circumstances that precipitated the disruption of the selfobject transference. Such an interpretive approach would aid the patient's cognitive grasp and permit gaining insight and would facilitate the acquisition of new psychic structures through transmuting internalizations. Herein lies the improved therapeutic leverage of this approach.

Reflecting on Mrs. B's treatment experience, our usual assumption would be that we have succeeded in reviving aspects of her central psychopathology, especially the distorted perception that the therapist had become just as emotionally unavailable to her as her mother was. We are accustomed to pay more attention to what we view as repetitions than to what we view as efforts at a new beginning in the transference. But can we now see how Mrs. B's particular transference also represents, perhaps even more forcefully, a reactivation of her thwarted need to grow? More particularly, can we recognize that her experience of improved psychic functioning, in a relatively undisturbed merger with the strength and power of the therapist, reflected her revived ability to borrow silently from her idealized selfobject-therapist that which she had been unable to acquire in her infancy and childhood? And does it not follow that the subsequent major disruption of her functioning, with the emergence of her helplessness, depression, and suicide attempt, were the consequences of the traumatic rupture of this selfobject transference that repeated the original trauma with her mother?

The answers to these questions lead to a deeper examination of Mrs. B's psychopathology. Her masochism and depression take on a different cast. Mrs. B's childhood solution to the emotional unavailability of her mother was to suffer silently and withdraw from her, since her mother herself would become intolerably agitated. And instead of calming Mrs. B., she would make things worse for her by closeting herself away from her child when she most needed her. Mrs. B's silent withdrawal and solitary head banging for self-stimulation was her childhood solution to feeling cut off from a desperately needed selfobject. Now, in the transference, this was slowly overcome by focusing on what was becoming a new mode of relating, rather than primarily or exclusively focusing on the repetitive aspects of the transference. Mrs. B. grew in her ability to express her rage directly in the transference, in response to its various and repetitive disruptions. Thereby she was able to establish a living, intense, albeit angry bond between herself and her therapist. And this did, indeed, represent the effort in the transference to resume a thwarted growth.

The point here is that psychic growth, structure building in childhood and in psychotherapy and psychoanalysis, can occur only within an empathically responsive selfobject milieu. When, in the course of treatment, the disruptions of a silent merger with the idealized therapist bring forth rage and destructive feelings or fantasies, the patient experiences the therapist differently from the original selfobject, the mother. If the therapist is, indeed, capable of *not* experiencing himself or herself as the target of the patient's rages and can stay focused upon the patient's subjective experience, then the therapist will be able to offer a reconstructive interpretation that will legitimize the rage within the transference. Such an interpretation, then, not only aids the reestablishment of the merger transference, but also aids the patient in accepting the demands of the childhood self.

What aspects of our theory of the transference and the nature of psychopathology and what aspects of our therapeutic techniques, we may now ask, might have interfered with our recognizing more clearly the presence and significance of this unextinguished developmental thrust, this thwarted need to complete a derailed or interrupted growth? Could it have been our emphasis on the indiscriminate repetitions and distortions, on the inappropriateness of these reactions, that is, our nearly exclusive focus upon pathology? Could these aspects have blocked our vision and interfered with our properly appraising the role and function of this thwarted need to grow as the motive force of both the selfobject transferences and of the therapeutic work within them? The need to complete the unfinished business of psychological growth and maturation is a stronger force and ally in therapy than we had been able to recognize before. Could we have improperly assumed the inevitability of repetition, the idea that we always approach each new situation with our repertoire of past modes of coping, and inferred a ubiquitous, hard-to-combat, *need* to repeat? Could this have made us less sensitive to a more profound "dread to repeat" and to the incessant search for a new beginning? Could it be, we may finally ask, that we have overgeneralized from those cases in which elaborate, archaic defensive structures make it continuously difficult or impossible for the patient to accept and use the analyst's empathy and, therefore, to dare to revive the thwarted developmental drive to grow?

The author's own answers to these questions are all in the affirmative. The interpretation should focus on what the patient is seeking (what might seem to the external observer as mere repetitions of the past), on what had originally traumatically interrupted and derailed his or her psychological growth, and on what might block its resumption in the transference. Such a focus would ultimately lead to the more or less extensive remobilization of the traumatically frustrated needs of infancy and childhood and prepare for the belated opportunity to acquire psychic structures within the two poles of the bipolar self.

CONCLUSION

This crucial methodologic shift in our mode of listening and observing entails sustained empathic immersion in the patient's transference experiences and thereby permits a consistent focus on the patient's inner world. The therapeutic effort consists of articulating what is thus perceived in the context of the treatment setting. Articulations take the form of understanding and explanation, the two layers of what we commonly refer to as "interpretation." The ensuing spontaneous emergence of the pathognomonic selfobject transference remobilizes a specific, hitherto thwarted childhood developmental thrust to grow, a thrust which was traumatically interrupted. Kohut and Wolf clearly and unambiguously stated the core issues of the psychoanalytic treatment of primary self pathology as follows:

> Faulty interaction between the child and his selfobjects results in a damaged self—either a diffusely damaged self or a self that is seriously damaged in one or the other of its constituents. If a patient whose self has been damaged enters psychoanalytic treatment, he reactivates the specific needs that had remained unresponded to by the specific faulty interactions between the nascent self and the selfobjects of early life—a selfobject transference is established (Kohut and Wolf, 1978, 414).

Chapter 34 An Ego Psychology and Object Relations Approach to the Narcissistic Personality
by Otto F. Kernberg, M.D.

What follows is a summary, expansion, and update of the author's understanding of the clinical characteristics of narcissistic personality disorders, the developments these patients present in the course of psychoanalytic treatment, and an outline of psychoanalytic technique geared to resolving their pathological character organization. A brief description of supportive psychotherapy for narcissistic patients functioning on an overt borderline level, where psychoanalysis or expressive psychotherapy is contraindicated, complements the outline of psychotherapeutic strategies with these patients.

Because limitations of space do not permit reviewing the pertinent literature here, the reader is referred to the published contributions of the author (Kernberg, 1975; 1976; 1980), and to the clinical observations of those who have influenced his work in this area (Abraham, 1919; Jones, 1913; Reich, 1953; 1960; Rosenfeld, 1964; 1971; 1975; 1978; Tartakoff, 1966; Van der Waals, 1965). By the same token, the reader is also referred to the alternative contemporary formulations regarding pathological narcissism, namely, Rosenfeld's, as mentioned, and the work of Kohut (1971; 1972; 1977; 1979; Kohut and Wolf, 1978; Goldberg, 1980; Stolorow and Lachmann, 1980).*

Elsewhere the author has proposed that a clinical diagnosis of narcissistic personalities may be made on the basis of descriptive and structural analysis of their psychopathology, and he has defined the various levels of severity of narcissistic pathology that have prognostic and therapeutic relevance (Kernberg, 1975).

Throughout the years, the author (Kernberg, 1975; 1976; 1980) has provided clinical material as well as theoretical considerations in support of three main viewpoints. (1) The specific narcissistic resistances of patients with narcissistic character pathology reflect a pathological narcissism that is different both from the ordinary adult narcissism and from normal infantile narcissism. (2) Pathological narcissism can be understood only in terms of the vicissitudes of libidinal and aggressive drive derivatives. Pathological narcissism does not simply reflect libidinal investment in the self in contrast to the libidinal investment in objects, but reflects libidinal investment in a pathological self structure. This pathological, grandiose self structure is an abnormal condensation of mental representations of the real self, the ideal self, and the ideal object. Devalued or aggressively determined self- and object representations are split off, repressed, or projected. The pathological grandiose self has defensive functions against underlying, libidinally invested and aggressively invested, primitive self- and object representations that reflect intense, condensed preoedipal-oedipal conflicts around both love and aggression. (3) The structural characteristics of narcissistic personalities cannot be understood simply in terms of fixation at an early level of development, or lack of development of certain intrapsychic structures. They are a consequence of development of pathological (in contrast to normal) differentiation and integration of ego and superego structures, derived from pathological (in contrast to normal) object relations.

Although normal narcissism reflects the libidinal investment of the self, the self actually constitutes a structure that includes both libidinally invested and aggressively invested components. In simple terms, integration of good and bad self-representations into a realistic self-concept, that incorporates rather than dissociates the various component self-representations, is a requisite for the libidinal investment of normal self. This also explains the paradox that integration of love and hate is a prerequisite for the capacity for normal love.

All these metapsychological considerations derive from Jacobson's (1964), Mahler's (Mahler and Furer, 1968; Mahler et al., 1975), and the author's own understanding that self- and object representations stem

*Preceptor's note: Kohut's views are outlined in the chapter by Cooper and more extensively elaborated in the preceding chapter by Ornstein.

simultaneously from a primary undifferentiated matrix. The author's understanding contrasts with the traditional psychoanalytic viewpoint stemming from Freud's (1914) pioneering examination of narcissism, according to which there first exists a narcissistic libido and later an object libido. It also contrasts with Kohut's (1971) view that narcissistic libido and object libido start out together and then evolve independently, and that aggression in narcissistic personalities is secondary to their narcissistic lesions. Rather, the author believes, the development of normal and pathological narcissism always entails the relationship of the self-representations to object representations and external objects, as well as instinctual conflicts involving both libido and aggression. If these formulations are valid, it would seem that the study of narcissism cannot be divorced from the study of the vicissitudes of both libido and aggression and of the vicissitudes of internalized object relations.

CLINICAL ASPECTS

For practical purposes, we may classify narcissism into normal adult, normal infantile, and pathological narcissism. Normal infantile narcissism is of importance here only because fixation at or regression to infantile narcissistic goals is an important feature of all character pathology. Such a fixation or regression is a relatively nonspecific type of narcissistic pathology and is characterized by a normal though excessively infantile self structure and a normal internalized world of object relations.

In contrast, in the case of pathological narcissism, we have an abnormal self structure that can be of two types. One type was first described by Freud (1914) as an illustration of "narcissistic object choice" in cases of male homosexuality. The patient's self is pathologically identified with an object, while the representation of the patient's infantile self is projected onto that object, thus creating a libidinal relation in which the function of self and object have been interchanged. This is quite frequently found in cases of male and female homosexuality. Again, while narcissistic conflicts are more severe here than in the case of ordinary character pathology of the normal infantile narcissistic type, these patients present a normally integrated self and a normal internalized world of object relations. A second and more severely distorted type of pathological narcissism is the narcissistic personality proper, a specific type of character pathology that centers around the presence of a pathological, grandiose self. The clinical characteristics are described very summarily in what follows.

The Spectrum of Narcissistic Pathology

Patients with narcissistic personality function along a broad range of social effectiveness. In *typical cases,* the surface functioning of these patients may show very little disturbance. Only on diagnostic exploration do they reveal an excessive degree of self-reference in their interactions with others, an excessive need to be loved and admired, and a curious contradiction between a very inflated concept of themselves and occasional feelings of extreme inferiority. In addition, they have an inordinate need for tribute from others, and their emotional life is shallow. They usually present an integration of a sort of their conscious self experience, which differentiates them from the typical patient with borderline personality organization. On the other hand, their capacity for an integrated concept of others is remarkably absent, they feel little empathy for others, and they present a predominance of the same primitive defensive operations that characterize borderline personality organization.

In their relation to other people, they tend to present inordinate envy, to idealize some people from whom they expect narcissistic supplies, and to depreciate and treat with contempt those from whom they do not expect anything (often their former idols). Their relations with others are frequently exploitative and parasitic, and, behind a surface that is often charming and engaging, one senses coldness and ruthlessness. They typically feel restless and bored when no new sources feed their self-regard. Because they need so much tribute and adoration from others, they are often considered to be excessively dependent. In fact, however, they are unable to depend on anybody because of their deep underlying distrust and devaluation of others and their unconscious "spoiling" of what they receive, which is related to conflicts around unconscious envy.

In psychoanalytic treatment, if and when the pathological grandiose self is systematically explored and resolved by means of interpretation, they evidence intense conflicts in which condensation of oedipal and preoedipal issues predominate. Preoedipal sources of aggression linked to their specific conflicts around envy are an overriding influence. In other words, they show, underneath the protective structure of the pathological grandiose self, the typical conflicts of borderline personality organization. The relative lack of object relations they show on the surface is a defense, at a deeper level, against intensely pathological internalized object relations.

The psychic structure of the narcissistic personality as described has relevance for treatment. It explains both the development of negative therapeutic reactions linked to unconscious sources of envy and the possibility of resolving, simultaneously with the pathological grandiose self, the pathology of their internalized object relations. This concept of psychic structure has important theoretical implications as well, since it is in contrast to the traditional psychoanalytic thinking. What the tradition holds is that severe narcissism reflects a fixation at an early narcissistic stage of development and a failure to develop object love. In contrast, what obtains in this concept of psychic structure is that an abnormal development of self-love coexists with an abnormal development in the love for others: narcissism and object relations cannot be separated from each other.

At the *highest level* of functioning of narcissistic personalities, we find patients without neurotic symptoms, with good surface adaptation, and with very little awareness of any emotional illness. These personalities do show a chronic sense of emptiness or boredom, an inordinate need for tribute from others and for personal success, and a remarkable lack of capacity for intuitive understanding, empathy, and emotional investment in others. Highly intelligent patients at this level of narcissistic personality functioning may appear to be quite creative in their fields. Careful observation of their productivity over a long period of time, however, will give evidence of superficiality and flightiness. Few of these patients come to treatment, unless they are suffering from some complicating neurotic symptom. Over the years, they tend to develop complications secondary to their narcissistic pathology, which worsens their functioning in middle and advanced age, but which paradoxically also improves their prognosis for psychoanalytic treatment in the middle years (Kernberg, 1980). At that stage of life, they tend to develop chronic depressive reactions, highly inappropriate use of denial and devaluation, and at times hypomanic personality traits to defend themselves against depression and an increasing sense of emptiness and of having wasted their lives.

The middle range of the spectrum of narcissistic psychopathology corresponds to the typical cases described earlier, and these cases are ideally indicated for standard psychoanalysis.

At the *most severe or lowest level* of the spectrum of narcissistic pathology, we find patients who, in spite of the defensive functions the pathological grandiose self provides for some continuity in social interactions, present overt borderline features. They lack impulse control and anxiety tolerance and manifest a severe crippling of their sublimatory capacities. In their interpersonal fields they are disposed to explosive or chronic rage reactions or to severely paranoid distortions. Many of these patients respond well to modified expressive psychotherapy rather than to psychoanalysis proper. The expressive psychotherapy coincides with that which the author outlined for borderline personality organization earlier in this volume, and it is modified in the light of the psychoanalytic technique described in what follows. When expressive psychotherapy is contraindicated, a supportive approach is recommended for these patients (see the last section of this chapter).

Aggression

One prognostically crucial dimension along which one can explore narcissistic personality structures is the extent to which aggression has been integrated into the psychic apparatus. Aggression may be integrated into the pathological grandiose self, or it may remain restricted to the underlying, dissociated, and/or repressed primitive object relations against which the pathological grandiose self represents the main defensive structure. One may in fact describe a developmental sequence of this integration of aggression into the psychic apparatus, including (1) primitive dissociation or splitting of aggressively invested object relations from libidinally invested object relations; (2) later condensation of such primitive aggressive object relations with sexual drive derivatives in the context of polymorphous perverse sexual strivings; and (3) predominant channeling of aggression into a pathological narcissistic character structure with direct investment of aggression by the pathological grandiose self. All three of these developmental fixations and/or regressions can be found in narcissistic personalities, each leading to different clinical characteristics.

When dissociated, aggressively invested part-object relations are directly manifest, we encounter the overtly borderline functioning narcissistic personality, with its generalized impulsivity and its proneness to paranoid developments and narcissistic rage. When condensation with partial sexual drives has taken place, sadistically infiltrated polymorphous perverse fantasies and activities are highly manifest. When primitive aggression has directly infiltrated the pathological grandiose self, a particularly ominous development occurs, perhaps best described as a characterological sadism.

In this last group, we find narcissistic patients whose grandiosity and pathological self-idealization are reinforced by the sense of triumph over fear and pain, achieved by inflicting fear and pain on others. We also find cases where self-esteem is enhanced by the direct sadistic pleasure of aggression linked with sexual drive derivatives. Some of these narcissistic personalities may pursue joyful types of cruelty. Some of them are self-mutilating and achieve a sense of superiority and triumph over life and death, as well as conscious pleasure, by their severe self-mutilation. Some of these narcissistic patients have a combination of paranoid and explosive personality traits, and their impulsive behavior, rage attacks, and blaming are a major channel for instinctual gratification. All such patients may reflect the condensation of aggression in the pathological grandiose self. They may find the treatment situation a welcome and stable outlet of aggression, which militates against their structured intrapsychic change.

In other narcissistic personalities, however, the grandiose self is remarkably free from directly expressed aggression, and repressive mechanisms protect the patient against the underlying primitive object relations that condense sexual and aggressive drive derivatives. In these cases, the "narcissistic rage" or paranoid reactions that develop in later stages of treatment, as part of the therapeutic process, have much less ominous implications.

In still other cases, some sublimatory integration of aggression has taken place, related more to that of neurotic character structures. When aggression has been integrated with existing superego structures, such cases present a clinically more favorable type of self-directed aggression and a capability for depression. Some of the highest-level functioning narcissistic personalities may have achieved sublimatory integration of aggression into relatively adaptive ego functions, pursuing ambitious goals with an appropriate integration of aggressive drive derivatives.

A relatively infrequent and particularly complicated type of narcissistic personality is the "as if" personality. This narcissistic personality differs from the usual type of "as if" personality with its chameleon-like, ever-shifting, pseudohyperemotional, and pseudoadaptive qualities. The "as if" qualities in these particular narcissistic patients reflect secondary defenses against a pathological grandiose self. These patients are reminiscent of Marcel Marceau miming the man who puts on one mask after another and finally, in despair, cannot tear the last one off. They shift from act to act, without knowing who the actor is, other than that he is a sum of impersonations. Usually, this character constellation protects the patient from very severe paranoid fears and, less frequently, against unconscious guilt.

Considering prognostically the integration of or the defenses against aggression as outlined, the most serious cases are those with a pathological infiltration of aggression into the grandiose self *per se*, and those where secondary, "as if" characteristics represent a defense against strong underlying paranoid traits.

A final factor that has crucial prognostic significance for the treatment of narcissistic personalities is the extent to which antisocial trends are built into the patient's narcissistic character pathology. The stronger the antisocial tendencies, the poorer the prognosis. Usually, such antisocial tendencies go hand in hand with a lack of integration of normal superego functions, and also with a lack of development of a modulated capacity for depressive reactions. The quality of object relations is also in an inverse relation to antisocial trends. Naturally, when antisocial trends are present in patients who also present a sadistic infiltration of the pathological grandiose self, or direct expression of severely sadistic sexual behavior, the prognosis significantly worsens.

The description of the Narcissistic Personality Disorder in DSM-III is satisfactory enough, except for the neglect of these patients' inordinate conflicts around envy, of the varying ways in which they integrate aggression, and of the spectrum of severity of this personality disorder.

OVERVIEW OF PSYCHOANALYTIC TECHNIQUE WITH NARCISSISTIC PERSONALITIES

All three contemporary psychoanalytic approaches to the treatment of narcissistic personalities—Kohut's self psychology, the Kleinian approach of Rosenfeld, and the ego psychology-object relations views the author is summarizing here—agree that psychoanalysis is the treatment of choice for these patients. In the author's view, however, narcissistic patients with overtly borderline functioning usually have serious contraindications for psychoanalysis proper and should be treated by psychoanalytic or expressive psychotherapy as outlined in the author's earlier chapter. Within this treatment some of the specific technical considerations that follow must be integrated to adapt it to the narcissistic personality. If psychoanalytic psychotherapy, in turn, is contraindicated, supportive psychotherapy is proposed as the treatment of choice (see the final section of this chapter).

The most important aspect of psychoanalytic technique in the treatment of narcissistic personalities is the systematic analysis of the pathological grandiose self that presents itself pervasively in the transference. What is unique about narcissistic character pathology is that the patient uses the pathological grandiose self in the transference precisely to avoid the emergence of the dissociated, repressed, or projected aspects of self- and object representations of the primitive object relations. When the grandiose self is activated in the psychoanalytic situation, the effect is a basic distance and an emotional unavailability. Subtly but chronically absent are the normal or "real" aspects of a human relationship between the patient and analyst, a relationship in which the patient treats the analyst as a specific, individualized person. In contrast, as the activation of a pathological self-idealization on the patient's part alternates with a projection of this self-idealization onto the analyst, the impression is that there is only one ideal, grandiose person in the room, and an admiring yet shadowy complement to it. Frequent role reversals between patient and analyst illustrate this basically stable transference paradigm.

Elsewhere, the author has described in detail the manifestations of this transference constellation—its recruitment, at its service, of primitive defense mechanisms, the analysis of the various aspects of this particular transference constellation, and the functions of the connected primitive defense mechanisms (Kernberg, 1975). Here, and in summary, the following issues are emphasized. In the course of psychoanalytic work with the narcissistic transference, the analyst has to interpret, among other things, the mechanism of omnipotent control by which the patient characteristically attempts to redesign the analyst to fit with the patient's own needs. The analyst must appear as brilliant and knowledgeable so that the patient will feel that he or she is in the presence of the greatest therapist of all times. Yet the analyst must not be too brilliant, presenting the patient with any knowledge or unexpected personality characteristics that might evoke the patient's envy and resentment. The analyst has to be as good as the patient—neither better, thus evoking envy—nor worse, thus provoking devaluation and the patient's sense of total loss.

When the analyst makes systematic efforts to help the patient understand the nature of this transference and does not fulfill the patient's expectations for admiration and reconfirmation of the grandiose self, the patient typically responds with anger or even rage, or a sudden devaluation of the analyst and his or her comments. Similar reactions of rage or devaluation characteristically follow times when the patient has felt important understanding and help coming from the analyst, understanding and help that painfully bring the patient to an awareness of the analyst's autonomous, independent functioning. The analyst's tolerance of such periods of rage or devaluation, and his or her interpretation of the reasons the patient activates such functions, gradually permit the patient to integrate the positive and negative aspects of the transference—idealization and trust with rage, contempt, and paranoid distrust.

Behind the apparently simple activation of narcissistic rage lies the activation of specific, primitive internalized object relations of the unconscious past. Typically these are of split-off self-representations with split-off object representations, reflecting condensed oedipal/preoedipal conflicts. In this context, periods of emptiness, and the patient's chronic feeling that "nothing is happening" in the treatment situation, may often be clarified as an active unconscious destruction of what the patient is receiving from the analyst, a reflection of the patient's lack of capacity to depend on the analyst as a giving maternal figure.

The patient's avid efforts to obtain knowledge and understanding from the analyst in order to incorporate them as something forcefully extracted, rather than something received with gratitude, contributes to the unconscious *spoiling* of what is received. First clarified by Rosenfeld (1964), this complex emotional reaction usually takes a long time to be understood and resolved. In a typical case, one finds lengthy periods of intellectual self-analysis, during which the patient treats the analyst as absent, which may elicit negative countertransference in the form of boredom in the analyst. These periods are followed by or interspersed with times when the patient eagerly expects and absorbs interpretations, attempts to outguess the analyst, and rapidly incorporates what he or she has received as if having known it all along, only once again to feel strangely empty and dissatisfied, as if not having received anything from this newly "metabolized" knowledge.

By the same token, in a typical case the patient by projection assumes that the analyst has no genuine interest in him or her and that the analyst is as self-centered and exploitative as the patient experiences him- or herself to be. The patient assumes that the analyst has no authentic knowledge or convictions but only a limited number of tricks and magic procedures which the patient needs to learn and incorporate. The more the superego corruption, and the more the patient needs to project devalued self- and object representations, the more he or she suspects the analyst of presenting similar corrupt and devalued characteristics. The gradual emergence or breakthrough of more primitive transferences may veer this overall picture into the expression of paranoid distrust and direct aggression in the transference. The apparent disruption of what may have earlier appeared as an "ideal" relation represents, in a deeper sense, the activation of a more real—though ambivalent and conflictual—relation in the transference, reflecting the activation of primitive object relations in it.

Advanced Stages of Treatment

During advanced stages of treatment, one often observes an oscillation between periods of idealization and overtly negative transference. In the course of this, the pathological narcissistic idealization already described is gradually replaced by higher levels of idealization. It is important to explore the changing nature of these periods of renewed idealization, which typically alternate with periods of intense negative transference. In the higher-level idealization, in contrast to narcissistic idealization, the patient no longer views the analyst as a projection of the patient's self-idealization. The analyst becomes an ideal parental (or combined parental) figure who has been able to tolerate the patient's aggression without counterattacking or being destroyed by it. This advanced type of idealization contains elements of guilt, expressing the patient's acknowledgment of his or her aggression. Elements of gratitude are also present and express the patient's understanding of the confidence and trust which the analyst has demonstrated through unwavering though tactful adherence to the truth of what has been going on in their relation.

Periods of predominantly negative transference are characterized by rage and the activation of a relation with a threatening, sadistic, dishonest, and manipulative mother or condensed mother/father figure. This may gradually evolve into the patient's alternately identifying with the sadistic parental image or with a complementary, persecuted one, the victim of parental aggression. The patient thus identifies him- or herself and the analyst alternately with previously dissociated or split-off self- and object representations. The analysis of the alternate activation of these self- and object representations of this particular "object relation unit" may then gradually be integrated with the dissociated or split-off idealized part-object relations referred to before. Consequently, self-representations may gradually coalesce into an integrated self, and object representations into an integrated concept of the parental objects.

Advanced stages of the treatment follow this systematic interpretation of the positive and negative transferences. Interpretation has thus permitted the integration of part-object into total-object relations, in other words, the achievement of object constancy. Good and bad self-representations are integrated, as are good and bad object representations. The dissolution of the pathological grandiose self and of the narcissistic resistances in general permit the emergence of normal infantile narcissism (the normal, regressed, infantile self) in the context of the analysis of condensed oedipal and preoedipal relations.

Certain typical issues emerge during advanced stages of the treatment of narcissistic personalities. A normal capacity to depend on the analyst gradually replaces the previous incapacity to depend on him or her. Now the patient may use interpretations to continue the self-exploration rather than as a starting point for greedily expropriating from the analyst hidden knowledge. The patient may now talk about him- or herself to the analyst rather than either talking to him- or herself alone or only to the analyst in a plea for gratification. The patient may now experience new sources of gratification and security from the certainty that he or she is able to learn about him- or herself, can creatively deal with difficulties, and above all, can maintain securely inside, in the the form of internalized good object representations, what he or she has received from the analyst.

The sense of internal wealth and gratification, stemming from the gratitude for what has been received, and the confidence in his or her own goodness typically brings about a decrease in the patient's envious reactions. The patient no longer needs to devalue what otherwise would trigger envy and may observe a parallel increase in the capacity for emotional and intellectual learning. The patient, in short, gradually feels free from internal emptiness, from the pathological driven quality of his or her ambitions, and from the previous, chronic experience of boredom and restlessness.

In the area of his or her sexual conflicts, the patient has experienced the activation and potential resolution of oedipal conflicts condensed with preoedipal issues. The patient may now tolerate and resolve the deepest, preoedipal roots of envy of the other sex. This prominent aspect of the sexual difficulties in narcissistic personalities relates to their homosexual conflicts and is a basic source of their unconscious rejection of a sexual identity that would have to be limited to "with one sex only." Grunberger (1979) first described the unconscious narcissistic fantasies of being both sexes simultaneously, which protect some narcissistic patients from the envy of the other sex. Clinically, change in this unconscious fantasy and the working through of envy influence the narcissistic patient's growing capacity to be able to fall in love and remain in love. In particular, these developments help the patient to establish a definite sexual commitment without chronic suspicions of losing out on all the other potential involvements available (Kernberg, 1976).

In the long run, when character analysis is systematically pursued, the paradoxical situation may emerge that patients find it much easier to talk about their past than about the unconscious aspects of their present relationship to the analyst. With the emphasis on analyzing the transference, the analyst may begin to wonder whether he or she is neglecting the exploration of the past. However, a careful working through of characterological resistances and a constant alertness should confirm the authenticity of psychoanalytic work. The analyst should be alert to whether the patient is changing his or her present experience of the psychoanalytic situation, thus indicating authentic shifts in predominant transference paradigms. But the analyst should also discern whether, in this context, there is a significant shift in the patient's emerging experiences of the past, thus expressing the working through of the transference. The analysis of the transference as a repetition of real experiences from the past, as fantasied experiences in the past, and as defenses against both is expressed, clinically, in the analysis of the unconscious aspects of the transference, as opposed to a premature deflection of it.

Modell (1976) and Volkan (1979) approach the analysis of narcissistic personalities within an ego psychology-object relations model that is quite closely related to the one underlying the author's technique. Unlike the author, they have proposed that, in the initial stage of analyzing these patients, the narcissistic idealization and the patient's incapacity to absorb interpretations should be respected, in a "holding"

(Winnicott, 1958) function that corresponds to a "cocoon" phase of the analysis. Gradually, however, in these authors' views, the analyst must interpret the narcissistic grandiose self and, in the process, facilitate the activation of the patient's primitive levels of internalized object relations in the transference. From that point on, the author believes, their approach largely corresponds to the one outlined in this section.

SUPPORTIVE PSYCHOTHERAPY WITH NARCISSISTIC PERSONALITIES

In an earlier section of this chapter, the author classified narcissistic personalities, according to the level of severity of their pathology, into overtly borderline cases and nonborderline-functioning cases. Psychoanalysis was the recommended treatment for the latter, in contrast to expressive psychotherapy for the former (see the author's previous chapter in this Part). But insofar as there are times when expressive psychotherapy is contraindicated, it becomes necessary to use supportive psychotherapy for these patients.

In addition to the general considerations presented earlier, a dominance of the following negative prognostic features would suggest that supportive psychotherapy would be preferable to the expressive type. First is the infiltration of the pathological grandiose self with aggression, so that the patient presents with conscious ideals of cruelty and destructiveness. These may be manifest in sadistic perversions or in conscious enjoyment of other people's suffering, in violence, and in severe forms of physical self-destructiveness. Other prognostically negative factors include severe antisocial features, chronic absence of actual involvements with other human beings—for example, a restriction of all sexual life to masturbation fantasies—characterologically anchored and rationalized chronic rage reactions, and transitory paranoid psychotic episodes. In all cases, it is advisable first to carry out an extensive evaluation with a probing, expressive approach and to decide on a supportive modality of treatment only by exclusion (see the author's earlier chapter in this volume). Again, as in all cases of supportive psychotherapy, common treatment goals should be set with the patient, his or her active cooperation expected, and work between psychotherapy sessions monitored.

Typical in these cases is the activation of certain defense mechanisms that are characteristic for narcissistic psychopathology and that need to be focused upon and worked with in noninterpretive ways. These patients' apparent development of intense dependency on the therapist may be a pseudodependency, rapidly punctured by radical devaluations of the therapist. It is important, therefore, to maintain a realistic therapeutic relationship. The therapist must focus on the patient's responsibilities in the treatment process and tactfully caution him or her against unrealistic idealizations of and expectations from the therapist, rather than directly feeding into the patient's apparently dependent relation. It is helpful to evaluate carefully the patient's disappointment reactions to the treatment hours in order to discern their implicit function of devaluing the therapist and their origins in prior developments in the psychotherapy hours.

For example, after the patient has received significant new understanding from the therapist, paradoxical disappointments (related to acting out unconscious envy) may be expected. These should be pointed out to the patient in terms of an observable sequence of behavior. The primitive pathological idealization typical for the narcissistic personality should be tactfully acknowledged, and its potentially negative effects on the patient's independent functioning brought up. The patient may see godlike qualities in the therapist. Such a patient should be helped to understand that it is difficult to identify oneself with such a godlike figure without running into serious problems in ordinary life, or that accepting the responsibility for independent living is difficult when a godlike therapist seems to be available for magically solving all problems. Naturally, the connection between primitive idealizations and the rapid spoiling of such idealizations by disappointment reactions and the underlying devaluation may also help the patient to acquire some distance from his or her own tendencies to idealize the therapist in unconsciously self-defeating ways.

Patients who present with intense rage reactions linked to frustration or narcissistic needs, particularly if these rage reactions evolve into microparanoid episodes, require a very active, painstaking evaluation. The therapist must evaluate all elements in the reality of the therapeutic interaction to determine what may have triggered the patient's rage and his or her paranoid distortions of the therapist. Under the effects of projective mechanisms, the patient's distortions of the reality of the therapeutic interactions must be carefully and tactfully clarified in order to reduce them. The problem here is that, under conditions of primitive rage reactions and paranoid distortions, the patient may experience any effort to clarify the immediate reality as blaming or sadistic accusations on the part of the therapist. The therapist must clarify, again and again, that he or she is not blaming the patient, and that, to the contrary, he or she is trying to help the patient understand the relation between the patient's perceptions and emotional reactions, regardless of whether or not these perceptions are realistic.

At times the reality of the interaction cannot immediately be clarified. In these circumstances the task is simply to acknowledge that patient and therapist may perceive reality in completely different ways without necessarily having to accept that one or the other of these perceptions is correct. In practice, the therapist might say, "I think I understand the way you are seeing my behavior, and I am not arguing with it; at the same time, I must tell you that I see it differently, although I acknowledge your perception as well. Do you think that you can tolerate our working together while each of us acknowledges to the other that our views are completely different?" Such a statement is often sufficient to continue work within a temporarily psychotic transference such as a microparanoid episode. In fact, the therapist's tolerance of a patient's narcissistic rage and paranoid distortion in the transference and his or her expressed acknowledgment of the patient's courage in maintaining their relationship may have longer-term benefits as well. The tolerance and acknowledgment in the light of such a stressful situation may lay the groundwork for later exploration of the patient's rage reactions and pathological character patterns in other interpersonal interactions.

At the same time, the analysis of what may be going on in other people's interactions with the patient, and the analysis of their hurt feelings or grandiose or derogatory reactions toward the patient as he or she describes them, may open the way for later exploration of similar reactive patterns in the patient him- or herself. The analysis of the grandiosity and depreciatory behavior the patient projects onto other people warrants much time because of its potential for leading to the study of similar reactions in the transference.

It is important to analyze the patient's sources of conscious and preconscious distrust in sexual relations, those sources derived from the unconscious envy of the other sex and the deep preoedipal pathology in relation to mother that contributes to narcissistic distortions of love relations. The careful exploration of conscious and preconscious sources of distrust and abandonment of sexual partners may have preventive value. By the same token, narcissistic patients with sexual promiscuity require a tolerant acceptance of their behavior. They must be helped to an awareness (and to remain tolerant of this awareness) of their incapacity to maintain stable sexual relations, and of their consequent loneliness and isolation.

This is an area where particular tact and patience are required. A grandiose male patient's search for the perfect unavailable woman, for example, and his relentless destruction of the valuable relations with women that he is temporarily able to achieve, represent, one might say, an existential tragedy. The therapist, by sharing with the patient his or her understanding of both the patient's needs and external reality, may make it possible for the patient to attempt new solutions to the problem, even though the therapist has not offered direct help. Under optimal circumstances, this approach may lead to a decrease in the patient's conscious expectations in his relations with the other sex, to a more careful behavior in his (or her) relations with partners, and to a tolerance of some frustrations in the light of the awareness of the alternative, namely, chronic loneliness. Unfortunately, supportive psychotherapy usually is much more limited in bringing about change in the psychosexual area than expressive modalities of treatment.

A patient's acting out of a need for omnipotent control in the therapy hours may restrict the therapist's independence of action. In subtle but deeply influential ways, the patient forces the therapist to attempt to be as good as the patient expects him or her to be, but without being better than or different from the patient, which would threaten the patient's self-esteem. In practice, this requires the therapist to become aware of the patient's controlling use of disappointment reactions in the treatment situation. The therapist must diagnose such disappointment reactions, ventilate them fully, and help the patient to tolerate his or her disappointments in the therapist and, correspondingly, in others. In this context, realistic exploration of such disappointments may lead to the patient's awareness of his or her excessive demands upon others and the social conflicts these bring about. Nonjudgmental evaluation of these issues may provide great help to patients who are unaware of how actively they are themselves destroying their opportunities in work and social life.

A major problem with some narcissistic patients who are functioning on an overtly borderline level is the discrepancy between their high ambitions and their incapacity to realize these ambitions. Many patients prefer to go on welfare rather than undergo the humiliation of working in what they consider an inferior job. The therapist's active exploration of this contradiction and his or her emphasis on how social ineffectiveness negatively affects self-esteem may help the patient to achieve compromise solutions between the relatively high levels of aspiration and the relatively low levels of capacity.

The narcissistic patients' tendency to "incorporate" eagerly what they have received from the therapist and to make it theirs is related to unconscious "stealing" from the therapist. Representing an effort to compensate for envy of the therapist and to reconfirm the patient's pathological grandiose self (Rosenfeld, 1964), this tendency may actually foster psychotherapeutic work in supportive psychotherapy. The patient may adopt the therapist's ideas and attitudes as his or her own and utilize them in daily life, while still reassuring him- or herself of the ability to do it all alone. If such an identification with the therapist has adaptive functions, even if it is based on pathological types of idealization, it should be tolerated and its strengthening of the patient's autonomy accepted. In fact, this mechanism has potentially strong positive effects in supportive psychotherapy of narcissistic personalities, counteracting the potentially negative effects of their unconscious envy.

Controversies regarding the treatment of narcissistic personalities are still unresolved, particularly the sharply contrasting approaches of Rosenfeld, Kohut, and the author. While these contrasts do demonstrate that the field of psychoanalytic modalities of treatment in this area is still open, the recent clinical observations and technical developments have nonetheless significantly improved the prognostic outlook for this prevalent and severely crippling personality disorder.

Bibliography for the Introduction

Kernberg, O. "The Structural Diagnosis of Borderline Personality Organization." In: *Borderline Personality Disorders*, edited by P. Hartocollis. New York: International Universities Press, 1977 87–121.

Kernberg, O. "Structural Interviewing." *Psychiatric Clinics of North America* 4 (1981): 169–195.

Stone, M. *The Borderline Syndromes*. New York: McGraw-Hill, 1980.

Bibliography for Chapter 28

Akiskal, H.S. "Subaffective Disorders: Dysthymic, Cyclothymic and Bipolar II Disorders in the 'Borderline' Realm." In *The Psychiatric Clinics of North America*, edited by M.H. Stone. Philadelphia: W.B. Saunders Co., April, 1981.

American Psychiatric Association, *Diagnostic and Statistical Manual of Mental Disorders, 3d ed.* Washington, D.C.: American Psychiatric Association, 1980.

Andrulonis, P.A., Glueck, B.C., Stroebel, C.F., Vogel, N.G., Shapiro A.L., and Aldridge, D.M. "Organic Brain Dysfunction and the Borderline Syndrome." In *The Psychiatric Clinics of North America*, edited by M.H. Stone. Philadelphia: W.B. Saunders Co., April, 1981.

Austin, V., Gunderson, J.G., and Madow, M. "Clinical Subtypes of Borderline Patients." Unpublished paper presented at the *Annual Meeting of the American Psychiatric Association*, San Francisco, 1980.

Baron, M., Asnis, L., and Gruen, R. "The Schedule for Schizotypal Personalities (SSP): A Diagnostic Interview for Schizotypal Features." *Journal of Psychiatry Research* 4 (1981): 213–228.

Bradley, S.J. *The Borderline Diagnosis in Children and Adolescents*. Unpublished manuscript, 1980.

Carpenter, W.T., Jr., Gunderson, J.G., and Strauss, J.S. "Considerations of the Borderline Syndrome: A Longitudinal Comparative Study of Borderline and Schizophrenic Patients." In *Borderline Personality Disorders: The Concepts, the Syndrome, the Patient*, edited by P. Hartocollis. New York: International Universities Press, 1977.

Carroll, B.J., Greden, J.F., Feinberg, M., Lohr, N., James, N., Steiner, M., Haskett, R.F., Albala, A.A., deVigne, J.P., and Tarika, J. "Neuroendocrine Evaluation of Depression in Borderline Patients." In *The Psychiatric Clinics of North America*, edited by M.H. Stone. Philadelphia: W.B. Saunders Co., April, 1981.

Cole, J.O. "Psychopharmacology Update: Drug Therapy of Borderline Patients." *McLean Hospital Journal* vol. 2, 1980.

Dickes, R. "The Concepts of Borderline States: An Alternative Proposal." *International Journal of Psychoanalytic Psychotherapy* 3 (1974): 1–22.

Feighner, J.P., Robins, F., Guze, S., Woodruff, R.A., Winokur, G., and Munoz, R. "Diagnostic Criteria for Use in Psychiatric Research." *Archives of General Psychiatry* 26 (1972): 57–63.

Grinker, R.R. "Diagnosis of Borderlines: A Discussion." *Schizophrenia Bulletin* 5 (1979): 47–52.

Grinker, R.R., Werble, B., and Drye, R. *The Borderline Syndrome*. New York: Basic Books, 1968.

Grinker, R.R., and Werble, B. *The Borderline Patient*. New York: Jason Aronson, 1977.

Gunderson, J.G. "Characteristics of Borderlines." In *Borderline Personality Disorders*, edited by P. Hartocollis. New York: International Universities Press, 1977, 173–192.

Gunderson, J.G. "Psychotic Regressions in Borderline Patients." Paper presented at the *Annual Meeting of the American Psychiatric Association*, San Francisco, 1980.

Gunderson, J.G., Carpenter, W.T., and Strauss, J.S. "Borderline and Schizophrenic Patients: A Comparative Study." *American Journal of Psychiatry* 132 (1975): 1257–1264.

Gunderson, J.G., and Kolb, J.E. "Discriminating Features of Borderline Patients." *American Journal of Psychiatry* 135 (1978): 792–796.

Gunderson, J.G., Kolb, J.E., and Austin, V. "The Diagnostic Interview for Borderlines (DIB)." *American Journal of Psychiatry* 138 (1981): 896–903.

Gunderson, J.G., Siever, L., and Spaulding, E. *The Search for a Schizotype: Crossing the Border Again*. Unpublished manuscript.

Gunderson, J.G., and Singer, M.T. "Defining Borderline Patients: An Overview." *American Journal of Psychiatry* 133 (1975): 1–10.

Guze, S.B. "Differential Diagnosis of the Borderline Personality Syndrome." In *Borderline States in Psychiatry*, edited by J.E. Mack. New York: Grune & Stratton, 1975, 69–74.

Kernberg, O.F. *Borderline Conditions and Pathological Narcissism*. New York: Jason Aronson, 1975.

Kernberg, O.F. "Borderline Personality Organization." *Journal of the American Psychoanalytic Association* 15 (1967): 641–685.

Kernberg, O.F. "The Structural Diagnosis of Borderline Personality Organization." In *Borderline Personality Disorders*, edited by P. Hartocollis. New York: International Universities Press, 1977, 87–121.

Kernberg, O.F. "Structural Interviewing." In *The Psychiatric Clinics of North America*, edited by M.H. Stone. Philadelphia: W.B. Saunders Co., April, 1981.

Kernberg, O.F. "Two Reviews of the Literature on Borderlines: An Assessment." *Schizophrenia Bulletin* 5 (1979): 53–58.

Kernberg, O.F., Goldstein, E.G., Carr, A.C., Hunt, H.F., Bauer, S.F., and Blumenthal, R. "Diagnosing Borderline Personality. A Pilot Study Using Multiple Diagnostic Methods." *Journal of Nervous and Mental Disease* 169 (1981): 225–231.

Kernberg, P. *Borderline Conditions: Childhood and Adolescent Aspects*. Unpublished manuscript, 1979.

Klein, D.F. "Psychopharmacological Treatment and Delineation of Borderline Disorders." In *Borderline Personality Disorders: The Concepts, the Syndrome, the Patient*, edited by P. Hartocollis. New

York: International Universities Press, 1977, 365–383.

Knight, F.P. "Borderline States." *Bulletin of the Menninger Clinic* 17 (1953): 1–12.

Kobele, S., Schulz, S.C., and van Kammen, D.P. *Diagnostic Interview for Borderlines Successfully Excludes Other Diagnoses.* Unpublished manuscript.

Koenigsberg, H. "A Comparison of Hospitalized and Non-Hospitalized Borderline Patients." *American Journal of Psychiatry*, in press.

Kolb, J.E., and Gunderson, J.G. "Diagnosing Borderline Patients With a Semistructured Interview." *Archives of General Psychiatry* 37 (1980): 37–41.

Kroll, J., Carey, K., and Sines, L. *Are There Borderlines in Britain? A Cross-Validation of U.S. Findings.* Unpublished manuscript.

Kroll, J., Pyle, R., Zander, J., Martin, K., Lari, S., and Sines, L. "Borderline Personality Disorder: Interrater Reliability of the Diagnostic Interview for Borderlines." *Schizophrenia Bulletin* 7 (1981a): 269–272.

Kroll, J., Sines, L., Martin, K., Lari, S., Pyle, R., and Zander, J. "Borderline Personality Disorder: Construct Validity of the Concept." *Archives of General Psychiatry* 38 (1981b): 1021–1026.

Leach, K.A. *MMPI Evaluation of Borderline Personality Disorder.* Unpublished manuscript.

Liebowitz, M.R., "Is Borderline a Distinct Entity?" *Schizophrenia Bulletin* 5 (1979): 23–28.

Mack, J.E. "Borderline States: A Historical Perspective." In *Borderline States in Psychiatry*, edited by J.E. Mack. New York: Grune & Stratton, 1975.

Mack, J.E., ed. *Borderline States in Psychiatry.* New York: Grune & Stratton, 1975.

Meissner, W.W. "Notes on Some Conceptual Aspects of Borderline Personality Organization." *International Review of Psychoanalysis* 5 (1978): 297–311.

Perry, J.C., and Klerman, G.L. "The Borderline Patient." *Archives of General Psychiatry* 35 (1978): 141–150.

Perry, J.C., and Klerman, G.L. "Clinical Features of the Borderline Personality Disorder." *American Journal of Psychiatry* 137 (1980): 165–173.

Perry, J.C., *Which Borderline? An Empirical Comparison of Clinical Descriptions.* Unpublished manuscript.

Robbins, M.D. "Borderline Personality Organization: The Need for a New Theory." *Journal of the American Psychoanalytic Association* 24 (1976): 831–853.

Sheehy, M., Goldsmith, L., and Charles, E. "A Comparative Study of Borderline Patients in a Psychiatric Outpatient Clinic." *American Journal of Psychiatry* 137 (1980): 1374–1379.

Siever, L.J., and Gunderson, J.G. "Genetic Determinants of Borderline Conditions." *Schizophrenia Bulletin* 5 (1979): 59–86.

Siever, L.J., Cohen, R.M., and Murphy, D.L. "Antidepressants and a_2-Adrenergic Autoreceptor Desensitization." *American Journal of Psychiatry* 138 (1981): 681–682.

Snyder, S., Pitts, W.M., Goodpaster, W.A., and Sajadi, C. *The MMPI Profile of the DSM-III Borderline Personality Disorder.* Unpublished manuscript.

Soloff, P.H. "Concurrent Validation of a Diagnostic Interview for Borderlines." *American Journal of Psychiatry* 138 (1981): 691–693.

Soloff, P.H. and Ulrich, R.F. "The Diagnostic Interview for Borderlines: A Replication Study." *Archives of General Psychiatry* 38 (1981): 686–692.

Spitzer, R.L., Endicott, J., and Gibbon, M. "Crossing the Border Into Borderline Personality and Borderline Schizophrenia." *Archives of General Psychiatry* 36 (1979a): 17–24.

Spitzer, R.L., Endicott, J., and Robins, E. *Research Diagnostic Criteria (RDC) for a Selected Group of Functional Disorders, 3d ed.* New York: New York Psychiatric Institute, 1977.

Spitzer, R.L., Forman, J.B.W., and Nee, J. "DSM-III Field Trials: I. Initial Interrater Diagnostic Reliability." *American Journal of Psychiatry* 136 (1979b): 815–817.

Stone, M.H. "The Borderline Syndrome: Evolution of the Term, Genetic Aspects and Prognosis." *American Journal of Psychotherapy* 31 (1977): 345–365.

Stone, M.H. "Assessing Vulnerability to Schizophrenia or Manic Depression in Borderline States." *Schizophrenia Bulletin* 5 (1979): 105–110.

Stone, M.H. *The Borderline Syndromes: Constitution, Adaptation and Personality.* New York: McGraw-Hill, 1980.

Werble, B. "Second Follow-up Study of Borderline Patients." *Archives of General Psychiatry* 23 (1970): 3–7.

Willett, A., Jones, A., Morgan, D., and Franco, S. "The Borderline Syndrome: An Operational Definition." Unpublished paper presented at the *Annual Meeting of the American Psychiatric Association*, Honolulu, 1973.

Bibliography for Chapter 29

Akiskal, H.S. "Subaffective Disorders: Dysthymic, Cyclothymic and Bipolar II Disorders in the 'Borderline' Realm." *Psychiatric Clinics of North America* 4 (1981): 25–46.

Akiskal, H.S., Djenderedjian, A.H., Rosenthal, R.H., and Khani, M.K. "Cyclothymic Disorder: Validating Criteria for Inclusion in the Bipolar Affective Group." *American Journal of Psychiatry* 134 (1977): 1227–1233.

Akiskal, H.S., Rosenthal, T.L., Haykel, R. F., Lemmi, H., Rosenthal, R.H., and Strauss, A.S. "Charactological Depressions. Clinical and Sleep EEG Findings Separating 'Subaffective Dysthymics' from 'Character Spectrum Disorders.'" *Archives of General Psychiatry* 37 (1980): 777–783.

American Psychiatric Association: *Diagnostic and Statistical Manual of Mental Disorders, 3rd ed.* Washington, D.C.: American Psychiatric Association, 1980.

Andrulonis, P.A. "Episodic Dyscontrol and Borderline Syndromes." Presented at the 134th *Annual Meeting of the American Psychiatric Association*, New Orleans, 1981.

Andrulonis, P.A., Glueck, B.C., Stroebel, C.F., Vogel, N.G., Shapiro, A.L., and Aldridge, D.M. "Organic Brain Dysfunction and the Borderline Syndrome." *Psychiatric Clinics of North America* 4 (1981): 47–66.

Baron, M., Asnis, L., and Gruen, R. "The Schedule for Schizotypal Personalities (SSP): A Diagnostic Interview for Schizotypal Features." *Psychiatry Research* 4 (1981): 213–228.

Baron, M., Levitt, M., and Perlman, R. "Low Platelet Monoamine Oxidase Activity: A Possible Biochemical Correlate of Borderline Schizophrenia." *Psychiatry Research* 3 (1980): 329–335.

Bleuler, E. *Textbook of Psychiatry*. Translated by A.A. Brill, New York: Macmillan Co., 1924.

Buchsbaum, M.S., Coursey, R., and Murphy, D.L. "The Biochemical High-Risk Paradigm: Behavioral and Familial Correlates of Low Platelet Monoamine Oxidase Activity." *Science* 194 (1976): 339–341.

Carroll, B.J., Feinberg, M., Greden, J.F., Tarika, J., Albala, A.A., Haskett, R.F., James, N. McI., Kronfol, Z., Lohr, N., Steiner, M., de Vigne, J.P., and Young, E. "A Specific Laboratory Test for the Diagnosis of Melancholia." *Archives of General Psychiatry* 38 (1981): 15–22.

Carroll, B.J., Greden, J.F., Feinberg, M., Lohr, N., James, N. McI., Steiner, M., Haskett, R.F., Albala, A.A., de Vigne, J.P., and Tarika, J. "Neuroendocrine Evaluation of Depression in Borderline Patients." *Psychiatric Clinics of North America* 4 (1981): 89–99.

Coursey, R.D., Buchsbaum, M.S., and Murphy, D.L. "Platelet MAO Activity and Evoked Potentials in the Identification of Subjects Biologically at Risk for Psychiatric Disorders." *British Journal of Psychiatry* 134 (1979): 372–381.

Cowdry, R.W., Pickar, D., and Davies, R. "Limbic Dysfunction in the Borderline Syndrome." New Research Abstracts No. NR32. Presented at the 133rd *Annual Meeting of the American Psychiatric Association*, San Francisco, 1980.

Davidson, J.R.T., McLeod, M.N., Turnbull, C.D., White, H.L., and Fever, E.J. "Platelet Monoamine Oxidase Activity and the Classification of Depression." *Archives of General Psychiatry* 37 (1980): 771–773.

Ekstein, R. "Vicissitudes of the 'Internal Image' in the Recovery of a Borderline Schizophrenic Adolescent." *Bulletin of the Menninger Clinic* 19 (1955): 86–92.

Essen-Moller, E. "Twenty-One Psychiatric Cases and Their MZ Co-Twins: A Thirty Year Follow-up." *Acta Geneticae Medicae et Gemallolagiae* 19 (1970): 315–317.

Federn, P. "Principles of Psychotherapy in Latent Schizophrenia." *American Journal of Psychotherapy* I (1947): 129–139.

Fischer, M. "A Danish Twin Study of Schizophrenia." *Acta Psychiatrica Scandinavica* Supplement 238 (1973): 9–142.

Frosch, J. "The Psychotic Character: Clinical Psychiatric Considerations." *Psychiatric Quarterly* 38 (1964): 81–96.

Gershon, E.S., Jargon, S.D., Kessler, L.R., Mazure, C.M., and Bunney, W.E., Jr. "Genetic Studies and Biologic Strategies in the Affective Disorders." *Progress in Medical Genetics, vol. 2*, edited by A.G. Steinberg, A.G. Bearn, A.G. Motulsky, and B. Childs. Philadelphia: W.B. Saunders Co., 1977.

Gottesman, I.I., and Shields, J. *Schizophrenia and Genetics: A Twin Study Vantage Point*. New York: Academic Press, 1972.

Grinker, R.R., Sr., and Werble, B. *The Borderline Patient*. New York: Jason Aronson, 1977.

Grinker, R.R., Sr., Werble, B., and Drye, R.C. *The Borderline Syndrome*. New York: Basic Books, 1968.

Gunderson, J.G. "The Relatedness of Borderline and Schizophrenic Disorders." *Schizophrenia Bulletin* 5 (1979): 17–22.

Gunderson, J.G., Carpenter, W.T., Jr., and Strauss, J.S. "Borderline and Schizophrenic Patients: A Comparative Study." *American Journal of Psychiatry* 132 (1975): 1257–1264.

Gunderson, J.G., and Kolb, J.E. "Discriminating Features of Borderline Patients." *American Journal of Psychiatry* 135 (1978): 792–796.

Gunderson, J.G., and Singer, M.T. "Defining Borderline Patients: An Overview." *American Journal of Psychiatry* 132 (1975): 1–10.

Hoch, P., and Polatin, P. "Pseudoneurotic Forms of Schizophrenia." *Psychiatric Quarterly* 23 (1949): 248–276.

Holzman, P.S., Kringler, E., Levy, D.L., and Haberman, S.J. "Deviant Eye Tracking in Twins Discordant for Psychosis." *Archives of General Psychiatry* 37 (1980): 627–631.

Holzman, P.S., Proctor, L.R., Levy, D.L., Yasillo, N.J., Meltzer, H.Y., and Hurt, S.W. "Eye Tracking Dysfunctions in Schizophrenic Patients and Their Relatives." *Archives of General Psychiatry* 31 (1974): 143–151.

Iacono, W.G., and Lykken, D.T. "Eye Tracking and Psychopathology: New Procedures Applied to a Sample of Normal Zygotic Twins." *Archives of General Psychiatry* 36 (1979): 1361–1369.

Inouye, E. "Similarity and Dissimilarity of Schizophrenia in Twins." *Proceedings of the Third International Congress of Psychiatry*. Montreal: University of Toronto Press, (1963): 524–530.

Jacobson, E. "Contribution to the Meta-Psychology of Cyclothymic Depression." *Affective Disorders*, edited by P. Greenacre. New York: International Universities Press, 1953.

Kernberg, O.F. *Borderline Conditions and Pathological Narcissism*. New York: Jason Aronson, 1975.

Kernberg, O.F. "Borderline Personality Organization." *Journal of the American Psychoanalytic Association* 15 (1967): 641–685.

Kernberg, O.F. "Two Reviews of the Literature on Borderlines: An Assessment." *Schizophrenia Bulletin* 5 (1979): 53–58.

Kety, S.S., Rosenthal, D., Wender, P.H., and Schulsinger, F. "The Types and Prevalence of Mental Illness in the Biological and Adoptive Families of Adopted Schizophrenics." *The Transmission of Schizophrenia*, edited by D. Rosenthal, and S.S. Kety. Oxford: Pergamon Press, 1968.

Kety, S.S., Rosenthal, D., Wender, P.H., Schulsinger, F., and Jacobsen, B. "Mental Illness in the Biological and Adoptive Families of Adopted Individuals Who Have Become Schizophrenics: A Preliminary Report Based on Psychiatric Interviews." *Genetic Research in Psychiatry*, edited by R. Fieve, D. Rosenthal, and H. Brill. New York: Johns Hopkins University Press, 1975.

Khouri, P.J., Haier, R.J., Rieder, R.O., and Rosenthal, D. "A Symptom Schedule for the Diagnosis of Borderline Schizophrenia: A First Report." *The British Journal of Psychiatry* 137 (1980): 140–147.

Knight, R.P. "Borderline States." *Bulletin of the Menninger Clinic* (1953): 1–12.

Kringlen, E. *Heredity and Environment in the Functional Psychoses*. London: Heinemann, 1967.

Kupfer, D.J., Foster, G., Coble, P., McPartland, R.J., and Ulrich, R.F. "The Application of EEG Sleep for the Differential Diagnosis of Affective Disorder." *American Journal of Psychiatry* 135 (1978): 69–74.

Liebowitz, M.K., and Klein, D.F. "Interrelationship of Hysteroid Dysphoria and Borderline Personality Disorder." *Psychiatric Clinics of North America* 4 (1981): 67–87.

Lipton, R.B., Levin, S., Holzman, P.S. "Horizontal and Vertical Pursuit Eye Movements, the Oculocephalic Reflex, and the Functional Psychoses." *Psychiatry Research* 3 (1980): 193–203.

Meehl, P.E. "Schizotaxia, Schizotypy, Schizophrenia." *American Psychologist* 17 (1962): 827–838.

Mirabile, C.S., and Glueck, B.C. "Motion Sickness Susceptibility and Patterns of Psychotic Illness." *Archives of General Psychiatry* 37 (1980): 42–46.

Murphy, D.L., and Weiss R. "Reduced Monoamine Oxidase Activity in Blood Platelets from Bipolar Depressed Patients." *American Journal of Psychiatry* 128 (1972): 1351–1357.

Murphy, D.L., and Wyatt, R.J. "Reduced Monoamine Oxidase Activity in Blood Platelets from Schizophrenic Patients." *Nature* 238 (1972): 225–226.

Noble, D. "A Study of Dreams in Schizophrenia and Allied States." *American Journal of Psychiatry* 107 (1951): 612–616.

Pollin, W., and Stabenau, J.R. "Biological, Psychological and Historical Differences in a Series of Monozygotic Twins Discordant for Schizophrenia." *The Transmission of Schizophrenia*, edited by D. Rosenthal, and S.S. Kety. Oxford: Pergamon Press, 1968.

Pollin, W., Stabenau, J.R., Mosher, L.R., and Tupin, J. "Life History Differences in Identical Twins Discordant for Schizophrenia." *American Journal of Orthopsychiatry* 36 (1966): 492–509.

Rado, S. "Dynamics and Classification of Disordered Behavior." *Psychoanalysis and Behavior, vol. 2*. New York: Grune & Stratton, 1962a, 268–285.

Rado, S. "Schizotypal Organization Preliminary Report on a Clinical Study of Schizophrenia." *Psychoanalysis and Behavior, vol. 2*. New York: Grune & Stratton, 1962b, 1–10.

Rieder, R.O. "Borderline Schizophrenia: Evidence of its Validity." *Schizophrenia Bulletin* 5 (1979): 39–46.

Rieder, R.O., Rosenthal, D., Wender, P.H., and Blumenthal, H. "The Offspring of Schizophrenics. Fetal and Neonatal Deaths." *Archives of General Psychiatry* 32 (1975): 200–211.

Rosenthal, D., Wender, P.H., Kety, S.S., Schulsinger, F., Welner, J., and Ostergaard, L. "Schizophrenics' Offspring Reared in Adoptive Homes." *The Transmission of Schizophrenia*. Oxford: Pergamon Press, 1968.

Rosenthal, D., Wender, P.H., Kety, S.S., Welner, J., and Schulsinger, F. "The Adopted-Away Offspring of Schizophrenics." *American Journal of Psychiatry* 128 (1971): 307–311.

Schildkraut, J.J., Orsulak, P.J., Schatzberg, A., Cole, J.O., Gudeman, J.E., and Rohde, W.A. "Elevated Platelet Monoamine Oxidase (MAO) Activity in Schizophrenic-Related Depressive Disorders." *American Journal of Psychiatry* 135 (1978): 110–112.

Siever, L.J. "Schizoid and Schizotypal Personality Disorders." In *Personality Disorders*, edited by J. Lion. Baltimore: Williams & Wilkins, 1981.

Siever, L.J., and Gunderson, J.G. "Genetic Determinants of Borderline Conditions." *Schizophrenia Bulletin* 5 (1979): 59–86.

Soloff, P.H., and Ulrich, R.F. "Diagnostic Interview for Borderline Patients." *Archives of General Psychiatry* 38 (1981): 686–692.

Spitzer, R.L. Endicott, J., and Gibbon, M. "Crossing the Border Into Borderline Personality and Borderline Schizophrenia. The Development of Criteria." *Archives of General Psychiatry* 36 (1979): 17–24.

Spitzer, R.L., Endicott, J., and Robins, E. *Research Diagnostic Criteria (RDC) for a Selected Group of Functional Disorders, 2d ed*. New York: New York Psychiatric Institute Biometrics Research Division, 1975.

Spitzer, R.L., Gibbon, M., and Endicott, J. *The Family Evaluation Form (F.E.F.)*. New York: New York Psychiatric Institute Biometrics Research Division, 1971.

Stone, M.H. "The Borderline Syndrome: Evolution of the Term, Genetic Aspects and Prognosis." *American Journal of Psychotherapy* 31 (1977): 345–365.

Stone, M.H. *The Borderline Syndromes*. New York: McGraw-Hill, 1980.

Stone, M.H. "Borderline Syndromes: A Consideration of Subtypes and an Overview, Directions for Research." *Psychiatric Clinics of North America* 4 (1981): 3–24.

Stone, M.H. "Genetic Aspects of Borderline Syndromes (Discussion of Siever and Gunderson's Article)." *Schizophrenia Bulletin* 5 (1979): 105–110.

Tienari, P. "Psychiatric Illnesses in Identical Twins." *Acta Psychiatrica Scandinavica* Supplement 171, (1963).

Tienari, P. "Schizophrenia and Monozygotic Twins." *Psychiatrica Fennica*, edited by K.A. Achte. Helsinki: Psychiatric Clinic of the Helsinki University Central Hospital, 1971.

Tulis, E.H. "Borderline Personality Disorder: Its Relation to the Major Psychoses and Other Genetic Factors." *Dissertation Abstracts International* 41 (1980): 382–B.

Wender, P.H., Rosenthal, D., Kety, S.S., Schulsinger, F., and Welner, J.J. "Crossfostering: A Research Strategy for Clarifying the Role of Genetic and Experiential Factors in the Etiology of Schizophrenia." *Archives of General Psychiatry* 30 (1974): 121–128.

Winokur, G., Clayton, P.J., and Reich, T. *Manic Depressive Illness*. St. Louis: C.V. Mosby, 1969.

Zilboorg, G. "Ambulatory Schizophrenics." *Psychiatry* 4 (1941): 149–155.

Bibliography for Chapter 30

American Psychiatric Association. *Diagnostic and Statistical Manual of Mental Disorders, 3d ed*. Washington, D.C.: American Psychiatric Association, 1980.

Bellak, L. (Ed.) *Psychiatric Aspects of Minimal*

Brain Dysfunction in Adults. New York: Grune and Stratton, 1979.

Brinkley, J., Beitman, B., and Freidel, R. "Low-Dose Neuroleptic Regimens in the Treatment of Borderline Patients." *Archives of General Psychiatry* 36 (1979): 319–326.

Cole, J.O. "Drug Therapy of Adult Minimal Brain Dysfunction (MBD)." *McLean Hospital Journal* 3 (1978): 37–49.

Dyrud, J.E. "The Treatment of Borderline Syndrome." In *Modern Psychiatry and Clinical Research*, edited by E. Offer, and D.X. Freedman. New York: Basic Books, 1972, 159–173.

Gunderson, J.G., and Kolb, J.E. "Discriminating Features of Borderline Patients." *American Journal of Psychiatry* 135 (1978): 792–796.

Gunderson, J.G., Kolb, J.E., and Austin, V. "The Diagnostic Interview for Borderlines (DIB)." *American Journal of Psychiatry* 138 (1981): 896–903.

Hedberg, D.L., Houck, J.H., and Glueck, B.C. "Tranylcypramine-Trifluoperazine Combination in the Treatment of Schizophrenia." *American Journal of Psychiatry* 127 (1971): 1141–1146.

Hoch, P., and Polatin, P. "Pseudoneurotic Forms of Schizophrenia." *Psychiatric Quarterly* 23 (1949): 248–276.

Huessey, H., Cohen, S., Blair, C., and Hood, P. "Clinical Explorations in Adult Minimal Brain Dysfunction." In *Psychiatric Aspects of Minimal Brain Dysfunction in Adults*, edited by L. Bellak. New York: Grune and Stratton, 1979, 19–36.

Kernberg, O. *Borderline Conditions and Pathological Narcissism*. New York: Jason Aronson, 1975.

Klein, D.F. "Delineation of Two Drug Responsive Anxiety Syndromes." *Psychopharmacologia* 5 (1964): 397–408.

Klein, D.F. "Importance of Psychiatric Diagnosis in Prediction of Clinical Drug Effects." *Archives of General Psychiatry* 16 (1967): 118–126.

Klein, D.F. *Psychiatric Case Studies: Treatment, Drugs, and Outcome*. Baltimore: Williams & Wilkins, 1972.

Klein, D.F. "Drug Therapy as a Means of Syndromal Identification and Nosological Revision." In *Psychopathology and Psychopharmacology*, edited by J. Cole, A. Freedman, and A. Friedhoff. Baltimore: Johns Hopkins University Press., 1973, 149–160.

Klein, D.F. "Psychopharmacological Treatment and Delineation of Borderline Disorders." In *Borderline Personality Disorders: The Concept, the Syndrome, the Patient*, edited by P. Hartocollis. New York: International Universities Press, 1977, 365–383.

Klein, D.F., Gittleman, R., Quitkin, F., and Rifkin, A. *Diagnosis and Drug Treatment of Psychiatric Disorders*. Baltimore: Williams & Wilkins, 1980.

Kolb, J.E., and Gunderson, J.G. "Diagnosing Borderline Patients With a Semistructured Interview." *Archives of General Psychiatry* 37 (1980): 37–41.

Last, U., Lowenthal, U., and Klein, H. "Borderline Patients in a Chronic Ward." *Archives of General Psychiatry* 28 (1973): 517–521.

Liebowitz, M. "Is Borderline a Distinct Entity?" *Schizophrenia Bulletin* 5 (1979): 23–28.

Lyskowski, J. and Tsuang, M. "Precautions in Treating DSM-III Borderline Personality Disorder." *American Journal of Psychiatry* 137 (1980): 110–111.

Monroe, R.B. *Episodic Behavioral Disorders*. Cambridge: Harvard University Press, 1970.

Ostow, M. *Drugs in Psychoanalysis and Psychotherapy*. New York: Basic Books, 1962.

Paykel, E. "Depressive Typologies and Response to Amitriptyline." *British Journal of Psychiatry* 120 (1972): 147–157.

Pennes, H. "Clinical Reactions of Schizophrenics to Sodium Amytol, Pervitin Hydrochloride, Mescaline Sulfate and LSD–25." *Journal of Nervous and Mental Disease* 119 (1954): 95–112.

Perry, J., and Klerman, G. "The Borderline Patient." *Archives of General Psychiatry* 35 (1978): 141–150.

Quitkin, F., Rifkin, A., and Klein, D. "Monoamine Oxidase Inhibitors." *Archives of General Psychiatry* 36 (1979): 749–764.

Rifkin, A., Levitan, S., and Galewski, J. "Emotionally Unstable Character Disorder: A Follow-up Study. I. Description of Patients and Outcome." *Journal of Biological Psychiatry* 4 (1972a): 65–79.

Rifkin, A., Quitkin, F., Curillo, C., Blumberg, A., and Klein, D. "Lithium Carbonate in Emotionally Unstable Character Disorders." *Archives of General Psychiatry* 27 (1972b): 519–523.

Schick, J.F.E., and Freedman, D.X. "Research in Non-Narcotic Drug Abuse." *American Handbook of Psychiatry, 2nd ed.*, edited by D.A. Hamburg, and H.K.H. Brodie. New York: Basic Books, 1974, 552–622.

Schmideberg, M. "The Borderline Patient." *American Handbook of Psychiatry*. New York: Basic Books, 1959, 398–416.

Shader, R., Jackson, A., and Dodes, L. "The Antiaggressive Effects of Lithium in Man." *Psychopharmacologia* 40 (1974): 17–24.

Sheard, M., Marini, J., Bridges, C., and Wagner, E. "The Effect of Lithium on Impulsive Aggressive Behavior in Man." *American Journal of Psychiatry* 133 (1976): 1409–1413.

Sheehan, D., Ballenger, J., and Jacobson, G. "Treatment of Endogenous Anxiety With Phobic, Hysterical and Hypochondriacal Symptoms." *Archives of General Psychiatry* 37 (1980): 51–62.

Stephens, J., and Shaffer, J. "A Controlled Study of the Effects of Diphenylhydantoin on Anxiety, Irritability and Anger in Neurotic Outpatients." *Psychopharmacologia* 17 (1970): 169–181.

Stewart, J., Quitkin, F., Liebowitz, M., McGrath, P., and Klein, D. "Efficacy of Desipramine in Mildly Depressed Patients: A Double-Blind Placebo-Controlled Trial." *Psychopharmacology Bulletin* 17 (1981): 136–138.

Tupin, J., Smith, D., Clanon, T., Kim, L., Nugent, A., and Groupe, A. "The Long-Term Use of Lithium in Aggressive Prisoners." *Comprehensive Psychiatry* 14 (1973): 311–317.

Vilkin, M.I. "Comparative Chemotherapeutic Trial in Treatment of Chronic Borderline Patients." *American Journal of Psychiatry* 120 (1964): 1004.

Wender, P., Reimherr, F., and Wood, D. "Attention Deficit Disorder (Minimal Brain Dysfunction) in Adults—Replication Study of Diagnosis and Drug Treatment." *Archives of General Psychiatry* 38 (1981): 449–456.

Wood, D., Reimherr, F., Wender, P., and Johnson, G. Diagnosis and Treatment of Minimal Brain Dysfunction in Adults." *Archives of General Psychiatry* 33 (1976): 1453–1460.

Zitrin, C., Klein, D.F., Woerner, M. "Behavior Therapy, Supportive Therapy, and Imipramine and Phobias." *Archives of General Psychiatry* 35 (1978): 307–316.

Bibliography for Chapter 31

Adler, G., and Buie, D.H. "The Psychotherapeutic Approach to Aloneness in the Borderline Patient." In *Advances in Psychotherapy of the Borderline Patient*, edited by J. LeBoit and A. Capponi. New York: Jason Aronson, 1979, 433–448.

American Psychiatric Association. *Diagnostic and Statistical Manual of Mental Disorders, 3d ed.*, Washington, D.C.: American Psychiatric Association, 1980.

Bibring, E. "Psychoanalysis and the Dynamic Psychotherapies." *Journal of the American Psychoanalytic Association* 2 (1954): 745–770.

Bion, W. *Second Thoughts: Selected Papers on Psychoanalysis*. New York: Basic Books, 1967.

Eissler, K. "The Effects of the Structure of the Ego on Psychoanalytic Technique." *Journal of the American Psychoanalytic Association* 1 (1953): 104–143.

Fairbairn, W.R.D. *An Object-Relations Theory of the Personality*. New York: Basic Books, 1954.

Frosch, J. "Psychoanalytic Considerations of the Psychotic Character." *Journal of the American Psychoanalytic Association* 18 (1970): 24–50.

Gill, M.M. "Psychoanalysis and Exploratory Psychotherapy." *Journal of the American Psychoanalytic Association* 2 (1954): 771–797.

Giovacchini, P. "The Many Sides of Helplessness: The Borderline Patient." In *Advances in Psychotherapy of the Borderline Patient*, edited by J. LeBoit and A. Capponi. New York: Jason Aronson, 1979a, 227–267.

Giovacchini, P. "The Psychoanalytic Treatment of the Alienated Patient." In *New Perspectives on Psychotherapy of the Borderline Adult*. New York: Brunner/Mazel, 1979b, 3–19.

Green, A. "The Borderline Concept." In *Borderline Personality Disorders*, edited by P. Hartocollis. New York: International Universities Press, 1977, 15–44.

Grinker, R. "Neurosis, Psychosis, and the Borderline States." In *Comprehensive Textbook of Psychiatry*, edited by A.M. Freedman, H.I. Kaplan, and B.J. Sadock. Baltimore: Williams & Wilkins, 1975, 845–850.

Heimann, P.A. "A Combination of Defense Mechanisms in Paranoid States." In *New Directions in Psycho-Analysis*, edited by M. Klein, P. Heimann, and R.E. Money-Kyrle. London: Tavistock Publications, 1955a, 240–265.

Heimann, P.A. "A Contribution to the Re-Evaluation of the Oedipus Complex: The Early States." In *New Directions in Psycho-Analysis*, edited by M. Klein, P. Heimann, and R.E. Money-Kyrle. New York: Basic Books, 1955b, 23–38.

Holzman, P.S., and Ekstein, R. "Repetition-

Functions of Transitory Regressive Thinking." *Psychoanalytic Quarterly* 28 (1959): 228–235.

Kernberg, O. *Borderline Conditions and Pathological Narcissism*. New York: Jason Aronson, 1975.

Kernberg, O. "Contrasting Approaches to the Psychotherapy of Borderline Conditions." In *New Perspectives of Psychotherapy of the Borderline Adult*, edited by J.F. Masterson. New York: Brunner/Mazel, 1978, 77–104.

Kernberg, O. *Internal World and External Reality*. New York: Jason Aronson, 1980a.

Kernberg, O. "Neurosis, Psychosis and the Borderline States." In *Comprehensive Textbook of Psychiatry*, edited by A.M. Freedman, H.I. Kaplan, and B.J. Sadock. Baltimore: Williams and Wilkins, 1980b, 1079–1092.

Kernberg, O. *Object Relations Theory and Clinical Psychoanalysis*. New York: Jason Aronson, 1976a.

Kernberg, O. "Supportive Psychotherapy with Borderline Conditions." In *Critical Problems in Psychiatry*, edited by J. Cavenar, and H.K.H. Brodie. Philadelphia: J.B. Lippincott, in press.

Kernberg, O. "Technical Considerations in the Treatment of Borderline Personality Organization." *Journal of the American Psychoanalytic Association* 24 (1976b): 795–829.

Kernberg, O., Burstein, E., Coyne, L., Appelbaum, A., Horwitz, L., and Voth, H. "Psychotherapy and Psychoanalysis: Final Report of the Menninger Foundation's Psychotherapy Research Project." *Bulletin of the Menninger Clinic* 36 (1972): 87–275.

Khan, M. *The Primacy of the Self: Papers on Psychoanalytic Theory Technique*. New York: International Universities Press, 1974.

Klein, M. "Notes on Some Schizoid Mechanisms." *International Journal of Psychoanalysis* 27 (1946): 99–110.

Knight, R.P. "Borderline States." In *Psychoanalytic Psychiatry and Psychology*, edited by R.P. Knight, and C.R. Friedman. New York: International Universities Press, 1954a, 97–109.

Knight, R.P. "Management and Psychotherapy of the Borderline Schizophrenic Patient." In *Psychoanalytic Psychiatry and Psychology*, edited by R.P. Knight, and C.R. Friedman. New York: International Universities Press, 1954b, 110–122.

Little, M. "Countertransference and the Patient's Response to It." *International Journal of Psycho-Analysis* 32 (1951): 32–40.

Little, M. *Transference Neurosis and Transference Psychosis*. New York: Jason Aronson, 1981.

Mahler, M. "Rapprochement Subphase of the Separation-Individuation Process." *Psychoanalytic Quarterly* 41 (1972): 487–506.

Mahler, M. "A Study of the Separation-Individuation Process and Its Possible Application to Borderline Phenomena in the Psychoanalytic Situation." In *Psychoanalytic Study of the Child*, Vol. 26. New York/Chicago: Quadrangle Books, 1971, 403–424.

Mahler, M., and Kaplan, L. "Developmental Aspects in the Assessment of Narcissistic and So-called Borderline Personalities." In *Borderline Personality Disorders*, edited by P. Hartocollis. New York: International Universities Press, 1977, 71–85.

Masterson, J. *From Borderline Adolescent to Functioning Adult*. New York: Brunner/Mazel, 1980.

Masterson, J. *New Perspective on Psychotherapy of the Borderline Adult.* New York: Brunner/Mazel, 1978.

Masterson, J. *Psychotherapy and the Borderline Adult: A Developmental Approach.* New York: Brunner/Mazel, 1976.

Modell, A. "The 'Holding Environment' and the Therapeutic Action of Psychoanalysis." *Journal of the American Psychoanalytic Association* 24 (1976): 285–307.

Money-Kyrle, R.E. "Normal Countertransference and Some of Its Deviations." *International Journal of Psycho-Analysis* 37 (1956): 360–366.

Racker, H. "The Meanings and Uses of Countertransference." *Psychoanalytic Quarterly* 26 (1957): 303–357.

Reider, N. "Transference Psychosis." *Journal of the Hillside Hospital* 6 (1957): 131–149.

Rey, J.H. "Schizoid Phenomena in the Borderline." In *Advances in Psychotherapy of the Borderline Patient,* edited by J. LeBoit and A. Capponi. New York: Jason Aronson, 1979, 449–485.

Rinsely, D.B. *Treatment of the Severely Disturbed Adolescent.* New York: Jason Aronson, 1980.

Romm, M. "Transient Psychotic Episodes During Psychoanalysis." *Journal of the American Psychoanalytic Association* 5 (1957): 325–341.

Rosenfeld, H. "Difficulties in the Psychoanalytic Treatment of Borderline Patients." In *Advances in Psychotherapy of the Borderline Patient,* edited by J. LeBoit and A. Capponi. New York: Jason Aronson, 1979a, 187–206.

Rosenfeld, H. (1963) "Notes on the Psychopathology and Psychoanalytic Treatment of Schizophrenia." In *Psychotic States.* London: Hogarth Press, 1965.

Rosenfeld, H. "Transference Psychosis in the Borderline Patient." In *Advances in Psychotherapy of the Borderline Patient,* edited by J. LeBoit and A. Capponi. New York: Jason Aronson, 1979b, 485–510.

Searles, H. "The Countertransference With the Borderline Patient." In *Advances in Psychotherapy of the Borderline Patient,* edited by J. LeBoit and A. Capponi. New York: Jason Aronson, 1979, 309–346.

Segal, H. *Introduction to the Work of Melanie Klein.* New York: Basic Books, 1964.

Sharpe, E.F. "Anxiety, Outbreak and Resolution." In *Collected Papers on Psycho-Analysis,* edited by M. Brierly. London: Hogarth Press, 1931, 67–80.

Stone, M. *The Borderline Syndromes.* New York: McGraw-Hill, 1980.

Stone, M. "Personality Type: Impact on Outcome in the Psychotherapy of Borderline Patients." Presented at "Dialogues on Borderlines." Earl D. Bond Symposium of the Institute of Pennsylvania Hospital, Philadelphia, April 3–4, 1981. (Unpublished)

Strachey, J. "The Nature of the Therapeutic Action for Psychoanalysis." *International Journal of Psycho-Analysis* 15 (1934): 127–159.

Ticho, E. "Termination of Psychoanalysis: Treatment Goals, Life Goals." *Psychoanalytic Quarterly* 41 (1972): 315–333.

Volkan, V. "The 'Glass Bubble' of the Narcissistic Patient." In *Advances in Psychotherapy of the Borderline Patient,* edited by J. LeBoit and A. Capponi. New York: Jason Aronson, 1979, 405–431.

Volkan, V. *Primitive Internalized Object Relations.* New York: International Universities Press, 1976, xiii–xvii.

Wallerstein, R.S. "Reconstruction and Mastery in the Transference Psychosis." *Journal of the American Psychoanalytic Association* 15 (1967): 551–583.

Winnicott, D.W. *Collected Papers: Through Paediatrics to Psycho-Analysis.* New York: Basic Books, 1958.

Winnicott, D.W. *The Maturational Process and the Facilitating Environment.* New York: International Universities Press, 1965.

Zetzel, E.R. "A Developmental Approach to the Borderline Patient." *American Journal of Psychiatry* 127 (1971): 867–871.

Bibliography for Chapter 32

American Psychiatric Association. *Diagnostic and Statistical Manual of Mental Disorders, 3d ed.* Washington, D.C.: American Psychiatric Association, 1980.

Bergler, E. *The Basic Neurosis.* New York: Grune & Stratton, 1949.

Buie, D.D. "Empathy: Its Nature and Limitations." *Journal of the American Psychoanalytic Association* 29 (1981): 281–308.

Erikson, E. *Childhood and Society, 2d ed.* New York: W.W. Norton & Co., Inc., 1963.

Fairbairn, W.R.D. *An Object-Relations Theory of the Personality.* New York: Basic Books, 1954.

Freud, S. "Female Sexuality" (1931). *The Standard Edition of the Complete Psychological Works of Sigmund Freud.* 21 (1961a): 225–246. London: The Hogarth Press and the Institute for Psychoanalysis.

Freud, S. "On Narcissism: An Introduction" (1914). *The Standard Edition of the Complete Psychological Works of Sigmund Freud.* 14 (1957): 69–102. London: The Hogarth Press and the Institute for Psychoanalysis.

Freud, S. "Three Essays on the Theory of Sexuality" (1905). *The Standard Edition of the Complete Psychological Works of Sigmund Freud.* 7 (1961b): 226, footnote 1920. London: The Hogarth Press and the Institute for Psychoanalysis.

Hartmann, H. "Comments on the Psychoanalytic Theory of the Ego." *Essays on Ego Psychology: Selected Problems in the Psychoanalytic Theory.* New York: International Universities Press, 1950, 113–141.

Horney, K. *New Ways in Psychoanalysis.* New York: W.W. Norton & Co., Inc., 1939.

Jacobson, E. *The Self and the Object World.* New York: International Universities Press, 1964.

Kardiner, A., Karush, A., and Ovesey, L. "A Methodological Study of Freudian Theory." *Journal of Nervous and Mental Disease* 129 (1959): 11–19; 133–143; 207–221; 341–356.

Kernberg, O. *Borderline Conditions and Pathological Narcissism.* New York: Jason Aronson, 1975.

Kernberg, O. "Contributions to the Technique of Character Analysis." Unpublished[a].

Kernberg, O. "Self Ego, Affects, and Drives." Unpublished[b].

Kohut, H. *The Psychology of the Self: A Casebook*, edited by A. Goldberg, et al. New York: International Universities Press, 1978.

Kohut, H. *The Restoration of the Self*. New York: International Universities Press, 1977.

Kohut, H. "Summarizing Reflections." In *Advances in Self Psychology*, edited by A. Goldberg. New York: International Universities Press, 1980.

Kohut, H. "The Two Analyses of Mr. Z." *International Journal of Psychoanalysis* 60 (1979): 3–27.

Laplanche, J., and Pontalis, J.B. *The Language of Psychoanalysis*. New York: W.W. Norton and Co., Inc., 1973.

Moore, B.E., and Fine, B.D., eds. *A Glossary of Psychoanalytic Terms and Concepts*. New York: The American Psychoanalytic Association, 1968.

Pulver, S. "Narcissism: The Term and the Concept." *Journal of the American Psychoanalytic Association* 18 (1970): 319–341.

Rado, S. "Hedonic Control, Action Self, and the Depressive Spell." In *Psychoanalysis of Behavior: Collected Papers*. New York: Grune & Stratton, 1956, 286–311.

Reich, W. *Character-Analysis, 3d ed.* translated by T.P. Wolfe. New York: Orgone Institute Press, 1949.

Schafer, R. "Generative Empathy in the Treatment Situation." *Psychoanalytic Quarterly* 28 (1959): 342–373.

Schwaber, E.A. "Self Psychology and the Concept of Psychopathology: A Case Presentation." *Advances in Self Psychology*, edited by A. Goldberg. New York: International Universities Press, 1980.

Spruiell, V. "The Self and the Ego." *The Psychoanalytic Quarterly* 50 (1981): 319–344.

Stein, M. "Book Review of *The Restoration of the Self* by Heinz Kohut." *Journal of the American Psychoanalytic Association* 27 (1979): 665–680.

Stone, L. *The Psychoanalytic Situation*. New York: International Universities Press, 1961.

Sullivan, H.S. *The Interpersonal Theory of Psychiatry*, edited by H. Swick-Perry and M. Ladd-Gowel. New York: W.W. Norton and Co., Inc. 1953.

Wallerstein, R.S. "The Bipolar Self: Discussion of Alternative Perspectives." *Journal of the American Psychoanalytic Association* 29 (1981): 377–394.

Winnicott, D.W. *The Maturational Processes and the Facilitating Environment: Studies in the Theory of Emotional Development*. New York: International Universities Press, 1965.

Bibliography for Chapter 33

Basch, M.F. "Selfobject Disorders and Psychoanalytic Theory: A Historical Perspective." *Journal of the American Psychoanalytic Association* 2 (1979): 337–353.

Kernberg, O. *Borderline Conditions and Pathological Narcissism*. New York: Jason Aronson, 1975.

Kernberg, O. *Internal World and External Reality*. New York: Jason Aronson, 1980.

Kernberg, O. *Object Relations Theory and Clinical Psychoanalysis*. New York: Jason Aronson, 1976.

Kohut, H. *The Analysis of the Self*. New York: International Universities Press, 1971.

Kohut, H. "Forms and Transformations of Narcissism." *Journal of the American Psychoanalytic Association* 14 (1966): 243–272.

Kohut, H. "The Psychoanalytic Treatment of Narcissistic Personality Disorders." *The Psychoanalytic Study of the Child* 23 (1968): 86–113.

Kohut, H. "Reflections on Self Psychology." In *Advances in Self Psychology*, edited by A. Goldberg. New York: International Universities Press, 1980.

Kohut, H. *The Restoration of the Self*. New York: International Universities Press, 1977.

Kohut, H. "The Two Analyses of Mr. Z. " *International Journal of Psychoanalysis* 60 (1979): 3–27.

Kohut, H., and Wolf, E.S. "The Disorders of the Self and Their Treatment: An Outline." *International Journal of Psychoanalysis* 59 (1978): 413–424.

Lampl-de Groot, J. "Ego Ideal and Superego." *The Psychoanalytic Study of the Child* 17 (1962): 94–106.

Lampl-de Groot, J. "Superego, Ego Ideal, and Masochistic Fantasies." In *The Development of the Mind*. New York: International Universities Press, 1965, 351–363.

Lichtenstein, H. "The Role of Narcissism in the Emergence and Maintenance of a Primary Identity." *International Journal of Psychoanalysis* 45 (1964): 49–56.

Lichtenstein, H. *The Dilemma of Human Identity*. New York: Jason Aronson, 1977.

Moore, B.E. "Toward a Clarification of the Concept of Narcissism." *The Psychoanalytic Study of the Child* 30 (1975): 243–276.

Ornstein, A. "Oedipal Selfobject Transferences: A Clinical Example." Unpublished paper presented at the Boston Psychoanalytic Society and Institute Symposium on "The Psychology of the 'Self.'" Boston, Mass., Oct. 31, 1980.

Ornstein, P.H. "On Narcissism: Beyond the Introduction, Highlights of Heinz Kohut's Contributions to the Psychoanalytic Treatment of Narcissistic Personality Disorders." In *The Annual of Psychoanalysis, vol. 2*. New York: International Universities Press, 1974, 127–149.

Ornstein, P.H., and Ornstein,A. "On the Continuing Evolution of Psychoanalytic Psychotherapy: Reflections and Predictions." In *The Annual of Psychoanalysis, vol. 5*. New York: International Universities Press, 1976, 329–370.

Rosenfeld, H. "On the Psychopathology of Narcissism." *International Journal of Psychoanalysis* 45 (1964): 332–337.

Sandler, J. "Actualization and Object Relationships." *Journal of the Philadelphia Association for Psychoanalysis* 3 (1976): 59–70.

Sandler, J. "Psychological Conflict and the Structural Model: Some Clinical and Theoretical Implications." *International Journal of Psychoanalysis* 55 (1974): 53–62.

Wallerstein, R.S. "The Bipolar Self: Discussion of Alternative Perspectives." *Journal of the American Psychoanalytic Association* 2 (1979): 377–395.

Wallerstein, R.S. "Self-Psychology and 'Classical' Psychoanalytic Psychology: The Nature of Their Relationship—A Review and Overview." Unpublished paper presented at the Boston Psychoanalytic Society and Institute Symposium on "The Psychology of the 'Self.'" Boston, Mass., Nov. 1, 1980.

Bibliography for Chapter 34

Abraham, K. (1919) "A Particular Form of Neurotic Resistance Against the Psychoanalytic Method." In *Selected Papers on Psycho-Analysis*, London: Hogarth Press, 1949, 303–311.

American Psychiatric Association. *Diagnostic and Statistical Manual of Mental Disorders, 3d ed.* Washington, D.C.: American Psychiatric Association, 1980.

Freud, S. "On Narcissism: An Introduction." (1914). *The Standard Edition of the Complete Psychological Works of Sigmund Freud*, vol. 14. London: The Hogarth Press and the Institute for Psychoanalysis, 1957, 69–102.

Goldberg, A. *Advances in Self Psychology.* New York: International Universities Press, 1980.

Grunberger, B. *Narcissism: Psychoanalytic Essays.* New York: International Universities Press, 1979.

Jacobson, E. *The Self and the Object World.* New York: International Universities Press, 1964.

Jones, E. (1913) The God Complex Essays. In *Applied Psycho-Analysis.* New York: International Universities Press, 1964, 244–265.

Kernberg, O. *Borderline Conditions and Pathological Narcissism.* New York: Jason Aronson, 1975.

Kernberg, O. *Internal World and External Reality.* New York: Jason Aronson, 1980.

Kernberg, O. *Object Relations Theory and Clinical Psychoanalysis.* New York: Jason Aronson, 1976.

Kohut, H. *The Analysis of the Self.* New York: International Universities Press, 1971.

Kohut, H. (1977) *The Restoration of the Self.* New York: International Universities Press, 1978.

Kohut, H. "Thoughts on Narcissism and Narcissistic Rage." *Psychoanalytic Study of the Child*, 27 (1972): 360–400.

Kohut, H. "The Two Analyses of Mr. Z." *International Journal of Psycho-Analysis.* 60 (1979): 3–27.

Kohut, H., and Wolf, E. "The Disorders of the Self and Their Treatment: An Outline." *International Journal of Psycho-Analysis*, 59 (1978): 413–426.

Mahler, M., and Furer, M. *On Human Symbiosis and the Vicissitudes of Individuation.* New York: International Universities Press, 1968.

Mahler, M., Pine, F., and Bergman, A. *The Psychological Birth of the Human Infant.* New York: Basic Books, 1975.

Modell, A. "The Holding Environment and the Therapeutic Action of Psychoanalysis." *Journal of the American Psychoanalytic Association*, 24 (1976): 285–307.

Reich, A. (1960) "Further Remarks on Countertransference." In *Psychoanalytic Writings.* New York: International Universities Press, 1973, 271–287.

Reich, A. (1953) "Narcissistic Object Choice in Women." In *Psychoanalytic Writings.* New York: International Universities Press, 1973, 179–208.

Rosenfeld, H. "A Clinical Approach to the Psychoanalytic Theory of the Life and Death Instincts: An Investigation into the Aggressive Aspects of Narcissism." *International Journal of Psycho-Analysis* 52 (1971): 169–178.

Rosenfeld, H. "Negative Therapeutic Reactions." In *Tactics and Techniques in Psychoanalytic Therapy, vol. II, Countertransference*, edited by P. Giovacchini. New York: Jason Aronson, 1975, 217–228.

Rosenfeld, H. "Notes on the Psychopathology and Psychoanalytic Treatment of Some Borderline Patients." *International Journal of Psycho-Analysis* 59 (1978): 215–221.

Rosenfeld, H. "On the Psychopathology of Narcissism: A Clinical Approach." *International Journal of Psycho-Analysis*, 45 (1964): 332–337.

Stolorow, R., and Lachmann, F. *Psychoanalysis of Developmental Arrests.* New York: International Universities Press, 1980.

Tartakoff, H. "The Normal Personality in our Culture and the Nobel Prize Complex." In *Psychoanalysis: A General Psychology*, edited by R.M. Lowenstein, et al. New York: International Universities Press, 1966, 222–252.

Van der Waals, H. "Problems of Narcissism." *Bulletin of the Menninger Clinic* 29 (1965): 293–311.

Volkan, V. "The 'Glass Bubble' of the Narcissistic Patient." In *Advances in Psychotherapy of the Borderline Patient*, edited by J. LeBoit, and A. Capponi. New York: Jason Aronson, 1979, 405–431.

Winnicott, D.W. *Collected Papers.* New York: Basic Books, 1958.

Index

phin hypothesis and, 141–42; enlarged ventricles and, 123–24, 149; environmental factors and, 88–89, 445; enzymes and, 125–29; families in, 103–06, 155; Frohman factor in blood and, 118, 119; genetic factors and, 96–97, 155, 445–52; gluten and, 145–46; hallucinogens and, 139–40; immunity and, 115, 118, 121–22; left hemisphere dysfunction in, 124; life stressors in, 103; L-γ-aminobutyric acid (GABA) deficits and, 138–39; lymphocytes and, 115; norepinephrine (NE) hypothesis and, 130–32; prostaglandins (PG) and, 146; serotonin hypothesis and, 129–30; serum levels of creatinine phosphokinase and, 128–29; social adjustment and, 89, 107–09, 167–68; socioeconomic factors, 98, 100; taraxein in blood and, 118–19; urinary phenylethylamine (PEA) and, 137–38, 149, 152; viral hypothesis and, 119–22; vitamin and mineral deficiencies and, 144–45.

Schizophrenia, psychotherapy with, 110, 160–66, 215–28; effect on symptoms, 216; group therapy, 170–72; therapeutic relationship in, 155–57; 162–65. *See also* Family therapy.

Schizophrenia, relapse in: and antipsychotics, 104, 168, 190, 195; and expressed emotion (EE), 103–06, 110–11, 172–74; functioning after, 223; and level of chronicity, 177; and life stressors, 102; and milieu therapy, 175; predictions as to, 396; and psychotherapy, 220; social skills and, 108; unemployment and, 176.

Schizophrenics, single-room occupancy hotels and, 107.

Schizophrenia, treatment of, 97, 159–60, 215.

Schizophrenia, symptoms of, 89, 97, 167; hallucinations, 149; negative, 167, 168, 172–78; positive, 173–178; thought disorder, 197.

Schizophrenia, unemployment and, 100, 103, 109–10, 176.

Schizophrenia, work and, 109–10, 176.

Schizophrenics, borderline relatives of, 450–452, 448.

Schizophrenics, hospitalization of, 225–27; readmission of, 176, 219, 227.

Schizophrenics, social support networks for, 106–07.

Schizophrenics, studies of: adoptive, 95–96, 445; measuring blood prolactin (PRL) in, 135–36; measuring growth hormone (GH) in, 135–36; twin, 126.

Schizotypal personality disorder, 428.

Self, concept of, 490, 493, 495–96, 500.

Selfobject, concept of, 492, 501–02, 509.

Selfobject: oedipal, 501, 503, 505; transference, 499, 503, 504, 507, 508–10.

Self psychology, 497–505.

Sentencing, role of psychiatry in, 392–95.

Separation, maternal, 51, 275.

17-item list, 424–25, 429, 432.

Sex therapy, 7, 8, 22, 27, 29–30, 32, 64; dual-, 21, 22.

Sexual activity: in the aging, 7, 45–47; in females, 47; postmarital, 43.

Sexual difficulties, narcissists', 519, 522.

Sexual disorders: in *International Classification of Disease*, ninth edition (ICD-9), 14; treating, 15, 24, 25–26, 34–35.

Sexual functioning, 35, 37.

Sexual identity, 49, 519.

Sexuality, 7, 14, 47.

Sexual patterns, psychosocial stressors and, 15.

Sexual phobias, 32, 36.

Sexual problems, secondary, 41–42.

Sexual response cycle, phases of, 15–16.

Sexual response, medication and, 8.

Sexual stimulation, 12–13.

Smooth-pursuit eye movement (SPEM), disordered, 453.

Stewart, Potter, 324.

Structural Interview, 432, 433, 434, 438–40, 454.

Suicide attempts, 51, 301.

Sullivan, Harry Stack, 85.

Supportive psychotherapy: with borderlines, 472; contraindications for, 481–82; goals of, 482–83, 485, 520; medication in, 484; with narcissistic personalities, 520–23; patient's responsibility, 485; technical neutrality and, 480–81; techniques of, 480, 483–85; therapist's role in, 483–85, 485–86, 520, 521, 522; transference in, 483, 485–86.

Supreme Court, 363, 364, 370, 373, 377, 378–79, 383, 386, 387, 390, 393–94.

Surgery, 38, 40, 48, 56.

Syndrome approach, 82–83.